Antiviral Mechanisms in the Control of Neoplasia

NATO ADVANCED STUDY INSTITUTES SERIES

A series of edited volumes comprising multifaceted studies of contemporary scientific issues by some of the best scientific minds in the world, assembled in cooperation with NATO Scientific Affairs Division.

Series A: Life Sciences

Recent Volumes in this Series

The series is published by an international board of publishers in conjunction with NATO Scientific Affairs Division

A	Life Sciences	Plenum Publishing Corporation
B	Physics	New York and London
C	Mathematical and Physical Sciences	D. Reidel Publishing Company Dordrecht and Boston
D	Behavioral and Social Sciences	Sijthoff International Publishing Company Leiden
E	Applied Sciences	Noordhoff International Publishing Leiden

Antiviral Mechanisms in the Control of Neoplasia

Edited by
P. Chandra

Center of Biological Chemistry
School of Medicine
University of Frankfurt
Frankfurt, Germany

PLENUM PRESS • NEW YORK AND LONDON
Published in cooperation with NATO Scientific Affairs Division

Library of Congress Cataloging in Publication Data

Nato International Advanced Study Institute on Antiviral Mechanisms for the Control
of Neoplasia, Corfu, 1978.
Antiviral mechanisms in the control of neoplasia.

(NATO advanced study institutes series: Series A, Life sciences; v. 20)
Includes index.
1. Viral carcinogenesis – Congresses. 2. Antiviral agents – Congresses. 3. Antineo-
plastic agents – Congresses. 4. Leukemogenic viruses – Congresses. I. Chandra, P. II.
North Atlantic Treaty Organization. III. Title. IV. Series.
RC268.57.N37 1978   616.9'94'079   78-10779
ISBN 0-306-40063-4

Proceedings of the NATO International Advanced Study Institute
on Antiviral Mechanisms for the Control of Neoplasia held on
Corfu Island, Greece, March 15–25, 1978

© 1979 Plenum Press, New York
A Division of Plenum Publishing Corporation
227 West 17th Street, New York, N.Y. 10011

Printed in the United States of America

Preface

The history of tumor virology that began at the turn of the century is most adequately depicted by the wisdom of Thomas Huxley's statement "Those who refuse to go beyond fact rarely get as far as fact". At that time, most of the pathologists and oncologists were influenced by Rudolf Virchow's dogma "Omnus cellula e cellula". He described the cell as the essential element of the living body and defined disease, which included cancer, as the cell's reaction to altered conditions. This dogma was the basis for the scientific community which completely opposed the concept of an infectious origin of cancer. Even Paul Ehrlich was of the opinion that there could be no transmissible agent involved in the etiology of cancer, since he was unable to induce tumors with cell-free filtrates of the murine mammary carcinoma that bears his name.

Seventy years have passed since the discovery of Ellerman and Bang that leukemia in chickens can be induced by a filterable agent. The discoveries by Rous (1911), Bittner (1936), Gross (1951), Friend (1956), Epstein et al. (1964), Jarrett (1964), Theilen et al. (1971), Kawakami et al. (1972), and a number of other investigators led to an outburst of scientific activity seeking to resolve the question of whether viruses were indeed involved in the genesis of cancer. Their oncogenic potential is today well established in a number of animal species, from mouse to non-human primates. The available data support the concept that the one indispensable element among all the elements in cancer may be a virus or viral genetic material, and that all other factors may only be secondary determinants. This position is reinforced by the fact that cancer cells often appear to have a new genetic input that allows them to make new and unique viral-specified antigens that are present in the cells and on their surfaces. Carcinogenic chemicals and physical agents, such as ionizing radiation, do not provide such genetic input - they only rearrange the output.

If it be true that virus infection is indispensable to cancer, then the target(s) of preventing viral infection or negating viral effect may permit one to dispense with the indispensable, thereby breaking the essential link in the neoplastic chain and making possible the prevention of cancer. This concept, then, is the primary basis for seeking to find the elusive viruses in cancer of man and for pursuing various means of their control. These are precisely the conceptual thoughts laid down in the present volume. This volume is based on a conference sponsored by the Scientific Division of the North Atlantic Treaty Organization (NATO) and the National Cancer Institute (U.S.A.) held on Corfu Island in Greece, March 15-25, 1978.

In 53 chapters we have tried to present an up-dated view on the genetics of cancer and the role of viruses in cancer (Sections I-III), and various mechanisms for their control (Sections IV-VI). To promote interchange at the conference, participants were invited from various fields including: genetics, epidemiology, molecular biology, chemistry, virology, biochemistry, pathology, immunology and cell biology. Thus, the interdisciplinary nature of this meeting set up a very enthusiastic atmosphere where participants could compare and discuss techniques, results and outlook for the near future.

It is clear that a great distance remains to be spanned before the dreams of today can be explored and analyzed. It is hoped however, that such interdisciplinary forums with possibilities of free exchange of thoughts will shorten this distance, so that we won't have long to wait before today's visions be turned into tomorrow's reality.

Prakash   Chandra

Acknowledgments

The conference from which this volume is compiled was financially supported principally by a grant from the Scientific Division of the North Atlantic Treaty Organization. The editor wishes to thank Dr. Tilo Kester of the Scientific Division of NATO for his support in obtaining this grant, and for his administrative guidance. Additional financial assistance was provided by the National Cancer Institute (U.S.A.) and I would like to thank Dr. Robert C. Gallo (National Cancer Institute, U.S.A.) for his help in obtaining this aid.

I am indebted to Drs. William A. Carter (Buffalo), Robert C. Gallo (Bethesda), George Klein (Stockholm), Fred Rapp (Hershey) and Robin A. Weiss (London) for acting as Section Convenors and for advice and guidance in compiling the scientific programme of this conference. In particular, I am grateful to Dr. Robert C. Gallo who, as a friend, was my principal guide in various phases of this conference.

The sessions were expertly moderated by the following Chairpersons: Drs. N. Teich, J. Sambrook, P. Bentvelzen, W.F.H. Jarrett, W.H. - Kirsten, D.P. Bolognesi, I. Witz, Eva Klein, M. Essex, F. Rapp, B. Roizman, K. Munk, D. Shugar, F. Bollum, P.H. Hoffschneider, M. Krim and D.C. Burke.

Last, but not least, I am grateful to many members of my Department for their very valuable assistance before and during the meeting. In particular I feel grateful to Dr. Uwe Ebener who, in his function as Secretary of the conference, has contributed significantly to the organization of this meeting.

Prakash   Chandra

Contents

SECTION II

THE ROLE OF RNA TUMOR VIRUSES IN
HUMAN CANCER

SECTION III

THE ROLE OF DNA TUMOR VIRUSES IN
HUMAN CANCER

SECTION IV

IMMUNOLOGICAL CONTROL MECHANISM OF
NEOPLASIA

SECTION V

MOLECULAR APPROACHES TO ACTIVE
INTERVENTION INTO ONCOGENESIS
BY TUMOR VIRUSES

CONTENTS

SECTION VI

HUMAN INTERFERONS: EFFECTS ON TUMOR VIRUSES AND ON HUMAN CANCER

SECTION I

Basic concepts in oncogenesis by tumor viruses

Convenor

Dr. Robin WEISS
Imperial Cancer Research Fund Laboratories
P. O. Box 123
Lincoln's Inn Fields
London, WC 2A 3PX

England

GENES, VIRUSES, AND CANCER

Robin A. Weiss

Imperial Cancer Research Fund Laboratories
P.O.B. 123, Lincoln's Inn Fields
London, WC2A 3PX, England

Much of the impetus for research in viral oncology has come from the search for viruses which may be etiological agents of human cancer. Potentially oncogenic DNA viruses of the herpes-, adeno-, and papovavirus families are known to be common infections in most human communities, and there is increasing evidence of retrovirus infection too. The natural history of human and animal infections with these viruses is discussed later in these proceedings. The first section is devoted to basic concepts of viral oncogenesis for which this article serves as a brief introduction. It is, perhaps, from these basic studies that viral oncology has reaped most benefit so far. The experimental induction of tumors and of cell transformation in vitro by tumor viruses has and will continue to play an important role in understanding mechanisms of carcinogenesis and the properties of neoplastic cells.

A unifying feature of cell transformation by tumor viruses is that the viral genome or a portion of it becomes inserted into host chromosomal DNA, so that the integrated viral genes become adopted by the host as extra genetic information. Integration is probably not the oncogenic event itself, but is the means by which viral genes may be heritably transmitted to daughter cells. It is becoming increasingly clear, at least for the smaller tumor viruses, that gene expression, probably the production of specific "transforming" proteins, is necessary for establishing and maintaining the neoplastic state of the virally transformed cell. However, we must be careful to distinguish between cell transformation and malignancy as well as between different criteria of cell transformation. Thus virologists working with Epstein-Barr virus (EBV) speak of transformation of B-lymphoblasts as the development of clones with indefinite proliferation potential (immortalization)

3

in vitro, though this is not sufficient to express full malignancy.
Transformation of fibroblasts by SV40 or by sarcoma viruses, on the
other hand, designates morphological and physiological changes in
the cells that do not pertain to the ultimate longevity of the
transformed clone. Transformation of hemopoietic cells by leukemia
viruses involves the emergence of cell populations with unbalanced
numbers of immature cells, although the cells can in many instances
be induced to differentiate further along normal pathways of
maturation. These examples of viral transformation of different
target cells are discussed in some detail by other contributors to
these proceedings.

     Little is known at present about the mechanisms of cell trans-
formation by viruses, but specific genes and the proteins which
they encode are being identified for papovaviruses and retroviruses. The "early region" of the genomes of SV40 and polyoma are not
only necessary for viral replication but for neoplastic transformation too. It has become apparent first from genetic studies of
mutants and more recently from the identification of different
mRNA and protein species that the early region codes for overlapping but distinct gene products which probably act at different
sites in the cell. Thus large T-antigen is a nuclear antigen which
binds to DNA and appears to have a strong affinity to sites of
origin of DNA replication. It is easy to imagine how this protein
might perturb the proliferation characteristics of infected cells.
Little t-antigen appears to be cytoplasmic and its function is as
yet unknown; polyoma virus also appears to encode a third protein
of the early region of the genome, "middle T-antigen," which
probably becomes located at the plasma membrane and perhaps
affects cell recognition mechanisms.

     Transforming genes of retroviruses are also becoming rapidly
unraveled. The classical one is the src (sarcoma) gene of non-
defective strains of Rous sarcoma virus, the only retrovirus transforming gene which is adequately defined by genetic techniques.
The isolation of deletion mutants and temperature-sensitive mutants
has shown that the src gene is not required for viral replication,
but is essential for fibroblast transformation and for sarcomagene-
sis. A protein of 60,000 daltons has been identified as a putative
src gene product and it is quite likely that other gene products,
as with the T-antigen family, may also be assigned to src. The src
gene of RSV appears to be derived from normal DNA sequences present
in chickens, and located in a different chromosome from endogenous
viral gene sequences. Apparently RSV has acquired this gene from
the host, and there is recent evidence that avian and murine sarcoma
viruses can be experimentally generated by a sort of viral trans-
duction mechanism whereby the host sequences are incorporated into
the viral genome. Indeed, most strongly-transforming viruses are
defective in replication, resembling defective-transducing bacterio-
phages in having substituted host genetic information in place of

viral genes essential for replication. Many kinds of host sequences
might be acquired, but only those with oncogenic potential will be
amplified by the generation of tumors and thus be identified and
selected for study by the viral oncologist. Acquisition of different "oncogenes" will confer on the virus different target specificities of cell transformation, explaining the wide variety, yet
specificity in any one virus strain, of tumors caused by strongly-
transforming retroviruses. How the gene products of these oncogenes exert a neoplastic effect and whether they have similar
mechanisms of action in their respective target cells is not known,
though one popular idea is that they may represent or mimic specific
mitogenic hormones.

The more weakly oncogenic lymphoid leukemia viruses do not
appear to insert new oncogenes in place of or in addition to viral
structural genes. However, there is growing evidence for the murine
viruses inducing thymic lymphomas that genetic recombination or
variation takes place in the env gene coding for the virus envelope
antigens. Variant envelope glycoproteins are generated which may
recognize and interact with different cell surface receptors, perhaps present only on certain T-lymphocytes; the glycoprotein-receptor
interaction may serve both as a mechanism for viral infection and as
a mitogenic stimulus.

The study of viral transformation systems highlight the concept
that the expression of a very small number of genes can be crucial
in causing neoplastic transformation. This concept is also implic-
itly assumed by proponents of the somatic mutation hypothesis of
chemical carcinogenesis, and by those who investigate neoplastic
expression by somatic genetic methods. Somatic cell hybridization
and more recently chromosome and DNA transfer experiments have been
usefully exploited in studying the malignant state. DNA transfection between cells of vertebrate species was first demonstrated by
the rescue of the proviral element of RSV in mammalian cells by
transfer of DNA to permissive chick cells and cell transformation
by fragments of papova- and adenovirus genomes has also been
demonstrated in this way. The transfer of the thymidine kinase (tk)
gene of herpes simplex virus to mutant tk⁻ mouse cells is demonstrated here by Minson, and Spandidos and Siminovitch discuss DNA transfer of markers of neoplastic transformation, such as the "rescue of
senescing cultures" and the ability of cells to proliferate when
suspended in soft agar. Whether the genetic information conferring
neoplastic properties apparent in experimental DNA transfer experiments and the "transducing" retroviruses are similar remains to be
investigated. Both systems, however, provide exquisite tools for
identifying the genes and functions involved in neoplastic transformation. How they relate to determinants of "household" and
differentiation functions of normal cells will be a fascinating
area of cancer research.

THE HERPES SIMPLEX THYMIDINE KINASE GENE AS A TRANSMISSIBLE GENETIC ELEMENT IN MAMMALIAN CELLS

A.C. Minson, K. Bastow and G. Darby

Department of Pathology

University of Cambridge

INTRODUCTION

It is well established that herpes simplex virus (HSV) contains a gene for the enzyme thymidine kinase (Kitt & Dubbs, 1963, 1965; Klemperer et al, 1967). The gene can be introduced into the genotype of mammalian cells which lack this enzyme either by infecting cells with virus inactivated with U.V. light (Munyon et al, 1971) or by inoculating cells with fragments of virus DNA (Bacchetti & Graham, 1977; Maitland & McDougall, 1977; Wigler et al, 1977). Following these treatments, cells which have acquired a thymidine kinase can be simply selected (Littlefield, 1964), and the enzyme can be shown to be virus-specific. Cells 'biochemically transformed' in this way have been shown to contain a small number of copies (1-5) of only part of the HSV genome (Kraiselbund, Gage & Weissbach, 1975; Davis and Kingsbury, 1976), but the stability of these newly acquired genes and of their expression varies from one cell line to another (Davidson, Adelstein & Oxman, 1973; Kauffman & Davidson, 1975; Bacchetti & Graham 1977). Cells of this type represent a model system with which to study the interaction of the herpes simplex virus genome with the genome of mammalian cells. This paper describes the isolation of cell lines carrying the herpes thymidine kinase gene and the detection in these lines of a number of non-selected virus-specific functions. DNA from these transformed cells has been used to 'transfect' further cells to a kinase-positive phenotype. The high efficiency of this phenomenon suggests that the DNA in transformed cells has different properties from the DNA in virus particles.

7

RESULTS

Transformation with Virus DNA

L-cells lacking the enzyme thymidine kinase (LTK⁻ cells) were seeded at 5×10^5 cells per 60 mm dish and after 24 h. were inoculated with 0.1 µg HSV-1 or HSV-2 DNA which had been sheared to a molecular weight of $10-20 \times 10^6$ by passage through a 21 gauge syringe needle. After 48 h. the cells were changed into selective medium containing methotrexate (Munyon et al, 1971), and colonies of cells appeared after 15 days. These experiments are essentially similar to those reported by Bacchetti & Graham (1977). Four clonally un-related cell lines were established from experiments using HSV-1 DNA and nine from experiments using type 2 DNA.

Thymidine Kinase Content of Transformed Cells

All the cell lines contained thymidine kinase activity which could be neutralised by anti-sera raised in rabbits against herpes infected cells (Thouless & Wildy, 1975). Table 1 shows the results of an enzyme neutralisation experiment using extracts of three cell lines transformed with type 1 DNA ($D1_2$, $D1_3$, $D1_4$) and four lines transformed with type 2 DNA ($D2_1$, $D2_3$, $D2_5$, $D2_6$). Anti-serum raised against type 1 or type 2 infected cells had no effect on the kinase in BHK cells or L-cells, but neutralised the kinase in

Table 1.   Inactivation of Thymidine Kinase by Specific Sera

Kinase Source	% Kinase Activity Remaining	
	Anti-Type 2 Serum	Anti-Type 1 Serum
$D1_2$	76	6
$D1_3$	81	9
$D1_4$	88	13
$D2_1$	15	33
$D2_3$	30	74
$D2_5$	8	25
$D2_6$	33	55
BHK	102	105
L-M	102	104
Type 1 Infected BHK	27	4
Type 2 Infected BHK	5	79

transformed cells. Anti–type 1 serum neutralised the enzyme
from type 1 transformed cells more efficiently than the enzyme from type 2 transformed cells. Anti type 2 serum exhibited the reverse specificity.

   Different cell lines contained different levels of thymidine kinase, but the enzyme level was characteristic for
any particular cell line and was stable to passage in selective medium for at least 50 generations. Simultaneous estimation of the enzyme levels in the type 2 transformed lines
is given in Figure 1. The levels are distributed over an
approximately four–fold range. Three cell lines ($D2_1$, $D2_5$,
$D2_6$) were passed for 50 generations in non–selective medium.
These also showed no detectable change in kinase levels. Taken together these results suggest considerable stability of
the kinase gene expression.

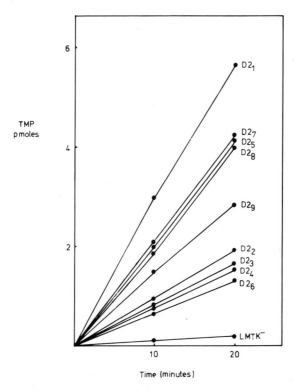

Figure 1. Thymidine Kinase Levels in Transformed Cells
   The cell lines were grown to confluence in selective
medium, harvested by trypsinisation and suspended at 4×10^7
cells/ml. Extracts were prepared by ultrasonic disintegra-
tion and assayed immediately. The data shown are thymidine
phosphorylated by extracts of 10^5 cells.

Non—Selected Virus—Specific Functions in Transformed Cells

Since these cell lines have been transformed by the introduction of HSV DNA fragments of $10-20 \times 10^6$ molecular
weight it is reasonable to suppose that in addition to the
selected kinase gene, other non—selected virus functions
should be carried by these cells. This was investigated by
testing the ability of cells transformed with type 2 DNA to
support the growth of temperature sensitive mutants of HSV
at the non—permissive temperature. A series of experiments
was first performed with four ts⁻ mutants of HSV type 1
designated N102, N103, B1 and B5. Cells were infected at
3 pfu per cell, incubated for 20 h. at 38.5° and the yield
of mutant virus was compared with the yield of the parental
wild type virus grown under identical conditions. The
results in Table 2 show that none of the cell lines gives
elevated yields of mutants B1 or B5 but that mutants N102
and N103 are efficiently complemented by cell line $D2_1$. The
variation in wild type yield from different cell lines is not
reproducible. No transformed line differs from any other or
from LTK⁻ cells in its ability to support the growth of wild
type virus.

Mutants N102 and N103 are DNA negative mutants which
fail to complement each other, but which complement efficiently with mutants B1 and B5. Mutants N102 and N103 are
therefore defective in the same function and the absence of
this function is compensated by an HSV type 2 function present in $D2_1$ cells. It is known that type 2 virus function

Table 2.   Complementation of HSV Type 1 Mutants by Cell Lines
            Transformed with HSV Type 2 DNA

Cell Line	Experiment 1 Yield (pfu x 10^{-5})			Experiment 2 Yield (pfu x 10^{-4})		
	Wild—type	N103	N102	Wild—type	B1	B5
LTK⁻	60	0.06	1.2	260	0.10	0.08
$D2_1$	25	6.0	35.0	260	0.05	0.15
$D2_2$	40	0.19	0.8	250	0.04	0.10
$D2_3$	180	0.27	1.2	180	0.08	0.12
$D2_4$	200	0.20	1.7	240	0.04	0.05
$D2_5$	120	0.28	1.4	380	0.12	0.10
$D2_6$	180	0.22	1.6	220	0.05	0.08
$D2_7$	20	0.05	1.0	ND	ND	ND
$D2_8$	27	0.05	ND	270	0.10	0.08
$D2_9$	130	0.18	1.3	ND	ND	ND

Table 3.   Complementation of HSV-2 ts Mutants by Type 2
            Transformed Cells

Cell Line	Virus Yield pfu x 10^{-3}	
	Wild-type	ts 208
LTK$^-$	47	0.8
D2$_1$	31	44
D2$_2$	14	<0.1
D2$_3$	45	1.3
D2$_4$	12	<0.1
D2$_5$	40	52
D2$_6$	19	<0.1
D2$_7$	36	<0.1
D2$_8$	16	0.1

will compensate the defect in ts N102 because this mutant has
been used to generate inter-typic recombinants of HSV (Morse
et al, 1977).

Similar experiments have also been done with HSV-2 ts
mutants, and one such mutant ts 208 is complemented by cell
lines D2$_1$ and D2$_5$ (Table 3). In addition a further mutant,
ts 178, is complemented by D2$_5$ but not D2$_1$. Finally, no
evidence was found of rescue of the virus genes resident in
transformed cells, since the progeny virus resulting from
complementation of N102, N103 and 208 was all of mutant
phenotype.

Revertant Cell Lines

Thymidine kinase-negative revertants of cell line D2$_1$
were obtained by plating 10^4 cells per dish in medium containing 50 µg/ml BUDR, and colonies from different dishes
were established as cell lines in non-selective medium
(D2$_1$R1, D2$_1$R2, D2$_1$R3). These cell lines contained no detectable thymidine kinase and failed to plate in methotrexate
(plating efficiency <10^{-4}). The revertant cells were tested
for their ability to support the growth of ts N103 at the
non-permissive temperature. The data in Table 4 show that
all three lines have lost this function, while their ability
to support the growth of wild type virus is unimpaired. Loss
of the thymidine kinase gene is therefore accompanied by loss
of the non-selected marker.

Table 4.   Growth of Mutant N103 in TK$^-$ Revertants of D2$_1$

Cell Line	Virus Yield (pfu x 10^4)	
	Wild-type	N103
LTK$^-$	300	0.1
D2$_1$	390	190
D2$_1$R1	200	0.15
D2$_1$R2	450	0.08
D2$_1$R3	440	0.18

Transfection

DNA was extracted from cell lines D2$_1$ and D2$_3$ and used to transform LTK$^-$ cells to a kinase-positive phenotype (Table 5).   In each instance the DNA was sheared to a molecular weight of 10-20 x 10^6 except in experiment 6 where DNA was used with a molecular weight of 20-30 x 10^6.   In four

Table 5.   Transformation of LTK$^-$ Cells with Transformed Cell DNA

Experiment	Source of DNA	Dose per dish (μg)	Proportion of Dishes with Colonies
1	HSV-2 virions	0.5	6/10
	D2$_1$ cells	10.0	9/10
	Salmon sperm	10.0	0/10
2	HSV-2 virions	0.5	10/10
	D2$_1$ cells	10.0	8/9
	Salmon sperm	10.0	0/10
3	HSV-2 virions	0.5	4/8
	D2$_3$ cells	10.0	5/8
	Salmon sperm	10.0	0/10
4	HSV-2 virions	0.5	8/10
	L-cells	10.0	0/10
5	HSV-2 virions	0.5	8/10
	HSV-2 virions	0.05	2/10
	D2$_1$R1 cells	10.0	0/10
6	HSV-2 virions	0.5	10/10
	D2$_1$ cells	10.0	9/10
	Salmon sperm	10.0	0/10

independent experiments inoculation of DNA from transformed cells resulted in the appearance of colonies in a majority of dishes, while L-cell DNA or DNA extracted from a kinase negative revertant of cell line $D2_1$ gave no transformants.

Five colonies from different dishes in experiment 1 were established as cell lines ($D2_1T1$, $D2_1T2$, $D2_1T3$, $D2_1T4$, $D2_1T5$). These cells contained HSV-2 specific thymidine kinase activity as judged by serological neutralisation. The enzyme level in each cell line was remarkably similar, and about half the level found in $D2_1$ cells (Figure 2). While transformation with virus DNA results in cells with very different kinase levels, transfection with transformed cell DNA yields cell lines which are uniform in this character.

To find whether transfection of the kinase gene was ac-companied by transfer of the non-selected markers, the trans-fected lines were infected at the non-permissive temperature with mutants ts N103 and ts 208. None of the transfected lines complemented either mutant (Table 6). A further five transfected lines were established from an experiment in which $D2_1$ DNA of molecular weight 20-30 x 10^6 was used as a source of the kinase gene (Table 5, experiment 6). These cell lines also failed to complement ts N103 or ts 208.

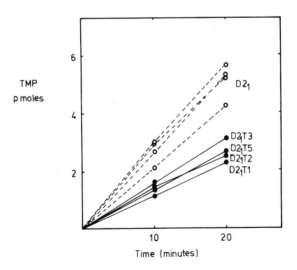

Figure 2. Thymidine Kinase Levels in Transfected Lines
        Conditions were as described in the legend to Figure 1. The data for $D2_1$ cell extracts were obtained on different occasions using cells at different passage numbers. Data for the transfected lines were obtained from parallel assays of extracts prepared from cells at passage 4.

Table 6.   Growth of ts⁻ Mutants in Cells Transformed with
D2$_1$ DNA

Cell Line	Experiment 1 Yield (pfu x 10^{-4})		Experiment 2 Yield (pfu x 10^{-4}	
	HSV-1	ts N103	HSV-2	ts 208
LTK⁻	300	0.10	47	0.7
D2$_1$	390	190	31	23.0
D2$_1$T1	760	0.05	43	0.1
D2$_1$T2	820	0.08	17	<0.1
D2$_1$T3	750	0.33	78	2.0
D2$_1$T4	420	0.08	11	0.1
D2$_1$T5	510	0.30	34	1.4

DISCUSSION

The experiments described here show that the thymidine
kinase gene of herpes simplex virus can be introduced into
the genotype of LTK⁻ cells using either virus DNA or transformed cell DNA as a gene source. The cell lines derived
from experiments using HSV-2 DNA as a transforming agent
contain a type 2 virus-specific kinase and two cell lines
carry non-selected virus-specific functions as judged by
their ability to complement HSV mutants. Kinase-negative
revertant cells do not contain these non-selected functions.
The simplest interpretation of this result is that the kinase
gene and the non-selected markers are introduced on the same
fragment of virus DNA and that selection against the kinase
gene results in the loss of the entire virus sequence or its
expression. Reversion to the kinase negative phenotype in
the instance of the D2$_1$R1 cell line presumably results from
gene loss since DNA from these cells cannot be used as a
source of the kinase gene in transfection experiments.

The transfer of the thymidine kinase gene to LTK⁻ cells
using transformed cell DNA (transfection) is surprisingly
efficient. The data given in Table 5, together with results
not shown here, demonstrate that 10 µg D2$_1$ DNA transforms at
least as efficiently as 0.1 µg HSV-2 DNA. Since 10 µg is the
DNA content of 10^6 cells and since 0.1 µg HSV DNA represents
10^9 genomes it follows that to account for the efficiency of
transfection by D2$_1$ DNA in terms of the kinase gene concentration, we would require each D2$_1$ cell to contain 10^3 gene
copies. This seems unlikely in view of the very small amounts

of virus DNA which have been found in HSV transformed cells (Kraiselbund et al, 1975; Davis and Kingsbury, 1976; Frenkel et al, 1976; Minson et al, 1976). An alternative is that the kinase gene in transformed cells is in a different physical state from the DNA extracted from virions, and transforms more efficiently in consequence. This view is supported by a comparison of the properties of transformed and transfected cells. The kinase levels in transfected cells are remarkably uniform compared with the distribution of enzyme levels found in transformed cells. Furthermore the transfected cells do not acquire the non-selected markers found in the donor transformed cell, even when the transfecting DNA is much higher molecular weight than the virus DNA initially used to produce the transformed cell. This implies a qualitative difference between transformation and transfection.

One possibility is that the virus DNA in transformed cells is integrated so that the virus sequences derived from such cells are flanked by host sequences. This is supported by preliminary evidence that the transfecting sequences derived from $D2_1$ cell DNA are of much lower density than the transforming sequences derived from virion DNA. If these flanking sequences were highly re-iterated in the recipient cell chromosomes, then integration of the donor genes might be facilitated by recombination of homologous sequences. This model would, however, predict that transfection would involve the transfer of the entire virus sequence present in the donor cell. In fact we have not observed co-transfer of the non-selected markers with the kinase gene. It is apparent that the resolution of this problem requires analysis of the physical properties of transfecting DNA and the determination of the HSV DNA sequences present in transformed and transfected cells.

ACKNOWLEDGEMENTS

We are grateful to Lynne Jeffrey and Susanne Bell for excellent technical assistance. We thank Dr. A. Buchan for type 1 ts⁻ mutants and Drs. K. Powell and D. Purifoy for type 2 ts⁻ mutants. We are also indebted to Professor P. Wildy for his interest and advice. This work was supported by the Cancer Research Campaign. K.B. receives a post graduate scholarship from the Medical Research Council.

REFERENCES

Bacchetti, S. & Graham, F.L. (1977). Proc. Nat. Acad. Sci. USA 74, 1590-1594.

Davidson, R.L., Adelstein, S.J. & Oxman, M.N. (1973). Proc.
    Nat. Acad. Sci. USA 70, 1912-1916.

Davis, D.B. & Kingsbury, D.T. (1976). J. Virol. 17, 788-793.

Frenkel, N., Locker, M., Cox, B., Roizman, B. & Rapp, F.
    (1976). J. Virol. 18, 885-893.

Kaufman, E.R. & Davidson, R.L. (1975). Somatic Cell Genet.
    1, 153-164.

Kit, S. & Dubbs, D.R. (1963). Biochem. Biophys. Res. Comm.
    11, 55-59.

Kit, S. & Dubbs, D.R. (1965). Virology 26, 16-27.

Klemperer, M.G., Haynes, G.R., Sheddon, W.I.H. & Watson,
    D.H. (1967). Virology 31, 120-218.

Kraiselbund, E., Gage, L.P. & Weissbach, A. (1975). J. Mol.
    Biol. 97, 533-542.

Littlefield, J. (1964). Science 145, 709-710.

Maitland, N.J. & McDougall, J.K. (1977). Cell 11, 233-241.

Minson, A.C., Thouless, M.E., Eglin, R.P. & Darby, G. (1976).
    Int. J. Cancer 17, 493-500.

Morse, L.S., Buchman, T.G., Roizman, B. & Schaffer, P.A.
    (1977). J. Virol. 24, 231-248.

Munyon, W., Kraiselbund, E., Davis, S. & Mann, J. (1971).
    J. Virol. 7, 813-820.

Thouless, M.E. & Wildy, P. (1975). J. Gen. Virol. 26,
    159-170.

Varmus, H.E., Vogt, P.I. & Bishop, J.M. (1973). Proc. Nat.
    Acad. Sci. USA 70, 3067-3071.

Wigler, M., Silverstein, S., Lee, L-S., Pellicer, A., Cheng,
    Y-C. & Axel, R. (1977). Cell 11, 223-232.

ON THE NATURE OF GENETIC CHANGE AS AN UNDERLYING CAUSE FOR THE ORIGIN OF NEOPLASMS

M. R. Ahuja

Genetisches Institut, Justus Liebig-Universität
6300 Giessen, West Germany

I. INTRODUCTION

Experimental studies with a variety of different organisms have shown that it is possible to induce neoplasms following treatment with radiation, chemicals and viruses. Although the mechanism(s) of transformation of a normal cell to a tumor cell is not yet understood, it seems highly plausible that these diverse agents singly or in combination may directly or indirectly affect the genetic apparatus of the cell by causing a certain genetic change. Regardless of what causes cancer, the end result of a transformed cell is nearly the same, namely, unrestrained cell reproduction accompanied by aberrant cell differentiation. This would imply that transformation of a normal to a neoplastic cell presumably affects a common cellular mechanism(s), which seems to be critical for cell reproduction and cell differentiation. Since the daughter cells exhibit traits similar to their progenitor cancer cells, and this cell heredity is maintained through subsequent cell reproductions, the cancer problem may, in the final analysis, be approached as a basic problem involving disorders at the biochemical and molecular genetic levels. It is suggested that neoplastic transformation may involve a genetic change(s) in specific genetic components of the cell genome, and this genetic change may be caused by external or internal factors, or through certain matings.

II. THE GENETIC COMPONENTS

A. Nature of the Tumor Information

In several different organism genes have been located which

17

are involved in the induction of neoplasms. There are distinct
melanophore spot patterns on the dorsal fin and skin of the
platyfish (Platypoecilus maculatus), and each pattern is controlled
in inheritance by a specific locus (Gordon, 1958; Anders, 1967;
Kallman, 1975). At least five well-investigated spot-specific
loci, Sd (spotted dorsal fin) (Fig. 1a), Sp (spotted), Sr (stripe
sided) (Fig. 1b), Li (lineatus), and Pu (punctatus), involved in
melanoma formation have been located near the end of the sex
chromosomes (Anders et al., 1973b). These loci subsequently
were named the Tu loci, or the tumor genes (Anders et al., 1974).
In the tobacco tumor system, Tu locus has located on an
autosome, which also carries genes for male sterility (Ahuja, 1962,
1971), although the precise location of the Tu on the autosome is
not known. In Drosophila tumorous head condition is caused by a
tumor gene (tu-3) placed at 58 map units from the left end of the
third chromosome (Gardner, 1970). In the AKR mouse the Akv-1 locus
involved in the induction of murine leukemia is located near the
centromere of chromosome 7 or in linkage group I with the
gene order centromere – Akv-1 – Gpi-1 –c (Rowe et al., 1972;
Chattopadhyay et al., 1975).

Based on observations of these and other animal model systems,
we have recently proposed (Ahuja and Anders, 1976, 1977) that cells
of the multicellular organisms carry in their genomes a potentially
tumor-inducing genetic information, designated "Tu", which in
most instances remains suppressed (one cannot rule out the possibility that there may not be specific Tu genes to cause cancer,
and it is equally plausible that certain genes normally involved
in cell reproduction and tissue differentiation, when impaired,
may lead to neoplastic development). It is speculated that Tu may
have certain functions in multicellular organisms. Partial
activation of Tu genes may possibly lead to bursts of cell division
in different tissues at different time periods during different

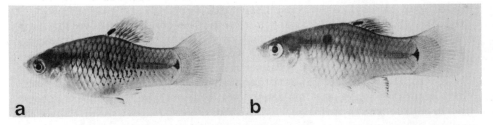

Fig. 1. Platyfish showing the expression of sex-linked spot pattern
Sd (spotted dorsal fin) and Sr (stripe sided body): a) male with
the genotype X Dr Sd, Y Ar Sr, which exhibits both Sd and Sr
expression, and b) female with the genotype X Dr Sd, X Dr Sd
exhibiting only Sd expression (Photographs courtesy Prof. F.
Anders).

stages of embryonic development. Some cell types during early
embryogeny of mammals, as for example, the trophoblast stem cells,
may even invade the surrounding cells, and thus may behave like
malignant cells (Manes, 1974). However, this invasive activity
is only temporary, and the trophoblast cell normally do not kill
its host. The trophoblast stem cells, under normal conditions,
undergo a degree of further differentiation under local or hormonal
influences, which limit their invasiveness and lead to an elaborate
capacity for endocrine function (Patillo et al., 1972); in the
absence of such influences, the primitive trophoblast cells can
indeed destroy the uterus (Kirby and Cowell, 1968) and behave in
humans as choriocarcinoma (Patillo et al., 1972). In the platyfish,
controlled Tu or Tu-associated manifestations can be detected in
the genetically determined spot-specific melanophore patterns on
the dorsal fin and the skin of the adult fish (Gordon, 1958;
Anders, 1967). These spot-specific melanophore patterns may play
a role in the sexual behavior and speciation of these fish.

B. The Regulatory Genes

We have recently proposed that Tu expression may be controlled
by different sets of cell type- or tissue-specific regulatory
genes (R-genes), which may be nonlinked and/or linked to the Tu
(Ahuja and Anders, 1976, 1977). In most instances, the Tu
information is repressed by the R-genes, and therefore, the host
tissues remain unharmed. On the other hand, a genetic change of
the R-genes (mutational or recombinational event) or permanent
disruption of the function of the R-genes, following exposure to
radiation, chemical carcinogens, or viruses, or certain matings,
could conceivably release the Tu from the restraint of suppression and trigger a chain of events which may eventually lead to
tissue-specific neoplasms. The conclusion that the regulatory
genes exist must be correct, because in all cancer a genetic change
in the regulatory genes results in a loss of control of cell
reproduction, but not in a loss of ability of the cells to grow
and divide (Prescott, 1973). Further, many neoplastically transformed cells remain incompletely differentiated, which may result
from a loss of control over a certain phase of cell differentiation,
an idea also consistent with the existence of the regulatory genes.
Evidence from the tumor systems suggest that there might be at
least three major types of regulatory controls of the Tu information in multicellular organisms. By and large the regulatory
genes may be diploid (Comings, 1973); however, variation from this
diploid nature may occur due to redundancy or duplication of the
regulatory genes.

1. Nonlinked Regulatory System. In the platyfish-swordtail
melanoma system two different loci, Sp and Sd may have relevance

to the nonlinked regulatory system. For example when sex linked locus Sp from a normal platyfish is introduced by selective matings into the genome of the normal swordtail (Xiphophorus helleri; which has neither Sp nor presumably its controlling genes), malignant melanomas are produced on the bodyside of 25 % of the backcross derivatives (Gordon, 1958; Anders, 1967; Anders et al., 1973a). On the other hand, when normal platyfish carrying the Sp locus are irradiated, only slightly enlarged spots or benign melanomas are produced in the treated animal or its progeny (Anders et al., 1971; Pursglove et al., 1971; Anders et al., 1973a). The same is true of another sex-linked locus, Sd. When Sd locus from the normal platyfish is introduced by selective matings into the genome of the swordtail, malignant melanomas develop on the dorsal fin of 25 % of the backcross derivatives. However, irradiation of the normal platyfish carrying the Sd locus did not lead to malignant melanoma formation, but only resulted in slight enhancement of the dorsal spot expression or benign melanoma formation in the treated animals or their progeny (Anders et al., 1973a). These genetic analyses on the fish indicate that the expression of Sp or Sd (both Tu loci) is mainly controlled by nonlinked R-genes which could be eliminated by appropriate matings; however, irradiation apparently did not delete or impair all the nonlinked R-genes controlling Tu expression.

In Drosophila the expression of tu-3, a semidominant gene which determines the tumorous head condition, seems to be modified by a nonlinked recessive gene tu-1 located approximately 64 map units from the left end of the X chromosome (Gardner, 1970). The expression of the Akv-1 locus (located in the linkage group I of the mouse), which is involved in murine leukemia virus production, is apparently controlled by a nonlinked regulatory gene Fv-1 located on linkage group VIII of the mouse genome. These observations are consistent with the hypothesis that Tu information for tumorous head in Drosophila and murine leukemia of the mouse may be controlled by nonlinked regulatory genes.

2. Linked/Nonlinked Regulatory System. Experiments on the platyfish-swordtail system have revealed (Anders et al., 1973a) that when Li-carrying X chromosome from the platyfish was introduced into the genome of the swordtail by selective matings, melanomas failed to develop on the backcross derivatives carrying the Li chromosome. Melanomas also did not develop on the Li-carrying purebred platyfish following X-irradiation, or treatment with a chemical carcinogen, N-methyl-N-nitrosourea (MNU) (Anders et al., 1973a; Schwab et al., 1978a). On the other hand, when hybrid derivatives carrying the Li locus in the swordtail genetic background were irradiated with X-rays or treated with MNU, melanomas developed on some of the treated animals (Anders et al., 1973a; Schwab

et al., 1978a and b). These results may be interpreted on the hypothesis that the Li (Tu) expression in the genome of the platyfish is probably controlled by tissue-specific linked and nonlinked R-genes, and in these experiments with fish the nonlinked R-genes were eliminated by selective matings to swordtail, and the remaining linked R-gene was impaired or deleted following exposure to irradiation or the chemical carcinogen, presumably due to a mutational event in a somatic cell. Since the swordtail is insensitive to MNU treatment, it is assumed that genetic information for the induction of melanomas may be rigidly controlled by a set of linked and/or nonlinked R-genes in the genome of the swordtail.

In a recent study the potential to develop neoplasms other than melanomas, for example sarcomas, was tested in specific genotypes of the fish (Schwab et. al. 1978). When normal platyfish carrying Li as a genetic marker was crossed to normal swordtail, no sarcomas developed in the F-1 animals or the backcross animals derived by backcrossing the F-1 to swordtail as a recurrent parent. Even when the platyfish with Li as a genetic marker, or the swordtail, or their F-1 was treated with the chemical carcinogen MNU, sarcomas failed to develop on the treated animals. On the other hand, when the animals from the backcross generations (BC 1, BC 4 from the above cross) were exposed to MNU, a small percentage (up to 8 %) of the backcross animals developed sarcomas (Schwab et. al. 1978a). This result is consistent with the hypothesis that tissue-specific linked and nonlinked R-genes suppress the Tu expression with respect to sarcomas in the genome of the platyfish, and therefore, the parental strain remains free from such a neoplasm. The untreated F-1 and the subsequent backcross generation animals did not develop sarcomas, presumably because by backcrossing to swordtail only the nonlinked R-genes could be eliminated, but the linked R-genes were transmitted along with the sarcoma Tu in the subsequent generations. Even following treatment with MNU the sarcomas did not develop on the parental strains and the F-1, because all the linked and unlinked R-genes specific for sarcomas were not impaired. On the other hand, sarcomas developed on the treated backcross animals presumably because the remaining linked R-gene was impaired due to a somatic mutational event.

3. Linked Regulatory System. One of the Tu loci, called Sr (stripe sided), is located on the distal end of the Y chromosome of a platyfish strain. Under normal conditions Sr determines the striped expression of the flank above the midlateral line and in front of the dorsal fin of the platyfish. Introduction of Sr from the platyfish into the genome of the swordtail by selective matings did not lead to melanoma formation on the bodyside of the F-1 hybrid or its backcross derivatives (Anders et al., 1973a).

On the other hand, by irradiation of the Sr platyfish two events
occur: a) the irradiated fish itself may produce somatic-condi-
tioned melanomas, which are not inherited, and b) the irradiated
fish irrespective of the fact whether or not they develop melanomas
may transmit germline conditioned melanomas to the progeny, and
this condition is transmitted as a Mendelian trait (Anders et al.,
1973a). **These results may be interpreted to imply that Sr (Tu)**
and its main R-gene are both closely linked. Selective matings
did not lead to melanoma formation in the hybrid descendants
because **Tu and its linked R-gene are both transmitted as a unit.**
Since no tumorous recombinants were recovered in the hybrid progeny,
it is implied that Sr (Tu) is very closely linked to its R-gene.
Melanomas developed on the irradiated platyfish or its progeny,
presumably due to a genetic change (mutational event) in the R-
gene, either in somatic or germline cells.

In principle, Tu may be present in homozygous condition in
the previous two subsystems. However, homozygosity of Tu and its
regulation will be briefly discussed with respect to the linked
regulatory system. The Tu may be controlled by its adjacent R-gene
or by the allelic R-gene on the homologous chromosome. Knudson
(1971) has provided data to suggest that retinoblastoma in man
is caused by two mutational events. According to him, the domin-
antly inherited form of retinoblastoma results from one mutation
inherited via the germinal cells and the second mutation that
occurs in the somatic cells. On the other hand, the nonhereditary
form of retinoblastoma results from two mutational events both
occurring in the somatic cells. Wilms' tumor of kidney, which may
be hereditary or nonhereditary, has also been interpreted on the
basis of the two-mutational model (Knudson and Strong, 1971). The
two mutational events may occur, according to Comings (1973), in
the regulatory genes controlling the retinoblastoma condition in
the germline and/or somatic cells.

Chronic myelogenous leukemia (CML) in man may have relevance
to the linked regulatory gene system. Most patients with CML
have a so-called Philadelphia chromosome (Nowell and Hungerford,
1960), which was presumed to be a deletion of about one half of
the long arm of chromosome 21 (Rudkin et al., 1964). Subsequently,
banding studies have shown that the Philadelphia chromosome
actually represented a chromosome 22 (Casperson et al., 1970).
It was suggested (Ohno, 1971) that a Philadelphia chromosome-
positive clone which eventually leads to the CML disease may
arise due to two mutational events: a) a loss due to deletion of
a chromosome segment from chromosome 22 carrying a leukemia-suppressing locus and b) a mutational event in the homologous leukemia-
suppressing locus. Recently, however, Rowley (1973, 1977) has
shown by a banding technique that the chromosome fragment from the
long arm of chromosome 22 is not lost due to a deletion, as was

previously thought, but the fragment from chromosome 22 is translocated onto the long arm of chromosome 9 in most cases with the
CML disease. Based on these observations, it has been suggested
(Comings, 1973; Ahuja and Anders, 1977) that altered regulation
of the leukemia-suppressing R-gene due to position effect by
translocation from chromosome 22 to 9, accompanied by a mutational
event of the homologous tissue-specific R-gene on chromosome 22,
presumably leads to the Philadelphia chromosome-positive leukemic
clone. Dr. R. C. Gallo (personal communication) has suggested
that there is a need to reconsider the acute phase ("Blast crisis")
of the CML disease, where a final and truly malignant transformation occurs. In this stage, additional and not so predictable
karyotypic changes may occur (see Rowley, 1977).

III. HOW MANY TUMOR GENES ?

In the platyfish-swordtail system genetic analysis has
revealed that a number of melanophore pattern loci, as Sd, Sp, Sr,
Li, and Pu, located on the sex chromosomes in different strains
of platyfish are involved in spot-specific melanomas (Anders et
al., 1973a and b). It was previously suggested (Anders et al.
1974; Ahuja and Anders, 1976) that these color genes represent
Tu loci (the possibility that Tu may be a constituent of these
melanophore pattern genes, or may even be closely linked to them,
is not excluded). The absence of genetic markers has so far
precluded a systematic analysis of neoplasms other than melanomas.
Recently, however, the influence of a melanophore pattern locus
Li (Tu) has been investigated on the induction of sarcomas
(Schwab et. al. 1978a). Specific genotypes of the fish with and
without the Li marker were treated with a chemical carcinogen MNU
for testing the potential of these genotypes to develop sarcomas.
The results of this study indicated that sarcomas developed on
animals regardless of the fact whether they carried Li (Tu) or
did not. This suggested that the tumor-inducing genetic information (Tu) for the sarcomas is located on a different chromosome
(probably an autosome) other than the Li-carrying X chromosome.
Therefore, it would appear that in the genome of the fish, and
perhaps other multicellular organisms, several Tu loci might be
present, and some of them may be tissue-specific.

IV. LOSS AND TRANSLOCATION OF THE TUMOR GENES

As mentioned earlier, several melanophore pattern loci, including Sd and Sr (Fig.1), involved in melanoma formation have been
located on the sex chromosomes of the platyfish. In addition to
the melanophore pattern loci, certain pterinophore pattern determining loci are also located on the sex chromosomes. In a certain

strain of platyfish, the X chromosome carries the Sd locus and a pterinophore locus Dr (red dorsal fin), while the Y chromosome carries Sr and another pterinophore locus Ar (red anal fin); the females are genotypically X Dr Sd, X Dr Sd, while the males are X Dr Sd, Y Ar Sr (Anders et al., 1973b; Kallman, 1975). Recently we have examined (Ahuja et al., unpublished data) the cytological nature of a deletion involving the Sd locus, and an X-Y translocation involving the Sr locus, and the genetic consequences of these sex chromosome aberrations on the tumor-forming potential and viability of the platyfish.

Karyotypic analysis of the normal platyfish has revealed (Fig. 2) that the X chromosome is metacentric, while the Y chromosome is acrocentric and nearly half the size of the X chromosome; the remaining 23 pairs of the autosomes are all acrocentric, as reported earlier (Foerster and Anders, 1977). The metacentric X chromosome showed 2 giemsa (G) bands on each arm (Fig. 3a), while the Y chromosome exhibited only 2 G-bands (Fig. 3b). Chromosome analysis of the platyfish with the Sd deletion has revealed a loss on one terminal G-band of the X chromosome (Fig. 3c). The genetic consequences of the deletion involving the Sd locus are that neither the platyfish females (X Dr -, X Dr -) or the males (X Dr -, Y Ar Sr) exhibit the black spot on the dorsal fin (Fig. 4), nor do these animals develop melanomas on the dorsal fin following exposure to MNU, or in the hybrids between the Sd deletion platyfish and the swordtail. On the other hand, loss of the Sd chromosome fragment leads to significant increase in the

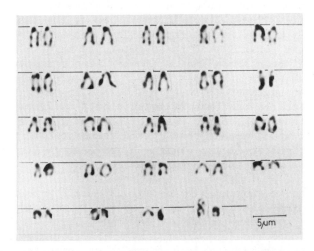

Fig. 2. Karyotype from a platyfish male showing 23 pairs of acrocentric autosomes, a metacentric X chromosome and an acrocentric Y chromosome.

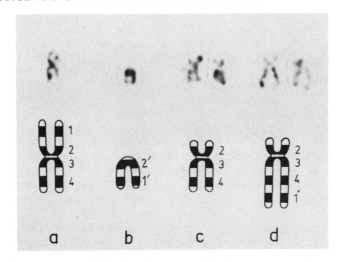

Fig. 3. Normal and aberrant sex chromosomes of platyfish (top row), pairs of chromosomes in (c) and (d) are derived from different individuals, and their schematic diagrams (bottom row); a) normal **metacentric X chromosome showing 4 G-bands, b) normal acrocentric Y chromosome showing 2 G-bands, c) Sd deletion X chromosome lack-ing a terminal G-band 1, and d) Sd deficient X chromosome, which lacks a terminal G-band 1, with an Sr translocation from the Y chromosome showing an extra terminal G-band 1' on the long arm of the X chromosome.** It would appear that Sd is located in or near the terminal G-band 1 and Dr in or near the G-band 2 of the X chromosome, while Sr is located in or near the terminal G-band 1' and Ar in or near the G-band 2' on the Y chromosome.

pterinophores determined by the Dr locus in the platyfish and its hybrids to swordtail (Henze et al., 1977). It is suggested that the Sd deletion segment may carry modifiers or regulator genes that control the expression of Dr, and their loss along with Sd leads to enhanced expression of Dr. Alternatively, the product of the Sd locus may, in some way, be inhibitory to the expression of Dr, and loss of Sd may lead to enhanced expression of the Dr gene. In the light of these observations, it would appear that Dr and Sd loci are located on the same arm of the X chromosome, but their precise linkage relationship cannot be specified. The effect of the Sd deletion segment on all life processes of the platyfish has not been thoroughly investigated. However, this deficiency of the X chromosome in the homozygous condition in the female or hemizygous state in the male has apparently no detectable effect on the viability of the platyfish.

The second chromosome abnormality involves an interchange between an X chromosome and a Y chromosome, in which a chromosome

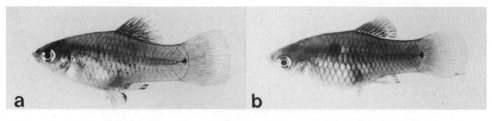

Fig. 4. Platyfish with the deletion of the S̲d̲ locus: a) male with
the genotype X D̲r̲ -, Y A̲r̲ S̲r̲, and b) female with the genotype
X D̲r̲ -, X D̲r̲ - . Note both sexes lack the S̲d̲ pattern (Photographs
courtesy Prof. F. Anders).

fragment carrying the S̲r̲ locus from the Y chromosome has been
translocated onto the S̲d̲ deficient X chromosome of the platyfish.
It was previously suggested (Anders et al., 1973b) that the S̲r̲
locus is translocated next to the D̲r̲ locus on the S̲d̲ deficient
X chromosome. However, the karyotypic analysis has revealed that
the S̲r̲ chromosome fragment is most likely translocated on the
end of the long arm of the X chromosome, and not on the short
deficient arm, since there was an additional terminal G-band on
the long arm of the X chromosome (Fig. 3d). Since in the translocation stock the S̲r̲ locus is present in the male (X S̲r̲ D̲r̲ -, Y A̲r̲ S̲r̲)
as well as the female (X S̲r̲ D̲r̲ -, X S̲r̲ D̲r̲ -), both sexes are stripe
sided (Fig. 5), whereas in the normal platyfish only the males are
stripe sided. Earlier studies have suggested (Anders et. al. 1973a)
that S̲r̲ expression is controlled by a linked R-gene, which when
impaired by irradiation leads to melanoma formation. In the S̲r̲
translocation melanomas did not develop on the platyfish females
or the males, and it would appear that the R-gene, which presumably
controls the expression of S̲r̲ (T̲u̲), is translocated along with S̲r̲,
and therefore must be closely linked to it. This is a confirmation
of a previous result. Further, the S̲r̲ translocation does not appear
to affect the viability of the platyfish females or the males.

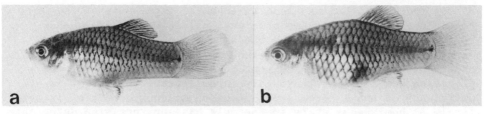

Fig. 5. Platyfish with the S̲r̲ locus translocated onto the S̲d̲ deficient X chromosome: a) male with the genotype X S̲r̲ D̲r̲ -, Y A̲r̲ S̲r̲,
and female with the genotype X S̲r̲ D̲r̲ -, X S̲r̲ D̲r̲ -. Note both sexes
exhibit stripe sided (S̲r̲) expression (Photographs courtesy Prof. F.
Anders).

In another study fish genotypes were treated for their potential to develop sarcomas in earlier and later backcross generations in a cross involving platyfish, carrying Li as a marker, and
the swordtail (Schwab et. al. 1978a). As mentioned in Section II B,
the parental strains, the F-1, and the backcross generation animals
did not develop sarcomas. However, sarcomas developed on specific
genotypes (with or without Li as a marker) following exposure a
chemical carcinogen, MNU. In the backcross generation 1 about
8 % (28/338) of the animals developed sarcomas, while in the backcross generation 4 only 4 % (13/316) of the animals developed
sarcomas following treatment with MNU (Schwab et al., 1978a). On
the other hand, none of the 344 MNU treated animals from the backcross generation 15, with or without Li as a marker, developed
sarcomas. These results may be interpreted to imply that during
backcrossing to swordtail, the sarcoma inducing Tu chromosome
from the platyfish was gradually eliminated, and the backcross 15
animals which essentially would have all swordtail chromosomes,
except those with the Li marker from the platyfish, may have lost
the sarcoma inducing Tu chromosome from the platyfish and consequently the potential to develop sarcomas. The genetic basis for
sensitivity of the swordtail to develop sarcomas has not been tested
due to lack of genetic markers. Since the swordtail is insensitive
to MNU treatment, it is assumed that the genetic information for
the induction of sarcomas may be rigidly controlled by a set of
linked and/or nonlinked R-genes in the genome of the swordtail.

In the framework of the present genetic model on carcinogenesis (Ahuja and Anders, 1976, 1977), impairment or deletion of the
R-genes, on the one hand, presumably leads to neoplastic development, whereas loss or impairment of the Tu genes would, on the
other hand, lead to loss of tumor-forming potential in a specific
tissue, and loss of Tu genes might represent a potential mechanism
involved in reversal from tumor to normal state.

V. CONTROL OF BENIGN AND MALIGNANT STATE

In the platyfish-swordtail system, benign or malignant melanomas can be produced by altering the genetic background of certain
Tu loci, as Sd or Sp, through appropriate genetic manipulations
(Anders et al., 1973a). Following selective matings of the platyfish carrying the loci Sd or Sp to swordtail, three phenotypically
distinguishable classes appeared in the backcross progenies in the
following proportions: 25 % benign melanoma, 25 % malignant melanoma, and 50 % nonmelanoma animals. It was later suggested (Vielkind
et al., 1974; Vielkind, 1976) that the benign or malignant nature
of the melanoma may be conditioned by the presence or absence of
another class of regulatory genes, the differentiation controlling
gene (R-Diff), which presumably operates in the already transformed

cells; backcross animals carrying the R-Diff develop benign melanomas, while those lacking R-Diff develop malignant melanomas
(Fig. 6). It is speculated that the mode of action of the R-Diff
might be through promotion of the density dependent regulation of
growth and/or through promotion of cell differentiation of already
transformed pigment cells.

Pigment cell differentiation has been extensively investigated in the platyfish-swordtail system (Tavolga, 1949; Gordon, 1959;
Humm and Young, 1956; Diehl, 1975; Vielkind, 1976; Vielkind et al.,
1977). Normal development of pigment cells begins in the stem cells,
the melanoblasts. The melanoblasts differentiate into dendritic
melanocytes, which are capable of synthesizing melanin. The melanocytes finally mature into nondividing melanophores, which store
melanin, but do not synthesize it.

Experiments with fish mutants, in which melanophore development is blocked at various stages of pigment cell differentiation,
have indicated that melanoblasts are the competent cell for neoplastic transformation. The transformed melanoblasts, called T-
melanoblasts, differentiate into T-melanocytes, which can be
distinguished cytologically from the normal melanocytes. In the
malignant melanoma, the frequency of T-melanoblasts and T-melanocytes increases considerably, and only a few may eventually mature
into T-melanophores. The benign and malignant melanomas differ
from each other in several cytological and biochemical attributes
(Vielkind, 1976; Vielkind et al., 1977). The benign melanomas,
which are conditioned by the R-Diff, consist of cells at various
degrees of differentiation. Besides, many large T-melanophores,
there are cells from transitional stages between melanoblasts and
melanocytes in the benign melanoma. On the other hand, malignant
melanomas, which lack the R-Diff locus, consist predominantly of
poorly differentiated cells; the T-melanoblasts are considerably
increased in number, while the T-melanocytes and T-melanophores

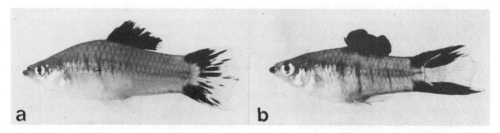

Fig. 6. Backcross segregants from a cross involving Sd platyfish
and swordtail (recurrent parent) showing: a) benign melanoma,
and b) malignant melanoma on the dorsal fin (Photographs courtesy
Prof. F. Anders).

are reduced to a minimum. The malignant melanoma condition is associated with high tyrosinase activity, which is several fold higher than that in the benign melanoma (Vielkind, 1976; Vielkind et al., 1977). Further, total lactate dehydrogenase activity was about two-fold higher in the malignant melanoma as compared to the benign melanoma (Schwab et al., 1976), although there were no qualitative differences in the lactate dehydrogenase isozymes in the benign and the malignant melanoma (Ahuja et al., 1975). Recent biochemical studies (Siciliano and Wright, 1976; Ahuja, 1978) have suggested linkage between R-Diff and a specific estrase locus, which is inherited from the platyfish (Ahuja et al., 1977) in the benign melanoma animals in the platyfish-swordtail melanoma system. Although, the chromosome location of the R-Diff locus has not been established in the Sp or Sd (both X linked loci) conditioned melanoma system, genetic studies suggest that genes similar to R-Diff may be located on one of the autosomes (Anders, 1967).

In mouse myeloid leukemia cell clones differ in their ability to be induced to differentiate by the protein inducer MGI (macrophage and granulocyte inducer): some clones are MGI$^+$ (can be induced to form rosettes), while others are MGI$^-$ (cannot be induced to form rosettes) (Azumi and Sachs, 1977). Chromosome studies of Azumi and Sachs indicate that mouse chromosomes 2 and 12 carry genes that control the differentiation of myeloid leukemic cells, and that inducibility by MGI is controlled by the balance between these. They have further suggested that chromosomes 2 and 12 also carry genes that control the malignancy of the mouse myeloid leukemic cells.

VI. NATURE OF THE HEREDITABLE CHANGE IN NEOPLASTIC TRANSFORMATION

Although all neoplastic cells exhibit cell heredity, that is, there is hereditary transmission of tumor properties to the descendants of a cancer cell, the nature of the primary event of cellular transformation remains an open question. Regarding the origin of neoplasms, it is possible to ask: Does the initial event of transformation result from an epigenetic change, that is, a change in the expression of a gene or activity of a gene product, which does not require an alteration in the gene structure? Or does neoplastic transformation results from an alteration of the genotype, that is, a genetic change (mutation) may be the underlying cause for the initiation of tumors? A mutation is defined according to Siminovitch (1976) as a heritable change in nucleotide sequence resulting from an alteration, deletion or rearrangement of primary structure of cellular DNA. This definition of mutation includes point mutation, deletion, chromosome rearrangements and chromosomal loss, as long as heritable change results (Siminovitch, 1976).

The capacity of mouse teratocarcinoma cells to give rise to
entirely benign progeny (Pierce, 1967), and rat squamous cell carcinoma to give rise to "pearls" of benign cells (Pierce and
Wallace, 1971), has led Pierce to suggest that malignant phenotype
may not require an alteration of the genotype, but may rather
result from an epigenetic change. In a recent study Mintz and
Illmensee (1975) and Illmensee and Mintz (1976) have demonstrated
that markers form malignant teratocarcinoma cells injected into
blastocytes subsequently show up in normal adult tissues, a result
which further lends support to the idea that neoplastic transformation results from a developmental aberration of gene expression
rather than a change in gene structure.

A number of studies with chemical and physical carcinogens,
on the other hand, suggest that neoplastic transformation is the
result of a genetic change. Most of the chemicals known to cause
cancer in animals are mutagenic, and in vivo and in vitro studies
indicate (Bridges, 1976) that the ultimate carcinogenic form of
the chemicals interact with DNA, and cause mutation in a bacterial
system (McCann et al., 1975; McCann and Ames, 1976). Somatic mutation as the basis of malignant transformation has been demonstrated
in hamster cells treated with chemical carcinogens (Bouck and
di Mayorca, 1976). By employing genetic markers, the relationship
between carcinogenesis and mutagenesis has been determined in
chinese hamster cells following exposure to chemical carcinogens
(Huberman and Sachs, 1976). Further, it was suggested (Huberman
et. al. 1976) that transformation of normal to cancer cells of
the golden hamster is due to somatic mutation in one out of a
small number of same or different genes. In the platyfish-swordtail system, we have recently investigated sensitivity to develop
neoplasms in 65 different genotype, including parental strains,
F-1 hybrids, and backcross derivatives from earlier and later
generations, following exposure to the chemical carcinogen MNU
and X-rays (Schwab et al., 1978a and b). Our results indicate
that the potential to develop neoplasms, for example, melanomas, sarcomas, neuroblastomas, etc., is dependent upon the genotype of
the host. These results further suggest that differential sensitivity of the genotypes is a function of the type of regulatory
control of the Tu information, and tissue-specific neoplasms develop
when R-genes controlling the Tu information in such tissues are
impaired or deleted by mutational events.

In man there are several neoplasms that have been associated
with specific gene abnormalities (see Knudson et al., 1973; Knudson,
1975). According to Knudson, there are two categories of genetic
disease associated with human cancer: a) genetic states predispos-
ing to cancer, which include chromosome abnormalities and Mendelian
conditions, and b) highly penetrant hereditary (autosomal dominant)
tumors. Knudson has proposed that autosomal dominant human tumors

(hereditary or nonhereditary) may arise as a result of two mutational events. In the genetic form one mutation is inherited via the germinal cells, while the second mutation occurs in the somatic cells. On the other hand, in the nonhereditary form both mutational events occur in the somatic cells.

Included in the first category are certain human neoplasms, which have been found to be associated with specific chromosome abnormalities. For example chronic myelogenous leukemia (CML) in man has been found to be associated with the Philadelphia chromosome, which arises by a translocation of the long arm of 22 to 9 (Rowley, 1973, 1977). Burkitt's lymphoma seems to be associated with a specific genetic change, probably involving a translocation of a terminal band from chromosome 8 to 14 (Manolov and Manolova, 1972; Zech, 1974). In meningioma there is a loss of one human chromosome 22 (mark, 1973). Based on studies on patients with the CML disease who are heterozygous for the X-linked enzyme locus for glucose-6-phosphate dehydrogenase (G-6-PD), Fialkow et al. (1967) have suggested that the CML disease, most likely, is a consequence of a rare event in a single somatic cell, thus supporting the mutational origin of CML. It has been suggested (Fialkow et al., 1970) that Burkitt's lymphoma may also have a clonal origin. Xeroderma pigmentosum, a recessive disorder, which predisposes its carriers to develop multiple cutaneous cancer following exposure to strong sunlight, is caused by a genetic defect in the enzyme system necessary for DNA repair of ultraviolet light-induced damage (Cleaver, 1968, 1969; Setlow et al., 1969).

Viruses have been shown to induce tumors in animals, and have been implicated in human cancer. Some have proposed that the oncogenic information may be present in the virogenes in the cell genome (Huebner and Todaro, 1969; Todaro and Huebner, 1972), while others have suggested that viruses must be introduced exogenously as infectious agents (Gross, 1970, 1974; Temin, 1972). According to the oncogene hypothesis of Huebner and Todaro, carcinogens, irradiation, and the normal aging process all favor the partial or complete activation, possibly through mutations, of the genes that control malignancy. On the other hand, following infection with an exogenous virus, the genotype of the infected cell is altered to give rise to a malignant phenotype, probably due to integration of partial or complete genome of the virus in the cellular DNA. Complete virus particles have been recovered from previously infected animal cells (Temin, 1974). However, only subviral components of the type C RNA viruses have been detected in the blood cells from many leukemic patients (Baxt et al., 1972, 1973; Gallo et al., 1973; Miller et al., 1974) and from the spleen of a patient with myelofibrotic syndrome (Chandra and Steel, 1977).

Tumor viruses may transform cells through several different

mechanisms. Some may transform cells by insertion of their transforming information into host cells, whose regulatory genes do
not suppress the transforming information (Comings, 1973). While
others might bring in some tissue-specific information that might
act as a carcinogen affecting the regulatory apparatus of the cell,
either directly impairing the R-genes, or indirectly, by causing
chromosome breaks at specific locations, by attaching to specific
sites on the chromosomes, which might lead to altered regulation
due to deletion and/or position effect of the tissue-specific R-
genes.

VII. CONCLUDING REMARKS

Evidence for the genetic control of tumor formation comes
from a wide variety of experimental systems, such as tobacco
(Ahuja, 1965, 1968; Smith, 1972), Drosophila (Gardner, 1970),
fish (Gordon, 1958; Anders, 1967; Anders et al., 1973a and b),
mice (see Heston, 1975), and hamster (Huberman and Sachs, 1976;
Azumi and Sachs, 1977). The observations from these experimental
systems suggest that neoplasms develop on individuals of specific
genotypes. These specific genotypes, prone to neoplastic development can be produced by genetic manipulations, or following exposure to chemical or physical carcinogens. Experimental evidence
from different systems suggest that a genetic change may be,
by and large, the underlying cause for neoplastic transformation,
although in some cases neoplastic transformation may result from
a developmental aberration. Data from the platyfish-swordtail
system suggest that the tumor-inducing information (Tu) may be
controlled in different ways in different tissues, and the potential to develop neoplasm in a specific tissue may be the function
of the type of regulatory control (R-genes) in that tissue. It
is proposed that mutational events may occur in the R-genes of a
specific tissue, which control the Tu information, and impairment
or deletion of the R-genes possibly leads to origin of neoplasms.
On the other hand, loss of Tu genes may lead to loss of potential
to form tumors. The role of viruses is considered to be one of
bringing in some information, which may directly or indirectly
cause a genetic change leading to neoplastic transformation. And
finally, human data on hereditary tumors, and neoplasms associated
with specific chromosome abonormalities, seem to be consistent with
the notion that a genetic change may trigger neoplastic development.

ACKNOWLEDGEMENTS

Author's research has been supported by grants from DFG, when
he was a Richard Merton Guest Professor, and subsequently from
SFB 103 (Marburg) through Prof. F. Anders. The author is grateful

to Prof. Anders for stimulating discussions. He also thanks Klaus
Lepper for excellent technical assistance.

REFERENCES

Ahuja, M. R., A cytogenetic study of heritable tumors in Nicotiana
species hybrids. Genetics 47, 865-880 (1962).

Ahuja, M. R., Genetic control of tumor formation in higher plants.
Q. Rev. Biol. 40, 329-340 (1965).

Ahuja, M. R., An hypothesis and evidence concerning the genetic
components controlling tumor formation in Nicotiana. Molec. gen.
Genet. 103, 176-184 (1968).

Ahuja, M. R., Genetic control of phytohormones in tumor and non-
tumor genotypes in Nicotiana. Ind. J. Exptl. Biol. 9, 60-68
(1971).

Ahuja, M. R., Linkage relationship between a regulatory gene R-Diff
and an esterase locus in the xiphophorine fish melanoma. Proc. XIV
Int. Congr. Genetics, Moscow, Abstract, in press (1978).

Ahuja, M. R. and Anders, F., A genetic concept of the origin of
cancer, based in part upon studies of neoplasms in fishes. Prog.
exp. Tumor Res. 20, 380-397 (1976).

Ahuja, M. R. and Anders, F., Cancer as a problem of gene regulation.
in Recent Advances in Cancer Research: Cell Biology, Molecular
Biology, and Tumor Virology, vol. I, Gallo, R. C. (ed.), pp. 103-
117, C. R. C. Press, Cleveland (1977).

Ahuja, M. R., Lepper, K. and Anders, F., Sex chromosome aberrations
involving loss and translocation of tumor-inducing loci of platyfish, Platypoecilus maculatus. (unpublished results).

Ahuja, M. R., Schwab, M. and Anders, F., Lactate dehydrogenase isozymes in xiphophorine fish melanoma conditioned by the locus Sd.
Experientia 31, 296-297 (1975).

Ahuja, M. R., Schwab, M. and Anders, F., Tissue-specific esterases
in the xiphophorine fish Platypoecilus maculatus, Xiphophorus
helleri and their hybrid. Biochem. Genet. 15, 601-610 (1977).

Anders, A., Anders, F. and Klinke, K.. Regulation of gene expression in Gordon-Kosswig melanoma system. I. The distribution of
controlling genes in the genomes of the xiphophorine fish,
Platypoecilus maculatus and P. variatus. in Genetics and Mutagenesis of Fish, Schroeder, J. H. (ed.), pp. 33-52, Springer,
Berlin (1973a).

Anders, A., Anders, F. and Klinke, K., Regulation of gene expression in the Gordon-Kosswig melanoma syste. II. The arrangement of
chromatophore determining loci and regulating elements in the
chormosomes of xiphophorine fish, Platypoecilus maculatus and
P. variatus. in Genetics and Mutagenesis of Fish, Schroeder, J.
H. (ed.), pp. 53-63, Springer, Berlin (1973b).

Anders, A., Anders, F., and Pursglove, D. L., X-ray induced mutations of the genetically-determined melanoma system of xiphophorine fish. Experientia 27, 931-932 (1971).

Anders, F., Tumor formation in platyfish-swordtail hybrids as a
   problem of gene regulation. Experientia 23, 1-10 (1967).
Anders, F., Anders, A. and Vielkind, U., Regulation of tumor expression in the Gordon-Kosswig melanoma system, and the origin of
   malignancy. XI Int. Cancer Congr. Florence, p. 305 (1974).
Azumi, J. and Sachs, L., Chromosome mapping of the genes that
   control differentiation and malignancy in myeloid leukemic cells.
   Proc. Natl. Acad. Sci. U.S.A. 74, 253-257 (1977).
Baxt, W., Hehlman, R. and Spiegelman, S., Human leukemic cells
   contain reverse transcriptase associated with a high molecular
   weight virus-related RNA. Nature new Biol. 240, 72-75 (1972).
Baxt, W., Yates, J. W., Wallace, H. J., Holland J. F. and Spiegelman, S., Leukemia-specific DNA sequences in leukocytes of the
   leukemic member of identical twins. Proc. Natl. Acad. Sci. U.S.A.
   70, 2629-2632 (1973).
Bouck, N. and di Mayorca, G., Somatic mutation as the basis for
   malignant transformation of BHK cells by chemical carcinogens.
   Nature 264, 722-727 (1976).
Bridges, B. A., Short term screening tests for carcinogens. Nature
   261, 195-200 (1976).
Caspersson, T., Gahrton,G., Lindsten, J. and Zech, L., Identification of the Philadelphia chromosome as a number 22 by quinacrine
   mustard fluorescence analysis. Exp Cell Res. 63, 238-240 (1970).
Chandra, P. and Steel, L. K., Purification, biochemical characterization and serological analysis of cellular deoxyribonucleic
   acid polymerases and a reverse transcriptase from spleen of a
   patient with myelofibrotic syndrome. Biochem. J. 167, 513-524
   (1977).
Chattopadhyay, S.K., Rowe, W. P., Teich, N. M. and Lowy, D. R.,
   Definitive evidence that the murine C type virus inducing locus
   Akv-1 is viral genetic material. Proc. Natl. Acad. Sci. U.S.A.
   72, 906-910 (1975).
Cleaver, J. E., defective repair replication of DNA in xeroderma
   pigmentosum. Nature 218, 652-656 (1968).
Cleaver, J. E., Xeroderma pigmentosum: a human disease in which an
   initial state of DNA repair is defective. Proc. Natl. Acad. Sci.
   U.S.A. 63, 428-435 (1969).
Comings, D. E., A general theory of carcinogenesis. Proc. Natl.
   Acad. Sci. U.S.A. 70, 3324-3328 (1973).
Diehl, H., Uber die Entwicklung des embryonalen Pigmentierung-
   smuster bei verschiedenen Genotypen von Xiphophorus (Pisces, Poe-
   ciliidae). Diplomarbeit, Giessen (1975).
Fialkow, P. J., Gartler, S. M. and Yoshida, A., Clonal origin of
   chronic myelogenous leukemia in man. Proc. Natl. Acad. Sci.
   U.S.A. 58, 1468-1471 (1967).
Fialkow, P. J., Klein, G., Gartler, S. M. and Clifford, P., Clonal
   origin for individual Burkitt tumours. Lancet 1, 384-386 (1970).
Foerster, W. and Anders, F., Zytogenetischer Vergleich der Karyo-
   typen verschiedener Rassen und Arten lebendgebärender Zahnkarpfen
   der Gattung Xiphophorus. Zool. Anz. 198, 167-177 (1977).

Gallo, R. C., Miller, N. R., Saxinger, W. C. and Gillespie, D., Primate RNA tumor virus-like DNA synthesized endogenously by RNA-dependent DNA polymerase in virus-like particles from fresh human acute leukemic blood cells. Proc. Natl. Acad. Sci. U.S.A. 70, 3219-3224 (1973).

Gardner, E. J., Tumorous head in Drosophila. Adv Genetics 15, 115-146 (1970).

Gordon, M., A genetic concept for the origin of cancer. Ann. N. Y. Acad. Sci. 71, 1213-1222 (1958).

Gordon, M., The melanoma cell as an incompletely differentiated pigment cell. in Pigment Cell Biology, Gordon, M. (ed.), pp. 215-236, Academic Press. New York (1959).

Gross, L., Oncogenic Viruses. 2nd ed. Pergamon Press, Oxford (1970).

Gross, L., Facts and theories on viruses causing cancer and leukemia. Proc. Natl. Acad. Sci. U.S.A. 71, 2013-2017 (1974).

Henze, M., Rempeters, G. and Anders, F., Pteridines in the skin of Xiphophorine fish (Poeciliidae). Comp. Biochem. Physiol. 56B, 35-46 (1977).

Huebner, R. J. and Todaro, G. J., Oncogenes of RNA tumor viruses as determinants of cancer. Proc. Natl. Acad. Sci. U.S.A. 64, 1087-1094 (1969).

Huberman, E. and Sachs, L., Mutability of different genetic loci in mammalian cells by metabolically activated carcinogenic polycyclic hydrocarbons. Proc. Natl. Acad. Sci. U.S.A. 73, 188-192 (1976).

Huberman, E., Mager, R. and Sachs, L., Mutagenesis and transformation of normal cells by chemical carcinogens. Nature 264, 360-361 (1976).

Humm, D. G. and Young, R. S., The embryonal origin of pigment cells in platyfish-swordtail hybrids. Zoologica 41, 1-10 (1956).

Illmensee, K. and Mintz, B., Totipotency and normal differentiation of single teratocarcinoma cells cloned by injection into blastocysts. Proc. Natl. Acad. Sci. U.S.A. 73, 549-553 (1976).

Kallman, K. D., The Platyfish, Xiphophorus maculatus. in Handbook of Genetics, vol 4, King, R. C. (ed.), pp. 81-132, Plenum Press, New York (1975).

Kirby, D. R. S. and Cowell, T. P., Trophoblast-host interactions. in Epithelial-Mesenchymal Interactions, Fleischmajer, R. and Billingham, R. E. (eds.), pp. 64-77, Williams and Wilkins Co., Baltimore (1968).

Knudson, A. G., Mutation and cancer: statistical study of retinoblastoma. Proc. Natl. Acad. Sci. U.S.A. 68, 820-823 (1971).

Knudson, A. G., Genetic influences in human tumors. in Cancer: A Comprehensive Treatise. I., Becker, F. F. (ed.), pp. 59-74, Plenum Press, New York (1975).

Knudson, A. G. and Strong, L. C., Mutation and cancer: a model for Wilms' tumor of the kidney. J. Natl. Cancer Inst. 48, 313-324 (1971).

Knudson, A. G., Strong, L. C. and Anderson, D. E., Heredity and cancer in man. Progr. Med. Genet. 9, 113-158 (1973).

Manes, C., Phasing of gene products during development. Cancer Res. 34, 2044-2052 (1974).

Manolov, G and Manolova, Y., Marker band in one chromosome 14 from Burkitt lymphomas. Nature 237, 33 (1972).

Mark, J., Karyotype patterns in human meningiomas. A comparison between studies with G- and Q-banding techniques. Hereditas 75, 213-220 (1973).

McCann, J. and Ames, B. N., Detection of carcinogens as mutagens in the Salmonella/microsome test: assay of 300 chemicals: discussion. Proc. Natl. Acad. Sci. U.S.A. 73, 950-954 (1976)

McCann, J., Choi, E., Yamasaki, E. and Ames, B. N., Detection of carcinogens as mutagens in the Salmonella/microsome test: assay of 300 chemicals. Proc. Natl. Acad. Sci. U.S.A. 72, 5135-5139 (1975).

Miller, N. R., Saxinger, W. C., Reitz, M. S., Gallagher, R. E., Wu, A. M., Gallo, R. C. and Gillespie, D., Systematics of RNA tumor viruses and virus-like particles of human origin. Proc. Natl. Acad. Sci. U.S.A. 71, 3177-3181 (1974).

Mintz, B. and Illmensee, K., Normal genetically mosaic mice produced from malignant teratocarcinoma cells. Proc. Natl. Acad. Sci. U.S.A. 72, 3585-3589 (1975).

Nowell, P. C. and Hungerford, D. A., A minute chromosome in human chronic granulocytic leukemia. Science 132, 1197 (1960).

Ohno, S., Genetic implication of karyological instability of malignant somatic cells. Physiol. Rev. 51, 496-526 (1971).

Patillo, R. A., Story, M. T., Hershman, J. M., Delfs, E. and Mattingly, R. F., Hormone control of differentiation and embryonic antigen in human placental tumor cells in vitro. in Embryonic and Fetal Antigens in Cancer, Anderson, N. G., Coggin, J. H., Cole, E. and Holleman, J. W. (eds.), pp. 45-71, USAEC Report, United States Dept. of Commerce (1972).

Pierce, G. P., Teratocarcinoma: model for developmental concept of cancer. in Current Topics in Developmental Biology, vol. 2, Moscona, A. and Monroy, A. (eds.), pp. 223-246, Academic Press, New York (1967).

Pierce, G. P. and Wallace, C., Differentiation of malignant to benign cells. Cancer Res. 31, 127-134 (1971).

Prescott, D. M., Cancer -- The Misguided Cell. The Bobbs-Merrill Co. Inc. New York (1973).

Pursglove, D. L., Anders, A., Döll, G. and Anders, F., Effects of X-irradiation on the genetically determined melanoma system of xiphophorine fish. Experientia 27, 695 (1971).

Rowe, W. P., Hartly, J. W. and Bremmer, T., Genetic mapping of murine leukemia virus-inducing locus of AKR mice. Science 178, 860-862 (1972).

Rowley, J. D., A new consistent chromosome abnormality in chronic myelogenous leukemia identified by quinacrine fluorescence and giemsa staining. Nature 243, 290-293 (1973).

Rowley, J. D., Are nonrandom karyotypic changes related to etio-
logic agents ? in Genetics of Human Cancer, Mulvihill, J. J.,
Miller, R. W. and Fraumeni, J. F. (eds.), pp. 125-136, Raven
Press, New York (1977).

Rudkin, G. T., Hungerford, D. A. and Nowell, P. C., DNA Content of
chromosome Ph[1] and chromosome 21 in human chronic granulocytic
leukemia. Science 144, 1229 (1964).

Schwab, M., Ahuja, M. R. and Anders, F., Elevated levels of lactate
dehydrogenase in genetically controlled melanoma of Xiphophorine
fish. Comp. Biochem. Physiol. 54b, 197-199 (1976).

Schwab, M., Abdo, S., Ahuja, M. R., Kollinger, G., Anders, A.,
Anders, A. and Frese, K., Genetic of susceptibility in the platy-
fish/swordtail tumor system to develop fibrosarcoma and rhabdomyosarcoma following treatment with N-methyl-N-nitrosourea (MNU).
Z. Krebsforsch. in press (1978a).

Schwab, M., Haas, J., Abdo, S., Ahuja, M. R., Kollinger, G., Anders,
A. and Anders, F., Genetic basis of susceptibility for development of neoplasms following treatment with N-methyl-N-nitrosourea (MNU) or X-rays in the platyfish/swordtail system. Experientia. In press (1978b).

Setlow, R. B., Regan, J. D., German, J. and Carrier, W. L., Evidence that xeroderma pigmentosum cells do not perform the first
step in the repair of ultraviolet damage to their DNA. Proc. Natl.
Acad. Sci. U.S.A. 64, 1035-1041 (1969).

Siciliano, M. J. and Wright, D. A., Biochemical genetics of the
platyfish-swordtail hybrid melanoma system. Prog. exp. Tumor Res.
20, 398-411 (1976).

Siminovitch, L., On the nature of hereditable variation in cultured somatic cells. Cell 7, 1-11 (1976).

Tavolga, W. N., Embryonic development of the platyfish (Platypoecilus), the swordtail (Xiphophorus) and their hybrids. Bull. Am.
Mus. Nat. Hist. 94, 163-229 (1949).

Temin, H. M., The RNA-tumor viruses, background and foreground.
Proc. Natl. Acad. Sci. U.S.A. 69, 1016-1020 (1972).

Temin, H. M., On the origin of genes for neoplasia. Cancer Res. 34,
2835-2841 (1974).

Todaro, G. J. and Huebner, R. J., The viral oncogene hypothesis:
new evidence. Proc. Natl. Acad. Sci. U.S.A. 69, 1009-1015 (1972).

Vielkind, U., Genetic control of cell differentiation in platyfish-
swordtail melanomas. J. Exp. Zool. 196, 197-204 (1976).

Vielkind, U., Vielkind, J. and Anders, F., Genetic control of melanoma cell differentiation. Proc. XI Int. Cancer Congr. Florence,
p. 306 (1974).

Vielkind, U., Schlage, W. and Anders, F., Melanogenesis in genetically determined pigment cell tumors of platyfish and platyfish-
swordtail hybrids: correlation between tyrosinase activity and
degree of malignancy. Z. Krebsforsch. 90, 285-299 (1977).

Zech, L. Nonrandom distribution of chromosome abnormalities in
tissues of neoplastic origin. Proc XI Int. Cancer Congr.
Florence, p. 644 (1974).

HIGH INCIDENCE ALIMENTARY CARCINOMA IN CATTLE ASSOCIATED WITH AN ENVIRONMENTAL CARCINOGEN AND VIRAL PAPILLOMAS

W.F.H. JARRETT

Department of Veterinary Pathology, University of Glasgow

Veterinary School, Bearsden, Glasgow, G61 1QH, Scotland

This paper deals with a possible bifactorial oncogenic situation in which a geographically sharply delineated area of high cancer incidence in cattle appears to be associated with the ingestion of bracken fern and infection by a papilloma virus. The interplay of the environmental chemical carcinogen and the virus has been partially worked out but the basic interactions involved present an interesting challenge in oncology, virology and immunology.

Carcinomas of the alimentary tract are not common tumours in cattle and several surveys have virtually failed to reveal their presence in abattoir material. In the last few years however we have found that there is a very high incidence of tumours of the alimentary tract and urinary bladder in the upland areas of Britain and in particular there is an extremely high occurrence rate of squamous carcinoma of the upper alimentary tract (Jarrett, 1973; Jarrett et al., 1978a). This has become one of the commonest diseases of beef cows and is a major feature in economic loss from farms. The disease is unknown in the neighbouring lowland areas both on dairy farms and beef farms. The incidence is very high and we estimate it to be about 2.5 to 5% of the population at risk but we have found as high an incidence as 20% in one herd in a period of observation of just over 1 year. Multiple case herds are common and cancer "storms" lead to the rejection of significant numbers of cows from the herds. The complex possibly ranks as the highest naturally-occurring cancer incidence known. We have carried out a detailed study of 80 cases of alimentary carcinoma from this area (Jarrett et al., 1978a). These cases were selected on clinical grounds for the syndrome associated with

squamous carcinoma of the upper alimentary tract. Four types of
alimentary tumours were found and their interrelationships are basically
the most interesting part of the complex and in particular to the possible
relationship to carcinoma of the intestine in man. The tumours found
were (1) squamous carcinoma, (2) papilloma of the upper alimentary
tract, (3) adenoma or polyposis and (4) adenocarcinoma of the intestine.
In the 80 cases, 165 squamous carcinomas of the alimentary tract were
found, of these 7% were on the tongue, 4% on the palate, 8% on the
pharynx, 41% in the oesophagus and 30% in the rumen. A very striking
feature of these cases was that 96% of them had concurrent papillomas
or warts of the squamous epithelium lining the upper alimentary tract.
These papillomas were distributed in exactly the same specific sites
as the carcinomas. Another noticeable feature was the occurrence
of obviously malignant tissue in pre-existing, clearly structured
papillomas which will be seen later to be of viral etiology. This change
was most noticeable when animals which were in the early stages of
the disease were examined. Such animals were purchased from
multiple incidence farms and slaughtered before they were in an
extreme clinical state. At this point one major carcinoma might be
present, several small carcinomas of 0.5 to 1 cm diameter, multiple
virus-induced papillomas and numbers of papillomas showing malignant
transformation. The carcinomas themselves ranged from 0.5 to 60 cms
in diameter and 36% of cases showed metastasis. Histological examination of the cases showed that there is no question that direct transformation
of papillomas gives rise to carcinomas but it naturally cannot be asserted
on histological grounds alone that all of the carcinomas originated from
virus papillomas because of the destructive nature of the malignant
lesions which obscured possible precursor papillomas.

It was of obvious importance to determine if the papillomas which
had the structure of typical warts were virus-induced or not. Virus
papilloma of the alimentary tract is not a condition that has been recognised
by meat inspectors or veterinary pathologists in Great Britain. In two
other localised areas of high incidence carcinoma of the oesophagus and
pharynx, papillomas had been noted but no virus could be observed or
extracted (Plowright et al., 1971, De The, Orth & Croissant, personal
communications, Dobereiner et al., 1967). As will be seen later, it is
easier to demonstrate productive virus infections in young tumours than
in old and with this possibility in mind we purchased young animals from
a high incidence cancer farm. These animals had palatine and oesophageal
papillomas and from these we isolated by maceration and density gradient
centrifugation a typical papilloma virus of 55nm diameter and a density
in CsCl of 1.36. The physical and morphological characteristics of this
virus are indistinguishable from those of the well known bovine cutaneous

papilloma virus (see review by Olson, 1969).   Olson and his collaborators were unable to infect the alimentary tract of cattle with cutaneous papilloma virus and did not recognise the condition we describe.

It should be stated at this point that we came to recognise three epidemiological variants of papilloma virus infection and tumour expression in cattle.   These are (1) cutaneous fibropapillomas which are very common and often go through a cycle of growth followed by rejection which lasts a few months, (2) alimentary papillomatosis of the type under discussion and (3) papillomas of the udder and teats.   These three lesion complexes behave in an epidemiologically distinct fashion which will be discussed in later publications.

It became necessary at this point in the study to carry out a large scale survey to determine the incidence and etiology of squamous papillomas of the alimentary tract of cattle from both the area in which carcinoma of the alimentary tract was unknown and from the high incidence area.   7,746 cattle of a wide range of ages were examined in Glasgow abattoir at the time of slaughter.   The overall incidence of alimentary papillomatosis was found to be 19%, 11% having mouth papillomas, 11% oesophageal papillomas and 3% having lesions in both their mouth and their oesophagus.   55% of these animals were below 2 years, 9% were 2 to 3 years and 36% were over 3 years.   There was no significant difference between the incidence in any age group and the figures are accurate reflections of the background population in terms of age.   A major finding here was that 89% of infected young cattle and 82% of aged infected animals had single alimentary papillomas.   11% of young and 18% of older animals had multiple tumours.   Again there was no significant difference between age groups.   The papillomas were found at exactly the same sites as the papillomas and carcinomas in the high incidence cancer area.   In addition the multiplicity of sites per animal was investigated and it was found that 95% of alimentary positive cases had tumours at one site only and only 5% had them at two sites. None had more.   This was in sharp contradistinction to carcinoma cases and "normal" animals from the cancer farms.   Of the former, 24% had papillomas at one site and 65% at more than one.   In the abattoir survey, 90% of the animals had less than 5 papillomas, 10% had more than 5 and none had more than 15.   In the cows from the high incidence farms, 15% had less than 5, 41% had more than 5 and 39% had more than 15.   We also clinically examined the mouths of 366 live cattle of all ages on 10 farms in the cancer area; there were papillomas in 39% of these compared with 11% in the survey of normal cattle.   It would appear, therefore, that there is marked difference in papilloma status between the cancer area and the non-cancer area.   The three major points are

(1) the overall incidence is much higher (2) the multiplicity of sites is increased and (3) the papilloma numbers per case are all increased in the high incidence cancer area. It is also obvious that there is an increase in the number of alimentary papillomas present in animals of all ages on the cancer farms. This indicates that an environmental factor is present on these farms which might be involved both in the amplification in incidence, sites and numbers of papillomas in the first 6 years of an animal's life and in the induction of carcinoma in the succeeding decade. Carcinomas are only seen from 7 years of age onwards, two-thirds occur below the age of 12 and they have been found in animals as old as 18 years.

The environmental factor which is thought to be involved is bracken fern as there is a very high infestation of grasslands with this plant in the upland areas. In general the higher the density of bracken geographically, the larger is the incidence of carcinoma and other tumours. Bracken fern contains a compound or compounds which have been demonstrated to be carcinogenic for laboratory animals (See Evans, 1972), is mutagenic and in high dose produces a disease known as acute bracken poisoning in cattle which has all the characteristics of radiomimetic toxicity. In the acute disease one sees agranulocytosis, aplastic anaemia, immunosuppression and widespread ulceration and haemorrhage. Bracken feeding has been shown to cause tumours of the urinary bladder in cattle (Pamukcu et al., 1976) and these particular tumours are found in the same herds as the squamous carcinoma cases (Jarrett et al., 1978a). Most of the farms in the carcinoma study had a history of outbreaks of acute bracken poisoning in the few years preceding the incidence of diagnosed carcinoma. Carcinoma of the alimentary tract in cattle has not yet been induced by feeding bracken although long-term experiments are in progress. We have infected animals with papilloma virus and subjected them to bracken in the diet. To date only one result is available. An animal, after 4 years of bracken feeding, had to be destroyed for other reasons. It had florid oesophageal papillomatosis of the type seen in young animals from the high cancer area.

The relationship of papilloma virus to the alimentary warts found in the abattoir survey is discussed in detail in Jarrett et al. (1978a) and Jarrett et al. (1978b) and the details of transformation of these papillomas is given in Jarrett (1978). Of the material from the abattoir survey, 100 unselected papillomas were taken for histological examination. 78 were true papillomas and 22 were basically fibromas and fibropapillomas. A detailed examination was made of a single section from each of these 100 cases for the presence of type A intranuclear inclusion bodies. No inclusions were seen in any fibroma but they were present in 13% of the papillomas. These cases when studied by electron microscopy showed large intranuclear crystalloid arrays of virus particles in the keratinising cells in the upper layers of the stratum spinosum. Seven of the 100 papillomas were chosen for further study. On examination of a single section, 4 were positive for inclusion bodies and 3 were negative. The virus-positive tumours were all large in size and histologically showed many mitotic figures. 100 serial sections were cut through each papilloma and every fifth section was studied in detail. All 20 sections in each inclusion body positive case were positive; all sections in the initially negative cases were negative. It was obvious, however, that many papillomas which had no fully developed type A inclusion bodies had nuclei which contained areas of amphophilic material of lower density than type A inclusions and which was quite distinguishable from normal chromatin. Study of such cases has revealed that the nuclei contain many typical virus particles. It was seen that certain tumours or individual subunits of tumours contained areas in which virtually every keratinising cell was productive or permissive of virus replication while other subunits of the same tumour might be completely negative for productive infection. There is also a great variability in the amount of virus which can be extracted by maceration and density gradient centrifugation from individual tumours. There would appear to be no doubt however that this condition is caused by a papilloma virus. Purified virus from these tumours has been used to induce papillomas in both the alimentary tract and the skin of susceptible calves (Jarrett et al. 1978a). Large amounts of virus have been obtained in this way. Studies are at present in progress to compare and contrast virus isolates from alimentary papillomas, skin warts and udder and teat warts by immunological molecular hybridisation and restriction endo-nuclease techniques. Results to date have shown differences between various virus strains but it is not yet clear if this reflects differences in individual virus isolates prepared from single tumours or different subgroups of bovine papilloma viruses with different organ site pre-dilections.

The situation in cattle therefore bears some similarities to humans with epidermodysplasia verruciformis and to the exacerbation of multiple cutaneous warts in patients subjected to prolonged immuno-suppressive therapy with azathioprene. Persistent papillomatosis has been reported in a bull with a deficiency of cell-mediated immunity (Duncan et al. 1975). The cattle situation also appears to have similarities with that of Shope papillomatosis in the cotton-tail rabbit where transformation of the virus-induced skin warts to malignancy is largely confined to the area of the Mississippi-Missouri basin. This epidemiology also suggests a geographical co-factor. Detailed investigations have yet to be made on a large number of individual papillomas from the cattle cancer cases to see if they are all associated with virus or whether the environmental factor can cause papillomas to proceed to carcinomas without the intervention of viral genetic material.

A surprising feature of the 80 cases of squamous carcinoma described was the finding that 56% had co-existent neoplastic lesions of the intestines including adenomas, polyposis, adenocarcinoma of the intestine and neoplasia of the Ampulla of Vater. In addition 30% of the cases had bladder tumours of which 23% were haemangiomas, 4% fibromas, 8% transitional cell carcinomas and 1% adenocarcinoma. It is obviously important to make an intensive study of the intestinal and bladder tumours particularly with hybridisation techniques to see if they contain identifiable DNA of papilloma virus origin. The results obtained to date are encouraging but a larger number of tumours will have to be studied by multiple techniques to preclude the presence of carrier virus in malignancies.

Scotland has the highest recorded incidence of human colorectal cancer and no reason for this has been adduced as yet. Since a large part of her water supply comes from bracken-infested drainage areas and since the radiomimetic toxin and carcinogenic factor from bracken can be passed in milk, it would seem worthwhile investigating these possibilities.

CONCLUSIONS

The various results presented here show that (1) warts or squamous papillomas are commonly found in the alimentary tract of all ages of cattle in Scotland, (2) the common picture in lowland areas is that each animal has a very small number of warts and that they are usually found at only one site, (3) in the upland areas there is a marked amplification in number of these papillomas in young animals and they are found at multiple sites, (4) the Highland area has a very high incidence of squamous carcinoma in female cattle over 6 years of age, (5) direct transformation of papillomas to carcinomas can be seen but it is not known whether carcinomas can arise de novo from normal epithelium, (6) all of the high incidence farms have in common the factor of severe infestation with bracken fern. This situation presents a challenge in the use of the range of molecular biological techniques which have been developed in viral and chemical oncology over the last few years in order to clarify the possibility in a naturally occurring high incidence tumour that an environmental agent which is a known mutagen and immunosuppressant may interact with an oncogenic virus to give rise to malignancy.

REFERENCES

1. JARRETT, W.F.H. Oesophageal and stomach cancer in cattle:
    A candidate viral and carcinogen model system and its possible
    relevance. Brit. J. Cancer 28, 93 (1973).

2. JARRETT, W.F.H., McNEIL, P.E., GRIMSHAW, W.T.R.,
    SELMAN, I.E. & McINTYRE, W.I.M. A high incidence area of
    cattle cancer with a possible interaction between an environmental
    carcinogen and a papilloma virus. Submitted for publication (1978a)

3. PLOWRIGHT, W., LINSELL, C.A. & PEERS, F.G. A focus of
    rumenal cancer in Kenyan cattle. Brit. J. Cancer 25, pp.72-80
    (1971).

4. DOBEREINER, J., TOKARNIA, C.H. & CANELLA, C.F.C.
    Occurrence of enzootic haematuria and epidermoid carcinoma
    of the upper digestive tract of cattle in Brazil. Pesq. agropec.
    bras. 2, pp.489-504 (1967).

5. OLSON, C., GORDON, D.E., ROBL, M.G. & LEE, K.P.
    Oncogenicity of Bovine Papilloma Virus. Arch. Environ. Health,
    19, pp.827-837 (1969).

6. EVANS, I.A. Proceedings 10th International Cancer Congress,
    Vol. V, Part A "Environmental Cancer". Year Book Medical
    Publishers Inc., Chicago, pp.178-195 (1972).

7. PAMUKCU, A.M., PRICE, J.M. & BRYAN, G.T. Naturally
    occurring and bracken-fern-induced bovine urinary bladder
    tumours. Vet. Pathol. 13, pp.110-122 (1976).

8. JARRETT, W.F.H., MURPHY, J., & O'NEIL, B.W. Virus-
    induced papillomas of the alimentary tract of cattle. In press
    (1978b).

9. JARRETT, W.F.H. Transformation of warts to malignancy in
    alimentary carcinoma in cattle. Bulletin of the French Cancer Soc.
    (1978).

10. DUNCAN, J.R., CORBEIL, L.B., DAVIES, D.H. SHULTZ, R.D.
    & WHITLOCK, R.H. Persistent papillomatosis associated with
    immunodeficiency. Cornell Vet. 65, No. 2, pp.205-211 (1975).

A PUTATIVE ROLE OF ENDOGENOUS C-TYPE VIRUS IN THE IMMUNE SYSTEM

C. Moroni, J. Stoye, J. DeLamarter, P. Monckton
and G. Schumann*

Friedrich Miescher-Institut, P.O.Box 273,
CH-4002 Basel, Switzerland
*Research Department, Pharmaceutical Division,
Ciba-Geigy Limited, CH-4002 Basel, Switzerland

Ever since it was realized that endogenous C-type viruses are components of normal vertebrate genomes the nature, origin and possible function of these viral genes have been a matter of speculation. As it seems that the known laboratory strains of leukemic C-type viruses are related to and presumably evolutionarily derived from endogenous viruses, one can wonder whether endogenous viruses are involved in cell division and, possibly, differentiation. If one believes that endogenous viral genes carry out a physiological function beneficial for their host, one could speculate that in cells which are the target cells for C-type leukemia viruses endogenous viruses are physiologically expressed.

For the last few years, we have been studying the induced expression of endogenous viruses in cells of the immune system. We reported in 1975 that lipopolysaccharide from E. coli, a B-cell mitogen, is a virus-inducer (1,2). Our results using a number of mitogens are summarized in Table 1. These studies revealed a fundamental difference between T- and B-cells with respect to virus expression. B-cells could be induced following mitogenic stimulation, whereas T-cells could not (3). Evidence from other workers supports this conclusion (4-6). Stimulation of DNA synthesis was found to precede and to be a necessary prerequisite for virus release (7 and unpublished). When BrdU, an effective inducer in fibroblasts,

47

TABLE 1: VIRUS INDUCTION BY MITOGEN

		Ref.
Inducing mitogens: (cell specificity)	lipopolysyccharide E.coli(B), lipoprotein E.coli (B), tuberculin (B), serum lipoprotein (?)	1,4,7, 8,17
Non-inducing mitogens: (cell specificity)	concanavalin A (T), phytohemagglutinin (T), dextran sulfate (B), pokeweed mitogen (T+B)	2,3,8
Inducible tissue:	spleen, lymph node	3
Inducible strain:	BALB/c, C57BL, DBA, AKR, C3H not inducible: 129	16
Type of virus:	BALB/c: selective induction of xenotropic virus	4,5,6
	AKR:induction of xenotropic virus and amplification of ecotropic virus	(unpublished, with Dr. N.Teich)
Mechanism:	virus induction depends on prior stimulation of DNA synthesis, induction involves de novo transcription	18,19

was added to mitogen-stimulated cells, B-cells released
more virus while T-cells remained negative (2,3). Interestingly, all virus inducing mitogens (e.g. lipopolysaccharide) from E. coli (1), lipoprotein from E. coli(8)
and tuberculin (10) trigger B-cell differentiation into
immunoglobulin secreting end cells (9,10). This fact that
mitogens mimick antigenic stimulation led us to hypothe-
size that the observed virus expression may reflect a
physiological process necessary in the generation of immunoglobulin-secreting cells. We have recently tested
this hypothesis by injecting mice with a rabbit antibody
directed against endogenous virus. Such animals showed

TABLE II: IMMUNOSUPPRESSION BY RABBIT ANTISERUM DIRECTED
AGAINST BALB/c ENDOGENOUS XENOTROPIC VIRUS

		References
Response suppressed:	sheep red blood cells, horse red blood cells, KLH-DNP, non specific polyclonal anti-DNP	11,12, and unpublished results with Dr. P. Erb
Strains suppressed:	BALB/c, C57BL, AKR, DBA, 129	12
Specificity:	effect absorbed by purified virus, no effect on cellular immunity	11,12, and unpublished results with A.Brownbill
Mechanism:	independent of complement, acts early during the immune response, possible blocking of T - B-interaction	12, and unpublished results

reduced numbers of immunoglobulin-secreting cells following antigenic stimulation (11). Experiments with this
immunosuppressive serum are summarized in Table II. Immunosuppression was observed with different antigens, in
all mouse strains tested and was also observed in in
vitro systems. Absorption experiments confirmed the viral
specificity of this phenomenon. Systems measuring the
cellular immune response were not affected. Surprisingly,
the antibody was only immunosuppressive when administered
early during the 4-5 day immune response against sheep
red blood cells (11,12). This suggested that it interfered with the events which lead to triggering the B-
cells to divide, possibly in T - B-cell cooperation. To
identify the target cell of the antiserum, experiments
using the KLH-DNP carrier-helper system were performed
in collaboration with Dr. Peter Erb. The results showed
that activated T-helper cells were one target of the
serum. A second target was the B-cell, since the serum
also suppressed the T-independent anti-DNP response
against bead-coupled DNP (unpublished results). These results are consistent with data by Wecker and coworkers

(13) who demonstrated the presence of viral glycoprotein gp70 on T- and B-cells participating in an anti-KLH-DNP response.

Since the serum does not act by cytotoxicity - F(ab')$_2$ fragments were equally effective in immunosuppression - it was concluded that blocking of viral structures present on T-helper cells and antigen reactive B-cells suppresses the immune response. Two alternative mechanisms can be proposed. Blocking of viral antigens could lead to steric hindrance of a functional structure. Alternatively, viral antigen itself represents a structure necessary for the generation of a humoral immune response. The present data does not allow one to distinguish between these two explanations, however, the latter is consistent with the hypothesis that endogenous viruses play a physiological role.

Since viral gene products are expressed on activated T-helper cells and antigen-reactive B-cells, we propose that they play a role in T-B-interaction. Gene products of the viral env and gag genes have been found expressed on the cell membrane (14,15). On T- and B-cells they could, for instance, be involved in cell-cell recognition. Alternatively, they could be secreted from the T-helper cell and deliver a biochemical signal necessary for B-cell activation. Should this hypothesis prove correct, it is conceivable that understanding how viral genes function in cell activation will also shed light on how leukemia viruses are involved in cell transformation.

References

1. Moroni, C. and Schumann, G. Nature 254, 60 (1975).
2. Moroni, C., Schumann, G., Robert-Guroff, M., Suter, E. and Martin, D. Proc. Natl. Acad. Sci. USA, 72, 535 (1975).
3. Schumann, G. and Moroni, C. J. Immunol. 116, 1145 (1976)
4. Greenberger, J.S., Phillips, S.M., Stephenson, J.R. and Aaronson, S.A. J. Immunol. 115, 317 (1975).
5. Phillips, S.M., Stephenson, J.R., Greenberger, J.S., Lane, P.E. and Aaronson, S.A. J. Immunol. 116, 1123 (1976).
6. Phillips, S.M., Stephenson, J.R. and Aaronson, S.A. J. Immunol. 118, 622 (1977).

7. Moroni, C. and Schumann, G. Virology 73, 17 (1976).
8. Moroni, C. and Schumann, G. J. gen. Virol. (in press) (1978).
9. Gronowicz, E. and Coutinho, A. Scand. J. Immunol. 4, 429 (1975).
10. Melchers, F., Braun, V. and Galanos, C. J. Exp. Med. 142, 473 (1975).
11. Moroni, C. and Schumann, G. Nature 269, 600 (1977).
12. Schumann, G. and Moroni, C. J. Immunol. (in press) (1978).
13. Wecker, E., Schimpl, A. and Hünig, T. Nature 269, 598 (1977).
14. Cloyd, M.W., Bolognesi, D.P. and Bigner, D.D. Cancer Res. 37, 922 (1977).
15. Snyder, H.W., Stockert, E. and Fleissner, E. J. Virol. 23, 302 (1977).
16. Schumann, G. and Moroni, C. Virology 79, 81 (1977).
17. Monckton, R.P. et al. (in preparation).
18. Stoye, J. et al. (in preparation).
19. DeLamarter, J.F. et al. (in preparation).

THE THYMIC EPITHELIUM IN LEUKEMOGENESIS

David R. Parkinson and Samuel D. Waksal

Cancer Research Center and Departments of Medicine and

Pathology, Tufts Univ. School of Med., Boston, MA 02111

The thymus gland has a central role in the development of lymphocytic leukemia in the mouse. The majority of these leuke-mias arise from cells that differentiate under the influence of the thymus, as shown by the presence of T cell markers on the leukemic cells. Neoplastic cells appear initially in the thymus, and thymectomy of young mice prevents the subsequent development of leukemia. In this paper we examine evidence that thymic epithe-lial (TE) cells influence the leukemogenic process in experimental murine systems. The implications of this information for human leukemias are discussed.

The Thymic Microenvironment

The epithelial cell network of the thymus arises in the embryo from the third and fourth pharyngeal pouches. Lymphoid precursor cells migrate from yolk sac or fetal liver to this epithelial structure during embryogenesis. After birth the precursors originate from bone marrow or spleen. In addition to lymphocytes and epithe-lial elements there are other cell types in the thymus.   Macro-phages are present, particularly near the corticomedullary boundary, and have recently been implicated in the differentiation of thymo-cytes* (Beller and Unanue, 1977). In some species occasional myoid (muscle-like) cells have been described (van de Velde and Friedman, 1970). The epithelial population may itself be heterogeneous, as

---

* A thymocyte may be defined as a lymphoid cell present in the thymus gland and differentiating under thymic influence, giving rise to those populations of mature T-lymphocytes subserving such cell mediated functions as graft rejection, graft-versus-host re-activity, and helper or suppressor activity.

Clark (1968) has presented autoradiographic evidence of secretory
activity by the medullary, but not cortical epithelial cells.

The Thymic Epithelial Cell and Normal Thymocyte Differentiation.

Concepts of the epithelial-mesenchymal interactions involved
in the differentiation of thymocytes have changed greatly in recent years. At one time lymphocytes were thought to arise directly
from the thymic epithelial network (Auerbach, 1961). We now know
that T-cells begin their process of differentiation when precursor
cells (termed prothymocytes) migrate to the thymus from bone marrow
and spleen (Kadish and Basch, 1976).

There is evidence for heterogeneity in this prothymocyte
population. Although a heterologous antiserum raised against mouse
brain (anti-BAT) recognizes both marrow and spleen prothymocytes
(Stout et al., 1976; Sato et al., 1976). prothymocytes from bone
marrow contain the DNA polymerase terminal deoxynucleotidyl transferase (TdT), whereas splenic prothymocytes do not. Ablation of
normal bone marrow by 89 strontium choride results in the appearance
within the spleen of a TdT-positive population of cells (Silverstone
et al. 1978 submitted for publication). This suggests that the
spleen may normally contain a population of cells which can be induced by appropriate signals to express TdT.

The ability of thymic epithelial cell monolayer cultures to
induce differentiation of prothymocytes in vitro has been demonstrated for both mice (Waksal et al., 1975) and humans (Pyke and
Gelfand, 1974). The TE cell is the probable source of soluble
thymic hormone (Dardenne et al., 1974); Mandi and Glant, 1973).
Although acquisition of thymic differentiation antigens (TL, Thy-1,
Lyt) can be demonstrated after in vitro incubation of prothymocytes
with a soluble product of the thymus (Komuro and Boyse, 1973),
direct contact with TE cells may be necessary for full functional
differentiation of the lymphocyte. The temporal relationship be-
bween acquisition of cell surface and of functional phenotypes remains largely unexplored. Besides fostering differentiation of prothymocytes, TE cells may control the number of prothymocytes in the
bone marrow, presumably by a humoral substance that exerts a negative feedback effect (Roelants and Mayor-Withey, 1977).

Certain precursor cells have different sensitivities to the
in vitro inductive influences of TE monolayers and soluble thymic
hormone (thymosin fraction V), when measured by the acquisition of
reactivity to alloantigens (Waksal, 1978). Prothymocytes from bone
marrow and spleens of athymic nu/nu mice were less responsive to the
influence of soluble thymic hormone than to cocultivation with TE
cell monolayers. By contrast, thymocytes, a population of immature
cells having already contacted the thymus, had the opposite pattern

of responsiveness. The inductive influence of contact with epithelial cells may therefore occur earlier in differentiation than the
hormonal effect.

The exact nature of the inductive influence of the TE cell is
unclear. Contact with the TE cell may initiate cell division in the
lymphocyte. Electron micrographic studies have suggested anatomic
associations between cortical epithelial cells and mitotic thymocytes (Mandel, 1969). Recent experiments by Zinkernagel and
colleagues (1978), indicate that the thymic epithelium imparts immunological specificity upon T cells. These investigators showed
that the generation of specific cytotoxic or helper T cells requires
shared I-region determinants between prothymocytes and the thymic
epithelium. Besides suggesting that the TE cell plays a critical
role in the development of the immunological repertoire of T-cells,
these experiments indicate that the prothymocyte-TE cell interaction
may involve cellular interaction molecules encoded by the I-region,
as originally proposed by Katz (1977) for other immune system interactions.

The sequential expression of differentiation antigens on the
surface of T-cells during their ontogeny has been studied in detail
(reviewed by Cantor and Boyse, 1977). Thymocyte maturation is associated with acquisition, loss, or intermediary quantitative change
in expression of specific thymocyte cell surface markers such as
TL, GIX, Thy-1, H-2, and Lyt alloantigens.

Large cells rich in Thy-1 and poor in H-2 antigens are present
in the subcapsular cortex; these cells are short-lived, rapidly
dividing, cortisone-sensitive, and immunologically incompetent. In
the deeper cortex there are small cells with intermediate amounts
of Thy-1. Immunologically mature thymocytes consisting of only
5-6% of the total thymocytes reside in the medulla. These cells
are cortisone resistant and possess relatively low amounts of Thy-1
but high amounts of H-2 antigens, as do peripheral T-cells. The
presence of characteristic Lyt phenotype profiles has been associated with specific T-cell functions. Both TL and GIX are alloantigens
acquired by prothymocytes after entry into the thymus, but lost with
further differentiation.

The association of different surface phenotypes with different
stages of differentiation allows investigation of leukemic T cell
stages of maturation. Study of the expression of Lyt 1, Lyt 2,
Thy-1, and TL differentiation antigens reveals various phenotypes
suggesting differentiation arrest at various stages   (Mathieson
et al., 1978).

The differentiation-linked expression of GIX is particularly
interesting (Boyse, 1977). This antigen is a type-specific antigenic
component of gp70, a glycoprotein coded for by retroviral genetic

information. The viral gene is integrated into the murine genome
and transmitted vertically in mendelian fashion. As a virus
structural protein gp70 plays a major role in the host range of the
virus, as well as its interference and neutralization properties.
Although this glycoprotein is the major coat protein of the retrovirus, it may be expressed independently of complete infectious
particles. Several antigenic variants of gp70 have been described
and more will be found in the future because of the polymorphic nature
of the glycoprotein (Elder et al., 1977; Del Villano et al., 1977).
It seems, therefore, that the expression of an endogeneous viral
genome is in some way linked to the differentiation of T cells.

The Thymic Epithelial Cell and Leukemogenesis

The fact that thymectomy sharply reduced the incidence of
leukemia in the high spontaneous leukemia strain AKR mouse (McEndy
et al., 1944) focussed attention on the role of the thymus in this
disease. These observations were extended for methylcholanthrene-
induced, radiation-induced, and virus-induced leukemias (Law and
Miller, 1950; Kaplan, 1950; Gross, 1959). In 1952 Law demonstrated
that fragments of thymus, from high leukemia incidence AKR mice,
when transplanted to thymectomized F_1 hybrids of high and low
leukemia incidence parents (AKR x C3H), resulted in an increased
incidence of leukemia (Law, 1952). Transplantation tests indicated
that the tumors were of host (hybrid) origin, and it was postulated
:hat the persisting thymic epithelial elements of the graft were in
some way responsible for the increased leukemia incidence.

Miller (1960) studied leukemogenesis in mice inoculated at
birth with Gross Passage A virus. He demonstrated that the leukemia
that usually followed injection of passage A virus into a C3H
substrain could be prevented by thymectomy. Susceptibility to
leukemia could be restored by grafts of normal thymuses into the
virus-infected mice, as late as six months after thymectomy. He
concluded that the thymic graft allowed expression of a leukemogenic potential still present in the virus-infected and thymectomized mice.

This thymic "leukemogenic factor", which could restore to
thymectomized hosts their susceptibility to leukemogenic agents,
was investigated by Furth and colleagues (1966). They prepared
lymphocyte-free epithelial cell cultures from newborn rat thymus.
When these cells were injected into the thigh muscle of neonatally
thymectomized, Passage A virus-infected rats, lymphomas developed
at the site of injection. Epithelial cell cultures were therefore
considered to be the source of the leukemogenic factor. The
suggestion was made that the epithelial cells themselves gave
rise to malignant lymphoid cells, consistent with the then-existing
concepts of normal lymphoid ontogeny. Serial histologic evidence

had earlier been interpreted to mean that malignant transformation
of thymic epithelial cells led directly to lymphoid leukemia (Siegler and Rich, 1963; Goodman and Block, 1963).

In 1966 Metcalf reported histologic changes in preleukemic AKR
mice. Cortical thinning and medullary enlargement, with the formation of lymphoid follicles in the medulla inverted the normal cortical-medullary pattern. The observation that grafts of neonatal
thymus placed into preleukemic hosts had normal thymic morphology
one month later was of particular interest. Conversely, preleukemic
thymuses grafted into young animals continued to evolve characteristic preleukemic histologic changes. In other words, the histology
of the transplanted thymus reflected the natural history of the donor,
and not the host. This implies the existence of an autonomous thymic
defect. Since Metcalf had already demonstrated that thymus epithelial
cells survived grafting, but that the lymphoid cells of the graft
were replaced completely within 3 weeks by cells of host origin
(Metcalf and Wakonig-Vaartaja, 1964), he postulated that the preleukemic thymic changes were due to abnormal function of TE cells.

Hays (1967) prepared "thymic epithelial remnants" by growing neonatal murine thymuses for 1 week in diffusion chambers planted intraperitoneally. She showed that these epithelial remnants, when used
as transplants, were able to restore immune functions of thymectomized
mice. She also obtained evidence for an important role for the TE cell
in leukemogenesis (Hays, 1968). AKR thymic epithelial cell remnants
were demonstrated to be as equally effective as whole thymus grafts
in restoring susceptibility to leukemia in thymectomized AKR mice.
C3H/HeJ thymic epithelial remnants could partially restore leukemia
incidence in Gross passage A virus-inoculated thymectomized mice. In
addition, AKR thymic remnants infected in vitro with virus could initiate leukemic transformation when grafted to syngeneic thymectomized
adult hosts. In a separate experiment Hays demonstrated that AKR
thymic remnant grafts placed into virus-infected, thymectomized C3H/HeJ
mice resulted in increased leukemia incidence with a shorter latent
period than intact mice given Gross virus alone. Tumor transplantation
studies showed the tumors to be of host (C3H/HeJ) origin. Hays postulated that it was the interaction between virus and thymic epithelial
cell which produced the leukemic transformation. She commented on the
possible differences between the epithelial cells of the low (C3H/HeJ)
and high (AKR) spontaneous leukemia strains, and speculated that the
TE cells from high leukemia strains provided a suitable environment
for viral replication.

In 1976 Waksal and colleagues showed that TE cell monolayer cultures prepared from AKR mice older than 24 weeks (i.e. preleukemic)
had the ability to transform young AKR thymocytes in vitro during 48
hours incubation. By contrast, monolayers prepared from thymuses of
young AKR animals, mouse embryo fibroblasts, or kidney epithelial cell
monolayers, did not possess this transforming capacity. By using AKR
strains differing phenotypically at the Thy-1 allele (AKR/J and AKR/Cu)

it was demonstrated that the co-cultivated donor thymocytes were in
fact the transformed cells. The occurrence of leukemia and the
duration of survival of the recipient mice were not changed when
the in vitro transformed cells were inoculated into thymectomized
hosts, suggesting that in vitro transformation event was complete.
Thymocytes from the low leukemia strain C3H were also transformed
by the AKR thymic epithelial monolayers (Waksal, 1978). All these
results suggested that the TE cell in the preleukemic AKR mouse has
a dual role: to bring the target cell into a state of differentiation that is susceptible to transformation, and to provide additional
factors such as oncogenic virus needed to initiate leukemogenesis.
Possible clues to the latter emerged from progress in the virology
of the AKR mouse.

    An age-dependent increase in leukemia virus antigens was demon-
strated in AKR thymus (Kawashima et al., 1976a). The increased expression of these antigens was not associated with an increased expression of ecotropic virus (classically thought to be the leukemogenic
virus). Rather, it was associated with the appearance of a xenotropic
virus that was expressed selectively in the preleukemic thymus (Kawashima et al., 1976b). By transplanting bone marrow from two or six-
month old animals into lethally irradiated hosts, it was found that
the radio-resistant thymic stroma, and not the cells in the bone
marrow, determined the increase in virus expression.

    An interesting but unexplained feature of these experiments was
the demonstration that preleukemic (6 month-old) thymic grafts induced
amplification of expression of murine leukemia virus antigen in the
thymuses of 2 month old recipients. Hays (Hays and Vredevoe, 1977),
studied the natural history of murine leukemia virus expression in AKR
mice and found a discrepancy between levels of XC plaque-forming virus
(the usual assay for ecotropic virus), and oncogenicity as measured by
lymphoma acceleration in virus-inoculated newborn animals. In addition,
supernatants from these virus-accelerated lymphomas were found to be oncogenic but XC plaque negative. Explanation for these phenomena came
with the demonstration of a new class of murine leukemia virus associated with the preleukemic AKR thymus (Hartley et al., 1977). This
virus had the host ranges of both ecotropic and xenotropic viruses, and
possessed properties that distinguished it from the three previously-
recognized classes of murine retrovirus. This mink cell focus-forming
class of virus (MCF) has been subsequently demonstrated, both by tryptic
peptide analysis (Elder et al., 1977) and by RNase-Tl resistant oligonucleotide mapping (Rommelaere et al., 1978), to be the result of recombinational events between constituent ecotropic and xenotropic
viruses in the env-gene (gp70) region. These MCF viruses are productively expressed by in vitro monolayer cell cultures of preleukemic
but not young AKR thymic epithelial cells (Waksal et al., 1978, submitted).

Haas (1977; Haas et al., 1977) extended Waksal's AKR in vitro transformation system to the C57B1/6 radiation induced leukemic model. Thymocytes were cocultivated on epithelial cell monolayers obtained from radiation leukemia virus (RadLV) - induced leukemic thymuses. Genetic markers confirmed the donor origin of the leukemic cells (Haas, 1978). Haas had previously demonstrated that the leukemogenic RadLV was thymotropic (Haas, 1974). He further showed that the TE monolayers obtained from RadLV-induced thymomas were infected with thymotropic RadLV virus. Co-cultivation of thymocytes on these virus-producing monolayers resulted in infection of the thymocytes by RadLV. This thymotropic RadLV has been shown to also be a recombinant virus within the envelope gene region (R.A. Lerner, personal communication).

Another experimental system, less intensively studied than the AKR or C57B1/6 RadLV systems, is the HRS/J (hairless) mouse. Homozygotes (hr/hr) for the recessive gene lose most of their body hair by 4 weeks of age and have a high (45% by 8 months) incidence of spontaneous thymic leukemia. Heterozygotes (hr/+) do not lose hair and have a lower (1%) incidence of thymic leukemia by the same age (Meier et al., 1969). Recently it was demonstrated that xenotropic virus is expressed at much higher titer in 8 month old homozygote mice. The increased expression of xenotropic virus was confined to the thymus and did not occur in hr/+ mice. Titers of ecotropic virus, although higher in older than younger animals, did not differ between heterozygote haired and homozygote hairless mice. Polytropic viruses with a dual host range, suggesting their recombinant origin, were identified only in preleukemic hr/hr thymuses (Hiai et. al. 1977). Thus, in this model, a single gene located on the fourteenth chromosome seems responsible for the virological events that precede the development of thymic leukemia. Thymic epithelial cell monolayer cultures from young animals have been found to express only ecotropic virus, while similar cultures from old animals yielded supernatant production of both ecotropic and xenotropic viruses and, in the case of the homozygote, preliminary results indicate the presence of polytropic virus (Parkinson et al., in preparation).

An additional intriguing aspect of the HRS/J system is the recent demonstration of a selective defect in the differentiation of T cells in the homozygote (Morrissey et al., in preparation). This occurs together with overt evidence of a generalized defect in the function of epithelial cells. The alopecia of the homozygote is a result of an epithelial defect leading to abnormal development of hair follicles. Females nurse poorly because of poor development of mammary glands. The epithelial cell defect, the T cell differentiation defect, and the selective thymic expression of xenotropic virus with the appearance of recombinant viruses all combine to make this an interesting model with which to explore the interrelationships of thymocyte differentiation, retrovirus expression, and thymic epithelial inductive influence.

TABLE 1

RETROVIRUS EXPRESSION IN THYMUSES OF OLD MICE

VIRUS TROPICITY

	ECOTROPIC	XENOTROPIC	POLYTROPIC	INCIDENCE
AKR	+	+	+	high
(AKR x NZB)F_1	-	+	-	low
HRS/J (hr/hr)	+	+	+	high
HRS/J (hr/+)	+	low	-	low

(references in text)

Possible Mechanisms

Abnormal cellular interactions which affect the differentiation of thymocytes appear during the latent period, prior to the onset of overt leukemogenesis. As AKR mice age, their thymocyte populations shift towards a greater number of cells with increased expression of H-2 antigens and decreased expression of Thy-1 (Waksal et al., 1976); Waksal, 1978). Preleukemic thymocytes also have decreased responsiveness to Con A and increased responses to PHA. These changes suggest a more mature thymocyte population, and correlate with Metcalf's histologic observations of preleukemic cortical-medullary inversion. We noted above that Metcalf found these morphologic changes to be a function of the thymic epithelial element. The evidence suggests that the TE cell participates in the abnormally accelerated, pre-leukemic differentiation of thymocytes, and permits changes in expression of retrovirus. TE cell cultures appear to reflect the natural history of the virology of the entire thymus. Whether the TE cell is the origin of xenotropic virus expression and recombinant virus formation is unknown. Another possibility is that the TE cell is secondarily infected by xenotropic virus or recombinant virus after inducing virus expression via its inductive influence during thymocyte differentiation. In (AKR x NZB)F_1 hybrid mice xenotropic virus is expressed in the thymuses of old mice in the absence of ecotropic virus. No MCF-like viruses were found in the thymuses of these mice (Datta and Schwartz, 1978, in press), which have a low incidence of spontaneous lymphoid leukemia (Holmes and Burnet, 1966). Despite expression of ecotropic and xenotropic virus together in spleen, bone marrow and lymph nodes no MCF-like viruses were found in those tissues.

TABLE 2

T-CELL DIFFERENTIATION, RETROVIRUS EXPRESSION, AND LEUKEMOGENESIS

EXPERIMENTAL SYSTEMS: A COMPARISON

MOUSE STRAIN	LEUKEMIA INCIDENCE	THYMUS VIROLOGY	T-CELL DIFFERENTIATION DEFECT
AKR	high	Ecotropic virus throughout life preleukemic xenotropic burst with appearance of MCF.	Accelerated thymocyte maturation in old thymuses.
(AKR x NZB)F$_1$	low	Xenotropic virus but no ecotropic virus in thymus—no recombinants found in old mice.	Not yet studied.
HRS/J (hr/hr)	high	Increasing ecotropic virus titers throughout life; preleukemic xenotropic burst and appearance of polytropic virus.	? epithelial cell inductive defect: increased prothymocyte population in spleen; defects in certain T-cell functions.
HRS/J (hr/+)	low	Similar ecotropic virus expression to homozygote; no equivalent xenotropic expression; no polytropic virus.	Differentiation relatively normal.
C57B1/6	high (post 175R per week x 4 wks).	Isolation from post radiation tumor tissue of thymoctropic RadLV.	? elimination of TdT positive thymocyte subpopulation by 175R/x4.

This fact suggests that somehow the thymus plays a central role in the formation of envelope gene recombinant viruses. A summary of retrovirus expression in thymuses of 8-10 month-old mice, related to relative incidence of leukemia, is seen in Table 1. The nature of the abnormal influence on differentiation exerted in the preleukemic thymus is unclear. Retrovirus infection or retrovirus-coded surface glycoprotein gp70 may be important in this interaction. Infection with RadLV has been shown to initiate increased synthesis of H-2 antigens within a few hours (Meruelo et al., 1978). Expression of Thy-1, Lyt 1 and Lyt 2 were unchanged, however, and the selectively greater increase in expression of H-2D as opposed to H-2 antigens was interpreted as a possible viral resistance mechanism rather than a disturbance in thymocyte differentiation.

The expression of gp70 on thymocytes as a differentiation antigen suggests a role for viral encoded information in normal differentiation. Epithelial cells at various sites of epithelial-mesenchymal interaction within the mouse, (the epididymis, gastrointestinal tract, and thymic medulla) express gp70 (Lerner et al., 1976). Therefore, if viral envelope gene products are related in some way to normal differentiation processes, the possibility arises that envelope gene recombinant gp70 molecules could be related somehow to the abnormal differentiation/proliferation states seen with leukemia. Detailed studies of the gp70's expressed on different murine T cell leukemias and on normal thymocytes would be of great interest. One recent study in this respect, using tryptic peptide mapping, suggests that normal AKR thymocyte membrane gp70's have ecotropic origin, whereas B6, B6-CIX$^+$ 129, and A strain mice membrane gp70's had xenotropic origin. Two A strain leukemias, however, were interpreted as having maps more consistent with ecotropic origin (Tung et al., 1978).

Different model systems with apparently different defects in T-cell differentiation share a high incidence of spontaneous leukemia (summarized in Table 2). Accelerated thymocyte maturation under thymus epithelial influence occurs in the AKR system. The homozygote HRS mouse, however, has impaired T-cell differentiation, with an increased splenic prothymocyte population. The leukemogenic radiation protocol in the C57B1/6 mouse is associated with the disappearance of a TdT-positive thymocyte population (J.N. Ihle, 1978 personal communication) until lymphoma develops. The fact that TdT-positive prothymocytes are normally present in bone marrow has already been discussed. These results taken together may bear relevance to the old observations that shielding one limb during radiation or transfusing syneneic marrow post-radiation (Kaplan et al. 1953) eliminates the subsequent development of leukemia.

Relevance of these Studies to Human Leukemia

Certain implications of these murine studies may be relevant to human leukemia. The high incidence of anterior mediastinal mass (almost 70%) among children with acute lymphoblastic leukemia (ALL) of T-cell type (Humphrey and Lankford, 1977) suggests the thymic origin of this neoplasm. This subgroup of ALL differs clinically from those forms of ALL with lymphoblasts lacking T-cell markers. In general, cases of the former type occur in boys older than 5 years, who present with thymic masses and very high white cell counts (Sen and Borella, 1975; Brunet et al., 1976). These children have a poor prognosis; remissions induced by chemotherapy are short, as is survival. Childhood lymphoblastic lymphoma (Sternberg's lymphoma) is a related neoplasm also associated with thymic masses and T-cell markers on the malignant cells (Smith et al., 1973). The disease invariably degenerates to a clinical picture of ALL within several months. Both the lymphoblastic lymphomas and the majority of childhood ALL's are TdT positive (Murphy and Mauer, 1977; McCaffrey et al., 1975). A more reliable indicator of thymic-associated malignant cell origin than T-cell rosetting is the acid phosphatase histochemical stain. This is suggested by the occurrence of positive acid phosphatase reactions in several cases of non T-cell ALL's associated with thymic masses (Catovsky et al., 1978). In addition it appears that acid phosphatase positivity appears earlier in the ontogeny of T-lymphocytes than positive sheep cell rosetting.

The T-cell markers and the association with thymic masses of these childhood lymphoid malignancies invite comparison with murine models of thymic leukemia. In the absence of definitely demonstrated infectious virus or integrated provirus information in human leukemia (Gallo et al. 1978), the comparison remains speculative. Nevertheless, the possibility of an abnormal inductive influence on thymocyte differentiation by thymic epithelial cells of the thymuses of these children should be considered. Possibly relevant in this respect are the two cases reported from Seattle involving girls with relapsed ALL who were transplanted with bone marrow from their histocompatibility antigen matched brothers (Fialkow et al., 1971; Thomas et al., 1972). In both cases the subsequent relapses were shown by karyotype analysis to involve leukemic cells of male (i.e. donor) origin. There were no cell surface marker studies published with these cases. The apparent in vivo leukemic transformation of these engrafted donor marrow cells suggest interesting parallels with both in vivo and in vitro thymic epithelial transformation studies already discussed.

The role of prophylactic thymectomy in children with thymus-associated ALL who are being considered clinically for bone marrow transplantation warrants investigation. Studies to determine the possible survival value of thymectomy post remission induction in childhood T-cell ALL and lymphoblastic lymphomas have already been initiated (S. Schlossman, 1978 personal communication).

CONCLUSION

Normal thymocyte differentiation occurs when genetic programs are induced by interaction of prothymocytes with the thymic epithelial matrix. Epithelial inductive influences therefore control normal differentiation via gene activation. The evidence for an abnormal thymic epithelial inductive influence in murine lymphoid leukemia has been reviewed. The question of how these abnormal interactions lead to neoplastic events is of prime importance. Retrovirus coded information, expressed either as complete virus particles or as cellular surface components, seems inextricably linked to thymocyte differentiation in the mouse. The viral envelope gene product gp70, a product of viral genome integrated into host genome, demonstrates great polymorphism. If viral products play any determinative role in normal thymocyte differentiation, abnormal (i.e. recombinant gp70) might play a role in abnormal differentiation or proliferation states. Abnormal thymic epithelial inductive influences may also exist in human thymic-related lymphoid malignancies.

ACKNOWLEDGEMENTS:

We would like to thank Drs. Robert S. Schwartz and Syamal K. Datta for useful discussion and critical review of this paper. The work on the HRS/J mouse was carried out in collaboration with P. Morrissey and Dr. H. Hiai. The manuscript was typed by Mrs. Bernice Kus. Work in this laboratory is carried out under Contract #N-OICB-74150 from the National Cancer Institute. Dr. David R. Parkinson is supported by a fellowship from the Medical Research Council of Canada.

REFERENCES

1. Auerbach, R., (1961) Dev. Biol. 3:336.
2. Beller, D.I. and Unanue, E.R., (1977) J. Immunol., 118:1780.
3. Boyse, E.A. (1977) Immunological Rev. 33:125.
4. Brunet, J.C., Valensi, F., Daniel, M.T., Flandrin, G., Preud'homme, J.L., Seligmann, M. (1976) Br. J. Haemat 33:319.
5. Cantor, H. and Boyse, E.A., (1977) Immunological Rev. 33:105.
6. Catovsky, D., Cherchi, M., Greaves, M.F., Janossy, G., Pain, C., and Kay, H.E.M. (1978) Lancet i, 749.
7. Clark, S.L., (1968) J. Exp. Med. 128:927.
8. Dardenne, M., Papiernik, M., Bach, J.F., and Stutman, O. (1974) Immunology 27:199.
9. Datta, S.K. and Schwartz, R.S. (1978) J. Exp. Med. in press.
10. Del Villano, B.C., Kennel, S.J. and Lerner, R.A. (1977) Cont. Topics Immunobiol. 6, 195.

11. Elder, J.H., Jensen, F.L., Bryant, M.L., and Lerner, R.A.
     (1977) Nature 267:23.
12. Elder, J.H., Gautsch, J.W., Jensen, F.C., Lerner, R.A.,
     Hartley, J.W., and Rowe, W.P., (1977) Proc. Natl.
     Acad. Sci. U.S.A. 74:4676.
13. Fialkow, P.J., Thomas, E.D., Bryant, J.I. and Neiman, P.E.,
     (1971) Lancet i, 251.
14. Furth, J., Kunii, A., Ioachim, H., Sanel, F.T., and Moy, P.
     (1966) in G.E.W. Wolstenholme (ed.) The Thymus, Ciba
     Foundation Symposium p. 288. Boston; Little, Brown,
     and Company.
15. Gallo, R.C., Ruscetti, F., and Gallagher, R.E. (1978) Cold
     Spring Harbor Symposium on Quantitative Biology in
     press.
16. Goodman, S.B., and Block, M.H., (1963) Cancer Res. 23:1634.
17. Gross, L., (1959) Proc. Soc. Exp. Biol. Med. 100:325.
18. Haas, M., (1974) Cell 1:79.
19. Haas, M. (1977) in "Radiation-induced Leukemogenesis and Re-
     lated Viruses." ed. J.F. Duplan. North-Holland Pub-
     lishing Company. Amsterdam, p. 149.
20. Haas, M., (1978) Int. J. Cancer 21, 115.
21. Haas, M., Sher, T., and Smolinsky, S., (1977) Cancer Res.
     37:1800.
22. Hartley, J.W., Wolford, N.K., Old. L.J., Rowe, W.P. (1977)
     Proc. Natl. Acad. Sci. U.S.A. 74:789.
23. Hays, E.F., (1967) Blood 29:29.
24. Hays, E.F., (1968) Cancer Res. 28:21.
25. Hays, E.F., and Vredevoe, D.L. (1977) Cancer Res. 37, 726.
26. Hiai, H., Morrissey, P., Khiroya, R., and Schwartz, R.S.
     (1977) Nature 270, 247.
27. Holmes,M.L. and Burnet, F.M. (1966) Aust. J. Exp. Biol.
     Med. Sci. 44:235.
28. Humphrey, G.B. and Lankford, J. (1976) Sem. Onc. 3:243.
29. Kadish, J.L. and Basch, R.S., (1976) J. Exp. Med. 143:1082.
30. Kaplan, H.S. (1950) J. Natl.Cancer Inst. 11:83.
31. Kaplan, H.S., Brown, M.B., and Paull, J. (1953). J. Nat.
     Cancer Inst. 14:303.
32. Katz, D.H. (1977) in "Lymphocyte Differentiation, Recognition
     and Regulation". Academic Press, N.Y., p. 589.
33. Kawashima, K., Ikeda, H., Stockert, E., Takahashi, T. and
     Old, L.J., (1976a) J. Exp. Med. 144:193.
34. Kawashima, K., Ikeda, H., Hartley, J.W., Stockert, E., Rowe,
     W.P., Old, L.J., (1976b) Proc. Natl. Acad. Sci. U.S.A.
     73:4680.
35. Komuro, L., and Boyse, E.A. (1973) Lancet i:740.
36. Law, L.W., (1952) J. Natl.Cancer Inst. 12:789.
37. Law, L.W., and Miller, J.H., (1950) J. Natl.Can. Inst. 11:425.
38. Lerner, R.A., Wilson, C.B., Del Villano, B.C., McConahey,
     P.J., and Dixon, F.J., (1976) J. Exp. Med. 143:151.
39. Mandel, T., (1969) Aust. J. Exp. Biol. Med. Sci., 47:153.
40. Mandi, B. and Glant, T. (1973) Nature New Biol. 246:25.

41. Mathieson, B.J., Campbell, P.W., Potter, M. and Asofsky,
      R.J. (1978) J. Exp. Med. 147: 1267.
42. McCaffrey, R., Harrison, T.A., Parkman, R. and Baltimore,
      D., (1975) N. Engl. J. Med. 292:775.
43. McEndy, D.P., Boon, M.C., and Furth, J., (1944) Can. Res. 4:377.
44. Meier, H., Myers, D.D. and Huebner, R.J. (1969) PNAS 63:759.
45. Meruelo, D., Nimelstein, S.H., Jones, P.P., Lieberman, M.,
      and McDevitt, H.O., (1978) J. Exp. Med. 147:470.
46. Metcalf, D., (1966) J. Nat. Cancer Inst. 37:425.
47. Metcalf, D. and Wakonig-Vaartaja, R., (1964) Proc. Soc. Exp.
      Bio. Med. 115:731.
48. Miller, J.F.A.P., (1960) Brit. J. Cancer 14:93.
49. Murphy, S.B., and Mauer, A.M. (1975) N. Engl. J. Med. 297:502.
50. Pyke, K.W. and Gelfand, E.W., (1974) Nature 251:421.
51. Roelants, G.E., and Mayor-Withey, K.S., (1977) Cellular
      Immunol. 34:420.
52. Rommelaere, J., Faller, D.V., and Hopkins, N. (1978) Proc.
      Natl. Acad. Sci. U.S.A. 75:495.
53. Sato, V.L., Waksal, S.D. and Herzenberg, L.A. (1976) Cellular
      Immunol. 24:173.
54. Sen. L. and Borella, K., (1975) N. Eng. J. Med. 292:828.
55. Siegler, R., and Rich, M.A., (1963) Can. Res. 23:1669.
56. Silverstone, A.E., Gordon, L., Baltimore, D., and Waksal,
      S.D. (1978) submitted for publication.
57. Smith, J.L., Barker, C.R., Clein, G.P., and Collins, R.D.
      (1973) Lancet i:74.
58. Stout, R.D., Waksal, D.S., Sato, V.L., Okumura, K., and
      Herzenberg, L.A. (1976) in Leucocyte Membrane Determi-
      nants Regulating Immune Reactivity ed. V.P. Eijsvoogel,
      D. Roos, and W.P. Zeijlemaker. Academic Press N.Y.,
      p. 173.
59. Thomas, E.D., Bryant, J.I., Buckner, L.D., Clift, R.A., Fefer,
      A., Johnson, F.L., Neiman, P., Ramberg, R.E., Storb,
      R., (1972) Lancet i:1310.
60. Tung, J.S., O'Donnell, P.W., Fleissner, E., and Boyse, E.A.,
      (1978) J. Exp. Med. 147:1280.
61. Van de Velde, R.L., Friedman, N.B. (1970) Am. J. Path. 59:347.
62. Waksal, S.D., Cohen, I.R., Waksal, H.W., Wekerle, H., St. Pierre,
      R.L., Feldman, M., (1975) Ann. N.Y. Acad. Sci. 241:492.
63. Waksal, S.D., Smolinsky, S., Cohen, I.R., St. Pierre, R.L.,
      and Feldman, M. (1976) Adv. Exp. Biol. Med. 66:141.
64. Waksal, S.D., Smolinsky, S., Cohen, I.R. and Feldman, M.,
      (1976) Nature 263:512.
65. Waksal, S.D. (1978) Cold Spring Harbor Symposium on Quantita-
      tive Biology, in press.
66. Zinkernagel, R., Callahan, G.N., Althage, A., Cooper, S.,
      Klein, P.A., and Klein, J., (1978) J. Exp. Med. 147:882.

STUDIES ON TRANSFER OF MuLV AND LYMPHOMA DEVELOPMENT

R. D. Barnes

Clinical Research Centre
Embryology & Foetal Development
Watford Road, Harrow, Middx. HA1 3UJ

Research into murine leukaemia was initiated in the 1930's by the development of inbred strains of mice bred up on the basis of tumour susceptibility. For twenty years murine leukaemia remained in the field of genetics. Gross' classic studies in the 1950's resulted in the introduction of virology. Twenty years later, with the definition of genetically determined host factors influencing permissiveness to murine leukaemia virus (MuLV) infection and to subsequent tumour development, genetics has re-emerged. The inter-relationship between oncogenic virus, host factors and subsequent tumour development is undoubtedly complex and although facts continue to emerge the story is far from complete. Here I wish to present data from several different studies performed in this laboratory that hopefully will complement existing knowledge.

INTRODUCTION

Although the incidence varies between sublines the susceptibility of the AKR to develop spontaneous lymphoma is well established. In contrast spontaneous lymphomas are uncommon in certain other strains including the CBA (1). With this knowledge the following studies were initiated.

1) TUMOUR SUSCEPTIBILITY VERSUS TUMOUR RESISTANCE

This was investigated in a group of early embryo aggregation AKR↔CBA/H-T6Crc chimaeras. In the chimaeras, lymphomas were not only delayed (2) but also the overall incidence was reduced (3). This observation was especially interesting when it was found that in spite of 'balanced' (3) coat colour composition and distribution of the gametes, each of the 18 chimaeras was essential AKR when analysed cytogenetically (3)(4) or by other cell product markers (5). Relative tumour resistance in this situation had to be attributed to the relatively minor cell CBA component or cell product in the chimaeras. This was a 'double' homozygote situation - each chimaera in fact presenting an admixture of AKR and CBA/H-T6Crc homozygote cells and related cell products. It was this observation that prompted us to investigate the situation in the naturally derived (AKRxCBA/H-T6Crc)F1.

2) THE (AKRxCBA)F1

CBA/H-T6Crc (CBA in text) and AKR/Crc (formerly AkR/J) were used to provide two groups of reciprocal crosses and these were examined with both AKR and CBA controls. One group was followed throughout their natural life span, a second group was investigated following elective sacrifice.

The main group of mice were studied to determine the data of onset and incidence of tumours. When signs suggestive of tumour development occurred, or occasionally following natural death, post mortem was performed and evidence of lymphoma sought macroscopically. On occasions when there was any doubt histology was performed upon haematoxylin and eosin stained sections. Various tissues were removed at autopsy not only of this group but also of the second group of electively sacrificed mice. Their tissues were screened by radioimmunoassay for levels of the group specific p30 MuLV associated antigen.

The radioimmunoassay for the group specific antigen p30 was a modification of a previously described method (6). In practice Rauscher p30 antigen was radiolabelled with ^{125}I (7).

The primary reaction consisted of incubating the ^{125}I labelled antigen together with an aliquot of the tissue extract with goat anti-AKR p30. Secondary precipitation of the primary antibody-antigen complex was achieved by adding pig anti-goat IgG. Subsequently after incubation and careful removal of the supernatant following centrifugation, radioactivity of the precipitate was determined.

In each case assay samples were examined in duplicate and levels of p30 were determined by extrapolation from a standard inhibition curve.

Values of p30 were expressed as ng/1.0 mg of tissue protein the latter determined using Lowry's method (8).

Results initially confirmed the presence of MuLV - moreover levels comparable with AKR; in spite of this tumours were delayed (9).

More recently in a further study it was seen that although lymphomas occurred in all the (AKRxCBA)F1, this was generally in the second year of life at a time when the majority of AKR controls had succumbed (Table 1).

TABLE 1

AGE OF ONSET OF LYMPHOMAS IN RECIPROCAL (AKRxCBA/H-T6Crc)F1

MICE (No)*		RANGE (wks)	MEAN	(S.E.)
(AKR x CBA)	(60)	40-113	86.55	(2.046)
(CBA x AKR)	(48)	33-99	82.90	(1.774)
AKR	(61)	30-86	61.06	(2.015)

*first strain = mother

Clearly tumours are delayed in the (AKRxCBA)F1, furthermore, this is independent of the viral load at least as determined by levels of the MuLV group specific associated antigen p30 (9). More recent findings shown here confirm this earlier view. (Table 2)

TABLE 2

LEVELS OF GROUP SPECIFIC MuLV ASSOCIATED ANTIGEN
p30 IN AKR AND (AKRxCBA)F1

	p30 LEVELS* IN SPLEEN		
	RANGE	MEAN	(S.E.)
AKR	7.72-59.49	31.20	(2.020)
(AKR x CBA) F1	40.40-58.03	33.91	(1.819)
CBA	2.22-18.18	6.26	(0.671)

In retrospect the high levels of MuLV in the F1 was not a surprising observation since the CBA like the AKR is also Fv-1 and hence permissive to N-tropic AKR MuLV infection (10). Therefore, in the (AKRxCBA) F1 Fv-1$^{n \times n}$ situation N-tropic AKR MuLV infection might be anticipated to be unrestricted. What was surprising was that the lymphomas originally appeared uncommon in the F1 (9) since it had hitherto been accepted that in general the incidence of lymphomas paralleled levels of MuLV in AKR crosses (11). Again the relative lymphoma resistance of (AKRxCBA) F1 appeared remarkable in respect of this being a H-2$^{k \times k}$ situation -H-2^k normally conferring susceptibility to virus associated tumour development (12).

Our original preliminary investigation of the (AKRxCBA)F1 (9) also suggested the possibility of differences in the incidence of tumours in reciprocal crosses and although not apparent in Table 1 examination was extended to a group of early embryo exchange derived hybrids.

3) EXAMINATION OF RECIPROCAL CROSSES

The experimental design involving exchange embryo trans-planation and summary of results is shown below:

EXCLUSION OF RECIPROCAL DIFFERENCES

(Genetic or Maternal?)

(AKRxCBA*) Incidence of tumours
$<$ (CBA*xAKR)F1[†]

Expt. Design

(AKRxCBA*)F1 ⟶ CBA*
(CBA*xAKR)F1 ⟶ AKR

        Embryo Transplantation

Result

  a) No difference in incidence of tumours

  b) No difference in viral load (p30)

No genetic (foetal heterosis) or maternal effect.

      *CBA/H-T6Crc
      † in each case
        first strain ♀

Basically embryos were obtained at the early blastocyst stage transplanted and uterine nurtured from the opposite mother. The experimental design is shown above, together with a summary of results.

So in conclusion our findings in the (AKRxCBA)F1 are:

(AKR x CBA/H-T6Crc) F1   (AKR x CBA/H-T6Crc) F1

1) Initial Findings   2) Subsequent Findings

   1) Reduced incidence of tumours   1) Delayed incidence of tumours

   2) ? Difference in incidence between reciprocal crosses - (AKR x CBA*) F1 ⟨ (CBA* x AKR) F1

   2) No difference between reciprocal crosses - early embryo exchange transplantation.

   3) In both cases in spite of a viral load (p30 & xc) comparable and occasionally in excess of AKR.

   3) **High viral load of both ecotropic MuLV (xc) and xenotropic MuLV (mink cells).**

     *CBA/H-T6Crc

To study the genetics further the corresponding CBA x (AKR x CBA) and AKR x (AKR x CBA) backcrosses have been set up and results are awaited. Meanwhile, it should be emphasised that throughout our studies we have used just one particular subline of the CBA and any extrapolation of our findings to other sublines of CBA are unwise. It should be noted that:

THE CBA/H-T6Crc

<u>Derived</u> from Harwell subline

<u>Gene status</u>

$Fv-1^n$; $Fv-2^s$; $H-2^k$ (Rgv-1) & Rgv-2

Pair of chromosome markers

<u>Virus status</u>

Ecotropic MuLV - negative -
(activation/co-cultivation)

Xenotropic MuLV - negative -
co-cultivation

Data with DNA probes awaited.

In contrast the viral status in the F1 is:

> Ecotropic MuLV - positive
>
> Xenotropic MuLV - positive
>
> Eco-xenotropic MuLV - unknown
> (recombinant)

The techniques for detection of infective ecotropic and
xenotropic were standard and will be described in full elsewhere -
with details of the cell lines investigated. Techniques were
basically co-cultivation of various tissue extracts on different
cell lines to determine host range restriction.

With the knowledge that both ecotropic and xenotropic MuLV
to date have failed to be demonstrated in the CBA/H-T6Crc, various
studies were initiated to study transmission of these viruses.
Materno→foetal transfer was investigated in several different
ways also the possibility of foeto→maternal transfer was studied.

4) FOETO→MATERNAL MuLV INFECTION

I earlier remarked upon the fact that levels of the group
specific MuLV antigen p30 were comparable in the (CBA/H-T6Crc
xAKR)F1 with the parental AKR (9). In retrospect this was not

surprising since in a $(Fv-1^n \times n)F1$ situation spread of N-tropic
AKR MuLV infection is to be expected. With this knowledge we
examined a group of CBA mothers used to derive MuLV positive
(CBA/H-T6CrcxAKR)F1 for evidence of foeto→maternal MuLV infection.
This possibility seemed particularly attractive since it is now
well established that foetal cells enter the maternal circulation
during pregnancy (13) (14). Another reasons for this investigation
was that to the best of our knowledge this has been the only
attempt to study foetal→maternal transfer of virus infection. CBA
mothers of such (CBAxAKR)F1 were examined here together with AKR
and CBA controls. An additional group of CBA controls were
included. These were sterile CBA females which had been
successfully mated (confirmed by the presence of a vaginal plug)
on one or more occasions with AKR males but after having Fallopian
tube ligation. The CBA mothers (of the F1) were killed at varying
ages after one or more successful pregnancies together with both
virgin and parous AKR and CBA controls - parity in the latter
situation incudced by mating within strains.

In the case of both the CBA mothers (of the F1) also the
controls, the uterus and spleen were screened for levels of the
MuLV group specific antigen p30 using a radioimmunoassay.   In
each case the tissues were frozen individually at -35^oC and
examined in radioimmunoassay for p30 described earlier.

Values of p30 were expressed as ng/1.0 mg of tissue protein -
the latter determined using Lowry's method (8)

Results are summarized in Table 3.   Here it can be seen that
although variable, levels of p30 in the uteri of CBA mothers of
the CBAxAKR hybrids were significantly higher levels than CBA
controls although not as high as in the AKR.   Levels of p30 in
the sterilized CBA mothers subsequently mated with AKR males was
no different to virgin or parous CBA mated with CBA.   The
implication of this result is that uterine infection is not a
consequence of mating alone - actual fertilization and subsequent
foetal development of the F1 is a pre-requisite of maternal
infection.   In contrast to the evidence that favours uterine
infection no significant increase in the levels of p30 was seen
in the spleens of F1 mothers.

Investigation of transplacental passage of virus has been
primarily concerned with materno→foetal transfer.   Not
surprisingly, this is of primary importance in considering the
effect of maternal infection upon foetal health.   However, for
reasons mentioned later the observations here concerning
foeto→maternal infection, hopefully, will not appear just of
academic interest.

TABLE 3

LEVELS OF GROUP SPECIFIC MuLV p30 ANTIGEN IN
MOTHERS OF (CBA/H-T6Crc x AKR)F1*

Groups	Strain (No.)	Age (Wks.)	Levels of p30[†] - Range (Mean $S.E.$)	
			Uterus	Spleen
	AKR (32)	12 - 20	22.58 - 271.96 (70.60; 10.70)	7.72 - 59.49 (31.20; 2.02)
Control	CBA/H-T6Crc[††] (25)	8 - 16	6.64 - 14.42 (10.45; 0.39)	1.42 - 11.41 (6.26; 0.67)
	CBA/H-T6Crc[†††] (5)	8 - 16	8.13 - 13.08 (8.41; 2.1)	n.t.
Experimental	CBA/H-T6Crc* F1 mothers (27)	12 - 19	7.70 - 33.08 (17.33; 1.16)	2.60 - 10.49 (6.20; 0.21)

* CBA/H-T6Crc mothers; [†] ng/mg tissue protein; [††] including group of post-parous CBA/H-T6Crc mothers used to derive CBA homozygote progeny; [†††] sterile mated with AKR.

Two factors prompted this investigation. Firstly, the failure to detect the group specific MuLV p30 antigen (9) and infective ecotropic MuLV in our CBA/H-T6Crc (Natalie Teich - personal communication). Secondly, finding high levels of p30 and infective ecotropic MuLV in the relatively lymphoma resistant (AKRxCBA)F1 (9). In retrospect, the latter finding was not surprising since as mentioned earlier, the CBA is like the AKR also $Fv-1^n$. The F1 presenting a $Fv-1^{n \times n}$ situation is permissive to the spread of N-tropic ecotropic AKR MuLV infection (10). It is, therefore, presumed that the AKR virus enters the (CBAxAKR)F1 upon the genome incorporated in the AKR sperm and in a permissive environment leads to high levels of p30 and infective virus. In the reciprocal (AKRxCBA) cross the virus would enter via the genome incorporated within the oocyte. Such is the situation in reciprocal CBAxAKR crosses. Results here examining the reverse passage show clearly that MuLV crosses in reverse from foetus to infect the mother. It was interesting to note that levels were not elevated in the sterile CBA mated with the AKR. This group was investigated because it is known that sperm can enter cells of the female genital tract (15) and the possibility of viral infection by this route had to be considered. In this respect evidence suggests that infection here occurs only from the foetus not the sperm.

The results were clear cut with respect to levels of p30 in the uterus. Although variable, levels were significantly higher in CBA mothers of the F1 than in CBA controls, however, levels were not as high in the AKR. Levels in the spleen,however, were not significantly higher than the CBA controls suggesting that infection might be confined to the uterus and systemic infection, at least involving the spleen is not a general phenomenon. If we accept that elevated levels of p30 reflect infection then the results suggest that infection once established persists after pregnancy.

It may well be argued that we have yet to confirm the nature of the virus, however, it seems most likely that the p30 detected here represents infective ecotropic MuLV. Xenotropic MuLV is an alternative possibility since both eco- and xenotropic MuLV have common p30 antigen specificity. However, the increased levels of p30 detected here are unlikely to represent xenotropic MuLV since this virus by definition does not normally grow on mouse cells, at least in vitro. Although there is the possibility that xenotropic MuLV may have been transmitted its replication in vivo seems an unlikely explanation for the elevated levels of p30 in the mothers of the (CBAxAKR)F1. Transplacental foeto→ maternal passage and resultant infection with ecotropic MuLV seems the most likely explanation for the increased levels of p30.

This aside, infection of Fl mothers is not surprising since the transplacental passage of foetal cells into the maternal circulation is a well established phenomenon (13) (14). However, in reverse the transplacental passage of maternal cells into the foetal circulation remains a controversy (16) (17) (18). Now lets consider materno → foetal infection. As mentioned above the transplacental passage of maternal cells into the foetal circulation remains a controversy (16) (17) (18) - however, this limitation does not necessarily effect studies of materno → foetal virus infection.

5) MATERNO —→FOETAL MuLV INFECTION

As shown below this has been studied in four different ways:

Germ line or non-germ line

A) Systems tested

a) Embryo transplantation studies.
b) Progeny of early embryo derived chimaera.
c) Progeny of naturally infected CBA mothers of (Fl).
d) Progeny of CBA x (AKR x CBA)

With respect to embryo transplantation, we noted that CBA born from the AKR following embryo transfer do not have elevated levels of virus at least as judged by the number of C-type particles observed on electron microscopy (19) - nor do they develop the AKR virus associated lymphomas (20). Naturally, these two factors might be related, this aside, the lack of elevated levels of p30 and infective ecotropic MuLV (21) in the group of CBA derived following early embryo transplantation and being born from AKR suggests materno → foetal infection of MuLV at or after the stage of implantation is not a general phenomenon. This conclusion has further support in the studies detailed below examining the progeny of AKR ↔ CBA chimaeras and the CBA homozygote progeny of naturally infected CBA mothers previously used to derive (CBA x AKR) Fl.

The rationale for examining the progeny of early embryo aggregation chimaeras and the preliminary results are summarized below.

B) **Progeny of early embryo aggregation**
    derived chimaeras

   a) One or other or both germ lines
       eg. in AKR↔CBA chimaeras.

   AKR   CBA germ lines

   b) Genital tract composed of AKR
       <u>and</u> CBA cells and cell products.

   c) Mating to CBA correspondingly would
       result in

       (CBA x AKR) F1 and
           (CBA x CBA)

   d) Results showed with respect to
       (Ec- & Xe- MuLV)

       a) positive (for both) in F1
           b) negative (for both) in homozygote

<u>Conclusion</u> - Transmission of both forms of MuLV
confined to germ line - genital tract environment
of no direct influence in respect of MuLV
transmission.

With the knowledge that 'reversed' foetal→maternal MuLV
infection occurs 'naturally' in CBA mothers of F1, we then mated
similarly infected mothers back with CBA males.   The aim here was
to examine their CBAxCBA progeny for presence of the virus.   The
rationale and summary of results is shown below.

C) **Progeny of naturally infected CBA mothers**

   a) (CBAxAKR)F1 have high levels of both
    Ec- & Xe- MuLV.

   b) Infection is derived from AKR sperm
    line transmission.

   c) CBA mothers of such F1 are also infected
    (p30) in reverse by the F1 foetus (the CBA
    being $Fv-1^n$ hence permissive to AKR N-tropic
    MuLV infection).

d) Mating of these 'naturally' infected
CBA mothers with CBA males resulted in
(CBAxCBA) homozygotes.

e) Results showed that these homozygotes were
non-infected with either Ec- or Xe- MuLV (p30)

Conclusion - transmission of both Ec- & Xe- MuLV
is via the germ line - generalized infection of
the mother not effective in transfer.

There is further evidence to support the above data and the
assumption that in respect of materno→foetal MuLV infection this is
confined to the germ line.   This evidence was gained in the
examination the CBAx(AKRxCBA) backcross.   The original rationale
for this examination is detailed below together with results.

D) The CBA x (AKR x CBA) backcross

Segregation towards tumour resistance
? controlled by a single gene.

Results:
a) incidence of tumours 50%
b) age of onset of tumours comparable with
     normally derived F1.
c) no statistical difference from normally
     derived F1 - no evidence of segregation
     towards tumour resistance.

These mice have subsequently been examined for MuLV infection
using both p.30 screening and levels of infective ecotropic MuLV.
Results were clear cut.   Levels were either high or negative -
moreover this corresponded to the genotype as defined by the
glucose phosphate isoenzyme (g.p.i.).

High levels of virus were found in the presence of both
a) and b) variants (g.p.i.) (AKRxCBA) cross whereas zero level of
virus was found in mice having only the b) g.p.i. (CBAxCBA) variant.

SUMMARY

Results expressed here show:

i) Lymphoma susceptibility is not invariably linked with high levels of MuLV (at least in the(AKRxCBA/H-T6Crc) F1)

ii) The CBA/H-T6Crc appears unusual in lacking to date detectable Ec- and Xe- MuLV

iii) Foeto→maternal MuLV infection occurs; knowledge led us to reconsider whether materno→foetal infection could occur independent of the germ line.   Results were clear cut.

iv) Materno→foetal MuLV infection is entirely confined to the germ line. This conclusion was drawn from the following studies involving investigating progeny obtained after:

   a) early embryo transplantation
   b) derived from tetraparental chimaera
   c) those derived from naturally ('reverse') infected CBA/H-T6Crc mothers and
   d) progeny of CBA x (AKR x CBA) backcross. In each situation all evidence points to materno→foetal infection being confined to the germ line.

REFERENCES

1. E.D. Murphy. In: Biology of Laboratory Mouse (Ed. by E.L.Green) The Blakiston Div/McGraw-Hill Book Co. New York (1966)

2. R.D. Barnes, M. Tuffrey & J. Kingman. Clin. Exp. Immunol. 12 : 541 (1972)

3. M. Tuffrey et al. Nature 243 : 207 (1973)

4. C.E. Ford et al. Differentiation 2: 321 (1974)

5. R.D. Barnes et al. Differentiation 2 : 257 (1974)

6. M. Strand, F. Lilly & J.T. August. Proc.Nat.Acad.Sci.U.S.A. 71: 3682 (1974)

7. R.D. Barnes & M. Simpson - in preparation.

8. O. H. Lowry et al. J.Biol. Chem. 193: 265 (1951)

9. R.D. Barnes et al. Cancer Res. 36 : 3622 (1976)

10. W.P. Rowe. J. Exp. Med. 136: 1272 (1972)

11. H. Meier et al. Proc. Nat. Acad. Sci. U.S.A. 70: 1450 (1973)

12. F. Lilly, M.L. Duran-Reynals, W.P. Rowe. J. Exp. Med. 141: 882 (1975)

13. C.G. Schmorl. Verhandl. Deut. Pathol. Ges. 8 : 39 (1905)

14. F. Cohen et al. Blood 23: 621 (1964)

15. C.R. Austin. Nature 183 : 908 (1959)

16. R.D. Barnes & M. Tuffrey. Adv. Biosci. 6: 457 (1970)

17. R. D. Barnes & J. Holliday. Blood 36: 480 (1970)

18. W. D. Billington et al. Nature 224: 704 (1969)

19. R.D. Barnes et al. Brit. J. Cancer 34 : 35 (1976)

20. R.D. Barnes & M. Tuffrey. Brit. J. Cancer 10: 35 (1976)

21. R.D. Barnes, M. Tuffrey & M.Simpson - in preparation.

S E C T I O N II

The role of RNA tumor viruses in human cancer

Convenor

Dr. Robert C. GALLO
National Cancer Institute
Laboratory of Tumor Cell Biology
Building 37, Room 6B04
Bethesda, Maryland 20014

U.S.A.

BIOCHEMICAL STUDIES ON ENZOOTIC AND

SPORADIC TYPES OF BOVINE LEUCOSIS

A. Burny[o,x], F. Bex[o], C. Bruck[o], Y. Cleuter[o], D. Dekegel[+],
J. Ghysdael[o,x], R. Kettmann[o,x], M. Leclercq[o],
M. Mammerickx[*] and D. Portetelle[o,x]

o Department of Molecular Biology, University of Brussels,
   67, rue des Chevaux, 1640, Rhode St-Genèse, Belgium.
x Faculty of Agronomy, 5800 Gembloux, Belgium.
+ Pasteur Institute, rue du Remorqueur, 1140 Bruxelles and
   Vrije Universiteit Brussel, 1050 Brussel, Belgium.
* National Institute for Veterinary Research, 99,
   Groeselenberg, 1180 Uccle-Bruxelles, Belgium.

Bovine leucoses are lymphoproliferative diseases (1). One
distinguishes essentially 2 types
- the enzootic type,
- the sporadic type.

1. ENZOOTIC BOVINE LEUCOSIS (EBL)
The basic features of this type of the disease are :
- it is contagious; it spreads within a herd through milk, contacts,
  saliva, ... and from herd to herd mainly through commercial
  exchanges;
- it is induced by Bovine Leukemia Virus (BLV) a retrovirus,
  exogenous to the bovine species (2);
- all animals infected by BLV develop a humoral response directed
  against the viral antigens (1);
- the disease can be easily transmitted by the virus to cattle or
  sheep. Experimental BLV infection (but no clinical disease, so
  far) has been obtained in goats and chimpanzees (1);
- it involves the B lymphocytes (3).

Enzootic bovine leucosis is a chronic d sease that develops
over a long period of time (several years generally) in which 3
phases can be distinguished :
- from birth to infection.
In natural conditions, very few cattle less than 2 years of age

83

harbor antibodies to BLV antigens (4). The same conclusion obtains
if BLV is searched for by its biological property of inducing
syncytia or early polykaryocytosis (5). If however, a search is
made among the offspring of BLV infected parents, it appears that
as much as 14 % of calves are infected at birth. As discussed in
(1), this situation reflects congenital infection by BLV and not
true vertical transmission;
- from viral infection to tumorous transformation this period can
  be very long, 10 years are not exceptional. It has, however, been
  experimentally observed that BLV infection may not persist (6).
  Persisting BLV infection is always accompanied by anti BLV antibodies, detectable by serological techniques. Infected animals
  may or may not develop persistent lymphocytosis. This hematological disorder is now proven to be a subclinical form of the
  disease (1,2). It clearly has a genetic background (7) being much
  more frequent in some families within a breed than in other
  families of the same breed;
- from tumor development to death. Age of tumor development is very
  variable. No breed is resistant and sex plays no role.

     Tumors may appear practically everywhere, in the digestive
tract, the respiratory tracts, in muscles, ... but they are always
lymphoïd. Most lymph nodes are enlarged, sometimes some of them
only.

2. SPORADIC BOVINE LEUCOSIS (SBL)

     As opposed to enzootic, sporadic means here that cases are
always isolated.
- No propagation within a herd has ever been observed.
- Transmission was never successful.
- No virus can be produced by short-term cultures of lymphocytes.
- Antibodies to BLV antigens are not detected.
- As illustrated below, molecular hybridization experiments show no
  detectable BLV proviral sequences.
- SBL tumors involve T lymphocytes (Jarrett, W.H.F., personal
  communication).

     Three main clinical types of Sporadic Bovine Leucosis tumors
are known :
- A multicentric type characterized by a general lymphadenopathy in
  calves 4 to 5 months old.
- A thymic type, involving a tumor of the thymus accompanied most
  often by a general lymphadenopathy. This type occurs mostly in 1
  year old animals.
- A cutaneous type characterized by skin tumors and eventually a
  general lymphadenopathy. It occurs in 1 year old animals.

     In the past, age has been a major criterion in distinguishing
between EBL and SBL. Now, presence of antibodies to BLV antigens is,

of course, the key criterion allowing clearcut distinction between
the two diseases. The factor age is of course, quite questionable.
Tumors may develop exceptionally early in EBL and exceptionally late
in SBL.

3. GEOGRAPHICAL DISTRIBUTION OF SBL AND EBL

SBL cases are uniformly distributed in a country whilst EBL
cases cluster. Infection of a herd by BLV can generally be traced
back to introduction of an animal carrying the virus.

4. ENZOOTIC BOVINE LEUCOSIS : THE AGENT : BLV

BLV is a retrovirus (8,9) produced by short term cultures of
bovine leukemic lymphocytes. It can also infect and be produced by
cell-lines as Fetal Lamb Kidney cells (10) or Tb₁Lu, a bat cell
line (11). Electron microscopy shows that BLV has a morphology
identical to other C types viruses except, that in many cases, the
particule matures while still attached to the producing cell. A
typical horse-shoe is rarely observed even in freshly released
particles.It follows that either maturation is rapid or release is
slow.

4.1 BLV Genome

The virus genome is a 60-70S RNA molecule associated with
reverse transcriptase. The latter exhibits DNA polymerizing activity
only in the presence of Mg ions. Mn^{++} is strictly inactive (9). DNA
complementary to the RNA genome has been synthesized using either the
endogenous BLV reverse transcriptase activity (9) or a reconstituted
system based on AMV reverse transcriptase (2).

The cDNA probe was then used to search for relatedness to BLV
among other retroviruses and to decide upon the exogenous or endogenous character of BLV versus the bovine genome. Answers to these
two questions are as follows :
- By molecular hybridization, BLV seems to be unrelated to any of
  the presently known retroviruses (1).
- BLV is clearly a retrovirus exogenous to the bovine species (Fig.
  2 and 3).

In Fig. 2 histograms represent the extent of hybridization of
BLV cDNA to DNA of various origins. It should be stressed here that
the BLV probe represented at least 60 % of the viral genome. Fig. 2
calls for the following comments :
  - If we take salmon sperm DNA as a control (histogram 11) it
    appears that normal bovine DNA hybridizes some 4 % better than
    the control. We now know that this is due to contamination of
    the 70S RNA used as template by some 28S ribosomal RNA.

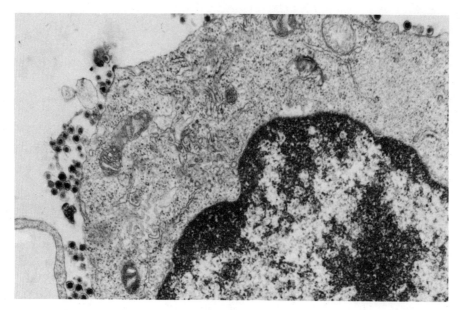

<u>FIG. 1A.</u>   Production of BLV by short—term cultures of leukemic
           lymphocytes.

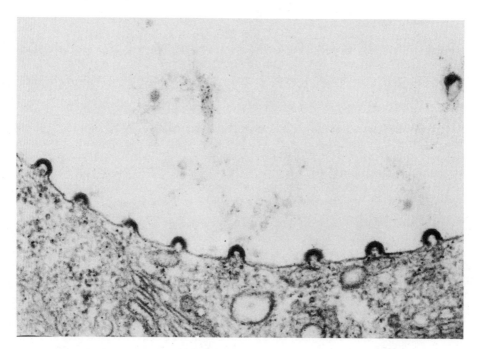

<u>FIG. 1B.</u>   Budding particles from infected FLK cells.

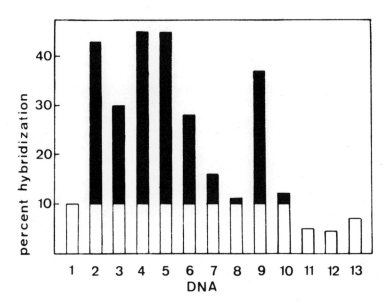

FIG. 2. Hybridization of BLV ^{3}H cDNA to various bovine, ovine
and human cellular DNAs. Hybridizations between 2400 cpm
of ^{3}H cDNA (specific activity : 1.8 x 10^7 cpm/μg) and
250 μg of cellular DNA were performed in 0.4 M phosphate
buffer (pH = 6,8) and 0,05 % SDS in a final volume of 85 μl
at 68°C. At a Cot value of 30.000, samples were assayed for
S_1 resistance.

Source of DNA :
1. Normal buffy coat cells.
2. FLK cell line.
3. Buffy coat cells from a cow in persistent lymphocytosis without
   tumors.
4. Buffy coat cells from a cow in persistent lymphocytosis with
   tumors.
5. EBL tumor.
6. Liver moderately infiltrated with lymphocytes (EBL).
7. Kidney slightly infiltrated with lymphocytes (EBL).
8. Tumorous lymphnode from an SBL case.
9. Cutaneous tumor from a sheep infected with BLV.
10. Liver from the same leukemic sheep.
11. Salmon sperm.
12. Human chronic lymphatic leukemia.
13. Human chronic lymphatic leukemia.

- DNAs from the producing cells FLK–BLV (histogram 2), from buffy coat cells of an animal in persistent lymphocytosis with tumor (histogram 4) and from bovine enzootic tumor (histogram 5) hybridize with a maximum of 45 % of the probe at a Cot value of 30.000. This result is compatible with 1 proviral DNA copy per haploid genome, if every cell contains the viral information.
- If a tissue is infiltrated with tumorous lymphocytes, its DNA hybridizes to BLV cDNA to an extent that is roughly proportional to the degree of infiltration (histograms 3, 6, 7).
- Sheep infected by BLV (histograms 9 and 10) show the same pattern of hybridization as cattle do.
- DNAs from human leukemic cells do not anneal to BLV cDNA.

In order to decide upon the exogenous or endogenous character of BLV and its possible involvement in Sporadic Bovine Leucosis, we ran a recycling experiment (Fig. 3). The principle of the operation is as follows : ^{3}H–BLV–cDNA is exhaustively hybridized to normal bovine DNA; the unannealed sequences are then recycled on Salmon sperm DNA, normal bovine DNA, EBL tumor DNA and SBL tumor DNA. As expected no hybridization occurred to Salmon sperm and normal bovine DNA, showing that the first round of hybridization was indeed exhaustive. Interestingly enough, no annealing was observed to sporadic bovine leucosis tumor DNA and as much as 22 % of the recycled probe hybridized to enzootic bovine leucosis tumor DNA.

These experiments have important consequences. They establish that BLV contributed to the leukemic cell genome sequences that are not detectable in normal DNA or SBL tumor DNA. This constitutes the biochemical proof that BLV is an exogenous agent, that EBL is an infectious disease. By the same token, these results suggest that eradication campaigns of EBL should be successful, if they are based upon the best method of detection of BLV infection (see below).

4.2 BLV Proteins (1)

Analysis of purified BLV preparations by polyacrylamide gel electrophoresis in the presence of sodium dodecylsulphate and immunological precipitation of ^{3}H–aminoacids labelled virus by sera of infected animals has led to the definition of 6 major viral polypeptides, two of them being glycosylated. There are 4 non–glycosylated polypeptides p24, p15, p12 and p10 and 2 glycoproteins gp60 and gp30. The two glycoproteins seem to be linked together within the knoblike structure by disulfide bonds. Indeed, analysis under reducing conditions reveals one glycosylated molecule of 94.000 daltons molecular weight. This value is in good agreement with the hypothesis of 1:1 complex of each polypeptide. The nonglycosylated virus polypeptides are internal antigens. In Fig. 4, p12 and p10 are not separated.

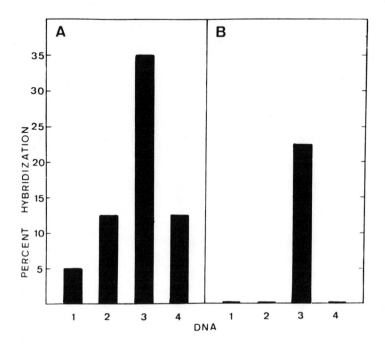

FIG. 3. Hybridization of BLV ^{3}H cDNA (panel A) and recycled BLV ^{3}H cDNA (panel B) to the following cellular DNAs :
1. Salmon sperm; 2. normal bovine buffy coat cells;
3. EBL tumor; 4. SL tumorous lymph node.
Twenty four hundred cpm of BLV ^{3}H cDNA (or recycled cDNA) and 250 µg of cellular DNA were hybridized in 0.4 M phosphate buffer (pH = 6,8) and 0.05 % SDS. At a cellular Cot value of 30.000 samples were assayed for S_1 resistance.

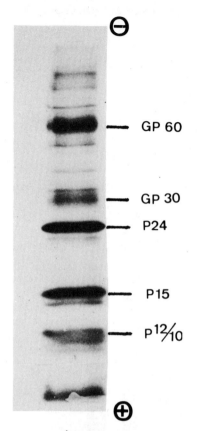

FIG. 4. Fluorograph of a 20 %-SDS containing-polyacrylamide slab
gel of (^{3}H) aminoacids labelled BLV proteins.

BLV structural proteins biosynthesis has been studied in the
Foetal Lamb Kidney cell line or in the Tb_1-Lu cell line infected
with and producing BLV, and in frog oocytes injected with the BLV
30-35D genome. Study of BLV protein synthesis in FLK-BLV line or in
frog oocytes, includes an immunoprecipitation step, viral protein
synthesis only representing about 1 % of total protein synthesis
(12).

Fig. 5 shows the outcome of an experiment including injection
of BLV 30-35S RNA into frog oocytes and analysis of polypeptides
precipitable by anti p24 antibody.

From our own experience, it appears that how short the pulse
can be, there are always 2 polypeptides appearing together, and
precipitable by antibody to p24. These precursors are called Pr70
and Pr45. Fingerprinting analysis of P70 and P45 precursors shows
that all 35S methionine containing peptides present in Pr45 are
also present in Pr70. Several hypotheses could explain these findings.

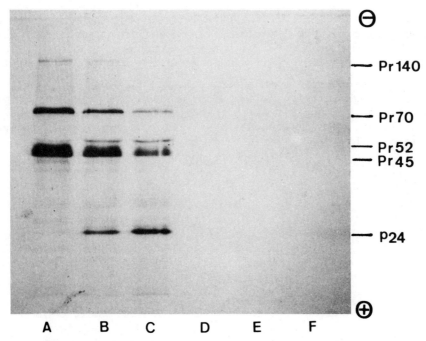

FIG. 5.   Fluorograph of SDS-polyacrylamide gel of immune precipitates.
Oocytes microinjected with a 1 mg/ml water solution of
30-40D BLV RNA were labelled for 20 hours in Barth medium
with 2 mCi/ml of (^{3}H) leucine, lysed immediately (A) or
chased in culture medium containing excess unlabelled
leucine for 100 hours (B) and 300 hours (C) and then lysed.
Non injected control oocytes were incubated in parallel
(D-F).
Direct immune precipitation is carried out on the same
amount of homogenate with 100 µl of monospecific anti p24
and 4 µg/ml of purified p24 as a carrier. The immuno-
precipitates were collected, washed, dissolved and subjected to electrophoresis on a 15 % polyacrylamide slab gel
in the presence of SDS.

Either there are several starting points or several termination
points or even there are two viruses. It is still too early to distinguish between these 3 possibilities.

    Both precursors are unstable in infected cells or frog oocytes
and maturation seems to occur as follows :
- Pr45 matures into p24;
- Pr70 gives slowly rise to a polypeptide of MW = 52.000 and perhaps
  to p24.

The same two precursors Pr45 and Pr70 are the only products synthesized in rabbit reticulocyte lysates depleted of endogenous activity by micrococcal nuclease treatment and programmed by BLV 30-35S RNA. Our present efforts are attempting at the separation of 2 putative classes of viral RNA molecules in the 30-35S population.

In a recent series of experiments BLV 60-70S RNA was melted and passed through an oligo dT cellulose column. The poly A containing fraction was then submitted to velocity sedimentation in glycerol gradients and the RNA present in each fraction was used to program protein synthesis in the reticulocyte lysate system (Fig. 6).

A clearcut picture arose from such experiments :
- 30-35S RNA codes for Pr45 and Pr70;
- 18-20S RNA codes for a 58.000 M.W. protein;
- 16S RNA codes for a 45.000 M.W. protein.

Whilst Pr70 and Pr45 share antigenic determinants with the major BLV internal antigen (p24) the 58.000 M.W., 45.000 M.W. and smaller products do not share any antigenic determinants with p24 or the major glycosylated BLV antigen (gp60).

It is, of course, very tempting to try to identify some at least of these products with the protein(s) responsible for trans-formation by BLV of hematopoietic cells but more work is clearly needed before such a conclusion can be drawn.

BLV reverse transcriptase has the peculiarity to require Mg^{++} (i). It sediments in glycerol gradients as a molecule of an apparent molecular weight of 70.000 (Fig. 7) and is probably synthesized -as in other systems- as a 140.000 M.W. read through product of the gag gene (Fig. 6).

5. DETECTION OF BLV INFECTION

As BLV is an exogenous agent inducing antibody synthesis in the infected host, detection of these antibodies by any suitable method constitutes at present, the basis of all seroepidemiological studies and eradication campaigns. Presence of BLV can be assessed directly through a syncytia inducing assay (5) but this may apparently lead to conflicting results (13).

BLV structural proteins gp60, p24 and p15 have been used as probes to detect BLV antibodies carriers. It seems that there is a fairly good agreement between all the research groups involved, to consider that BLV gp60 is the antigen of choice (1). Antibodies to BLV reverse transcriptase have also been detected in leukotic animals (14). Their titer does not necessarily parallel anti gp or p24 titers. Recently, J. Zavada designed a biological test based on VSV pseudotypes VSV (BLV) to detect antibodies to BLV (R. Weiss, personal communication). It will be quite informative in the near future to compare the most sensitive radioimmunological test

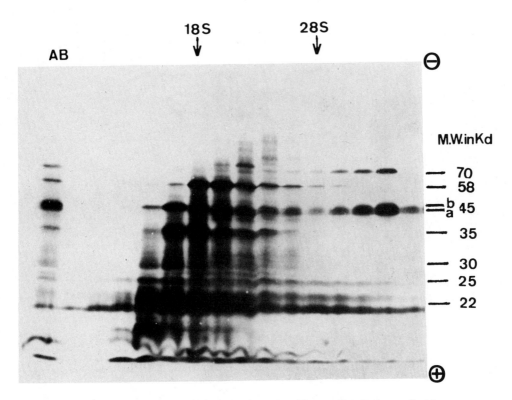

FIG. 6. Fluorograph of SDS-polyacrylamide gel of translation
products of fractionated BLV virion RNA.
Heat denatured (95°C; 45 sec. in Tris 10^{-2}M, pH 7,4,
EDTA 10^{-3}M) BLV 60-70S RNA (80 µg) was fractionated by
oligo (dT) chromatography and the poly A containing
fraction (25 µg) was sedimented on a linear 15-30 %
glycerol gradient in Tris 10^{-2}M, pH 7,4, NaCl 0,1 M;
EDTA 0,01 M in a SW 41 rotor at 40.000 rpm for 4 hours
at 20°C.
The RNA of each gradient fraction was precipitated twice
with ethanol, calf liver tRNA being added as a carrier.
One fourth of the RNA of each fraction was used to program protein synthesis in a messenger dependent reticulocyte cell-free lysate. Analysis of translation products
is made on a 15 % SDS polyacrylamide slab gel.
Track A : complete translation products of the poly A
          containing BLV RNA.
Track B : control; no added RNA.

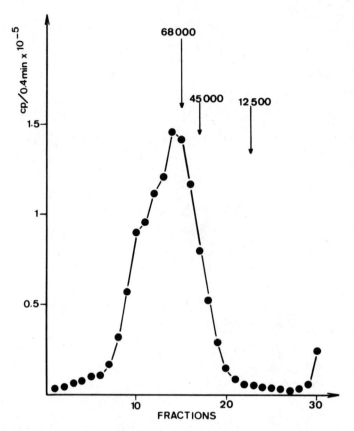

FIG. 7. Sedimentation velocity of BLV reverse transcriptase in 10-30 % (v/v) glycerol gradients in potassium phosphate 0,125 M, pH = 8.0; dithioerythritol 0,005 M. Centrifugation was for 20 hours at 1° C and 49.000 rpm in the Spinco 50-1 rotor. Enzyme activity was assayed with dG_{12-18} : rC as template. Molecular weight markers were bovine serumalbumin, ovalbumin and cytochrome c.

(^{125}I BLV-gp RIA) to the best biological tests, VSV (BLV) plaque inhibition or Early Polykaryocytosis inhibition, as far as sensitivity, specificity, feasibility, flexibility and field efficacity.

Table 1 details the results obtained when comparing gp60 and p24 RIAs to gp60 immunodiffusion, a method of choice for field studies.

TABLE 1

Tests	Number of animals
Total Population	296
Positive in the BLV p24 RIA	64
Positive in the BLV gp immuno-diffusion test.	64
Positive in the BLV gp RIA	66

It should be emphasized that the methodology used to derive the numbers of Table 1, implies that antibodies to be detected are IgGs. Experiments dealing with IgM   detection are presently on the way.

BLV gp60, p24, p15 and reverse transcriptase have also been used in competition radioimmunoassays in order to detect any possible relatedness of BLV to other presently known retroviruses (1, 3). So far, such experiments have invariably lead to negative results. No hypothesis can be made at present about the origin of this virus.

6.   HOST-VIRUS INTERPLAY

The incoming of BLV antigens into a host immediately induces an antibody response; the intensity of which probably depends on age of the host and its genetic make-up, virus dose, ... We already stressed (see above) that infection may just not take (6) but this issue fortunate for the host seems to be rather rare.

Fig. 8 and 9 display our first results (15) dealing with the problem : host-virus relationship.

In Fig. 8, the case of sheep n° S 328 is illustrated. The animal was experimentally infected in 1973. Antibodies to BLV p24 and gp60 were followed by RIA since February 1975 until death of the animal in November 1977. It can be seen that in this case antibody titer to p24 remained more or less constant whilst antibody titer to gp60 increased steadily until February 1977.

We then tested the cytotoxicity of these antibodies versus FLK cells infected with and producing BLV but most probably not transformed by the virus.

Fig. 9 illustrates the outcome of complement dependent cytotoxicity assays. As a base of comparison, bovine serum n° R 2123 is included in the assays. This bovine serum is one of our best positive reactors in the cytotoxic reaction conditions used. Five different sera of sheep n° S 328 were tested at the same time. They cover the time period elapsed from 04/02/73 to 11/28/77, at the death of the animal.Clearly the cytotoxicity of the sera increases with time. From the analyses we could perform, so far, it is established that immunoglobulins active in the cytotoxic reaction belong to the IgG$_1$ class.

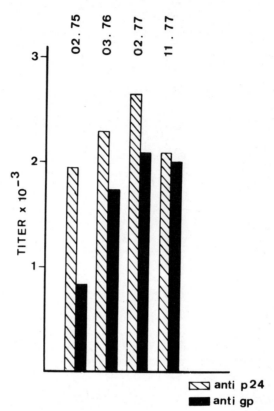

<u>FIG. 8.</u> Evolution of antibody titers during the last 2 years of
life of a BLV infected sheep developing tumors.
            antibody titer to BLV p24.
            antibody titer to BLV gp.

7. CONCLUSIONS

In conclusion, enzootic bovine leucosis is induced by a retrovirus, exogenous to the bovine species and unrelated to the presently
known RNA oncogenic viruses. Infection of the recipient animal
induces a humoral response, including synthesis of IgG, antibodies,
cytotoxic to BLV producing cells. No trace of anti-BLV antibodies
has so far been found in man. Sporadic types of bovine leucosis are
not related to BLV infection. Sporadic bovine leucosis tumors do
not contain any BLV proviral sequences.

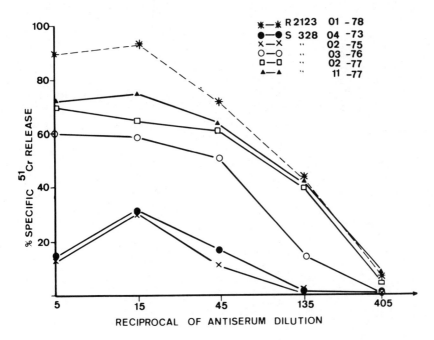

FIG. 9.   Evolution of cytotoxic activity of a sheep serum (same
animal as in Fig. 8) during the last two years of the
animal's life. Target cells were Fetal Lamb Kidney cells
infected by and producing BLV. (These cells are most
probably no transformed by BLV). One of our best cytotoxic bovine sera (R 2123) was used here as a reference.

REFERENCES

1. BURNY, A., BEX, F., CHANTRENNE, H., CLEUTER, Y., DEKEGEL, D.,
   GHYSDAEL, J., KETTMANN, R., LECLERCQ, M., LEUNEN, J., MAMMERICKX,
   M. and PORTETELLE, D. 1978. Bovine Leukemia Virus Involvement in
   Enzootic Bovine Leucosis.
   Adv. in Cancer Res., 28, in press.

2. KETTMANN, R., BURNY, A., CLEUTER, Y., GHYSDAEL, J. and
   MAMMERICKX, M. 1978. Distribution of Bovine Leukemia Virus Pro-
   viral DNA Sequences in Tissues of Animals with Enzootic Bovine
   Leucosis.
   Leukemia Res., 2, in press.

3. POMEROY, K.A., PAUL, P.S., WEBER, A.F., SORENSEN, D.K. and
   JOHNSON, D.W. 1977. Evidence that B Lymphocytes Carry the Nuclear
   Pocket Abnormality Associated with Bovine Leukemia Virus Infection.
   J. Natl. Cancer Inst., 59, 281-283.

4. MAMMERICKX, M., BURNY, A., DEKEGEL, D., GHYSDAEL, J., KETTMANN, R.
   and PORTETELLE, D. 1977. Comparative Study of Four Diagnostic
   Methods of Enzootic Bovine Leukemia, pp. 209-221. In "Bovine
   Leucosis. Various Methods of Molecular Virology".(A. Burny, ed.)
   Commission of the European Communities, Luxembourg.

5. FERRER, J.F., PIPER, C.E. and BALIGA, V. 1977. Diagnosis of BLV
   infection in Cattle of Various Ages, pp 323-336. In "Bovine
   Leucosis : Various Methods of Molecular Virology". (A. Burny, ed.)
   Commission of the European Communities, Luxembourg.

6. MILLER, J.M. and VAN DER MAATEN, M.J. 1976. Serologic Response
   of Cattle Following Inoculation with Bovine Leukemia Virus.
   Bibl. Haemat., 43, 187-189.

7. ABT, D.A., MARSHAK, P.R., FERRER, J.F., PIPER, C.E. and BHATT, D.M.,
   1976. Studies on the Development of Persistent Lymphocytosis and
   Infection with the Bovine C-type Leukemia Virus (BLV) in Cattle.
   Vet. Microbiol., 1, 287-300.

8. KETTMANN, R., PORTETELLE, D., MAMMERICKX, M., CLEUTER, Y.,
   DEKEGEL, D., GALOUX, M., GHYSDAEL, J., BURNY, A. and CHANTRENNE, H.
   1976. Bovine Leukemia Virus : An Exogenous RNA Oncogenic Virus.
   Proc. Nat. Acad. Sci. USA, 73, 1014-1018.

9. CALLAHAN, R., LIEBER, M.M., TODARO, G.J., GRAVES, D.C. and
   FERRER, J.F. 1976. Bovine Leukemia Virus Genes in the DNA of
   Leukemic Cattle.
   Science, 192, 1005-1007.

10. VAN DER MAATEN, M.J., MILLER, J.M. and BOOTHE, A.D. 1974.
    Replicating Type-C Virus Particles in Monolayer Cell Cultures
    of Tissues from Cattle with Lymphosarcoma.
    J. Nat. Cancer Inst., 52, 491-497.

11. Mc DONALD, H.C. and FERRER, J.F. 1976. Detection, Quantitation
    and Characterization of the Major Internal Virion Antigen of the
    Bovine Leukemia Virus by Radioimmunoassay.
    J. Nat. Cancer Inst., 57, 875-882.

12. GHYSDAEL, J., HUBERT, E. and CLEUTER, Y. 1977. Biosynthesis of
    Bovine Leukemia Virus Major Internal Protein (p24) in Infected
    Cells and X. laevis oocytes Microinjected with BLV 60-70S RNA.
    Arch. Int. Physiol. Bioch., in press.

13. VAN DER MAATEN, M.J. and MILLER, J.M. 1977. An Evaluation of
    the Syncytium Assay for the Detection of Bovine Leukemia Virus
    in Peripheral Blood Leukocytes. pp 299-309. In "Bovine Leucosis :
    Various Methods of Molecular Virology".(A. Burny, ed.)
    Commission of the European Communities, Luxembourg.

14. WUU, K.D., GRAVES, D.C. and FERRER, J.F. 1977. Inhibition of the
    Reverse Transcriptase of Bovine Leukemia Virus by Antibody in
    Sera from Leukemic Cattle and Immunological Characterization of
    the Enzyme.
    Cancer Res., 37, 1438-1442.

15. PORTETELLE, D., BRUCK, C., BEX, F., BURNY, A., DEKEGEL, D. and
    MAMMERICKX, M. 1978. Detection of Complement Dependent Lytic
    Antibodies in Sera from Bovine Leukemia Virus Infected Animals
    by the Chromium-51 Release Assay.
    Arch. Int. Phys. Bioch., in press.

ROLE AND CONTROL OF RECOMBINANT VIRUSES IN MURINE LEUKEMIA

Peter J. Fischinger

National Cancer Institute

Bethesda, Maryland 20014

For a number of years the prevalent ecotropic murine C type oncornaviruses were thought to have been the causative agents of natural and induced murine leukemia (1-3). Further investigation revealed in the DNA of all mouse cells multiple proviral copies, some of which could be induced by various means to yield both eco- and xenotropic mouse leukemia virus (MuLV) isolates (4, 5). More recently, further complexity became evident by the isolation of nondefective, amphotropic viruses which were shown to be recombinants of eco- and xenotropic (MuX) variants (6, 7). Based on phenomena in preleukemic states of natural disease in the high leukemia incidence AKR mouse strain, it was conjectured that it was the recombinant rather than the ecotropic virus that was the causative agent in the disease process (7). The isolation of such a recombinant virus (HIX) in pure form from Moloney (M-) MuLV stocks allowed the demonstration that the recombinant virus was oncogenic by itself in the absence of detectable ecotropic virus (8). HIX virus induced lymphomas contained ample amounts of only HIX virus which even after cloning was able to induce de novo lymphomas in mice, thus fulfilling the accepted postulates of causality (9). Analogous recombinant viruses were isolated from lymphomas of AKR mice; these were described as mink cell cytopatic agents (MCF) (7). From functional and structural points of view, HIX and MCF viruses are analogous, but they originated from different parental viruses (9, 10). Although it has been demonstrated that HIX and MCF are "intragenic" recombinants, recently further viruses were isolated which were recombinants encompassing a substitution of whole genes (our unpublished data). The well-known defective recombinant subgroups of MuLV derived oncogenic

101

agents such as the various isolates of murine sarcoma virus (MSV) or the Friend spleen focus-forming virus (SFFV) represent further variations of oncogenic murine C type agents. What is clear from the above is that extensive variation in the MuLV derived group of viruses is quite common and that both defective and nondefective recombinant variants occur frequently. It is of interest that essentially all such oncogenic isolates were found to be recombinants in the general area of the envelope gene region of viral RNA. Because pseudotyping of several of these oncogenic variants such as MSV or SFFV is a common phenomon, treatment modalities would have to take into account potentially significant variations in susceptibility. A murine recombinant, nondefective leukemogenic virus isolate was recently found to exhibit the particularly interesting phenomenon of "genomic masking" by which the oncogenic variant subjected to survival pressure adopted the attending ecotropic virus envelope, against which the natural host defense mechanisms were inadequate. The following description encompasses the identification and the structure of the recombinational event, various aspects of in vivo survival pressure resulting in masking, and the implications as well as the reasons for success of anti-viral therapy. Specific materials and methods have been described in various publications (6, 8, 9, 11).

Composition of Nondefective Amphotropic Recombinant Viruses. The initial distinctive description of this group of recombinant viruses was that even after sequential steps of limiting dilution isolation in various cell systems, the progeny virus possessed stable properties of both eco- and xenotropic MuLV's (6, 7). A compilation of these properties is presented in Table 1 which specifically describes the HIX isolate. Host range was very broad in that HIX virus could avidly replicate in both mouse cells as well as in cells of most mammalian species. Preinfection of mouse or other mammalian cells with HIX virus rendered those cells insusceptible to transformation by its homologous MSV pseudotype-MSV(HIX), yet those cells remained susceptible to transformation by MSV(MuLV) and MSV(MuX) pseudotypes. MSV(HIX) could bypass ecotropic MuLV or its gp70 preinfection interference but could not enter cells preinfected with MuX. Accordingly the nature of HIX relationship to MuX is unique in its "one-way" interference pattern. The determinants on the gp70 polypeptide of HIX which are reactive with neutralizing antibody were found to be most closely related to those found on M-MuLV. Anti M-MuLV gp70 sera neutralized either HIX or M-MuLV with about an equal efficiency. Antisera directed against MuX gp70 or Friend MuLV gp70 were partially effective. Anti AKR gp70 specific antisera were not at all neutralizing, an observation which clearly distinguishes HIX from the MCF group of recombinants (7, 8).

Table 1.   Properties and Makeup of HIX Oncornavirus, a Recombinant
           Derived from Moloney MuLV and Murine Xenotropic Virus

Properties	HIX Virus (grown in mouse or heterologous cells)
Host range	: Amphotropic (mouse, rat, human, cat, mink, rabbit)
Interference spectrum	: Completely with self One way with MuX No interference with ecotropes (and their gp70's)
Susceptibility to neutralizing antibody	: Susceptible to anti M-MuLV gp70 Partly susceptible to anti MuX gp70 Susceptible to MSF
Viral genes, immunology and structure	:
"gag" p12	: M-MuLV type, by RIA
p15	: M-MuLV type, by RIA, peptide maps
p30	: M-MuLV type, by peptide maps
p10	: Group specific only, by RIA
"pol"	: Type specificity unknown
"env" gp70	: Not M-MuLV, by type specific RIA : Not MuX, by type specific RIA Unique by peptide maps
Oncogenicity	: T cell lymphomas in several strains of mice, no response in cats

    Both competition radioimmunoassays and tryptic peptide
mapping were used to determine the origin of individual viral
polypeptides of HIX.   Salient differences were found in the gp70
polypeptide.   Neither type specific antiserum reactive with M-MuLV
gp70 nor the type specific anti MuX gp70 serum could be competed
with HIX gp70 in respective homologous RIA's.   Tryptic peptide
maps of HIX virus showed specific oligopeptides associated with
xenotropic viruses and a group of peptides presumably originating
from M-MuLV.   Again the peptide maps of HIX are clearly different
from MCF recombinants because their respective ecotropic MuLV
derived oligopeptides are different (10, 11).   The individual
products of the "gag" gene near the 5' end of viral RNA were
similarly analyzed.   The highly type specific phosphorylated p12

was clearly derived from M-MuLV as seen by an exact and complete
competition RIA. This was also true for the p15 of the "gag"
region. Both the competition RIA and a tryptic peptide map showed
identity of HIX p15 with M-MuLV p15. The main reactive determinants of p30 and p10 are group specific and thus competition RIA's
were not helpful relative to the identification of origin.
However, the tryptic peptides of p30 of HIX also showed complete
congruity with M-MuLV. The origin of the reverse transcriptase
is as yet unknown. A final but very pertinent property of HIX is
that it is oncogenic in that it induces T cell lymphomas in
several strains of mice after a $\sim$2 month latent period. In
contrast, despite high titer virus inoculation of HIX grown in
cat embryo cells, no tumors were induced in newborn kittens in
the past two years of observation.

Survival Pressure and Genomic Masking of Recombinant Viruses.
Two basic observations are relevant to understanding the oncogenicity of HIX in vivo: (1) HIX recombinant virus as well as MCF are
acutely susceptible to mouse serum factor (MSF) which inactivates
xenotropic and recombinant viruses. This factor is found in
essentially all strains of mice. (2) Most stocks of M-MuLV have
no detectable free recombinant virus even when tested by most
sensitive assays available. The above observations led to the
question whether and how HIX virus could induce tumors in mice,
and secondarily whether HIX virus was the causative agent in
M-MuLV induced mouse lymphomas.

A number of M-MuLV induced lymphoma extracts obtained from
several strains of mice were compared with M-MuLV grown in mouse
tissue culture cells relative to the quantity of ecotropic M-MuLV
and to potential presence HIX or MuX viruses. The above extracts
were further compared to extracts of lymphomas induced by HIX
virus and to tissue culture derived HIX virus. All M-MuLV
induced tumor extracts had high titers of ecotropic virus ($\geq 10^6$
focus-inducing units (FIU)/ml). Tumor extracts from NIH Swiss
mice, whose serum has no detectable MSF, also contained 10^2-10^3
FIU of HIX virus. Passage of such NIH Swiss lymphoma extracts
into BALB/c mice also resulted in typical lymphomas which
contained $\geq 10^6$ FIU of ecotropic M-MuLV. In contrast these BALB/c
mouse derived lymphoma extracts had no detectable HIX or MuX
whatsoever. To examine whether recombinant virus could arise
de novo, several hundred limiting dilution foci were examined
individually to determine whether their progeny was composed of
a mixture of M-MuLV and HIX and/or MuX. It was surprising that
a number of limiting dilution foci from mouse S+L- cells yielded
progeny composed only of HIX and no M-MuLV. This was based on
the amphotropic host range and complete susceptibility of progeny

virus to MSF.   The probability of having found such foci in the
original stock calculated from the direct assays of ecotropic and
recombinant viruses indicated that there had to be much more
recombinant virus than was immediately obvious.   To examine the
possibility of masking of HIX by ecotropic M-MuLV, blind dilution
analysis was also carried out in mouse cells.   Dilutions of M-MuLV
stocks were made in mouse S+L- cells and the first cycle progeny
assessed for the appearance of recombinant virus now presumably
coated with the recombinant envelope.   The endpoint dilution at
which such recombinant virus would become obvious should roughly
correspond to analysis of individual foci.   As seen in Table 2,
five stocks of M-MuLV or HIX were examined.   In summary, both
methods of analysis demonstrated that regardless of the actual
amount of recombinant virus $\geq$99% of HIX virus was masked in M-MuLV
induced lymphomas whether MSF was present in a given strain or not.
More free as well as masked HIX virus was present in NIH Swiss
mouse lymphomas than in BALB/c lymphomas.   It was surprising that
when the BALB/c lymphoma derived virus mixture was grown in mouse
3T3 cells for several years, about 90% of HIX virus was still
masked by the M-MuLV envelope.   In contrast cloned HIX virus,
either from tissue culture or in pure form from HIX induced
lymphomas, had no other detectable envelope contributions.   When
ecotropic M-MuLV was cloned and passed in culture no de novo
appearance of HIX virus was noted.   The specific quantitative
aspects of the above phenomena are detailed elsewhere (6, 8, 9).

Susceptibility of Masked Virus and Discussion of Control
Measures.   The virological and immunological status of mice
bearing M-MuLV and HIX induced tumors was assessed not only by
the examination of the presence of virus(es) but also whether
free antibody was detectable in sera and whether any changes
occurred in the quantity of MSF.   Secondarily, the susceptibility
of detectable virus in tumors to MSF and to type specific anti
M-MuLV gp70 antibody was also of interest.   The results are
compiled in Table 3.   It was clear that no tumored animal serum
contained any neutralizing antibody for either M-MuLV or AKR
viruses.   Because MSF is normally not detectable in normal NIH
Swiss mice, a lack of MSF in tumored NIH Swiss mouse sera was
expected.   Normal BALB/c mice do have about 1000 units of MSF/ml.
The BALB/c mice with M-MuLV induced tumor which had no free HIX
and only about 400 masked HIX infectious units/ml of extract had
free MSF.   Although not shown, AKR mice with lymphomas also had
adequate amounts of MSF in their sera.   The exception was that
the serum pool of mice carrying HIX virus induced lymphomas had
very little free factor left in the presence of >10^4 infectious
units of free HIX virus.   Apparently actively replicating HIX
virus in some way abrogated MSF activity.

Table 2. Predisposition to Genomic Masking of Recombinant Virus
            by Ecotropic Envelopes

	Proportion of free recombinant to masked recombinant virus	
Virus and source	Blind dilution[a] analysis	Individual focus progeny analysis[b] ($\geq$50 foci examined)
M-MuLV NIH Swiss lymphoma	0.01	0.01
M-MuLV (ICB-3T3-77) Mouse 3T3 cells	0.16	0.05
M-MuLV	$\leq$0.003	None of 50 foci
HIX BALB/c or NIH Swiss lymphoma	1.0	1.0
HIX Cat FEF cells	1.0	1.0

[a]Virus stock was passed as half log dilutions in replicate plates of mouse S+L- cells for four days. Progeny virus was assayed for xenotropic type variants by focus assays of resulting pseudotype in cat embryo cells and by helper assay in cat S+L- cells. Titer was calculated as the dilution at which half the plates were positive for recombinant virus. Value represents titer on direct assay in cat S+L- cells/endpoint dilution value.

[b]An m.o.i. of 0.3 infectious units/well of Falcon microtiter plates resulted in appropriate Poisson distribution of foci. Each focus was picked and its progeny assayed in mouse S+L- cells with and without MSF and also assayed in cat S+L- cells (9). Value represents titer on direct assay in cat S+L- cells/titer of recombinant calculated from the number of foci yielding recombinant virus.

Table 3. Susceptibility of Detectable Viruses in Moloney Type Mouse Lymphomas to Two Control Modalities

Pooled tumor extract, mouse strain and lymphoma inducing virus	Presence of MSF units/ml[a]	Presence of free neutralizing antibody[b]	Susceptibility of Tumor Derived Viruses, (Vn/Vo)[c]:			
			to MSF		to antibody	
			M-MuLV	Recombinant (unmasked)	M-MuLV	Recombinant (unmasked)
NIH Swiss, M-MuLV	<10	0	>0.5	0.005	0.02	0.04
NIH Swiss, HIX	<10	0	No ecotrope	<0.008	No ecotrope	0.03
BALB/c, M-MuLV	500	0	>0.5	<0.01	0.01	0.03
BALB/c, HIX	<50	0	No ecotrope	0.005	No ecotrope	0.05

[a]MSF units, given as 50% inhibitory doses per ml.

[b]Tested against M-MuLV and AKR viruses.

[c]Vn/Vo, virus surviving fraction, MSF is STU normal mouse serum at a 1:100 final dilution, antibody is rabbit anti M-MuLV gp70 serum prepared by J. Ihle and previously described relative to its potency and type specificity (11).

Because further changes could have occurred in tumor derived viruses, each stock was subjected to treatment with MSF or type specific anti M-MuLV gp70 serum. It was clear that M-MuLV in tumors was not susceptible to MSF and that HIX virus from any of the tumors was as susceptible to MSF as the original input virus. Unmasking of HIX from M-MuLV induced tumors was achieved by a single passage through mouse cells followed by one passage through cat embryo cells. The susceptibility of either M-MuLV or HIX to anti M-MuLV gp70 type specific sera was as expected.

Based on the above phenomena, plans for specific antiviral therapy of virus induced neoplasms have to include the probability of envelope changes. Analogous phenomena have been observed in the induction of sarcomas in AKR mice by the Moloney MuLV pseudotype of MSV. There the tumors that did come up were all progressor tumors. The animal had made type specific antibody to M-MuLV. The tumors were full of virus, but all of the MSV was coated with the AKR virus envelope (12). Thus treatment of Moloney MSV with type specific anti M-MuLV sera would have been useless. Further specific analogy to the present system involving genomic masking can be found in the natural AKR lymphomas. Free recombinant virus cannot be found, and preliminary experiments have detected low levels of masked recombinant in some of the tumors tested. It is of interest that successful serotherapy has been reported in AKR mice with sera prepared against Friend MuLV gp70 which had a very strong group specific neutralizing antibody (13). Further extrinsic envelope changes have to be considered as possible with the initiation of specific therapeutic regimens. The presence of MSF as a lethal factor for recombinant virus seemed to have forced the recombinant to adopt the insusceptible ecotropic envelope. Evolution apparently favored recombinant with such ability because even in tissue culture mixed HIX and M-MuLV virus stocks exhibited the phenomenon that the majority of HIX virus was in M-MuLV envelopes. In addition to the above, the documented recombinational ability of this group of viruses could lead to further genotypic variants as well.

REFERENCES

1. Gross, L., Proc. Soc. Exp. Biol. Med. 76, 27-33 (1951).

2. Friend, C., Ann. N.Y. Acad. Sci. 68, 522-541 (1957).

3. Moloney, J. B., J. Natl. Cancer Inst. 24, 933-951 (1960).

4. Lowy, D. R., Rowe, W. P., Teich, N. M., and Hartley, J. W., Science 174, 155-156 (1971).

5. Chattopadhyay, S. K., Lowy, D. R., Teich, N. M., Levine, A. S.,
Rowe, W. P., Cold Spring Harbor Symp. Quant. Biol. 39, 1085-1101
(1974).

6. Fischinger, P. J., Nomura, S., Bolognesi, D. P., Proc. Natl.
Acad. Sci. USA 72, 5150-5155 (1975).

7. Hartley, J. W., Wolford, N. K., Old, L. J., Rowe, W. P.,
Proc. Natl. Acad. Sci. USA 74, 785-792 (1977).

8. Fischinger, P. J., Ihle, J. N., deNoronha, Fernando, and
Bolognesi, D. P., Med. Microbiol. Immunol. 164, 119-129 (1977).

9. Fischinger, P. J., Dunlop, N. M., and Blevins, C. S., J. Virol.
(in press).

10. Elder, J. H., Gautsch, J. W., Jensen, F. C., Lerner, R. A.,
Hartley, J. W., and Rowe, W. P., Proc. Natl. Acad. Sci. USA 74,
4676-4680.

11. Fischinger, P. J., Frankel, A. E., Elder, J. H., Lerner, R. A.,
Ihle, J. N., and Bolognesi, D. P. (Virology, submitted).

12. Chieco-Bianchi, L., Colombatti, A., Collavo, D, Sendo, F.,
Aoki, T., and Fischinger, P. J., J. Explt. Med. 140, 1162-1179
(1974).

13. Schäfer, W., Bolognesi, D. P., de Noronha, F., Fischinger, P.
J., Hunsmann, G., Ihle, J. N., Moennig, V., Schwarz, H., and
Thiel, H.-J., Med. Microbiol. Immunol. 164, 217-229 (1977).

THE NATURAL OCCURRENCE

OF FELINE LEUKAEMIA VIRUS INFECTIONS

Oswald Jarrett and William Jarrett

Department of Veterinary Pathology, University of Glasgow

Veterinary School, Bearsden, Glasgow, G61 1QH, Scotland

The leukaemia-lymphosarcoma complex (LLC) constitutes the most common group of malignancies in the cat and the absolute incidence of these tumours is very high, probably in excess of 5 times the incidence of leukaemia in man. Feline leukaemia virus (FeLV) is the etiological agent of a large proportion of these cases and infection by this virus can cause, directly or indirectly, a number of other diseases, the combined incidence of which is probably many times that of frank neoplasia. FeLV is therefore a major pathogen in the cat.

Feline leukaemia viruses

FeLV is a retrovirus (oncornavirus) with C-type morphology and chemical composition. Three subgroups of FeLV are known (A, B and C) and these are defined by interference properties (Sarma and Log, 1971). The relationship of the subgroups to each other is unique to the cat and is discussed in detail below. Cultured cells of several species can be infected by FeLV: in general the growth of viruses of subgroup A (FeLV-A) is restricted to feline cells while viruses of subgroups B and C have a wider host range (O. Jarrett et al. 1973). Although FeLV can cause leukaemia in dogs experimentally, there is no evidence that transmission and tumour induction in any species other than the feline occurs in nature.

The cat also has an endogenous oncornavirus the prototype of which is RD114 (McAllister et al. 1972). This virus has little genetic relationship with FeLV and is not known to be involved in any disease process. In addition, other nucleotide sequences which are distantly related to FeLV are present in feline cellular DNA (Okabe et al. 1976).

111

Diseases caused by FeLV

The wide range of haemopoietic neoplasms associated with FeLV
are given in detail in Jarrett and Mackey (1974). In addition a number
of other serious illnesses follow infection with FeLV (Hardy et al. 1976a).
Some of these such as haemobartonellosis, feline infectious peritonitis
and a variety of severe viral and bacterial infections which might otherwise be trivial are probably consequent upon immunosuppression.
Others, including glomerulonephritis, osteosclerosis and reproductive
failure, result directly from virus infection. Since oncornaviruses
are moderate and non-lytic in their host-cell relationship it is often
assumed that the diseases resulting from infection are associated with
cell proliferation and not destruction. Table 1 illustrates the probable
relationship between infection of the various cells of the haemopoietic
system and the ensuing diseases. It will be seen that there is evidence
for infection of all basic haemopoietic cell types and that the disease
produced might result from either proliferation or ablation of that cell
type. This is not to suggest that a directly lytic virus cycle occurs:
such effects could be mediated by immunological or other means. It
is probable, however, that in the general population the number of cats
suffering diseases of the ablation type is much greater than the number
of animals with neoplasia.

Detailed work on the putative specific cytotropism of different subgroups and serotypes within subgroups is in progress in an attempt to
clarify the virological and pathological pictures outlined above.

Association of FeLV with the leukaemia-lymphosarcoma complex

It is not emphasised frequently enough that FeLV is isolated from
only a proportion of cats with LLC. For example, in our series the
figure is 50%; but this proportion varies depending on the types of
tumour which constitute any given series. The three main pathological
types of lymphosarcoma are thymic, multicentric and alimentary
(W. Jarrett and Mackey, 1974). The proportion of these which yield
FeLV is about 90% of the thymic, 70% of the multicentric and 30% of the
alimentary cases and the total proportion of FeLV-negative tumours in
any one series reflects the frequency of alimentary cases in it (Hardy
et al. 1976a). These cases need more detailed study to determine
their relationship, if any, to FeLV. This is being investigated by
examining the tumour cells for FeLV-specific genetic information
(Okabe et al. 1976; Levin et al. 1977) and gene products (Hardy et al.
1977) and by defining the epidemiology of FeLV-negative cases of
leukaemia. It will be seen below that in FeLV-infected multiple cat

TABLE 1

Diseases Associated with FeLV Infection

Cell Type	Proliferation	Ablation
T-cell	Leukaemia Thymic lymphosarcoma	Immunosuppression (Runting; enhancement of infectious diseases)
B-cell	Leukaemia Alimentary lymphosarcoma Multicentric lymphosarcoma	Immunosuppression
Myeloblast	Myeloid leukaemia Monocytic leukaemia	Agranulocytosis Myelofibrosis
Erythroblast	Acute erythraemia Polycythaemia vera	Aplastic anaemia
Erythrocyte		Acquired haemolytic anaemia

households, the feline inmates are usually either positive for FeLV or
have antibodies associated with FeLV infection. We have recently
found a FeLV-negative case of thymic lymphosarcoma in a household
in which the other cats were all negative for virus and for antibodies.
Since horizontal transmission is the rule in association with FeLV
expression, there exists an area of feline LLC of which the epidemiology
and cause is unknown and this may be of specific relevance to the human
situation.

Natural transmission of FeLV

The original transmission experiments leading to the discovery of
FeLV were carried out after finding a cluster of 8 lymphosarcoma
cases in a short period of time among a number of unrelated cats in a
single household (W. Jarrett et al. 1964a). This natural situation
predicated horizontal transmission and experimentally it was accomplished by needle passage in neonatal kittens (W. Jarrett et al. 1964b).
Subsequently Rickard et al. (1969) found FeLV infection in 3 uninoculated
animals which were in contact with experimentally inoculated animals
and Brodey and his colleagues found strong circumstantial evidence of
horizontal transmission instituted by the transference of FeLV-infected
breeding cats between households (Brodey et al. 1970). Hardy found
FeLV-specific antigen in the saliva of cats and Gardner et al. (1971)
observed FeLV particles budding from salivary gland secretory cells.
W. Jarrett et al. (1973) showed that horizontal transmission took place
in experimental situations both between kittens and kittens, between
kittens and adults and from adult to adult. Transfer of infection was
demonstrable within a month of mixing and transmission of virus in this
way could lead to the development of tumours in cats exposed both as
kittens and as adults. A wide variety of tissues was examined by
electron microscopy to determine the possible routes of excretion of
FeLV. Virus was most commonly found in the trachea and oral mucosa
but was also found in the urinary tract, the alimentary tract and the
pancreas. Much recent epidemiological work has proven beyond doubt
that FeLV in the form in which it has been conventionally recognised
up until now is transmitted horizontally. The subject is well reviewed
by Hardy et al. (1973; 1976a).

Epidemiology of FeLV

Two main epidemiological situations exist: the randomly mixed
urban cat society; and the relatively closed enzootic multiple cat
household (MCH).

Rogerson et al. (1975) studied over 1,500 cats in Glasgow, a large industrial town, and in the surrounding rural environment. The households from which these originated contained single cats which were allowed to roam freely and mix with other cats. The degree of roaming and the density of the cat population is, in the urban locale, roughly proportional to the socio-economic group of the relevant human population. Two major parameters have been measured to date: first, viraemia by cultivation of plasma virus and secondly, antibodies to the feline oncornavirus-associated cell membrane antigen (FOCMA) (Essex et al. 1971); more recent studies have involved the use of virus neutralising antibody tests. The general situation was that over 70% of urban strays, 30% of urban pets and only 5% of urban kittens (below 5 months of age) had anti-FOCMA antibodies. Over 400 rural farm cats of all ages showed an antibody prevalence of only 4%. An age structured study of this population revealed that significant infection rates started at 5 months, the time that cats begin to mix socially. There was then a linear rise of antibodies with age until the surprisingly high prevalence of over 70% was reached at 3 years of age. There were no differences in antibody titre between the age groups indicating possible frequent re-exposure to virus. Subsequently we studied 400 urban cats and found 5% to be excretors of virus (P. Rogerson, W. Jarrett and O. Jarrett, unpublished results). This epidemiological situation therefore reflects a widespread infection by horizontal transmission and may be roughly summarised thus: of every 1,000 urban cats, 500 have been infected with FeLV and have antibodies, 50 are virus excretors and 1 develops LLC.

In the closed house epidemiological situation, several cats are usually kept in the same household and many of these are of the pedigree breeds. In these households there is often a history of both LLC and of other diseases which are known to be associated with FeLV infection. In a study of a large number of households of this type Hardy et al. (1973) showed that about one-third of the apparently healthy cats were viraemic and had a risk of developing leukaemia of about 1,000 times that of a cat in the general population. This is almost certainly caused by the prolonged exposure to cats in enzootic households to large quantities of FeLV which are excreted orally by viraemic animals in the same house and to some extent to congenital infection from infected mothers. FeLV-positive cats had a range of low anti-FOCMA antibody titres but little or no virus neutralising antibodies whereas the FeLV-negative cats frequently had high titres of both FOCMA and serum neutralising antibodies and these titres were highly correlated (Hardy et al. 1976a; Russell and Jarrett, 1978b).

Pathogenesis of FeLV infection

FeLV-infected cats excrete virus and cats can be infected by the naso-pharyngeal route (Francis et al. 1977; Hoover et al. 1972; O. Jarrett and Russell, 1978).   This apparently simple pattern of transmission has been verified in several large scale epidemiological studies.   However, much greater complexities are now emerging. The study of the relationship of virus infection to time, organ, virus subgroup, differential excretion of subgroups, phenotypic mixing and possible genetic recombination is beginning to reveal a situation of great interest.

FeLV-related diseases occur in cats with persistent FeLV infections which may be detected by the demonstration of virus in the blood (O. Jarrett et al. 1968; Hardy et al. 1973).   The incubation period between infection and the appearance of clinical disease, especially leukaemia, may be very long and during this time the cat appears to be healthy although it will be excreting virus continuously (Francis et al. 1977; O. Jarrett and Russell, 1978).   It is obvious that it is often difficult to establish a clear cause-and-effect between exposure of a cat to FeLV and the development of disease in the field in the absence of virological and serological investigation.

It is likely that the outcome of FeLV infection in individual cats is determined by the balance between the extent of early virus replication and the capacity of the cats to mount an immune response to FeLV. This in turn is influenced by two main factors: the age at which the cat is infected with FeLV and the dose of virus to which the cat is exposed.

The proportion of cats which develops persistent infection varies according to the age at which the cat is exposed.   When a cat is infected early in life, either in utero or in the neonatal period, the outcome is always a persistent viraemia with no detectable immune response and these cats have a very high risk of developing FeLV-related disease. Between the age of 12 and 20 weeks there is a transitional period in which most kittens exposed to FeLV become persistently infected, but some become immune and thereby have a much lower risk of disease. From about 16 weeks of age onwards the majority of cats become immune following FeLV infection (Hoover et al. 1976).

Another important determinant of susceptibility is virus dose which is often a function of how the cats are maintained.   As described above, free range cats hardly ever become persistently infected with FeLV while a high proportion of cats kept in closed communities in which

FeLV is enzootic develops chronic infections. The basis of this
difference in response is probably that in closed communities a high
dose of virus is transmitted which often leads to persistent infection
while the low dose to which free range cats are exposed tends to
immunise.

Recently we have found that the prevalent FeLV subgroup also
influences the extent of persistent infections in multicat households.
The 3 FeLV subgroups, A, B and C, are not found randomly in FeLV-
infected cats. Sarma and Log (1971) and O. Jarrett et al. (1978) found
that they occurred in combinations in which A was always present:
all isolates contained FeLV-A; a high proportion also had FeLV-B;
virus of subgroup C was rare and occurred only in the combinations AC
and ABC. The relative prevalence of the subgroups differed in LLC cats
and healthy carriers (O. Jarrett et al. 1978). Of the LLC cats, 42%
had FeLV-A and 58% had FeLV-AB. No obvious correlation was found
between the type of disease and the subgroup present. However, in one
cat with thymic lymphosarcoma, FeLV-A alone was isolated from the
plasma, bone marrow and spleen while FeLV-A and B were found in the
thymic tumour, suggesting the possibility of cell tropisms of different
subgroups. In healthy carrier cats, 65% had FeLV-A and 33% had
FeLV-AB. FeLV of subgroup C was found only in cats with disease:
one with LLC and two with severe anaemia. Experimentally, infection
of cats with FeLV-C alone has been shown to be associated with aplastic
anaemia (Mackey et al., 1975).

The study of multiple cat households revealed two distinct situations
which were designated MCH-A in which the carrier cats had only
FeLV-A, and MCH-AB in which cats with either subgroup A or AB were
present. In MCH-AB half of the cats had FeLV-A and half FeLV-AB.
The proportion of cats in all MCHs which were viraemic was 42% but
there was a marked difference in the prevalence of carrier cats in each
type of household: in MCH-A 28% were FeLV-positive while in MCH-AB
53% were viraemic. The development of this situation was observed in
a series of experiments in which cats were infected with subgroups A
and B singly and together (O. Jarrett and Russell, 1978). In most cats
virus appeared quickly in the blood and oropharynx after FeLV-A
infection but following infection with FeLV-B only a small proportion
developed viraemia and this only after a long interval. There was
also no evidence that FeLV-B was transmitted by contact. It is
possible that the growth of FeLV-B is restricted to relatively few cells
in the cat and this may be relevant to the pathogenesis of disease
caused by FeLV of different subgroups in that different cells in
different organs may be infected by viruses with distinct cytotropisms.

Out of 56 cats inoculated as newborns with FeLV-B, only 8 became persistently viraemic and 2 of these have developed thymic lympho-sarcoma.

When cats were infected with phenotypic mixtures of FeLV-A and B it appeared that, to a large extent, each virus operated independently in that FeLV-A was recovered from the plasma first and FeLV-B appeared later (but not in all cats). However, there was evidence of interaction between the viruses: the proportion of cats which were viraemic with FeLV-B was greater following FeLV-AB infection than after infection with FeLV-B alone. Also FeLV-B was transmitted by contact from cats which were excreting FeLV-AB. One reason for the possible enhancement of FeLV-B by FeLV-A is that the mixing of subgroups A and B in an infection confers an expansion of the cell range of FeLV-B by phenotypic mixing with FeLV-A. FeLV-B might then be able to replicate in normally non-permissive cells and might consequently be found in the blood. Phenotypic mixing might also explain the fact that cats viraemic with FeLV-AB can transmit FeLV-B horizontally while cats infected with FeLV-B alone do not.

The difference in proportion of viraemic cats in MCH-A and MCH-AB was possibly due to susceptible cats being originally infected with a higher dose of virus when exposed to a cat excreting FeLV-AB compared to a cat excreting FeLV-A: cats viraemic with FeLV-AB, as described above, have a well-established infection and excrete maximum quantities of virus. The apparent "over-representation" of FeLV-AB in leukaemic cats compared to healthy carriers is probably a related situation and it will be important to determine prospectively if more cases of FeLV-related disease develop in MCH-AB than in MCH-A.

The primary events in leukaemogenesis in the cat are as obscure as in any other species. It is now obvious that immunodepression particularly of humoral antibodies in the first few days after infection is virtually a prerequisite for ultimate neoplasia. About 75% of LLC cats have no antibodies to virus or FOCMA and the remaining 25% have low levels. Viral thymectomy and CMI deficiency occur subsequently (Anderson et al. 1971; Perryman et al. 1972). The relationship between infection (with prolonged viraemia) and the transformation event or target cell strike is also unknown. Some virus strains have a median time to tumour of a month or two while others may have a median of over 4 years with a large standard deviation. Both B cell and T cell lymphoid neoplasms are found and the transformed cells disseminate throughout the body in a distribution that is similar to the immunological traffic system of the appropriate cell of origin; this is responsible for the distinct pathological types of LLC such as thymic, alimentary and multicentric lymphosarcoma and the lymphoid leukaemias. Again studies on the nature of virus cytotropism, transformation permissiveness and subsequent malignant potential are required.

Immunity to FeLV

At the moment it is clear that at least two operationally defined immune systems are important in FeLV infections and although much is known about these and about vaccination against the disease (by utilising either of these systems or both), the basic immune mechanism remains obscure.   The two systems of antibodies are first, virus neutralising (VN) antibodies directed against antigenic determinants on the viral envelope; and secondly, those directed against antigen(s) on the surface of cells transformed by FeLV (but more rigorously defined as antigens expressed on cells of the FL74 line (Theilen et al. 1969) which is a tumour-derived lymphoblastoid cell line infected with FeLV of subgroups A, B and C). These cells express a high density of so-called FOCMA on their surfaces.   This antigen-antibody system was defined and is normally measured by an indirect immunofluorescence assay on live cells (Essex et al. 1971).

Over the last few years a few working, but now questionable, assumptions have been common among workers on FeLV.   These are: (1) VN antibodies are directed against a determinant of the major glyco-protein of the virus envelope, gp71; (2) VN antibodies probably define the subgroups in a similar fashion to interference tests, i.e. serotypic specificity is a reflection of subgroup specificity; (3) cats with VN antibodies do not have viraemia; and (4) FOCMA is a cell surface antigen coded for by FeLV but not a virion structural protein. Antibodies to FOCMA are cytotoxic (Grant et al. 1977) and animals with moderately high titres are resistant to the emergence and proliferation of clones of virus-transformed tumour cells.   Thus VN antibodies protect against reinfection with FeLV and FOCMA antibodies appear to ablate virus transformed cells and act as an immune surveillance mechanism.

The position can no longer be visualised in such simple terms but the approximations are partially correct.   The historical situation concerning VN antibodies is reviewed by Russell and O. Jarrett (1978a). Sarma et al. (1974) found naturally occurring VN antibodies to the three FeLV subgroups, A, B and C, and Hardy et al. (1976a) found VN antibodies in 5% of free-range cats, in no cat with LLC tumours and in

30% of healthy cats from FeLV-infected multicat households. Russell
and O. Jarrett (1978a, 1978b) examined the antigenic specificities of VN
antibodies and their occurrence in various cat populations. FeLV-A
virus isolates were monotypic but, by contrast, there was antigenic
variation within subgroups B and C and there was also some evidence of
cross-reactivity between subgroups. An important finding was that
within subgroup C, one isolate was indistinguishable from the standard
C strain but another two were very similar to A so that serotypic
specificity revealed by neutralisation did not correspond to subgroup
classification based on interference. It was also found that the prevalence
of anti-FeLV-A antibodies was related to the frequency of isolation of
FeLV-A in any given population except leukaemic cats. Thus, they
were found in 4% of free-range cats and in 42% of the cats in MCHs.
In individual cats in MCHs there was a strong correlation between the
presence of anti-FeLV-A antibodies and the absence of viraemia,
although this was not absolute and occasional animals were found in
which both were present. Similar animals seen experimentally have
often been in the process of conversion from a virus-positive to a virus-
negative state. Anti-FeLV-B antibodies were not encountered as
frequently as one would have expected from the prevalence of FeLV-B
virus isolates and it was postulated that this was due to the restricted
growth of FeLV-B in cats. The most surprising result however was
the prevalence of anti-C antibodies: 11% of free-range cats, 51% of
those in MCHs and 40% of leukaemic cats had such antibody. None was
found in SPF cats. They were found more or less equally in viraemic
and non-viraemic animals. These results were paralleled by the
findings in a number of reconstruction type experiments designed to
mimic the various field situations. FeLV-C is rarely isolated from
cats and it was surprising that such a high proportion of cats in nature
had neutralising antibodies of this specificity. Russell and O. Jarrett
(1978a) have suggested that it is unlikely that these antibodies are
produced in response to exogenous infection with viruses of subgroup C.
Experimentally it was found that some animals which were exposed to
FeLV-A subsequently developed antibodies to subgroup C. They also
thought it unlikely that all of the anti-FeLV-C activity was directed
against an antigenic determinant shared between A and C largely
because the anti-C activity was not absorbed in vivo in many cats which
are viraemic with FeLV-A. They suggested that the antibodies might
be induced by an antigen which is expressed in cats during infection
with FeLV-A and might be derived from a recombination event between
FeLV-A and endogenous FeLV-like genes present in cat cells (Okabe
et al. 1976).

In another article in this publication FOCMA is discussed in detail by M. Essex. Until the antigen is purified and compared with all the FeLV gene products which are precursors of, or are, viral structural proteins of all three subgroups, its nature must remain obscure. It is clear, however, that FOCMA represents a major protective system against LLC.

Vaccination against FeLV

It has been shown by W. Jarrett et al. (1974, 1975) that it is possible to vaccinate cats against FeLV infection and to produce high anti-FOCMA titres and VN antibodies using live killed transformed cells. The addition of adjuvants enabled numbers as small as 10^6 cells, on which the antigenicity had been fixed by paraformaldehyde treatment, to be effective. The vaccine is at present under trial for field use.

Control of FeLV infections in multiple cat households

A highly effective method of control of the disease in enzootic households is in widespread use. The development of a simple slide fluorescent antibody test to detect viraemia ensured the practicability of the system under field conditions (Hardy et al. 1973). The method consists of essentially four stages: (1) test and removal of all FeLV-positive sick cats; (2) test the other cats in the household and remove all FeLV-positive cats; (3) after 3 months test the remaining population to ensure that all are FeLV-negative; and (4) subsequently test all new cats before introducing to the household. Using this system Hardy et al. (1976b) have demonstrated that FeLV, and also the risk of FeLV-related disease, may be eliminated.

It would therefore appear that one could envisage that in the not too distant future practical control measures will be available for both of the major epidemiological situations found in the FeLV infection. However, as a model system cat leukaemia has several unique features and also several aspects, the solution of which might have considerable relevance to leukaemia in man.

ACKNOWLEDGEMENTS

The work carried out in this laboratory was supported by a grant from the Cancer Research Campaign.

REFERENCES

ANDERSON, L.J., JARRETT, W.F.H., JARRETT, O., and LAIRD, H.M. (1971). J. Nat. Cancer Inst. 47, 807-817.

BRODEY, R.S., McDONOUGH, S.K., FRYE, F.L. and HARDY, W.D. Jr. (1970). In R.M. Dutcher (ed.) Comparative Leukaemia Research 1969, pp.333-342, Karger, Basel.

ESSEX, M., KLEIN, G., SNYDER, S.P., and HARROLD, J.G. (1971). Int. J. Cancer 8, pp.384-390.

FRANCIS, D.P., ESSEX, M., and HARDY, W.D. Jr. (1977). Nature 269, pp.252-254.

GARDNER, M.B., RONGEY, R.W., JOHNSON, E.Y., DeJOURNETT, R., and HUEBNER, R.J. (1971). J. Nat. Cancer Inst. 47, 561-568.

GRANT, C.K., WORLEY, M.B., and De BOER, D.J. (1977). J. Nat. Cancer Inst. 58, 157-161.

HARDY, W.D., Jr., OLD, L.J., HESS, P.W., ESSEX, M., and COTTER, S.M. (1973). Nature 244, pp.266-269.

HARDY, W.D., Jr., HESS, P.W., MacEWAN, E.G., McCLELLAND, A.J., ZUCKERMAN, E.E., ESSEX, M., COTTER, S.M. and JARRETT, O. (1976a). Cancer Res. 36, pp.582-588.

HARDY, W.D. Jr., McCLELLAND, A.J., ZUCKERMAN, E.E., HESS, P.W., ESSEX, M., COTTER, S.M., MacEWAN, E.G. & HAYES, A. (1976b). Nature 263, 326.

HARDY, W.D. Jr., ZUCKERMAN, E.E., MacEWAN, E.G., HAYES, A.A. and ESSEX, M. (1977). Nature 270, 249.

HOOVER, E.A., OLSEN, R.G., HARDY, W.D. Jr., SCHALLER, J.P., and MATHES, L.E. (1976). J. Nat. Cancer Inst. 57, 365-369.

HOOVER, E.A., McCULLOUGH, C.B., and GRIESMER, R.A. (1972). J. Nat. Cancer Inst. 48, 973-983.

JARRETT, O., LAIRD, H.M., CRIGHTON, G.W., JARRETT, W.F.H. and HAY, D. In H.J. Bendixen (ed) Leukemia in Animals and Man, pp. 244-254, Karger, Basel (1968).

JARRETT, O., LAIRD, H.M., and HAY, D. (1973). J. Gen. Virol. 20, 169-175.

JARRETT, O., HARDY, W.D. Jr., GOLDER, M.C., and HAY, D. (1978). Int. J. Cancer 21, 334-337.

JARRETT, O., and RUSSELL, P.H. (1978). Int. J. Cancer (in press).

JARRETT, W.F.H., MARTIN, W.B., CRIGHTON, G.W., DALTON, R.G., and STEWART, M.F. (1964b). Nature 202, 566-567.

JARRETT, W., JARRETT, O., MACKEY, L., LAIRD, H., HARDY, W.D. Jr., and ESSEX, M. J. Nat. Cancer Inst. 51, 833-841 (1973).

JARRETT, W., MACKEY, L., JARRETT, O., LAIRD, H.M. and HOOD, C. (1974). Nature 248, 230-232.

JARRETT, W.F.H., and MACKEY, L.J. (1974). Bull. Wld. Hlth. Org. 50, 21-34.

JARRETT, W., JARRETT, O., MACKEY, L., LAIRD, H., HOOD, C and HAY, D. (1975). Int. J. Cancer 16, 134-141.

LEVIN, R., RUSCETTI, S.K., PARKS, W.P., and SCOLNICK, E.M. Int. J. Cancer 18, 661-671 (1976).

MACKEY, L., JARRETT, W., JARRETT, O., and LAIRD, H. (1975). J. Nat. Cancer Inst. 54, 209-217.

McALLISTER, R.M., NICHOLSON, M., GARDNER, M.B., RONGEY, R.W., RASHEED, S., SARMA, P.S., HUEBNER, R.J., HATANAKA, M., OROSZLAN, S., GILDEN, R.V., KABIGTING, A., and VERNON, L. (1972). Nature (New Biol.) 235, 3-6.

OKABE, H., TWIDDY, E., GILDEN, R.V., HATANAKA, M., HOOVER, E.A., and OLSEN, R.G. (1976). Virology 69, 798-801.

PERRYMAN, L.E., HOOVER, E.A., and YOHN, D.S. (1972). J. Nat. Cancer Inst. 49, 1357-1365.

RICKARD, C.G., POST, J.E., NORONHA, F., and BARR, L.M. (1969). J. Nat. Cancer Inst. 42, 987-1014.

ROGERSON, P., JARRETT, W., and MACKEY, L. (1975).
Int. J. Cancer 15, 781-785.

RUSSELL, P.H., and JARRETT, O. (1978a).   Submitted for
publication.

RUSSELL, P.H., and JARRETT, O. (1978b).   Submitted for
publication.

SARMA, P.S., and LOG, T. (1971).   Virology 44, 352-358.

SARMA, P.S., SHARAR, A., WALTERS, V., and GARDNER, M.
(1974).   Proc. Soc. Exptl. Biol. Med. 145, 560-564.

THEILEN, G.H., KAWAKAMI, T.G., RUSH, J.D., and MUNN, R.G.
(1969). Nature 222, 589-590.

FOCMA: A TRANSFORMATION SPECIFIC RNA SARCOMA VIRUS ENCODED PROTEIN

M. Essex,[1] A. H. Sliski,[1] and W. D. Hardy Jr.[2]

[1]Dept. of Microbiology, Harvard Univ. School of Public Health, [2]Memorial Sloan-Kettering Cancer Center [1]Boston, Massachusetts 02115, [2]New York, New York 10025

INTRODUCTION

It is clear that horizontally acquired Oncornaviruses and Herpesviruses cause certain hematopoietic malignancies in several species of lower animals under natural conditions. It is not yet apparent whether or not such viruses are etiologically associated with the same types of tumors in man. If viruses representative of these groups also cause pathologically related tumors in man, we must assume that they neither replicate from the tumor tissues nor synthesize virus structural proteins in the tumor cells, at least in the vast majority of cases.

In the case of RNA tumor viruses, human tumor tissues have occasionally been reported as positive for such virally-related markers as reverse transcriptase, antibodies to reverse transcriptase or other viral proteins, and sequences of DNA that show relatedness to known oncorna proviruses of primate or rodent origin (Gallo and Gillespie, 1977; also see other articles in this volume). If the RNA tumor viruses ever do cause cases of hematopoietic tumors in man we must assume one or more of the following conditions; (1) the agents must be able to maintain the transformed phenotype in the tumor cells without allowing the synthesis of cross reactive virus structural protein antigens, and/or (2) the agents must be able to induce and maintain the transformed phenotype in the tumor cells without retaining either major portions of the provirus DNA sequences in most of the cells and/or alternatively, full copies in more than a minor portion of the cells, and/or (3) the hypothetical agents associated with malignancies in man must be only very distantly related to existing RNA tumor viruses of rodents, cats, gibbons, and baboons.

125

In lower animal species such as chickens and mice, the RNA
tumor viruses that cause lymphoma and leukemia replicate efficiently from the tumor cells. A clear model where RNA tumor viruses
can be used to produce "virus negative" (VN) leukemias and/or lymphomas, especially tumors that are "genome negative" or "partially
genome negative" is thus far lacking in the rodent and gibbon species. In the feline species we know that most cases of naturally
occurring leukemia or lymphoma are caused by horizontally acquired
feline leukemia virus (FeLV) that replicates extensively in the
tumor cells (Hardy et al., 1973; Jarrett et al., 1973; Essex, 1975a;
Essex et al., 1977a). Yet, one-fourth or one-third of the field
cases of these feline malignancies are VN (Essex et al., 1975a)
and "genome negative" (Levin et al., 1976; Koshy et al., 1978)
as are the human malignancies. Are these VN feline tumors caused
by FeLV? If so, an understanding of how FeLV caused the VN feline
tumors might be an important approach to an understanding of the
disease in man. From the practical standpoint it might reveal
how the limited number of viral gene(s) and/or the virus-directed
gene products initiate and maintain the transformed phenotype.

FELINE LEUKEMIA AND SARCOMA VIRUSES

The FeLV and feline sarcoma viruses (FeSV) are typical C-type
oncornaviruses (Essex, 1975a,b). Hypothetically, and by analogy
with the avian and murine viruses we would predict a gene order
of 5'-gag-pol-env-onc-3' for virion RNA's that possess both replicative and transforming potential (Kurth et al, 1978; Stephenson
et al, 1978). The gag gene codes for a polyprotein which undergoes post-translational cleavage to become virion core structural
polypeptides of 15,000, 12,000, 30,000, and 10,000, respectively.
They are designated p15, p12, p30, and p10 and they probably occur
in that order progressing from the 5' end of the RNA to the pol
gene (Khan and Stephenson, 1977). The pol gene codes for reverse
transcriptase. The env gene codes for a polyprotein which becomes
the virion envelope glycoprotein knobs (gp70), which serve as a
target for virus neutralizing antibody, and a small protein (p15e)
which becomes the backbone of the virion envelope. Further detail
on both the functional and biochemical aspects of these proteins
has been recently reviewed (Stephenson et al, 1978).

The onc gene exists to code for the transforming protein which
would initiate and/or maintain the malignant phenotype. In the
case of most sarcoma viruses (e.g. FeSV) the onc sequences (designated src or sarc) occur at the expense of one or more of the genes
needed for replication and/or assembly. Thus, most sarcoma viruses,
which are "transformation-competent" for fibroblasts, are replication-defective. To overcome this, such defective sarcoma viruses
occur in the presence of replication-competent helper viruses which
provide these functions in the cell. Sarcoma virus (including

FeSV) transformed cells can be selected that have lost the ability
to replicate virus (i.e., nonproducer cells) (Henderson et al.,
1974). From work with the avian and murine systems it is apparent
that the src sequences are closely related to genes that occur
in chicken or rodent cells, presumably becoming linked to viral
sequences by recombinational events that occur quite infrequently,
except in an evolutionary sense (Stephenson et al., 1978). Naturally occurring fibrosarcomas with or without associated sarcoma
viruses occur very rarely if at all in chickens and rodents. This
suggests that the transformation competent RNA sarcoma viruses
derived in the laboratory, whether defective or competent for replication, probably play little if any role in the natural causation
of cancer in these species. In the cat, however, naturally occurring fibrosarcomas are infrequent but not rare (Essex, 1975b).
Furthermore, most of the multicentric fibrosarcomas that occur
in young cats readily yield transformation competent FeSV's (Snyder,
1971, Essex and Snyder, 1973).

LEUKEMIA AND LYMPHOMA

Although conceptually valuable, it is not clear that an understanding of sarc genes and sarcoma viruses can be easily extrapolated
to an understanding of how RNA tumor viruses cause leukemias and
lymphomas, the tumors that occur most frequently in association
with these agents under natural conditions. At least two general
hypotheses can be considered. First, FeLV's and leukemia viruses
of other species that are truly leukemogenic might possess a leuk
gene analogous to the sarc gene. This virus population might be
replication defective, existing in the presence of an excess of
replication competent non-leukemogenic helper virus. Alternatively,
strains of FeLV that are "leukemia-competent" might also be replication competent. A second hypothesis might be that none of the
FeLV's contain a leuk gene as part of the virion RNA, but cause
leukemia by turning on such a "leuk" gene in lymphoid cells (e.g.,
by integrating the provirus next to such a gene and derepressing
it). With either model one might imagine that the leuk gene might
be related to the sarc gene as part of a family of tissue differentiation genes and thus the gene products might be serologically
related. Lymphoid cells and fibroblasts are both derived from
the same germ layer.

FELINE ONCORNAVIRUSES ASSOCIATED CELL MEMBRANE ANTIGEN (FOCMA)

FOCMA was initially described on the basis of an antibody
activity which occurred in cats inoculated with FeSV. Cats which
resisted the development and/or progression of fibrosarcomas developed high titers of antibody which reacted with the surface of FeLV-
producer lymphoma cells (Essex et al., 1971, Essex and Snyder,

1973). In subsequent studies FOCMA was shown to be the target
of an effective immunosurveillance response which occurred in cats
with both FeSV induced fibrosarcoma and FeLV induced leukemia and
lymphoma (see Essex et al., elsewhere in this volume).

Studies with FeSV transformed fibroblasts revealed that FOCMA
was expressed only on transformed cells, but expressed regardless
of whether or not the cells were replicating FeLV (Sliski et al.,
1977). See Table 1. Non-transformed fibroblasts that produced
FeLV did not express FOCMA, nor did the same fibroblasts when they
were transformed with murine sarcoma viruses.

Serologic analyses were undertaken to compare the titers of
antibody to FOCMA to the titers of antibody to the known virion
gene products. Cats exposed to FeLV were often discordant when
comparing antibody titers to FOCMA to antibody titers to any of
the gag gene products, p30, p15, p12, and p10 (Charman et al.,
1976; Essex et al., 1977a,b; Stephenson et al., 1977a,b). Discor-
dance was also seen between titers to FOCMA and titers to the major
env product gp70 or titers of virus neutralizing antibody, which
are directed to gp70 (Schaller et al., 1975; Stephenson et al.,
1977a). In the above cases for example, persistently viremic healthy
cats often had significant FOCMA antibody titers. Such cats however never had detectable free antibody to the virus structural
proteins, presumably because of adsorption that might occur by
the situation of antigen excess. Very recent studies indicated
that FeLV-exposed cats also have significant levels of antibody
to reverse transcriptase, the product of the pol gene, but that
some animals have anti-FOCMA in the absence of detectable antibodies
to reverse transcriptase (Jacquemin et al., 1978).

When FeSV is used to transform cells of non-feline origin,
the cells still express FOCMA (Sliski et al., 1977). This strongly
suggests that FOCMA is encoded by FeSV. Nonproducer (NP) mink
cells that have been transformed by FeSV also express FOCMA, in
amounts that appear equal to that expressed by the same cells superinfected with helper virus. These NP cells make no gp70, nor
p30, so we must obviously consider the possibility that FOCMA is
coded for by sarc, and functioning as a "transforming protein."
Some of the FeSV transformed NP mink cells make p15 and p12, in
addition to FOCMA. (Stephenson et al., 1977b).

When the FOCMA positive NP cells were examined for molecular
species containing the FOCMA activity, two classes of molecules
were found (Stephenson et al., 1977b). The first was in the size
range of 80,000 - 100,000 daltons (85K). In addition to FOCMA,
it contained the 5' terminal gag gene products p15 and p12. The
second species containing FOCMA activity was about 60,000 - 65,000
daltons (65K). Serologically the 65K species contained FOCMA activity but not FeLV p15 or p12. The same cells also contained free
p15 and p12, and a p25 precursor species which contained both p15

TABLE 1. CORRELATION BETWEEN EXPRESSION OF FOCMA, EXPRESSION OF VIRION ANTIGENS, AND TRANSFORMED PHENOTYPE IN CULTURE CELLS

Cell Culture	Description	Antigens Present			Virus Release	Transformed Phenotype
		FOCMA	FeLV gp70	FeLV p30		
F174, F422	Feline lymphoma origin	+	+	+	+	+a
CCC-81	Feline kidney, S+L− with MuSV	−	−	−	−	−
CCC-81 (FeLV)	Above infected with FeLV	−	+	+	+	+
F1f-3	Normal feline control	−	−	−	−	−
F1f-3 (FeLV)	Above infected with FeLV	−	+	+	+	−
F1f-3 (FeSV)	Above infected with FeSV	+	+	+	+	+
CCL64	Normal mink control	−	−	−	−	−
CCL64 (FeLV)	Above infected with FeLV	−	+	+	+	−
64 F3 C17	FeSV infected cloned nonproducer CCL64	+	−	−	−	+
64 F3 (FeLV)	Above infected with FeLV	+	+	+	+	+
64 J1	CCL 64 transformed with murine sarcoma virus	−	−	−	−	+

aLymphoblastoid lines grown in suspension; all others are adherent monolayer lines unless of transformed phenotype.

and p12. None of the latter molecules contained FOCMA activity.
By pulse chase experiments the 85K species was observed to become
the 65K, p15, and p12 entities.

The 85K species, containing FOCMA, p15 and p12, was also present in transforming FeSV particles that were rescued by superin-
fecting the NP cells with a poorly replicating helper virus (e.g.,
the xenotropic mouse or baboon viruses) (Sherr et al., 1978).
When good ratios of transforming viruses were present in the resulting rescued virus, the particles contained only FOCMA, p15 and
p12 as proteins related to FeSV. All p30, p10, and gp70 found
in the virions was due to the helper virus. FOCMA was not present
in those FeLV helper viruses checked.

FOCMA IN LYMPHOID TUMOR CELLS

As opposed to the FeSV transformed NP mink cells, which contain
p15 and p12, biopsied NP lymphoid tumor cells from FeLV negative
cats contain none of the FeLV structural proteins. Such cells
are still FOCMA positive, even when lacking at least part of the
FeLV DNA provirus sequences (Hardy et al., 1977; Essex et al.,
1978b). (Table 2). FeLV producing normal lymphoid cells do not
express FOCMA, but malignant lymphoid tumor cells express this
antigen regardless of whether they are of T or B origin, or in
thymic, lymph node, bone marrow, or other tissues. If cats are
inoculated with a strain of highly leukemogenic FeLV which produces
thymic lymphomas, FOCMA containing lymphoid tumor cells appear
first in the thymus, and only start to appear at 12-16 weeks, just
before the clinical signs of lymphoma become apparent (Essex et
al., 1978a) (Table 3). Conversely, lymphoid cells containing
gag and env products p30 and gp70 were detected at the earliest
time checked, at four weeks after inoculation with FeLV. Furthermore, the virion structural proteins were expressed in equal amounts
in normal lymphoid cells that occurred in sites distant from the
tumor target tissue (Essex et al., 1978a,b).

Thus, regardless of whether or not FOCMA is encoded by leukemogenic FeLV, or turned on in the cell by FeLV transformation, the
FeLV associated FOCMA is serologically related to the FeSV associated FOCMA. Whether leukemic cell FOCMA is FeLV coded or induced
could be answered by two approaches. First, FeLV induced lymphomas
could be induced in non-feline species and analyzed for FOCMA expression. Secondly, lymphomas could be induced in cats with irradiation
or chemicals, and subsequently analyzed for FOCMA expression.

Aside from the expression of FOCMA, at least one other observation suggests an association between FeLV and VN leukemias: such
tumors often cluster along with FeLV positive leukemias in FeLV
exposure environments. (Hardy, Francis, and Essex, unpublished
observations.)

TABLE 2. EXPRESSION OF FOCMA AND FeLV PROTEINS ON FRESHLY BIOPSIED LYMPHOID CELLS FROM CATS WITH NATURAL EXPOSURE TO FeLV.

Category	Presence of FeLV	Presence of FOCMA on Cells from:		FeLV gp70 and p30
		Tumor	Normal[a] Tissues	
Lymphoma	+	51/51[b]	0/18	+
Lymphoma	–	16/16	0/6	–
Leukemia	+	6/6	0/3	+
Healthy	+		0/29	+
Healthy	–		0/31	
T cell lymphoma		27/27		
B cell lymphoma		6/6		
Thymic lymphoma		18/18		
Multicentric lymphoma		20/20		
Alimentary lymphoma		7/7		

[a]Buffy coat, spleen, mesenteric lymph node, bone marrow and/or thymus mononuclear (primarily lymphoid) cells from tissues judged normal at time of histopathology.

[b]Number of positive over number tested. To be judged positive, at least 40% of mononuclear cells in lymphoid cell suspension reacted with FOCMA antiserum. Tissues judged malignant at time of histopathology.

TABLE 3. EXPRESSION OF FOCMA AND FeLV PROTEINS ON FRESHLY BIOPSIED LYMPHOID CELLS FROM CATS INOCULATED WITH FeLV

Time after inoculation (weeks)	Disease Status	Nonthymic lymphoid cells[a]			Thymic lymphoid cells		
		FeLV (infectious centers)	Presence of FOCMA	Membrane FeLV gp70 and p30	FeLV (infectious centers)	Presence of FOCMA	Membrane FeLV gp70 and p30
4	normal	4/4[b]	0/4	4/4	4/4	0/4	4/4
8	normal	4/4	0/3	3/3	3/3	0/3	3/3
12	normal	2/3	0/3	3/3	2/3	1/3	3/3
16	normal	1/1	0/1	1/1	1/1	1/1	1/1
16	leukemic	2/2	0/2	2/2	2/2	2/2	2/2
20-24	leukemic	6/6	2/6	6/6	6/6	6/6	6/6

[a]Cells from bone marrow, spleen, mesentric lymph nodes, and buffy coat were tested from each cat. All cells from different organs of the same animal (other than thymus) gave the same result. The only exception was the presence of a significant population of FOCMA positive cells in the spleens of 2 of 6 leukemic animals even though less than 10% of the cells in the bone marrow, buffy coat, or mesentric lymph nodes of the same animals were FOCMA positive.

[b]Number positive over number tested.

CONCLUSIONS AND SPECULATION

In the case of both lymphoid and fibroblastoid tumors caused by feline RNA tumor viruses, common tumor specific protein antigens are expressed. Learning about how these antigens function in relation to specific mechanisms of transformation will presumably tell us how cells become malignant. This seems to be of particular importance in the case of the lymphoid tumor cells because (a) such tumors are the class most frequently associated with viruses, including RNA tumor viruses, under natural conditions, and (b) such tumors are often at least partially negative for the FeLV DNA provirus. Accordingly, if the FOCMA in VN lymphoid tumors is actually encoded by FeLV, we would have to assume that the FOCMA gene must be selectively retained. One hypothesis that we have proposed to explain how in vivo selection pressure could enhance the development of VN tumors involves the FeLV gp70-directed immune response (see Essex et al. elsewhere in this volume). The central question of whether or not tumor virus associated transforming protein genes can be introduced and maintained in the absence of sequences that code for viral structural proteins is not unique to oncornaviruses. In the case of cancer of the human uterine cervix, for example, an attractive seroepidemiologic association has been observed between exposure to Herpes simplex type II and disease development. Yet, nucleic acid hybridization experiments failed to reveal significant levels of virus-specific DNA in the tumor cells (Rawls and Adam, 1977). Further studies on the identity of the limited sequences of FeLV related gene(s) in VN feline lymphoma cells may help to resolve this general issue.

That FeSV codes for a FOCMA containing protein which is covalently linked to p15 and p12 might seem hard to rationalize along with the general assumption that sarc is positioned at the 3' end of the virion RNA. This has only been clearly established in the rare case of those avian sarcoma viruses that are competent for both replication and transformation. In the case of the replication defective mammalian sarcoma viruses the sarc gene must be defined primarily on the basis of operational functions rather than topographical position. Defective DNA proviruses might lack all but the 5' end of gag and sarc, due to some earlier recombinational event. If so, representative straightforward transcription of mRNA would code for the observed 85K protein. Alternatively, a more complete representation may be present in the provirus, with such mechanisms as gene splicing or "read-through" accounting for translation products that are subsequently observed. Answers to these questions seem within reach, and could be approached, for example, by fingerprinting both the virion and cellular mRNA species, and hybridization using selected restricted fragments of RNA or cDNA. Such results could be coordinated with protein studies to compare virion and FOCMA-cellular peptides obtained

by tryptic and chymotryptic peptide mapping and/or in vitro translation.

In conclusion, it seems too early to rule out the possibility
that viruses, including RNA tumor viruses, might funciton as etiologic agents in some cases of human leukemia and/or lymphoma.
Our existing knowledge should be adequate cause for optimism and
sufficient rationale for perseverance.

SUMMARY

FeLV and FeSV are typical RNA tumor viruses. They cause lymphomas, leukemias, and fibrosarcomas under both natural and manipu-
lated laboratory conditions. FOCMA is a transformation specific
antigen that is expressed on both FeSV-transformed cells and tumorous
lymphoid cells. The antigen is FeSV coded, expressed on transformed
NP cells, and distinct from the known gag, pol, and env gene products. Serologically indistinguishable FOCMA is also present on
lymphoid tumor cells that make none of the FeLV structural proteins.
Since this antigen is tumor specific for both FeLV and FeSV NP
cells the FOCMA model may be valuable for studying mechanisms of
leukemogenesis and transformation. Since FOCMA positive NP lymphoma cells lack complete copies of the DNA provirus, the feline
model may be uniquely appropriate in our pursuit toward understanding "virus negative" leukemia of man.

ACKNOWLEDGEMENTS

Work done in the laboratories of the authors was supported
by National Cancer Insitute grants CA-13885, CA-18216, CA-16599,
CA-18488, and CA-08748, contract CB-64001 from the National Cancer
Institute, grant DT-32 from the American Cancer Society, and a
grant from the Cancer Research Institute. W. D. Hardy, Jr. is
a Scholar of the Leukemia Society of America.

REFERENCES

Charman, H.P., Kim, N., Gilden, R.V., Hardy, W.D., Jr., and Essex,
     M., Humoral immune responses of cats to feline leukemia virus:
     Comparison of responses to the major specific cell membrane anti-
     gen (FOCMA), J. Natl. Cancer Inst. 56:859.

Essex, M., 1975a, Horizontally and vertically transmitted oncorna-
     viruses of cats, Advan. Cancer Res. 21:175.

Essex, M., 1975b, Tumors induced by oncornaviruses in cats,
     Pathobiol. Ann. 5:169.

Essex, M., and Snyder, S.P., 1973, Feline oncornavirus associated
    cell membrane antigen. I. Serological studies with kittens
    exposed to cell-free materials from various feline fibrosarcomas,
    J. Natl. Cancer Inst. 51:1007.

Essex, M., Klein, G., Snyder, S.P. and Harrold, J.B., 1971, Feline
    sarcoma virus (FSV) induced tumors: Correlations between humoral
    antibody and tumor regression, Nature 233:195.

Essex, M., Jakowski, R.M., Hardy, W.D., Jr., Cotter, S.M., Hess, P.,
    and Sliski, A., 1975a, Feline oncornavirus associated cell mem-
    brane antigen. III. Antibody titers in cats from leukemia cluster
    household, J. Natl. Cancer Inst. 54:637.

Essex, M., Cotter, S.M., Hardy, W.D., Jr., Hess, P., Jarrett, W.,
    Jarrett, O., Mackey, L., Laird, H., Perryman, L., Olsen, R.G.,
    and Yohn, D.S., 1975b, Feline oncornavirus associated cell mem-
    brane antigen. IV. Antibody titers in cats with naturally occur-
    ring leukemia, lymphoma and other diseases, J. Natl. Cancer Inst.
    55:463.

Essex, M., Cotter, S.M., Sliski, A.H., Hardy, W.D., Jr., Stephenson,
    J.R., Aaronson, S.A., and Jarrett, O., 1977a, Horizontal trans-
    mission of feline leukemia virus under natural conditions in a
    feline leukemia cluster household, Int. J. Cancer 19:90.

Essex, M., Stephenson, J.R., Hardy, W.D., Jr., Cotter, S.M., and
    Aaronson, A.S., 1977b, Leukemia, lymphoma, and fibrosarcoma of
    cats as models for similar diseases of man, Cold Spring Harbor
    Proc. on Cell Proliferation 4:1197.

Essex, M., Hoover, E.A., and Hardy, W.D., Jr., 1978a, manuscript
    in preparation.

Essex, M., Sliski, A.H., Hardy, W.D., Jr., Cotter, S.M., and
    Noronha, F. de, 1978b, Feline oncornavirus associated cell mem-
    brane antigen: Specificity for transformation or tumor induction,
    in Comparative Leukemia Research, in press.

Essex, M., Sliski, A.H., and Hardy, W.D., Jr., FOCMA: A transfor-
    mation specific RNA sarcoma virus encoded protein, this volume.

Gallo, R.C., and Gillespie, D.H., 1977, The origin of RNA tumor
    viruses and their relation to human leukemia, in: The Year in
    Hematology (R.D.Silber, A.S. Gordon, and J. LoBue, eds.), p. 305,
    Plenum Press, New York.

Hardy, W.D., Jr., Old, L.J., Hess, P.W., Essex, M., and Cotter,
    S.M., 1973, Horizontal transmission of feline leukemia virus in
    cats, Nature 244:266.

Hardy, W.D., Jr., Zuckerman, E.E., MacEwen, E.G., Hayes, A.A., and Essex, M., 1977, A feline leukemia virus- and sarcoma virus-induced tumor-specific antigen, Nature 270:249.

Henderson, I.C., Lieber, M.M., and Todaro, G., 1974, Mink cell line MvlLu (CCL-64): Focus-formation and the generation of "nonproducer" transformed cell lines with murine and feline sarcoma viruses, Virology 60:282.

Jacquemin, P., Saxinger, C., Gallo, R.C., Hardy, W.D., Jr., and Essex, M., 1978, An immune response in serum of cats to feline leukemia virus reverse transcriptase, submitted for publication.

Jarrett, W., Jarrett, O., Mackey, L., Laird, H.M., Hardy, W.D., Jr., and Essex, M., 1973, Horizontal transmission of leukemia virus and leukemia in the cat, J. Natl. Cancer Inst. 51:833.

Koshy, R., Wong-Staal, F., Hardy, W.D., Jr., Gallagher, R., Essex, M. and Gallo, R.C., 1978, manuscript in preparation.

Khan, A.S., and Stephenson, J.R., 1977, Feline leukemia virus: Biochemical and immunological characterization of gag gene-coded structural proteins, J. Virol. 23:599.

Kurth, R., Fenyo, E.M., Klein, E., and Essex, M., 1978, Tumor cell surface antigens induced by RNA tumor viruses, Nature, in press.

Levin, R., Ruscetti, S.K., Parks, W.P., and Scolnick, E.M., 1976, Expression of feline type C virus in normal and tumor tissues of the domestic cat, Int. J. Cancer 18:661.

Rawls, W.E., and Adam, E., 1977, Herpes simplex viruses and human malignancies, Cold Spring Harbor Conf. on Cell Prolif. 4:1133.

Schaller, J., Essex, M., Olsen, R.G., and Yohn, D.S., 1975, Feline oncornavirus-associated cell membrane antigen. V. Humoral immune response to virus and cell membrane antigens in cats inoculated with Gardner-Arnstein feline sarcoma virus, J. Natl. Cancer Inst. 55:1373.

Sherr, C.J., Sen, A., Todaro, G.J., Sliski, A., and Essex, M., 1978, Pseudotypes of feline sarcoma virus contain an 85,000 dalton protein with feline oncornavirus-associated cell membrane antigen (FOCMA) activity, Proc. Natl. Acad. Sci. 75, in press.

Sliski, A.H., Essex, M., Meyer, C., and Todaro, G., 1977, Feline oncornavirus-associated cell membrane antigen: Expression in transformed non-producer mink cells, Science 196:1336.

Snyder, S.P., 1971, Spontaneous feline fibrosarcomas: transmissibility and ultrastructure of associated virus-like particles,
J. Natl. Cancer Inst., 47:1079.

Stephenson, J.R., Essex, M., Hino, S., Aaronson, S.A., and Hardy,
W.D., Jr., 1977a, Feline oncornavirus-associated cell-membrane
antigen (FOCMA): Distinction between FOCMA and the major virion
glycoprotein, Proc. Natl. Acad. Sci. 74:1219.

Stephenson, J.R., Khan, A.S., Sliski, A.H., and Essex, M., 1977b,
Feline oncornavirus-associated cell membrane antigen (FOCMA):
Identification of an immunologically cross-reactive feline
sarcoma virus-coded protein, Proc. Natl. Acad. Sci. 74:5608.

Stephenson, J.R., Devare, S.G., and Reynolds, F.H., 1978, Translational products of Type C RNA tumor viruses, Advan. Cancer
Res., in press.

EXPERIMENTS WITH A TYPE C VIRUS FROM A HUMAN CELL STRAIN (HEL-12)

S. Panem, E. V. Prochownik and W. H. Kirsten

Departments of Pathology and Pediatrics, The University of Chicago
Chicago, Illinois 60637

This overview is concerned with HEL-12 virus and its possible relationship to human diseases.

In 1975, we observed the release of a type C virus from cultures of the human embryonic lung cells (HEL-12) which had been propagated for 4-6 months (1). The HEL-12 virus has the typical morphology and buoyant density of retroviruses, contains 70S RNA, and its RNA-dependent DNA polymerase utilizes both polyadenylate-oligodeoxythimidylate as well as virion RNA as templates. As determined by indirect cytoplasmic immunofluorescence and double immunodiffusion tests, the HEL-12 virus is antigenically related to simian sarcoma virus (SiSV) and baboon endogenous virus (BaEV), but not to feline or mouse leukemia viruses, or Rous sarcoma virus. Furthermore, the reverse transcriptase of the HEL-12 virus is markedly and specifically inhibited by antiserum to the respective enzymes of gibbon ape lymphosarcoma virus suggesting a relatedness to antigens of certain subhuman primate-tye C viruses.

Subsequent to the chance observation of spontaneous virus release from HEL-12 cells, we have used several frozen seed stocks of this diploid human fibroblast strain to confirm the original observations. Virus release has been consistently observed from over 15 separate cultures established from frozen HEL-12 cells. The experimental details and results are summarized elsewhere (2,3). The salient features of these experiments are as follows. Expression of cytoplasmic antigens and production of HEL-12 cells are not demonstrated during the initial 20-30 days after HEL-12 cells are grown from frozen seed stocks. However, such early passage cells contain DNA sequences which hybridize with ^{125}I-HEL-12 viral RNA (4), indicating that early-passage cultures contain the proviral

139

genome prior to the expression of type-C viral antigens or spontaneous virus release. The early passages are followed by an antigen-positive interval which extends from approximately 30-80 days of in-vitro growth. Cytoplasmic antigens cross-reactive with an antiserum to SiSV are detected first, followed by the expression of antigens related to the RD-114/CCC group of type C viruses in an increasing number of HEL-12 cells. Extracellular HEL-12 virus cannot be demonstrated during this intermediate interval. Between 80-120 days of continuous in-vitro propagation extracellular virus is easily recovered from the culture fluids and cytoplasmic immunofluorescence against type-C viral antigens is maximal. Following 120 days, virus production ceases, and only cytoplasmic antigens can be detected before the HEL-12 cells become senescent and die (2, 3). As expected, late-passage HEL-12 cells contain DNA sequences homologous to HEL-12 viral RNA (4). The HEL-12 virus productively infects lines of human, rhesus monkey, dog and rabbit cells (3). The infectivity experiments have revealed two antigenically distinct virion components by the use of antisera to SiSV and the RD-114/CCC virus group. The two major antigenic components in the HEL-12 virus population have not been analyzed in detail. The temporal restriction of spontaneous antigen expression and virus release in HEL-12 cell cultures was confirmed by studying clones of HEL-12 cells derived from single cells (5). Five of seven cell clones expressed antigens and released HEL-12 virus in a temporal sequence similar to mass cultures.

Additional evidence for the presence of HEL-12 viral sequences in early passage cultures has been obtained by growing cells in medium containing the glucose analog 2-deoxy-D-glucose and the halogenated pyrimidine iododeoxyuridine (2, 6, 7). Several series of experiments have shown that HEL-12 cells are inducible to release a type C virus during 20-80 days of in-vitro growth, whereas the inducing agents did not enhance yield during the spontaneous, virus production interval (Prochownik et al; unpublished).

A relationship between human diseases and HEL-12 virus or subhuman primate type C viruses is suggested by several lines of evidence: First, nucleic acid sequences homologous to the RNAs of SiSV were detected in the spleen (but not the liver or the primary tumor) of a boy who died from osteogenic sarcoma (4). Homologous DNA sequences were also found in the spleen of a patient with myelogenous leukemia, whereas several other patients with this disease, acute lymphatic leukemia or nasopharyngeal carcinoma were negative. Second, from the plasma of two patients with myeloid leukemia was isolated an antibody (IgG) which inhibited the uptake of radioactive precursor by the purified reverse transcriptases of SiSV, HEL-12 virus and BaEV, but no significant inhibition of the reverse transcriptases of Rous sarcoma virus or Gross leukemia virus was noted (8). These findings have recently been extended and confirmed in a larger number of patients with leukemias or lymphomas. Third, a relationship between HEL-12 virus and a human disease has come from recent observations on the nature of immune complex deposition in patients with systemic lupus erythematosus (9). Over 30 biopsies from lupus kidneys contained antigens which reacted with HEL-12 virus antiserum by indirect immunofluorescence. The intensity of immunofluorescence with several HEL-12 virus antisera correlated with the extend of immune complex deposition, whereas renal biopsies from patients with diseases other than lupus nephropathy or normal tissues did not react with the anti-HEL-12 virus serum. An antibody eluted from one kidney with lupus nephropathy also reacted with human or dog cells infected with HEL-12 virus, but not with uninfected control cells. Immunofluorescence in samples of immune complex nephropathies was not demonstrated with several other viruses, except the BK virus (Panem et al., unpublished). The evidence for an involvement of HEL-12 virus in the immune complex deposits of systemic lupus is not confined to the kidneys. Lupus lesions of the heart, lung, spleen, eye and skin also reacted with the HEL-12 virus antiserum, suggesting that viral antigens related to HEL-12 virus are contained in most, if not all immune complex deposits of systemic lupus erythematosus.

HEL-12 virus, despite its uncertain origin, has proven a useful tool to study some aspects of the pathogenesis of diseases of man. Only further work will show whether this and related viruses are involved in the causation of these diseases.

Acknowledgements

This work was supported by USPHS Grants No. CA 14898 and CA 14599 from the National Cancer Institute

References

1. Panem, S., Prochownik, E. V., Reale, F. R. and Kirsten, W.H. Isolation of type C virions from a normal human fibroblast strain. Science 189:297-298, 1975.

2. Panem, S., Prochownik, E.V. and Kirsten, W.H. Kinetics of type C virion release from a human diploid fibroblast strain. In Comparative Leukemia Research, Biblio. Haematology. 43:572-573, 1976.

3. Panem, S., Prochownik, E.V., Knish, W.M. and Kirsten, W.H. Cell generation and type C virus expression in the human embryonic cell strain HEL-12. J. Gen. Virol. 35:487-495, 1977.

4. Prochownik, E.V. and Kirsten, W.H. Nucleic acid sequences of primate type C viruses in normal and neoplastic human tissues. Nature 267:175-177, 1977.

5. Panem, S., Spontaneous Type C virus expression in human embryonic lung cells (HEL-12): comparison of cloned and mixed population. In Animal Virology, pp 409-417. Edited by D. Baltimore, A. Huang and C. F. Fox. New York: Academic Press.

6. Lowy, D.R., Rowe, W.P., Teich, N.M. and Hartley, J.W. Murine leukemia virus: High frequency activation in vitro by 5-iodo-deoxyuridine. Science 174:155-156, 1971.

7. Prochownik, E.V., Panem, S. and Kirsten, W.H. Induction of type C virions from normal rat kidney cells by 2-deoxy-D-glucose. J. Virology 17:219-226, 1976.

8. Prochownik, E.V. and Kirsten, W.H. Inhibition of reverse transcriptase of primate Type C viruses by 7S immunoglobulin from patients with leukaemia Nature 260:64-67, 1976.

9. Panem, S., Ordonez, N.G., Kirsten, W.H., Katz, A. I. and Spargo, B.H. C-type virus expression in systemic lupus erythematosus. N. Eng. J. Med. 295:470-475, 1976.

10. Ordonez, N.G., Panem, S.., Aronson, A., Dalton, H., Katz, A.I., Spargo, B.H. and Kirsten, W.H. Viral immune complexes in systemic lupus erythematosus. Virch. Arch. B. Cell Path. 25: 355-366, 1977.

ON THE POSSIBLE VIRAL ETIOLOGY OF CHILDHOOD LEUKEMIA

Peter Bentvelzen

Radiobiological Institute of the Organization for Health
Research TNO
151 Lange Kleiweg, 2288   GJ   RIJSWIJK, The Netherlands.

Cancer is usually a disease associated with aging. Childhood
neoplasia therefore presents to the oncologist a bizarre but highly interesting phenomenon. Like in some animal models (1-3) a
genetic propensity to the early development of specific forms of
cancer might be assumed. Several well-defined gene-mutations are
known in man, which are associated with an increased risk of
cancer at a young age, in particular leukemias and lymphomas (4).
Some of these mutations are also linked with chromosomal
instability like in the case of Fanconi and Bloom's syndromes (5).
Possibly, such a condition of chromosomal instability enhances the
chance for that somatic mutation, which underlies the neoplastic
alteration of a cell.
Several hereditary immunodeficiencies like Bruton's agamma-
globulinemia, the Wiskott-Aldrich syndrome or ataxia teleangiectasia show a very highly increased incidence of leukemias and
lymphomas (6), a situation similar to that of immunosuppressed
renal transplant patients. Quite remarkably is the low incidence
of bone tumors or nephroblastomas in children with a inherited
immunodeficiency. Probably immunosurveillance only strongly
operates in the case of hematological malignancies.
Although several gene-mutations are responsible for an
increased risk of leukemia or lymphoma, the heretability of these
neoplasms is generally low. The concordance rate of leukemia in
monozygotic twins is only 25 %. Most of the cases, in which both
twins are afflicted, occur in the first year of life, while the
peak of childhood leukemia is between 3 and 5 years of age. It is
a reasonable assumption, that the cases of concordance are due to
vascular anastomosis during fetal life. Malignant transformed
hemopoietic cells would then be transferred from one fetus to the
other (7).

Viral aspects of human leukemia
    Spontaneous tumors, which arise at a young age in animals,
usually have a viral etiology. This certainly holds for leukemias
and lymphomas (8). However, research on a possible viral etiology
of human leukemia has been mostly performed on the disease in
adults. The highlight of these investigations is certainly the
repeated isolation of type-C oncoviruses from an aged patient with
acute myelogenous leukemia (9-11). The emphasis on the disease in
adults is probably due to the higher incidence and the better
availability of clinical specimens, such as bone marrow,
peripheral blood cells and spleens.
    In Spiegelman's laboratory highly elegant molecular biological
studies have been performed on monozygous twins, which were dis-
concordant with regard to leukemia. In the leukemic cells, so-
called biochemical particles are found which have many properties
in common with RNA tumor viruses, like high-molecular weight RNA
and the enzyme reverse transcriptase. In an endogenous reaction a
DNA copy is prepared of the particle-associated RNA. This probe is
then "absorbed" for sequences, which might also occur in normal
human DNA, by hybridizing with DNA isolated from normal
lymphocytes of the unafflicted twin. The recycled probe did not
hybridize with normal human cellular DNA but still gave a significant reaction with DNA from leukemic cells. These data indicate
the acquisition of new sequences in the DNA of the leukemic child,
most likely due to an infectious virus (12).

Cocultivation studies with the rat tumor XC cell line
    In our laboratory, Dr. Kees Nooter initiated a study on the
isolation of type-C oncoviruses from bone marrow cells of leukemic
children by cocultivation with animal indicator cells. First were
used the rat cell line XC, derived from a tumor induced by the
avian Rous sarcoma virus. This cell line produces syncytia after
having been in contact with cells producing murine or primate
type-C viruses. Bone marrow cells from one leukemic child produced
a few typical type-C particles after in vitro stimulation with PHA
(13). Cocultivation of the patient's leukemic cells with the XC
cell line yielded a very large number of syncytia. This co-culture
produced initially large quantities of type-C oncovirus on the
basis of reverse transcriptase and syncytia-assay, but upon
further passage this gradually declined (Table I). By means of
immunofluorescence a relationship of the isolate with the simian
sarcoma virus-gibbon ape leukemia virus group was established, as
far as the major internal protein p30 is concerned (13). However,
also a weak reaction was noticed with antisera to p30 of the
feline endogenous virus RD114 (14). It is an attractive hypothesis
that this reaction is due to the presence of a virus related to
the baboon endogenous virus, which is also present in other human-
derived type-C oncovirus isolates (15-17).
    The virus propagated in XC cells could be transferred to human
embryonic kidney cells. It could be reisolated from the same child

Table I

SYNCYTIA ASSAY IN XC CELLS OF A TYPE–C ONCOVIRUS DERIVED FROM A
LEUKEMIC CHILD

Donor cells	No. of syncytia per dish	Electron microscopy (type-C particles
None	17*	–
Normal human bone marrow	10*	–
Leukemic bone marrow	393	+
2nd passage cocultivation with XC	520	+
3rd passage cocultivation with XC	465	+
4th passage cocultivation with XC	606	+
12th passage cocultivation with XC	13*	–
Human embryonic kidney cells (HEK)	14*	–
HEK + irradiated infected XC cells	352	+
HEK + irradiated control XC cells	18*	–
Human embryonic fibroblast line FB 289	9*	–
FB 289 + supernatant infected XC	120	+
FB 289 cocultivated with peripheral blood cells	53	+

*only small syncytia with less than four nuclei.

by cocultivation of its peripheral white blood cells with human
embryonic fibroblasts. In both cases virus production was low, as
determined by reverse transcriptase assay. Unfortunately, both
human cell lines with the human–derived virus were lost due to an
accident. Since the XC line ceased to produce the human derived
virus (18), this human isolate is not available any longer.

Cocultivation of XC cells with bone marrow cells from two other
leukemic children did not yield any positive results, not did the
combination of XC cells with bone marrow samples from 4 normal
donors, 2 patients with acute myelogenous leukemia, 2 with chronic
myelogenous leukemia, 1 with chronic lymphatic leukemia, 1 with
aplasia and 1 with secondary polycythemia vera.

The use of the XC cell line was abandoned because it produced
low levels of endogenous type–C oncovirus. The rat endogenous type-
C viruses show some relationship with primate viruses, and therefore complicate these studies.

History of the SKA21–3 cell line and its virus
The XC cell line was substituted by the canine cell line A7573,
which was known to be permissive to the so–called HL–23V isolate
(10), obtained by Gallagher and Gallo from an old patient with
acute myelogenous leukemia (9). Cocultivation of two bone marrow

samples from leukemic children with this cell line resulted in
transient production of a retrovirus as determined by reverse
transcriptase assay. The cocultures from which the human cells had
disappeared were then mixed with the K-NRK cell line (19), which is
a rat cell line, non-productively transformed by Kirsten murine
sarcoma virus (Ki-MuSV). This resulted in the release of a transforming entity, which could morphologically alter rat embryonic
fibroblasts, human kidney cells and the rabbit cornea cell line
SIRC, but not any mouse cell (20). The transforming activity of
these pseudotypes of K-MuSV and human-derived helper viruses could
be neutralized by an antiserum to the simian sarcoma virus (SiSV),
kindly provided by Doctors C. Bergholz and F. Deinhardt. The
antiserum mainly reacts with the envelope proteins of this primate
virus.

From bone marrow cells of two leukemic children such a helper
virus to the replication-defective Ki-MuSV could be isolated.
Despite repeated attempts, such a virus could not be obtained from
normal human bone marrow cells (20).

Several of the foci of transformed cells were cloned. Some
clones proved to produce rapidly growing tumors after subcutaneous
inoculation into nude mice. One of these clones (SKA 21-3; for its
derivation see fig. 1) unexpectedly started to produce large
quantities of virus as determined by reverse transcriptase assay.
Inoculation of SKA cells (21) or cell-free supernatants (22) into
newborn rats and rabbits resulted in the rapid development of
generalized sarcomatous lesions in many organs like brain, liver
and thymus. Inoculated mice remained disease-free during a one-
year observation period. This negative finding corresponds with
the observed refreactoriness of mouse cells in vitro to SKA 21-3.

By cocultivation of a rat lymph node infiltrated by typical
sarcoma cells induced by SKA 21-3, with A7573, a virus was
isolated with exactly the same properties as SKA 21-3 (23).

The Ki-MuSV transforming principle was eliminated from SKA
21-3 by endpoint dilution. The infected A204 cell line produced a
type-C virus, which was able to produce syncytia in the XC cell
line but unable to produce foci of transformed cells in a variety
of cell lines (21). Inoculation of this virus into newborn rats
resulted into the development of leukemia, predominantly lymphatic
ones, but not into the appearance of sarcomatous lesions (21, 24).
The oncogenic activity of the Ki-MuSV-free virus preparation,
which is assumed to contain "pure" human-derived type-C oncovirus,
might be due to the bestowment of the "innocuous" human virus with
a lymphatic leukemia gene from Ki-MuSV by genetic recombination.
This seems to be a remote possibility, as no indications have been
obtained for the presence in Ki-MuSV of a gene causing lymphoblastic leukemia (21, 22).

From the leukemias induced by this Ki-MuSV-free virus preparation a virus could be obtained by cocultivation of a tumorous
lymph node with A7573. This virus had no transforming activity in
vitro but could induce syncytia in the XC cell line. The Sepharose

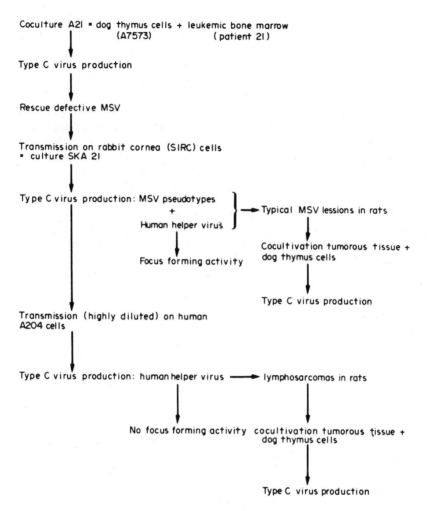

Fig. 1.   *Scheme of isolation procedure and subsequent passages of a human tissue-derived C-type oncornavirus.*

bead immunofluorescence assay, as developed in our laboratory (25), revealed that the viruses isolated from lymph nodes infiltrated by either sarcomatous or leukemic cells, contained an internal antigen closely related to the p30 of the simian sarcoma virus-gibbon ape leukemia virus group (23). Both SKA 21-3 and the derived virus-stock, free of Kirsten murine sarcoma virus, have been analyzed in the laboratory of Dr. R.C. Gallo, National Cancer Institute, Bethesda, Md., USA. By means of competitive radioimmunoassay it was found that p30 and p12 of both SiSV and baboon endogenous virus could be found in the cytoplasm of either cell line producing these viruses. Also competitive molecular hybridization revealed the presence of RNA molecules, with a great degree of homology to either primate virus in these cell lines.

Immunofluorescence studies on co-cultures of A7573 and human bone
marrow cells

In our laboratory experience was obtained in the detection of
primate virus-related antigens in cultures of human mesenchymal
tumors by means of fixed-cell immunofluorescence (26). Cocultures
of bone marrow cells from a variety of human donors and the A7573
line were screened at the 8th - 10th passage for the presence of
virus-related antigens by rabbit antisera raised against the p30
of Rauscher murine leukemia virus of simian sarcoma virus. As we
have repeatedly found, using the Sepharose bead immunofluorescence assay (25), all rabbit sera raised against purified viral
proteins have a high reactivity with fetal calf serum. After
absorption with this material, the antisera specifically reacted
with only virus-producing cell lines but not uninfected control
cells (27). For instance, the antisera did not react with A7573,
SIRC, BALB/3T3 and rat embryonic fibroblasts nor with several
human cell lines like R970 and A204 and skin fibroblast lines
derived from seven individuals. As far as the virus infected cell
lines are concerned, antisera usually gave in homologous systems a
titer (endpoint dilution) of 1 : 320, while in the heterologous
systems the titer was only 1 : 40. In each experimental series as
controls were used normal rabbit serum absorbed with fetal calf
serum, and cells incubated with only phosphate buffered saline in
order to estimate the autofluorescence background. As the indirect
immunofluorescence technique was used, an additional control was
incubation with only fluorescein-conjugated goat antiserum to
rabbit immunoflobulins.

Only results of those cocultures, which have been subjected to
the same protocol, are presented in Table II. Results obtained
with other indicator cells than A7573 or screening at later
passages than 8 to 11, have been omitted.

In the cocultures of A7573 and human bone marrow cells with
A7573, a positive reaction was never obtained with the antisera to
the p30 of the murine virus. In several instances, a weak but
clearly positive reaction (titers 1 : 40 or 1 : 80) was found with
the antiserum to the p30 of the simian sarcoma virus (Table II).
Only one adult, scored positive in this test. It might be accidental that this positive case was leukemic. Of the 7 positive
children, 5 were found in the group of leukemic patients. There
seems to be a clearly positive association between the presence of
an antigen, related to the p30 of simian sarcoma virus, and childhood leukemia. In view of the employed technique, the detection of
this antigens at the 8th passage or later indicates the transfer
of a principle, related in some way to the simian sarcoma virus,
from the leukemic bone marrow cells to A7573.

General considerations

The repeated isolation of type-C oncovirus, related to the
simian sarcoma virus-gibbon ape leukemia virus group, from hemopo-

Table II

DETECTION OF AN ANTIGEN RELATED TO P30 OF SIMIAN SARCOMA VIRUS BY
MEANS OF FIXED-CELL IMMUNOFLUORESCENCE IN COCULTURES OF HUMAN BONE
MARROW CELLS AND THE CANINE THYMUS CELL LINE A7573

Bone marrow donors	No. of donors	No. of patients for viral antigens
Adults:		
normal subjects	4	0
patients with no hematological malignancies	7	0
patients with lymphoma	1	0
leukemic patients	9	1
Children:		
normal subjects	5	1
patients with aplastic anemia	2	0
patients with lymphoma	2	1
leukemic patients	9	5

ietic cells of leukemic children; as well as the prevalence of
antigens, related to the p30 of this virus group, in cocultures of
bone marrow cells from leukemic children and A7573 in contrast to
the results obtained with cocultures of bone marrow samples from
other groups of donors, suggest this virus to be etiologically
involved in childhood leukemia. The leukemogenicity of the SKA
21-3 isolate, when free of Ki-MuSV, supports this idea.

The presence of a virus, related to the baboon endogenous
virus in SKA 21-3, and possibly also in our first isolate, cannot
be mere coincidence as it has also been found in other isolates
from human material (15-17). Its possible role in leukemogenesis
in man remains completely unclear to me, however.

So far, most laboratories have been unsuccessful in detecting
footprints of SiSV in human leukemia. It might be rewarding to
look for such footprints in specimens from leukemic children.

Epidemiological data do not provide convincing evidence for
the infectious nature of childhood leukemia. Rarely, does one find
families with more than one afflicted child. The few reported
cases of clustering can be regarded on a statistical basis as just
accidental. The apparent conflict between the virological data
obtained in our laboratory and the epidemiological data can be
solved by the assumption of a wide-spread distribution of the
virus in the human population. Like in cats (28), immunosurveillance mechanisms usually prevent the development of malignant
disease. In view of the usually good prognosis of the disease in

children (29), it is not likely that the occasional emergence of leukemia is due to an innate immunodeficiency, however.

Seroepidemiological studies somehow support the concept of a wide distribution of both SiSV and baboon endogenous virus in the human population (30). In view of the difficulty in detecting these viruses in man, the horizontal transmission of the virus remains a mystery. A very scrutinous examination of excretion products like saliva, milk or seminal fluid might reveal that occasionally virus particles are released. The detection of primate viruses in some human embryonic cells lines (17, 31) suggest that in utero infection might take place, as has been described for a murine oncovirus (32).

Acknowledgements

Dr. Kees Nooter is the great motor in our laboratory with regard to human tumor virus research. Infatiguably he initiated several biological investigations, which often caused huge dis-appointments but have been rewarding in the end.

Dr. Chris Zurcher made immunofluorescence a very reliable technique in our laboratory, due to his critical attitude. The investigations on which this review is mostly based, have been supported to a large extent by the Koningin Wilhelmina Fonds (the Netherlands Organization for the Fight against Cancer) and the Netherlands Organization for Fundamental Medical Research FUNGO.

References
1. MacDowell, E.C. et al., Cancer Res. 5 (1945) 65.
2. Eker, R. and Mossige, J., Nature 189 (1961) 858.
3. Bentvelzen, P. and Daams, J.H., J. Nat. Cancer Inst. 43 (1969) 1025.
4. Mulvihill, J.J., In: Genetics of Human Cancer, Progr. Cancer Res. Therapy, vol. 3, Raven Press, New York. (1977) p. 137.
5. German, J. Progr. Med. Genetics 8 (1972) 61.
6. Gatti, R.A. and Good, R.A., Cancer 28 (1971) 89.
7. Zuelzer, W.W. and Cox, D.E., Seminars Hematol. 6 (1969) 228.
8. Tooze, J., The Molecular Biology of Tumor Viruses (Cold Spring Harbor Laboratory, New York, 1974).
9. Gallagher, R.E. and Gallo, R.C., Science 197 (1975) 350.
10. Teich, N.M. et al., Nature 256 (1975) 551.
11. Gallagher, R.E. et al., Proc.Nat.Acad. Sci. USA 72 (1975) 4127.
12. Baxt, W. and Spiegelman, S., Proc. Nat. Acad. Sci. USA 69 (1972) 3737.
13. Nooter, K. et al., Nature 256 (1975) 595.
14. Van Pelt, F.G., unpublished results.
15. Okabe, H. et al., Nature 260 (1976) 264.
16. Chan, E. et al., Nature 260 (1976) 266.
17. Panem. S. et al., J. Gen. Virol. 35 (1977) 487.
18. Nooter, K. et al., Bibl. Haemat. 43 (1976) 574.

19. Klement, V. et al., Nature New Biol. 234 (1971) 12.
20. Nooter, K. et al., Int. J. Cancer 19 (1977) 59.
21. Nooter, K. et al., Int. J. Cancer 21 (1978) 27.
22. Bentvelzen, P., unpublished results.
23. Koch, G. et al., Europ. J. Cancer 13 (1977) 1397.
24. Nooter, K. and Zurcher, C., unpublished results.
25. Haaijman, J.J. and Brinkhof, J., J. Immunol. Methods 14 (1977)
    213.
26. Zurcher, C. et al., Nature 254 (1975) 457.
27. Zurcher, C. et al., In: Advances in Comparative Leukemia
    Research 1977 (Bentvelzen, P., Hilger, J. and Yohn, D.S., eds.)
    Elsevier/North-Holland, Amsterdam, p. 144 (1978).
28. Essex, M. et al., Science 190 (1975) 790.
29. Pinkel, D. et al., Cancer 39 (1977) 817.
30. Kurth, R. et al., Proc. Nat. Acad. Sci. USA 74 (1977) 1237.
31. Zurcher, C. and Bentvelzen, P., unpublished results.
32. Andervont, H.B., J. Nat. Cancer Inst. 31 (1963) 261.

STUDIES IN HUMAN HEMATOPOIETIC CELLS:

CELLULAR AND VIROLOGICAL ASPECTS

R. C. Gallo, M. S. Reitz, W. C. Saxinger, P. Jacquemin, and F. W. Ruscetti

Laboratory of Tumor Cell Biology
National Cancer Institute

Bethesda, Maryland 20014

INTRODUCTION

RNA tumor viruses have only rarely been reported to be isolated from human tissues as complete replicating entities, and the status of the various isolates is not yet clear. Despite this, we have invested considerable effort in finding so called "footprints" of these viruses in humans. There are a number of considerations which lead us to believe that such studies are important: 1) RNA tumor viruses can produce leukemia in a wide variety of animals; 2) We have recently shown that some RNA tumor viruses can transform fresh human blood cells in vitro. The viruses which can do this are those that are leukemogenic in gibbon apes (gibbon ape leukemia virus, or GaLV), the very closely related simian sarcoma virus (SiSV) isolated from a spontaneous sarcoma of a pet woolly monkey), and the virus we call HL23V, isolated from human leukemic cells a few years ago, and which is also very closely related to these viruses of subhuman primates; 3) In every species where the cause of naturally occurring leukemia is known for a sizable fraction of the cases, it involves an RNA tumor virus. Species for which this is true now include chickens, wild mice, cats, cows, and the previously mentioned gibbon apes, which is the species closest to man for which an animal model of leukemia is available; 4) RNA tumor viruses can sometimes transform a cell and never be seen again as a whole replicating virus, thus making it necessary to ascertain their presence by detection with biochemical or immunological probes; 5) Some studies have shown that these viruses can pick up cellular sequences and these sequences may be important to growth and/or differentiation. Such

153

cellular sequences may be altered in leukemogenesis whatever the
cause and the alteration might be detected with specific viral
probes.

It is worth describing briefly the first RNA tumor viruses to
be isolated from primates, collectively called the woolly monkey
(simian) sarcoma virus (SiSV)-gibbon ape leukemia virus (GaLV)
group. GaLV was isolated from a colony of gibbons in Thailand used
for experimental malaria research (1). Several of these animals
developed leukemia and GaLV was isolated. This virus was shown to
be able to produce a myeloproliferative disease after infection of
some newborn or young gibbon apes (T. Kawakami, personal communication). Two types of leukemias have been observed in gibbons,
chronic myelogenous leukemia, resembling the disease in man, and an
acute lymphatic leukemia. Other isolates of GaLV included viruses
from leukemic gibbons in a San Francisco zoo (2), from the brains
of animals inoculated with human brain extracts (3), and most
recently, from a leukemic gibbon from Hall's Island, Bermuda (4).
SiSV, isolated from a woolly monkey, has been shown by Deinhardt
and colleagues to produce fibrosarcomas or malignant brain tumors
on inoculation into marmosets (5). Several interesting facts have
emerged from studies with these viruses. It has been shown in several laboratories that the so-called woolly monkey virus is closely
related to the various strains of GaLV. In fact, SiSV is about as
closely related to different isolates of GaLV as are the different
isolates of GaLV to each other (3,4). It is clear that they are
exogenous, i.e., there is little or no homology of nucleic acid
sequences in the RNA genome of GaLV or SiSV with DNA of uninfected
normal primates (6-8). Some studies have indicated that these
viruses originated in rodents, probably mice, and entered these two
primates by interspecies transmission sometime in the past. Thus,
it appears then that a mouse type-C virus has been able to enter at
least two phylogenetically distinct primates.

As described by the leading investigators in the field elsewhere in this symposium (See 9 and 10), leukemia in outbred cats
may be of even greater interest as a model for leukemia in man,
inasmuch as the epidemiology of feline leukemia has been extensively
studied and shown to involve feline leukemia virus (FeLV) as an
etiologic agent in about half of the cases. FeLV is a common infectious agent in free-roaming populations of cats. Apparently, infection with FeLV usually produces only minor clinical symptoms. In
rare instances (approximately 1%), however, after a latent period
of three months to five years, infection can result in a leukemia
similar to acute lymphocytic leukemia of children, a lymphoma
resembling Burkitt's lymphoma, and other forms of leukemia.

Since infection is so common but leukemia so rare, and usually
then only after a long latent phase, it was difficult to establish
FeLV as the etiologic agent. One type of evidence was the induction

of the disease with cell-free filtrates from tumored cats. Serologic
data also provided evidence for the etiologic role of this virus in
cat leukemia. Cats can respond immunologically to both virus and
to virus-induced tumor cells. Thus, antibodies to viral proteins
are detectable in virus-resistant cats, and these antibodies inactivate infectious virus. In tumor-resistant cats, antibody to a
virus-coded cell neoantigen (FOCMA) is present, and is apparently
the determinant of tumor resistance.

   In a sizable number of feline leukemias, however, not only is
there an absence of infectious virus, but also a lack of viral
nucleic acid sequences above the levels found in "normal" cats and
a lack of detectable antibody to FeLV proteins. Even in these
"virus-negative" cats, however, Essex has emphasized that the disease
may still be caused by the virus (11). This is suggested by two
results: First, in cat households where FeLV is present, there may be
an equally increased risk for FeLV-positive and FeLV-negative tumors.
Second, the virus negative tumor cells themselves express FOCMA,
which is apparently FeLV-coded or specifically induced by FeLV.
Thus, virus-negative leukemias in cats provide an example in nature
of an apparently virus-induced neoplasm where virus and antibodies
to that virus are not directly detectable, although presumably
enough viral genetic material for transformation and FOCMA production remain present. If human leukemias are in some way associated
with RNA tumor viruses, it is likely to be in a manner analogous to
the "FeLV-negative" leukemias and lymphomas. We have been attempting
therefore to develop probes which will permit the indentification
of subviral molecules, and to study proviral nucleic acid sequences
through the use of restriction endonucleases.

ANALYSIS OF HUMAN DNA FOR VIRUS-RELATED SEQUENCES

   We have tested a number of DNA samples prepared from human
tissue (both leukemic and non-leukemic) using labelled viral RNA
or labelled DNA transcripts of viral RNA (cDNA) from various type-C
viruses for the presence of virus-related sequences as assayed by
thr formation of complexes resistant to digestion by single-strand-
specific nucleases.

   When SiSV-SiSAV from the marmoset tumor cell line 71AP1 is
used as a source of probe, some human DNA samples hybridize a greater
amount of the probe than others. The kinetics of formation of the
nuclease-resistant complexes and their thermal stabilities are
consistant with the presence of sequences related but not identical
to a fraction of sequences obtained in SiSV-SiSAV (71AP1) cDNA,
ranging up to about 35% of the probe (normalized for its hybridization to homologous DNA). The higher values are more often obtained
with leukemic DNA samples than non-leukemic, and this particularly at
true of DNA from chronic myelogenous leukemia (CML) patients. This
data is summarized in Figure 1, which presents percentage of DNA

DISTRIBUTION OF HUMAN DNA SEQUENCES
HYBRIDIZABLE TO SiSV cDNA

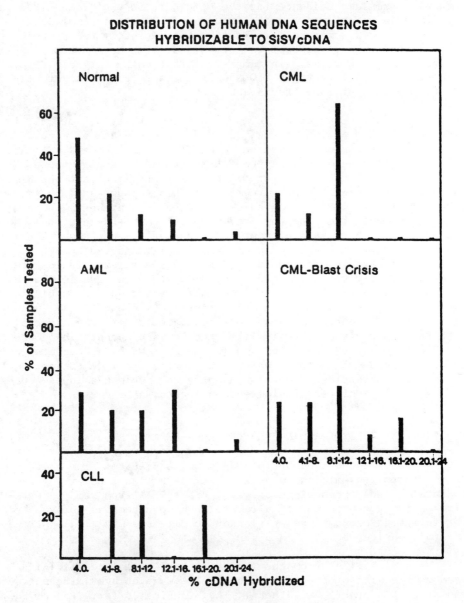

Figure 1. Hybridization of SiSV ^{3}H–cDNA to DNA from leukemic or non-leukemic tissue as assayed by S1 nuclease digestion. The percentage of DNA samples in each group which hybridize the indicated amount of cDNA is shown.

samples within each group which hybridize a given percentage of SiSV cDNA. The same pattern is observed when SiSV-SiSAV(71AP1) ^{125}I-RNA is used as the probe, except that the overall percent hybridization is lower (not shown).

Probes prepared from Rauscher murine leukemia virus (MuLV-R) or a wild mouse leukemia virus (SC-185) behave in the same way as those from SiSV-SiSAV(71AP1). DNA samples from leukemic patients, particularly CML, tend to hybridize more probe than non-leukemic samples. In contrast, we have observed neither high levels of hybridization nor a difference in hybridization between normal and leukemic DNA samples when probes from endogenous rat virus (V-NRK), the Hall's Island strain of gibbon ape leukemia virus (GaLV-H), or the Rickard or Theilen strains of feline leukemia virus (FeLV) are used as the source of probes. Data obtained with V-NRK or GaLV-H cDNA, which are typical of this type of result, are shown in Figure 2.

Whether these data indicate the presence of complete or partial viral genomes in some humans is at present hard to determine with certainty because of the low level of the observed hybrid formation and the reduced thermal stability of the hybrids. Work is presently underway to prepare and use probes which are specific to defined regions of viral genomes, in order to characterize more precisely the nature of the apparently extra DNA sequences observed in some human DNA samples.

SURFACE IMMUNOGLOBULINS ON LEUKEMIC CELLS

DNA polymerases resembling viral reverse transcriptase in their biochemical (12) and serological (13) properties have been detected sporadically in human leukemic tissue. Since this is the only viral protein we have been able to detect thus far, we have looked for the presence of naturally-occurring antibody to reverse transcriptase in humans. In addition, recent evidence has shown the presence of antibody to reverse transcriptase in naturally-occurring animal leukemias in the absence of detectable virus (14). Attempts to find similar antibodies in human serum have been negative in our hands. Since there is precedent for various tumor cell bound antibodies which can be eluted from the cell surface, we decided to look at the surface of the leukemic cells themselves for antibodies specific for reverse transcriptase from different animal viruses.

Buffy coat white blood cells are incubated 12 hours at 37° to elute surface IgG. The crude eluate is then further purified by $(NH_4)_2SO_4$ precipitation, DEAE-agarose chromatography, and fractionation on a goat anti-human IgG affinity column. Two bands corresponding in size to human IgG light and heavy chains are evident after SDS gel electrophoresis (Figure 3).

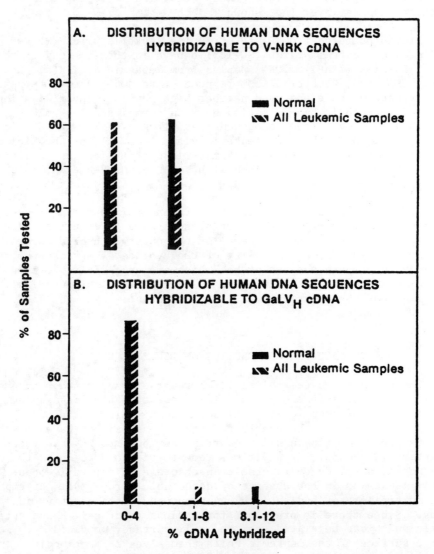

Figure 2. Hybridization of V-NRK and GaLV-H cDNA to DNA from leukemic or non-leukemic tissue as assayed by S1 nuclease digestion.
The percentage of DNA samples of each group which hybridize the
indicated amount of cDNA is shown.

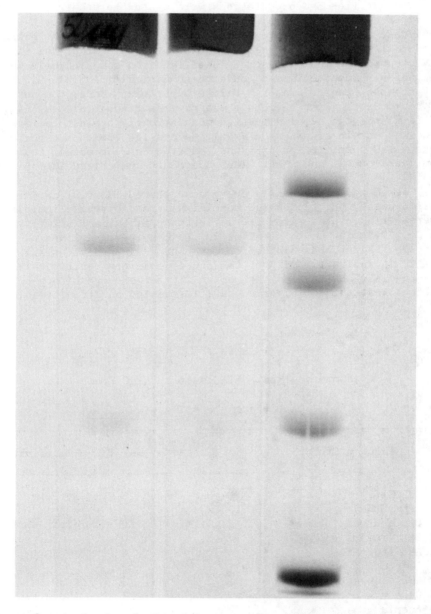

Figure 3. Analysis of eluted human antibody by polyacrylamide gel
electrophoresis. Left gel, authentic human IgG; center gel, eluted
human surface antibody from cells of patient with chronic myelogenous
leukemia in blast crisis; right gel, molecular weight standards:
bovine serum albumin - 68,000, ovalbumin - 45,000, chymotrypsinogen -
25,000, pancreatic ribonuclease - 13,000.

The purified IgG preparations were tested for their ability to
inhibit the activity of reverse transcriptase from different viruses.
Consistent with previous reports on the presence in human leukemic
blood cells of reverse transcriptase related to that of the SiSV-
GaLV group of primate viruses, eluted IgG from some leukemic and
some normal blood cells was found to specifically inhibit SiSV and
GaLV reverse transcriptases. Unlike hyperimmune sera, the natural
IgG could distinguish between these reverse transcriptases. All
tested normal IgG samples reacted most strongly against the San
Francisco strain of GaLV (GaLV-SF), as did IgG from CML chronic
phase. IgG specific for SiSV was observed in four out of ten samples
from cases of AML and AMML. These data are summarized in Table 1.

Unexpectedly, in nearly every case tested (8 of 9) of CML
blastic phase, the eluted IgG specifically and strongly inhibited
reverse transcriptase from FeLV. That the inhibitory activity is
due to IgG acting on this enzyme is shown by several lines of
evidence. First, the biochemical and physical properties are those
of IgG, including the size of the proteins in the purified eluate,
the non-dialyzability and thermostability of the inhabitory activity,
the fact that the inhibitor co-purifies as IgG on affinity columns,

Table 1

Summary of Anti-RT Results of IgG From
Blood Leukocyte Surfaces From
Different Specimens

	Source of IgG	No. Tested	No. +	Specificity
1.	CML (BC) (Ph+,TDT-)	9	8	8 FeLV
2.	CML (chronic phase)	4	2	Both GaLV
3.	CML (remission)	2	0	
4.	AML and AMML (untreated or relapse)	10	4	4 SSV
5.	AUL (untreated)	2	0	
6.	Diserythropoietic Anemia	3	2	Both FeLV
7.	Polycythemia Vera	4	1	SSV
8.	ALL	3	0	
9.	CLL	3	0	
10.	Normal Blood Donors (randomly selected)	24	6	GaLV

and the presence and positive activity of $F(ab^1)_2$ fragments in the
purified eluate after pepsin digestion. Second, we could find no
known inhibitors of DNA polymerase in the purified eluate, including
proteases, nucleases and phosphatases. Further evidence includes
the specificity of inhibition (an example is shown in Figure 4),
the removal of inhibitory activity by incubation with goat anti-
human IgG, an increase in the sedimentation velocity of the reverse
transcriptase in the presence of the eluted IgG, and specific
binding of the reverse transcriptase in question to sepharose beads
containing the IgG. It is perplexing that despite the presence of
antibodies reactive with FeLV reverse transcriptase in a large fraction of CML blast crisis cells, that FeLV-related sequences are not
detected in the DNA or RNA of these cells. However, as discussed
above and elsewhere in this symposia, leukemia in virus-negative
cats is associated with FeLV by epidemiology and the presence of
FOCMA, and yet do not have detectable viral nucleotide sequences (15).
It may be that the amount of information present in the DNA is too
small to detect with our currently available probes, yet important
pathologically. In humans, the antibody on the cell surface would
be originating from tissue other than the cells in question. Alternatively, the antibody may be directed against reverse transcriptase
of a different but related virus or even to a non-viral but coinci-
dentally structurally closely related protein, or we do not have
nucleic acid probes of the right specificity. Thus, these data at
this time are stimulating for further studies but in our opinion,
cannot be taken as conclusive evidence for an anti-viral immune response. This can be determined if a viral-specific antigen is
identified.

GROWTH OF HUMAN HEMATOPOIETIC CELLS IN VITRO

We have been concerned with the development of long-term suspension culture systems for various types of human hematopoietic cells.
Development of these systems was undertaken for three reasons:
First, to determine whether the use of DNA from cloned leukemic
hematopoietic cells will allow the more consistent detection of
viral information; Second, to determine the effect of Type-C viral
infection on human hematopoietic cells; and Third, to be able to
grow the large quantity of cells needed for biochemical analysis not
only of viral information, but also for studying growth regulators,
cell surface changes particularly receptors, and other biochemical
markers which may be important in understanding the phenotype of the
leukemic cells.

Some of the results presented above on surface immunoglobulins
suggest that acquired retrovirus information could be present in
human hematopoietic cells more frequently than indicated by molecular
hybridization analyses. As mentioned, one possiblity is that viral

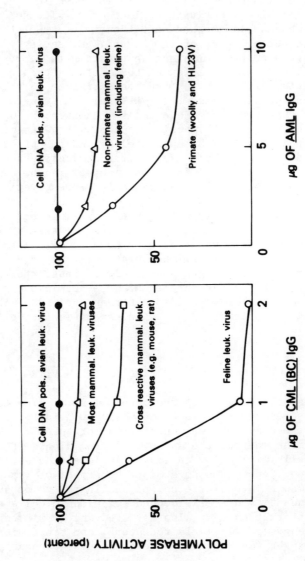

POLYMERASE ACTIVITY (percent)

μg OF CML (BC) IgG

Cell DNA pols., avian leuk. virus

Most mammal. leuk. viruses

Cross reactive mammal. leuk. viruses (e.g. mouse, rat)

Feline leuk. virus

μg OF AML IgG

Cell DNA pols., avian leuk. virus

Non-primate mammal. leuk. viruses (including feline)

Primate (woolly and HL23V)

Figure 4.   Specificity of myloid leukemia surface leukocyte IgG for reverse transcriptase.

information could be present in only a sub-population of cells in
the primary tissues. One way to test this is to selectively grow
in tissue culture specific cell types from the heterogenous primary
tissue. In practice, this has involved attempts to propagate cells
in liquid suspension culture, since established methods of growing
myeloid cells in semi-solid medium (16,17) yield inadequate quantities of viable cells and since our attempts to propagate these
cells on alternative materials, e.g., diffusion chambers in vitro,
hollow fiber culture devices, etc., have failed to produce sustained
leukocyte growth.

However, as previously described (18), we have found that by
using conditioned medium from certain "feeder" cell cultures it is
possible to grow select leukocyte cell types in suspension culture.
From myelogenous leukemia cells, we have succeeded in growing mixed
populations of leukemic myeloid cells for periods of several weeks
in numerous instances (18). This growth of myeloid leukemic cells
was stimulated only by conditioned media from human embryonic materials. Only a small fraction (5/53) of CM from embryonic sources was
active. Positive results with two sources of whole human embryo
(WHE) conditioned media (CM) are summarized in Table 2. Two different

Table 2

Growth of Myelogenous Leukemic Cells

Conditioned Medium Source	Leukemic Specimen	Growth[a]	Cell[b] Maturation
WHE-1	AML[c]	6/6	2/6
	CML/BC	2/2	1/2
	AMML	4/4	1/4
	Other	4/4	4/4
	normal marrow	0/20	–
WHE-2	AML	7/27	7/7
	CML/BC	13/16	8/13
	AMML	0/3	–
	normal marrow	0/17	–
None	AML	0/23	–
	CML/BC	2/16	0/2

[a]Three cell doublings/week for at least three weeks.
[b]Determined by differential leukocyte count.
[c]Abbreviations are, AML (acute myelogenous leukemia), CML/BC
(chronic myelogenous leukemia in blast crisis), AMML (acute
myelomonocytic leukemia), "Other" includes various myeloproliferative syndromes.

patterns of response were observed. Using WHE sample number 1
as a source for CM, the logarithmic growth of peripheral blood
leukocytes was stimulated from 16 cases of myelogenous leukemia (19).
Leukocyte growth remained dependent upon CM, even after 300 days
in culture. Two of the cultures have chromosome markers indicating
the proliferation in vitro of leukemic myeloid cells. However, only
a portion of the metaphases contained the marker chromosome,
indicating either the growth of different clones of leukemic cells
or a mixture or normal and leukemic cells. The differentials of
the cells growing varied from case to case (19). All contained a
sub-population of blast cells which presumably accounted for the
self-renewal capability of these cultures. Some cultures contained
the whole spectrum of myeloid and monocytoid cells. Histochemical
stains and functional tests verified the predominant myeloid nature
of the cultures.

The other active preparation, also derived from CM of embryonic
human cell strains, we call WHE-42 CM. Only a portion of the
leukocyte specimens responded to this CM, and the magnitude and the
duration were more limited. The cells in culture developed a
declining growth fraction and a longer doubling time after a few
weeks. This was usually coincident with an increasing degree of
cell differentiation to mature granulocytes. The embryonic sources
of active CM selectively stimulated growth of myeloid leukocytes
from leukemic patients with no effect on myeloid cells from bone
marrow of normal people, and did not support the growth of myeloid
colonies in semi-solid media.

The release of active CM was in every case restricted to early
passage, unfrozen cellular materials, limiting our ability to
purify and characterize these factors. Attempts to recover this
activity by biochemical fractionation of more abundant but poorly
active CM from later passaged cultures have so far been unsuccessful.
Nevertheless, the results allow some conclusions: (a) leukemic
myeloid cells can be grown in suspension culture; (b) many human
leukemic cells can be stimulated to mature into non-dividing
granulocytes; and, (c) specific leukemic cell stimulating factors
exist and/or that cell membranes of myeloid leukemia cells may
preferentially recognize fetal growth and differentiation promoting
factors.

In only one of 38 cases of myelogenous leukemia cells which
actively replicated in culture for more than six weeks, have we
observed production of virus. This was the type-C virus produced
by three different cultured strains derived from AML patient HL23,
as previously reported (20).

During attempts to grow myelogenous leukemia cells in vitro, it
was discovered that conditioned medium from phytohemagglutinin-
stimulated mixed lymphocyte cultures (Ly-CM) selectively stimulated

growth of a sub-population of lymphoid cells rather than myeloid
cells. Subsequent studies indicated that these lymphoid cultures
consist entirely of thymus-derived lymphocytes, i.e., T-cells (21).
Successful cultures have been started from human bone marrow, peripheral blood and spleen. Cultures have been continuously maintained
for more than one year with a 5 to 10-fold increase in cell number
every 3 to 4 days. These cells can be distinguished from permanently
transformed lymphoblastoid cell lines by their: (1) dependence for
growth upon the continuous presence of protein factor(s) in Ly-CM;
(2) lack of detectable EBV; and (3) exhibition of immunologic reactivities not associated with transformed lymphoblastoid cells.
These T-cell cultures can be grown from both leukemic and normal
people and appear to be normal colonies of cells as judged by
morphology and functional response.

ESTABLISHMENT OF A HUMAN MYELOID CELL LINE (HL-60)

We recently showed that peripheral blood leukocytes from a
patient (HL-60) with acute promyelocytic leukemia grew in the presence but not in the absence of CM from an embryonic lung fibroblast
culture. However, in contrast to our previous experience with
myeloid cell cultures, once growth started the CM was no longer
needed. This led to the establishment of a continuously growing
cell line with distinct myeloid characteristics (23). As in the
fresh leukemic blood from this patient, the predominant cell type
in the culture is a promyelocyte with distinct azurophilic granules
(Figure 5), although small numbers of more mature myeloid cells are
also present as are a low percentage of myeloblasts. A striking
feature of the cells is their histochemical staining properties (23).
Apparently all of the cells are positive for myeloperoxidase, chloroacetate esterase, and Sudan black B, assays specific for myeloid
leukocytes (24). The cells also contain lysozyme and acid phosphatase. Five to 10% of the leukocytes spontaneously differentiate
to metamyelocytes or beyond, including a rare neutrophil.

Chromosome studies of HL-60 cells reveal aneuploidy with the
majority of the metaphases having 44 chromosomes and the remainder
ranging from 43 to 47 in number (23). These results are similar to
chromosomal analysis of the fresh cells (Gallagher et al., in
preparation) and indicate that the cultured cells are of leukemic
origin.

INDUCTION OF LEUKOCYTE MATURATION (HL-60)

The addition of 1.25% dimethylsulfoxide (DMSO) to the HL-60
culture induces a striking morphological change in the majority of
the cells resembling the terminal differentiation stages of myeloid
cells (25). The induced cells exhibit the following changes:

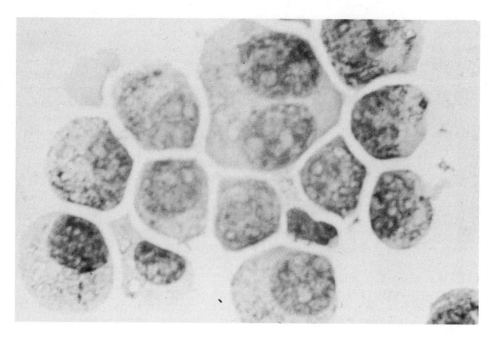

Figure 5.   Morphology of Human Myeloid Cell Line HL-60.

smaller size, decreased nuclear/cytoplasmic ratio, less prominent
cytoplasmic granules, disappearance of nucleoli, marked indentation,
convolution, segmentation of the nuclei and inability to synthesize
DNA and to divide (Figure 6).   Clones of HL-60 have been developed
in which more than 99% of the cells differentiate in the presence
of DMSO.   Metamyelocytes and neutrophilic bands rather than segmented
neutrophils, the final cells in the myeloid series, predominate in
the culture 5-7 days after induction.   This pattern is analogous
to that seen in induced Friend mouse erythroleukemia cells in which
complete erythroid differentiation with the extrusion of nuclei
and progression to the most mature red blood cells is infrequent (26).

     Growth of HL-60 cells begins to plateau at day five after treat-
ment with DMSO concentrations of 1.25% and below.   Concentrations of
1.5% or higher completely inhibit cell growth.   Maximum differentiation of the cells occurs 5-7 days after addition of DMSO (Figure 7).
The concentration of DMSO which gives maximum induction of maturation
without inhibition of cell replication is approximately 1.3%.

     Although DMSO has been the most widely studied inducing com-
pound, numerous other low molecular weight, polar, freely diffus-
sible compounds exist which induce differentiation of Friend mouse

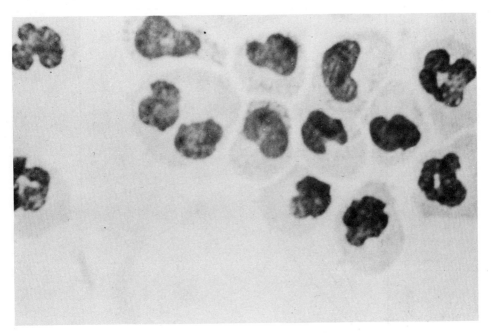

Figure 6. Morphology of HL-60 Cells Induced for Differentiation with DMSO.

erythroleukemia cells at molar concentrations significantly less than that required for DMSO (25). We have tested some of these compounds, and all of those tested also induce myeloid differentiation of the HL-60 cells. The kinetics of induction and extent of morphological differentiation are similar to those described above for DMSO. Although the optimal molar concentrations of the polar inducers in the HL-60 system are 40-60% less than the concentrations used in the Friend mouse system (25), the relative potency of the compounds in inducing differentiation is the same in both. These striking similarities in the behavior of Friend and HL-60 cells in the presence of these compounds suggest that similar mechanisms may be involved in the terminal differentiation of both. All the compounds that are active in inducing differentiation of HL-60 cells share certain structural similarities (Figure 8). These compounds can alter many biological activities such as membrane function, cell transport and nucleic acid structure, but it is not clear by what mechanism they induce cell differentiation.

After treatment with DMSO, the HL-60 cells differentiated not only as judged by morphological but also by functional criteria. The latter was assessed by assays for phagocytosis. Uninduced and

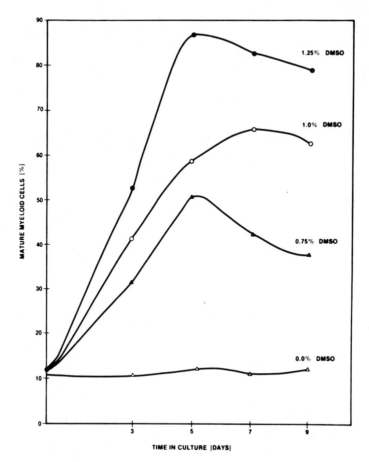

<u>Figure 7</u>. Maturation of HL-60 cells in the presence of different
concentrations of DMSO

induced HL-60 cells were incubated with <u>Candida albicans</u>. After
incubation with 1.25% DMSO for 7 days, 85-90% of the cells were
positive for phagocytosis of the yeast, while only 5-10% of the
uninduced were capable of phagocytosis. Those cells in the uninduced
cultures capable of phagocytosis were the spontaneously differentiating mature cells; clearly identifiable promyelocytes were not
capable of phagocytosis. Other hyman hematopoietic cell lines such
as T-lymphocytes stimulated by lymphocyte CM (22), B-lymphocytes,
and K-562, exhibited no rise in phagocytic capacity when similarly
incubated with DMSO. This indicates that the induction of phagocytosis in HL-60 cells is not merely a non-specific membrane
phenomenon generated by DMSO and that functional as well as morphological maturation has occurred in the myeloid HL-60 cells. If the
number of cells capable of phagocytosis is determined as a function

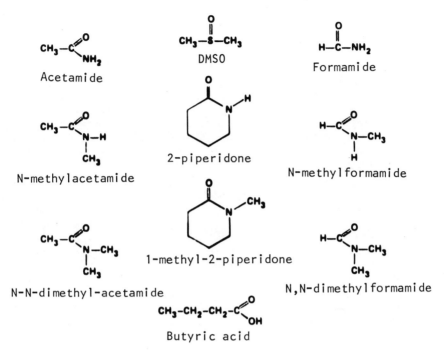

<u>Figure 8</u>. Agents inducing terminal differentiation of HL-60 human myeloid cells.

of the length of time the cells have been exposed to DMSO, it correlates with the kinetics of appearance of mature cells in the cultures. The maximum number of cells capable of phagocytosis appear after seven days in culture. These cells also respond to chemotactic stimuli as a result of DMSO induced differentiation. However, these myeloid cells are not completely functional because they lack alkaline phosphatase, probably indicating incomplete secondary granule formation.

The presence of a cell culture that shows some spontaneous differentiation and complete differentiation in response to DMSO, raises questions about the presence in these cultures of colony-stimulating factor (CSF), thought to be the normal myelopoietic regulator. Numerous attempts to find myeloid stimulatory activity in HL-60 CM have failed to indicate any stimulation of normal or leukemic myeloid cell growth in semi-solid medium or liquid suspension culture. In this regard, it is important to point out that in the HL-60 culture, the commitment of cells to myelogenous differentiation has already been made. CSF may primarily affect an early undifferentiated cell, called the colony forming cell, which is not a recognizable myeloid cell (27). Thus, it is not clear that CSF

is required for the sequence of late differentiative events of the
HL-60 leukocytes.

Despite the inability to detect CSF in HL-60 cell cultures, we
asked whether these cells are capable of responding to an exogenous
source of CSF, as is the case for certain mouse myeloid leukemic
cell lines (29). HL-60 cells are capable of forming colonies in the
absence of any added factor with a plating efficiency of approximately 0.5%, but the addition of exogenous sources of CSF to the
culture results in a 5-30 fold increase in the number of colonies
formed (Table 3). Partially purified CM from human placenta, kindly
provided by Dr. Tony Burgess, stimulated a 10-fold increase in colony
formation over control. If one looks at the morphology of individual
colonies stimulated by CSF, there are several different types. These
include: 1) promyelocytes; 2) promyelocytes in center of colonies
with more mature metamyelocytes and bands around the outside of the
colony; 3) mononuclear cell colonies with the cytoplasm more mature
than the nucleus; and, 4) entirely mature colonies consisting mainly
of metamyelocytes and bands with an occasional segmented neutrophil.
Does this very heterogenous response to CSF indicate that the HL-60
cell culture has a heterogenous population of cells as defined by
their differentiation potential? Cloning experiments are in progress
attempting to develop cell lines with a more uniform response to
these factors. The fact that HL-60 cells can be made to grow and
differentiate in semi-solid media when stimulated by CSF may mean
that these cells possess a receptor for CSF. The availability of the
line may make it feasible to isolate such receptors.

Table 3

Colony Formation of HL-60 Cells

Source of CSA[a]	Colonies[b]		
Cells plated:	5×10^3	10^4	5×10^4
Human placenta	222	564	>2500
Activated lymphocytes	1311	341	2270
Leukocyte feeder layer	681	1486	>2500
None	2	51	293

[a]Conditioned medium of human placenta (30) and activated
lymphocytes (31) were prepared as previously described, as were
leukocyte underlayers (32).

[b]Number of colonies per number of cells plated as indicated
were counted in triplicate plates at days 7, 10, 14, 21. The
colony count did not change appreciably after day 10.

PHENOTYPIC ALTERATIONS OF HL-60 CELLS INDUCED BY VIRAL INFECTION

The availability of established human hematopoietic cell lines
of different types allows a study of the effects of type-C viral
infection on specific cell types. We tested the effect of various
viruses on HL-60 cells and observed a remarkable change 10-30 days
after productive infection of HL-60 cells with either SiSV, HL23V,
or BaEV. The morphological changes in the infected cells are con-
trasted with the uninfected cells in Figure 9. The nuclei, containing multiple (2-6) small nucleoli, are frequently indented and
folded, giving the infected cells a more monocytoid appearance than
the uninfected cells with their predominantly round or oval nuclei.
The cytoplasm is gray-blue and the prominent azurophilic granules
seen in the uninfected cells are absent. In marked contrast to
the uninfected cultures, over 99% of the infected cells are negative
when stained for myeloid-specific stains, such as myeloperoxidase
and chloroacetate esterase. In addition, these infected cells were
negative for surface immunoglobulin, Epstein-Barr viral nuclear
antigen, complement receptor, sheep erythrocyte (E-rosette) receptor transferase, α-napthylacetate esterase, lysozyme production
and F_C receptor. Thus, the cells have converted from promyelocytes
to less differentiated blast cells. The growth kinetics of these
infected cells possessing these marked cellular changes did not
appreciably change from the HL-60 control cells. The doubling time
of the infected cells ranged from 36-46 hours, while the doubling
time for HL-60 cells is 40-44 hours.

Upon the addition of appropriate concentrations of DMSO, the
vast majority of HL-60 cells undergo morphological and maturational
changes characteristic of terminal differentiation of myeloid cells.
However, the addition of DMSO in a wide range of concentrations to
the infected cells does not result in any detectable myeloid differentiation. All other inducing agents like dimethylformamide and
butyric acid also have no effect. The infected cells do not phago-
cytize yeast or respond to chemotactic stimuli. Uninfected HL-60
cells will form colonies in methycellulose in the presence of CSA.
The infected cells will not form colonies, but grow as single cells.

The characteristics of HL-60 cells after induction with DMSO
are compared with virus infected cells in Table 4. The main observation is that the infected cells lose all recognizable myeloid
characteristics, resemble undifferentiated blast cells, and are
blocked from responding to differentiation promoting molecules.
Karyotypic analysis shows that these cells contain two marker
chromosomes present in the differentiated HL-60 cell line.

After productive infection of HL-60 cells, certain cell characteristics were followed daily until the altered phenotype of the
cells developed. The cell viability remained above 85% during the

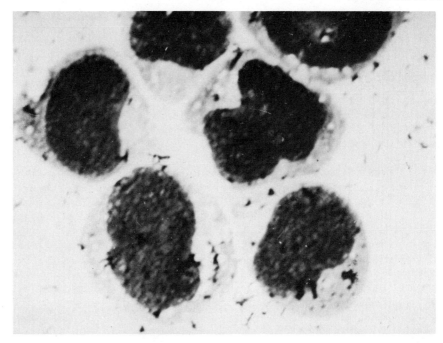

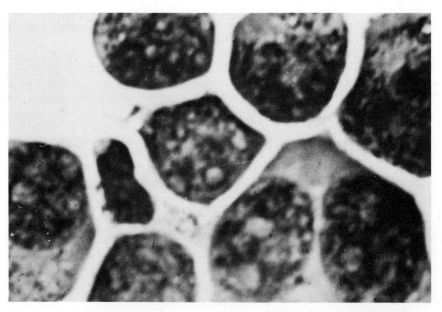

Figure 9. Morphologic changes in HL-60 cells after exposure to SiSV.
Top panel, cells not exposed to SiSV. Bottom panel, cells exposed
to SiSV.

Table 4

Characteristics of HL-60 Cells in Culture

Characteristics	HL-60	Me$_2$SO Induced HL-60	Type-C Viral Infected HL-60
Cellular morphology	promyelocyte	neutrophil	undifferentiated blast
Doubling time	40-44 hrs.	–	36-46 hrs.
Myeloid-specific cytochemistry	positive	positive	negative
Phagocytosis	negative	positive	negative
Agar colony formation	positive	negative	negative
Differentiative response to Me$_2$SO	positive	–	negative
Granule formation	immature	mature	negative

whole time.   The dense staining peroxidase particles were gradually reduced and finally disappeared as did the azurophilic granules. The ability of these cells to be induced to terminally differentiate in the presence of DMSO is lost three days before the visible alterations of the morphological characteristics.   These morphological and functional changes in the cells seem to occur as an all or nothing effect, suggesting that cell change and not cell selection is occurring after type-C viral infection.   Our hypothesis is that specific primate type-C viruses may induce blocks in differentiation by modifying receptors for growth and differentiation regulating molecules or result in production of new factors which complex to receptors and induce growth without normal differentiation and prevent binding of the normal regulator molecules.   Both concepts are testable and under study.

REFERENCES

1.   Kawakami, T., and Buckley, P.M., 1974.   Transplant. Proc. 6, pp. 193-196.

2.   Kawakami, T.G., Huff, S.D., Buckley, P.M., Dungworth, D.C., Snyder, J.P., and Gilden, R.V., 1972.   Nature New Biol. 235, pp. 170-177.

3. Todaro, G.J., Leiber, M.M., Benveniste, R.E., Sherr, C.J., Gibbs C.J., and Gajdusek, D.C., 1975. Virology 67 pp. 335-357.

4. Gallo, R.C., Gallagher, R.E., Wong-Staal, F.W., Aoki, T., Markham, P.D., Schetters, H., Ruscetti, F., Valerio, M. Walling, M., O'Keefe, R.T., Saxinger, W.C., Smith, R.G., Virology 84, pp. 359-373.

5. Wolfe, L.G., Deinhardt, F., Theilen, G.H., Rabin, H., Kawakami, T., and Bustad, L.K., 1971. J. Natl. Cancer Inst. 47, pp. 1115-1120.

6. Wong-Staal, F., Gallo, R.C., and Gillespie, D., 1975. Nature (London) 256, pp. 670-672.

7. Scolnick, E.M., Parks, W., Kawakami, T., Kohne, D., Okabe, H., Gilden, R., and Hatanaka, M., 1974. J. Virol.13, pp. 363-369.

8. Benveniste, R.E., Heinemann, R., Wilson, G.H., Callahan, R., and Todaro, G.J., 1974. J. Virol. 14, pp. 56-57.

9. Jarret, W., this symposium.

10. Essex, M., et al., this symposium.

11. Francis, D.P., and Essex, M., 1978. Infect.Dis., in press.

12. Sarngadharan, M.G., Sarin, P.S., Reitz, M.S., and Gallo, R.C., 1972. Nature N. Biol. 240, pp. 67-72.

13. Todaro, G.J., and Gallo, R.C., 1973. Nature (London), pp.206-207.

14. Jacquemin, P., Saxinger, C., and Gallo, R.C., submitted for publication.

15. Wong-Staal, F.W., et al., submitted for publication.

16. Pluznik, D.H., and Sachs, L. 1965. J. Cell Comp. Phys. 66, pp. 819-824.

17. Bradley, T.R., and Metcalf, D. 1966.Aust. J. Exp. Biol. Med. Sci, 44, pp. 287-300.

18. Gallagher, R.E., Salahuddin, S.Z., Hall, W.T., McCredie, K.B., and Gallo, R.C., Proc. Natl. Acad. Sci., 72, pp. 4137-4144.

19. Gallagher, R.E., Ruscetti, F., Collins, S. and Gallo, R.C., 1977. *Advance in Comparative Leukemia Research*. P. Bentvelzen *et al.* (eds.) Elsevier/North Holland Biomedical Press, Amsterdam, pp. 303-306.

20. Gallagher, R.E., and Gallo, R.C. 1975. *Science 187*, pp. 350-352.

21. Morgan, D.A., Ruscetti, F. and Gallo, R.C., 1976. *Science*, pp. 1007-1008.

22. Ruscetti, F.W., Morgan, D.A., and Gallo, R.C. 1977. *J. Immunol. 199*, pp. 131-138.

23. Collins, S.J., Gallo, R.C., and Gallagher, R.E. 1977. *Nature 270*, pp. 347-349.

24. Yam, L.T., Li, C.Y., and Crosby, W.H. 1971. *Am. J. Pathol, 55* pp. 283-290.

25. Collins, S.J., Ruscetti, F.W., Gallagher, R.E., and Gallo, R.C. 1978. *Proc. Natl. Acad. Sci.* 78, pp. 2458-2462.

26. Friend, C., Scher, W., Holland, J.G., and Sato, T. 1971 *Proc. Natl. Acad. Sci. 68*, pp. 378-381.

27. Moore, M.A.S., Williams, N. and Metcalf, D., 1974. *J. Cell Physiol., 79*, 283-294.

28. Lozzio, D.C., and Lozzio, B.B. 1974. *Blood 45*, pp. 321-334.

29. Klein, E., Ben-Bassat, H., Neumann, H., Ralph, P., Zeuthen, J. Pillcock, P., and Vansky, F. 1976. *Int. J. Cancer 8*, pp. 421-434.

30. Burgess, A.W., Wilson, E.M.A. and Metcalf, D. 1977. *Blood 49*, pp. 573-585.

31. Ruscetti, F.W., and Chervenick, P.A. 1975, *J. Clin Synet. 55*, pp. 520-527.

32. Robinson, W.A., and Pike, B.L. 1970 *J. Cell Physiol 76*, pp.77-84.

EXPRESSION OF c-TYPE VIRAL INFORMATION IN TISSUES OF PATIENTS WITH
PRELEUKEMIC DISORDERS: MYELOFIBROSIS AND GRANULOCYTIC SARCOMA ASSO-
CIATED WITH ACUTE MYELOMONOCYTIC LEUKEMIA (A.M.M.L) IN CHILDREN

P. Chandra, L.K. Steel, H. Laube and B. Kornhuber

Zentrum der Biologischen Chemie, Abteilung für Molekular-
Biologie,Theodor-Stern-Kai 7, Frankfurt 70, W. Germany

THE role of c-type RNA tumor viruses in leukemias and lymphomas of birds, mice and cats is now well understood. Type c
viruses have also been observed in naturally occuring tumors of subhuman primates (Theilen et al., 1971; Kawakami et al., 1972 and
Snyder et al., 1973).

In man, however, the morphological identification, or the biological activity has not yet provided a definite basis for demonstrating viruses in cells from patients with malignant diseases.
However, as a result of progress in the understanding of molecular
biology of RNA tumor viruses it has been possible to detect molecular components of these viruses in several human malignant cells
and tissues. The detection of oncornaviral reverse transcriptase
(RTase) provided the first tangible evidence for the presence of
an oncornavirus in human neoplasia (see Gallo et al., 1976). Later
its capacity to make DNA copies of the genomic RNA yielded probes
to test for the presence of viral-related RNA in a variety of human
malignant tissues. The improved methodology (Lewis et al., 1974)
has been a decisive advance in obtaining highly purified preparations of RTase, and to study their immunological behavior towards
the cellular DNA-polymerases and their relatedness to other DNA-
polymerases from RNA tumor viruses (Gallo et al., 1974).

This report describes the purification, biochemical characterization and serological analysis of a reverse transcriptase from
the spleen of a child with myelofibrosis. The fact that myelofibrosis has a preleukemic tendency was of particular interest for
us. Analogous to these studies we have found high levels of RTase
activity in the orbital tumor of a child with acute myelomonocytic
leukemia (A.M.M.L.). This tumor has been reported to be associated

177

to A.M.M.L. in children in some regions of Turkey (Cavdar et al., 1971). The tumor consists of primitive white blood cells with supportive connective tissue, stroma, and vessels. Since these tumors were devoid of the characteristic green color, and no periosteal or other bone changes were present the authors (Cavdar et al., 1971) suggest the term granulocytic sarcoma to be more appropriate than the chloroma. The striking feature is the occurence of ocular lesions before the onset of A.M.M.L., varying from 20 days to 8 months (Cavdar et al.,1971). Viral probe carried out on one orbital tumor revealed the presence of a group-specific (GS-3) antigen, previously observed in murine cells as an expression of type-c viruses (Dr. A. Cavdar, personal communication). This motivated us to look for the presence of oncornaviral RTase in these orbital tumors.

Materials and Methods
    Labelled deoxynucleoside triphosphates were from NEN-Chemicals G.m.b.H., Dreieichenhain, Germany; non-labelled deoxynucleoside triphosphates were from Calbiochem A.-G., Lucerne, Switzerland, or Boehringer Mannheim, Tutzing, Germany. Anti-(reverse transcriptase) IgG from gibbon-ape leukemia virus, simian (woolly monkey) sarcoma virus, Rauscher leukemia virus and avian myeloblastosis virus were from Litton Bionetics, Kensington, Maryland, U.S.A. Activated DNA (salmon sperm) was prepared by the method of Schlabach et al. (1971). DEAE-cellulose (DE 23) and phosphocellulose P were from Serva Chemicals, Heidelberg, Germany. DEAE-cellulose (DE 52) was obtained from Whatman Biochemical, Maidstone,Kent, U.K. DNA-cellulose was prepared from cellulose powder (2200 ff; Machery, Nagel & Co., Düren,Germany) by the method of Alberts and Herrick (1971). All operations were performed at 4 °C. Salt concentrations were determined by conductimetry.

    Spleen (1.45 kg) from a patient with osteomyelofibrosis was obtained from a girl of 2.5 years. The patient was subjected to splenectomy as part of therapeutic treatment. The spleen was immediately sectioned and frozen at -70 °C.

    Orbital tumor (9.1 g) was obtained from the Hematology Division of the Department of Pediatrics (Prof. A.O. Cavdar), Ankara University, Turkey; from a child with A.M.M.L. The tumor was immediately frozen and maintained at -70 °C until isolation procedures commenced.

    Isolation and purification of DNA polymerases: Cellular DNA polymerases, and the reverse transcriptase were extracted from tissue homogenates by the procedure of Lewis et al. (1974). The ezymes were separated by subjecting the appropriate fractions (Fig. 1) to a set of chromatographic columns, as mentioned elsewhere (Chandra and Steel, 1977).

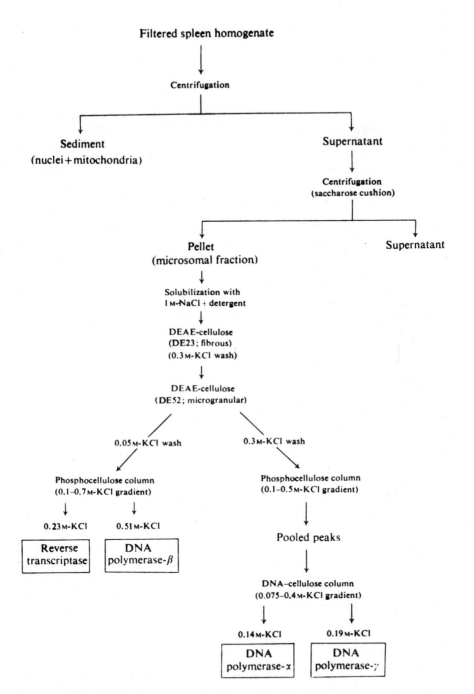

Fig. 1: Methods used to separate and isolate the DNA polymerases from human tissues (adapted from Lewis et al., 1974).

DNA polymerase assay system: Stages in the isolation and purification of the DNA polymerases were characterized by their response to various template-primer systems. Fractions were assayed for the presence of DNA polymerase activity by adding 0.25 ml of the test fraction to a volume of 0.225 ml containing 0.05M-Tris/HCl (pH 7.5 or 7.8), 1mM-dithiothreitol, 0.01 M-MgCl$_2$ or 1mM-MnCl$_2$, 0.06M- or 0.125 M- KCl, 1 uCi of ^{3}H-dGTP (192 c.p.m./pmol; for oligo dG. poly rC-primed reactions) or 1 uCi of ^{3}H-dTTP (1279 c.p.m./pmol), unlabelled 0.4 mM- dATP, -dCTP and -dGTP (0.4 mM-dTTP for oligo dG.poly rC-primed reactions) and 1 ug of the indicated template-primer (2 ug in the case of "activated" DNA). Reaction mixtures were incubated for 60 min at 37 °C (MgCl$_2$ present) or 30 °C (MnCl$_2$ present) and stopped by the addition of 0.36 mg of bovine serum albumin (BSA) and 3 ml of cold 10% (w/v) trichloroacetic acid. Acid-precipitable material was collected on Whatman glass-fibre paper discs, washed three times with 5 ml of 5 % (w/v) trichloroacetic acid, dried at 100 °C for 30 min, then suspended in 10 ml of toluene scintillator fluid (Quickszint; Zinsser, Frankfurt, Germany) and counted for radioactivity in a liquid-scintillation spectrometer.

Molecular-weight determination: Molecular weights of DNA-polymerases were estimated by ultracentrifugation using glycerol- (5-20 %), or sucrose-gradients (5-20 %). Three external protein standards, ovalbumin (mol. wt. 45,000), bovine serum albumin (mol. wt. 67,000) and aldolase (mol. wt. 147,000), were prepared at concentrations of 1 mg/ ml, and layered on parallel gradients. The gradients were centrifuged at 4 °C for 24h at 200,000g, then fractionated in 0.3 ml portions from the top by using ISCO density-gradient fractionator. DNA polymerase activity of the fractionated enzyme samples was assayed by the standard DNA polymerase assay system.

Preparation of antisera: Antiserum against the purified spleen reverse transcriptase was prepared in two female goats. Each was initially given 70 ug of enzyme emulsified with Freund´s adjuvant and injected intramuscularly. Three subsequent booster injections of 35 ug of enzyme and adjuvant were given intramuscularly at 2-week intervals. Then 10 days after the last injection, blood was obtained, IgG salt precipitated and purified on a column of Sephadex G-200. Normal goat serum IgG was assayed as a control in the enzyme neutralization assays.

RESULTS

Fig. 1 outlines the overall technique of DNA polymerase separation from myelofibrotic human spleen. DEAE-cellulose (DE 23) chromatography of the solubilized microsomal extracts removed most of the nucleic acids, as determined by the A$_{254}$ of input and effluent materials.

DEAE-cellulose (DE 52) chromatography of the effluent from DEAE-cellulose (DE 23) chromatography resulted in the elution of DNA polymerase-β and reverse transcriptase in the column void volume and 0.05 M-KCl wash, as determined by assay of samples in the DNA-polymerase assay system. DNA polymerase assay of a sample of the 0.3M-KCl wash showed the activities of DNA polymerase-α and-γ .

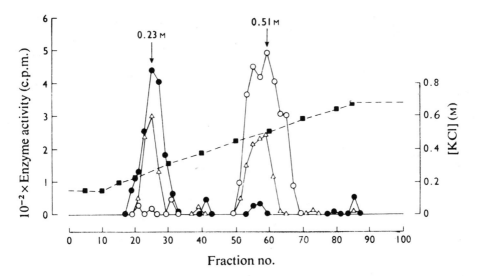

Fig.2. Phosphocellulose chromatography of material eluted from the the DEAE-cellulose (DE 52) column with the 0.05M-KCl wash.

DNA-polymerase activity was measured utilizing poly rA.oligo dT (filled circles), poly dA.oligo dT (open circles) or poly-dA-poly dT (open triangles) as template-primer with Manganese ions and 0.06M-KCl present. Resolution of the RTase (eluting at 0.23M-KCl) and DNA polymerase-ß (eluting at 0.51M-KCl) was was achieved; KCl concentration is depicted by the hatched line (filled squares).

When the 0.05M-KCl wash was chromatographed on phosphocellulose, adequate separation of DNA polymerase-β and reverse transcriptase was achieved. DNA polymerase assay of fractions (Fig. 2) indicated two distinct peaks of activity: reverse transcriptase was eluted at 0.23M-KCl concentration and DNA polymerase- β was eluted at 0.51M-KCl.

Phosphocellulose chromatography of the 0.3M-KCl-wash from DEAE-(DE 52) chromatography resulted in two overlapping peaks of activity

DNA polymerase assay of samples indicated that DNA polymerase-α and -γ were eluted at a concentration of 0.27–0.40 M-KCl. The peaks were pooled and further chromatographed on DNA-cellulose. The DNA polymerase assay of samples from the DNA-cellulose column is shown in Fig.3. Resolution of the two enzymes was achieved: DNA polymerase - α was eluted at a concentration of 0.13 M-KCl and DNA polymerase-γ was eluted at 0.19M-KCl.

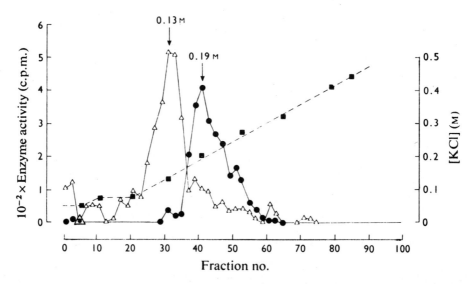

Fig.3. DNA-cellulose chromatography of the 0.34M-KCl peak (DNA-polymerases α andγ) from the phosphocellulose column.

DNA polymerase activity was measured with "activated"DNA (magnesium ions and 0.06M-KCl present) open triangles; or poly rA. oligo dT (Manganese ions and 0.125M-KCl present) filled circles. DNA polymerase-α (eluted at a concentration of 0.13M-KCl) and DNA polymerase-γ (eluted at a concentration of 0.19M-KCl) were adequately separated; KCl concentration is depicted by the hatched line (filled squares).

Molecular-weight determination: Results of the glycerol-gradient centrifugation of the purified spleen reverse transcriptase and three protein standard markers are shown in Fig.4. The apparent molecular weight of the enzyme, assuming a globular shape, is approx. 70,000. Disc-gel electrophoresis of the enzyme demonstrated a mobilitycorresponding to that of bovine serum albumin, further varifying the glycerol-gradient value of 70,000 daltons for the enzyme.This determination agrees with the reported molecular weight of reverse transcriptases isolated from other mammalian type-c viruses(Grandgenett et al., 1972; Tronick et al., 1972; Abrell and Gallo, 1973;

Gallo et al., 1975; Mondal et al., 1975; Witkin et al, 1975)and from
human breast cancer particles (Ohno et al., 1977).However, in contrast
with the reverse transcriptase of leukemic cells, where two size
classes of 70,000 and 130,000 daltons have been reported (Mondal et
al., 1975), only one molecular species of 70,000 daltons could be detected in the human myelofibrotic spleen.

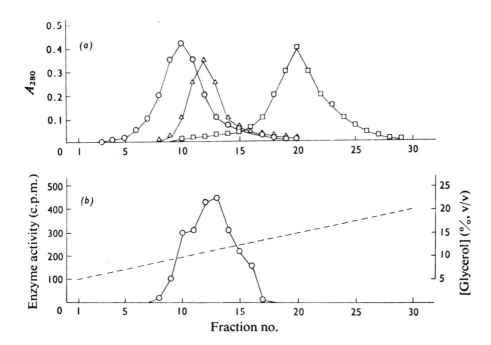

Fig.4. Velocity sedimentation of the reverse transcriptase isolated
       from spleen and three protein markers on a glycerol gradient.

*About 30 equal fractions were collected from the top of the
tube for each gradient. (a) A_{280} of protein standard fractions.
circles:Ovalbumin (mol.wt. 45,000); triangles:bovine serum
albumin (mol.wt. 67,000); squares: aldolase (mol.wt. 147,000).
(b) ^3H-dGMP incorporation in the DNA polymerase assay system
(details given in the text); Glycerol concentration in the
gradient is depicted by the hatched line (b)-*

        Molecular-weight determination of the cellular DNA polymerases
is shown in Fig. 5. The sucrose - gradient centrifugation of DNA
polymerase-β indicated a mol. wt. of approx. 40,000. Other labora -
tories (Smith and Gallo, 1972; Sedwick et al., 1972; Chang, 1973;
Lewis et al., 1974) have reported mol. wts. of 40,000- 45,000 for
the enzyme. DNA polymerase - γ sucrose-gradient centrifugation indicated a mol. wt. of 100,000 - 110,000. Lewis et al. (1974) have

reported a value of approx. 10^5 daltons for this enzyme isolated from human lymphoblastoid cells. DNA polymerase - α demonstrated an approx. mol. wt. of 150,000. Similar findings for this enzyme have been reported by Sedwick et al. (1972), Smith and Gallo (1972), Lewis et al. (1974 a) and Loeb (1974).

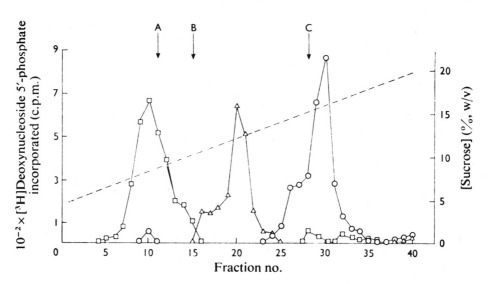

Fig. 5. Velocity sedimentation of the cellular DNA polymerases isolated from spleen on sucrose gradients.

About 40 equal fractions were collected from the top of the tube for each gradient. DNA polymerase- α (circles) was assayed with "activated" DNA; DNA polymerase-ß (squares) assayed with poly dA.oligo dT; and DNA polymerase-γ assayed with poly rA.oligo dT (triangles). A, Ovalbumin (mol. wt. 45,000); B, bovine serum albumin (mol. wt. 67,000); C, aldolase (mol. wt. 147,000).

BIVALENT CATIONIC, IONIC AND TEMPLATE REQUIREMENTS: Table 1 summarizes the preferences of the cellular polymerases and reverse transcriptases for magnesium or manganese cations in the presence of various template-primers. DNA polymerase -α required "activated" DNA in the presence of magnesium ions, and poly (dA-dT) with either bivalent cation. This specificity of deoxyribose-template systems is a characteristic of the response in vitro of this enzyme, i.e. it preferentially transcribes poly (dA), and poorly poly rA, or poly rC (Sedwick et al., 1972; Loeb, 1974; Lewis et al., 1974).DNA polymerase - α was also sensitive to high ionic strength and pH. The

TABLE 1

Bivalent cation and template specificities of the cellular DNA polymerases and reverse transcriptase isolated from human myelofibrotic spleen

Reactions were performed as described for the DNA polymerase assay system. Reactions containing the reverse transcriptase enzyme were carried out at pH 7.5, with DNA polymerase-α at pH 7.5 and DNA polymerase-β and -γ at pH 7.8. All reactions with DNA polymerase-α and those with the template-primer 'activated' DNA contained 0.06 M-KCl; all others contained 0.125 M-KCl.

Template	Bivalent cation	[³H]Deoxynucleoside 5'-phosphate incorporated (pmol mg of protein)			
		Reverse transcriptase	DNA polymerase-α	DNA polymerase-β	DNA polymerase-γ
Poly(rA)·(dT)$_{12}$	Mn^{2+}	1355.0	16.9	13.1	1015.0
	Mg^{2+}	1714.0	10.1	6.3	770.1
Poly(dA)·(dT)$_{10}$	Mn^{2+}	7.9	0.1	572.4	0.1
	Mg^{2+}	0.1	37.1	553.5	424.6
Poly[d(A–T)]	Mn^{2+}	38.5	503.2	94.4	710.3
	Mg^{2+}	224.5	597.6	173.0	188.7
Poly(rC)·oligo(dG)	Mn^{2+}	2060.1	24.0	0.1	56.1
	Mg^{2+}	1628.3	0.1	0.1	37.4
'Activated' DNA	Mg^{2+}	30.8	1844.4	36.7	728.6

enzyme functioned best at pH 7.5 and at 60 mM-KCl. This agrees with
the findings of Bollum (1960), who found DNA polymerase-α to function
optimally at pH 7.0 - 7.5 and at low ionic strength.

DNA polymerase-β preferentially transcribed poly dA.oligo dT,
and showed a preference for high ionic st-ength and pH, which agrees
with the higher pH optima and stimulation by high ionic strength reported by Sedwick et al. (1972 a). The template - primer specificities of DNA polymerase-γ are similar to those reported by Fridlender et al. (1972), Loeb (1974) and Lewis et al. (1974).

The reverse transcriptase from myelofibrotic spleen showed a
strong preference for poly rC.oligo dG and poly rA. oligo dT,chara-
cteristic for mammalian c-type oncornavirus DNA polymerase (Baltimore
and Smoler, 1971). Optimal activities were obtained when the KCl
cncentration was 60 - 125 mM at pH 7.5. Variations in the manganese
cation concentration showed optimal activities between 0.8 and 1.0 mM.
The magnesium cation concentration was also tested (0-18 mM) and the
optimal concentration was found to be 8 - 12 mM.The absence of terminal transferase activity in the purified enzyme preparation was indicated by the RNase-digestion experiments, and the inability of oligo-
dG, or oligo-dA alone to catalyze the incorporation of ^{3}H-dGMP.Varying
the concentration of template-primer poly rC.oligo dG, the K_m-value
of this reverse transcriptase obtained was 1.82×10^{-5}M.

The purified reverse transcriptase was able to transcribe the
heteropolymeric regions of a 70s RNA from R(Mu)LV, as shown in Table
2.

T A B L E   2

TRANSCRIPTION OF HETEROPOLYMERIC REGIONS OF A 70 S-
RNA FROM R(MU)LV

| Template-Primer | ^{3}H-dNMP Incorporation into DNA by (pmoles/ 60 min./mg protein) | | | |
| | Polymerase (γ) | | Rev.-Transcript. | |
	dGMP	dTMP	dGMP	dTMP
70s RNA	0.01	13.70	4.90	74.70
70s RNA + oligo dT	0.01	0.01	43.40	146.40
Oligo dT	0.01	0.01	0.01	0.01

R (Mu)LV= Rauscher murine leukemia virus

T A B L E   3

RESPONSES OF THE DNA-POLYMERASES ISOLATED FROM SPLEEN
TO MYELOFIBROTIC SPLEEN ANTI-(REVERSE TRANSCRIPTASE)IgG

Myelofibrotic spleen anti-(reverse transcriptase) IgG and pre-immune (control) IgG were prepared to concentration of 8,16,32 and 64 ug in 0.05M-Tris/HCl, pH 7.8. A portion (0.025 ml) of each polymerase was preincubated with an equal volume of IgG for 40 min. at 4 °C, and subsequently assayed for the enzyme activity, as described under "materials and methods".

Spleen anti-rev.transcriptase IgG (µg)	Percentage of Inhibition[x] of enzyme activity			
	α	β	γ	RTase
8	O	O	O	35.7
16	O	O	1.7	49.0
32	O	O	12.8	71.2
64	O	O	15.0	78.1

(x) *Data expressed as the percentage of inhibition of the DNA polymerase tested with immune IgG compared with the same quantity of preimmune (control)IgG.*

SEROLOGICAL STUDIES WITH THE SPLEEN REVERSE TRANSCRIPTASE:

Table 3 summarizes the responses of the cellular DNA polymerases and reverse transcriptase when challenged with various concentrations of the anti (spleen reverse transcriptase)IgG. DNA polymerases α and β showed no inhibition at concentrations of 8-64ug of IgG, whereas DNA polymerase-γ was inhibited slightly (15% with 64 ug of IgG). Splenic reverse transcriptase was strongly inhibited by the anti-(spleen reverse transcriptase) IgG (78.1 % inhibition with 64 ug of IgG). These results support the idea that the isolated reverse transcriptase is a unique, immunologically distinct, DNA polymerase of the human spleen from a patient with myelofibrotic syndrome.

Table 4 shows the results of antibody inhibition studies with reverse transcriptases isolated from simian sarcoma virus,gibbon-ape leukemia virus and avian myeloblastosis virus utilizing antisera against the spleen reverse transcriptase.

T A B L E 4

Responses of reverse transcriptase from other sources to the myelofibrotic spleen anti-(reverse transcriptase) IgG

Pre-immune (control) and immune anti-(myelofibrotic spleen reverse transcriptase) IgG were prepared at concentrations of 4–64 μg per 0.025 ml of 0.05 M-Tris/HCl, pH 7.5. Gibbon-ape leukaemia virus reverse transcriptase and avian myeloblastosis virus reverse transcriptase were prepared at concentrations of 1 μg per 0.025 ml of 0.05 M-Tris/HCl. pH 7.5. Simian sarcoma (woolly monkey) virus reverse transcriptase was prepared at a concentration of 0.032 μg per 0.025 ml of Tris/HCl, pH 7.5, and myelofibrotic spleen reverse transcriptase was prepared at a concentration of 0.5 μg per 0.025 ml of Tris/HCl, pH 7.5. Each reverse transcriptase was incubated for 16 h at 4 C with an equal volume (4–64 μg) of pre-immune or immune IgG. Remaining activity was measured in a DNA polymerase assay as described in the text (total incubation volume 0.15 ml).

Source of reverse transcriptase	Template-primer	Spleen anti-(reverse transcriptase) IgG (μg)	Percentage of inhibition*				
		...	4	8	16	32	64
Simian sarcoma virus	Poly(rA)·(dT)$_{12}$		4.2	11.8	30.2	54.0	51.0
Gibbon-ape leukaemia virus	Poly(rA)·(dT)$_{12}$		0	0	5.7	12.6	22.2
Avian myeloblastosis virus	Poly(rA)·(dT)$_{12}$		0	0	1.1	6.7	7.7
Human spleen	Poly(rC)·oligo(dG)		19.8	35.7	49.0	71.2	78.1

* Data expressed as the percentage of inhibition of the reverse transcriptase tested with immune IgG compared with the same quantity of pre-immune (control) IgG.

The data (Table 4) show inhibition of the simian sarcoma virus
and gibbon-ape leukemia virus enzymes of 51 % and 22.2 % respectively,
at 64 ug of IgG. Avian myeloblastosis virus reverse transcriptase
was not significantly inhibited. It would appear that the reverse
transcriptase isolated from human spleen is antigenically related
to the simian sarcoma virus enzyme, and the gibbon-ape leukemia virus
enzyme to a lesser extent. This was supported by experiments done
with anti-reverse transcriptase IgG fractions from simian sarcoma
virus, gibbon-ape leukemia virus and other tumor c-type viruses (see
for details, Chandra and Steel, 1977). The anti-reverse transcriptase
IgG from simian sarcoma virus inhibited the splenic enzyme by 76.3 %
with 64 ug of IgG, whereas gibbon-ape leukemia virus anti-reverse
transcriptase IgG inhibited the splenic reverse transcriptase by
60.4 % with 64 ug of IgG. The anti-reverse transcriptase IgG from
two non-primate sources, avian myeloblastosis virus and Rauscher
leukemia virus, had a very low inhibitory effect.

Data from other laboratories further support these observations.
Reverse transcriptase isolated from human acute-myeloblastic-leukemia
cells has shown cross-reactivity only with gibbon-ape leukemia virus
and simian sarcoma virus (Todaro and Gallo, 1973). Simian sarcoma
virus was found to be the closest to, but not identical with Hl23V-1,
a human leukemia virus purified from long-term cultures of myeloid
cells from a leukemic patient (Teich et al., 1975).

Anti-reverse transcriptase IgG to myelofibrotic spleen was
able to partially neutralize the reverse transcriptase activity from
human leukemic cells (unpublished results). Gallo et al. (in this
volume) have isolated, from plasma membranes of blood and bone marrow
cells of patients with acute myelogenous leukemia, natural antibodies
that consistently react very strongly with reverse transcriptase from
HL23-virus, isolated from an acute myelogenous leukemia patient.
Using our enzyme, they found that these antibodies have a very strong
neutralizing effect on the splenic reverse transcriptase. This again
suggests that the reverse transcriptase from an acute myelogenous
leukemia patient, and our reverse transcriptase from a patient with
a preleukemic disease, are antigenically similar.

SEROLOGICAL IDENTIFICATION OF REVERSE TRANSCRIPTASE IN LEUKEMIC CELLS
FROM PATIENTS, USING ANTI-(REVERSE TRANSCRIPTASE) IgG FROM MYELOFIBRO-
TIC SPLEEN.

An examination of leukemic cells from a large number of patients
for reverse transcriptase activity showed that only some of them,
approx. one-third, contained detectable amounts of the enzyme activity (Bhattacharyya et al., 1973). Using a more sensitive assay procedure for reverse transcriptase by semi-automated chromatography
through a multiple column system, the same laboratory reported the

presence of reverse transcriptase activity in white blood cells of
eight patients out of twelve having acute myelogenous leukemia (
Gallo et al., 1976). The success in detecting reverse transcriptase
activity in leucocytes of leukemic patients indirectly by the simultaneous detection test is even higher (Spiegelman, 1976); of the
23 patients examined, 22 showed clear evidence for the presence of
reverse transcriptase activity. It was therefore,of interest to
examine the presence of reverse transcriptase activity in leukemic
cells of patients immunologically, using antibodies to reverse transcriptase from the myelofibrotic spleen.

Fig. 6.   Immunofluorescence of reverse transcriptase in bone
marrow cells of an ALL patient (Sandwich technique).

    Leukemic patients studied were children (2 - 15 years) ad-
mitted to the Department of Pediatric Oncology, Frankfurt University Medical School, Germany. The bone marrow smears were fixed with
formaldehyde and acetone. The smears were covered with a suspension
containing anti-(reverse transcriptase) IgG from myelofibrotic spleen,
and left for one hr at room temperature. The suspension was decanted,
and the smears were washed with phosphate-buffered saline. The smears
were then covered with a suspension containing rabbit-anti goat(IgG)
conjugated to FITC (RAG-FITC), and left at room temperature for one
hr. The suspension was decanted, and the smears were washed again
with phosphate buffered saline. These smears were examined under a

fluorescence microscope (Fig. 6). Of the 25 patients examined in the active phase of the disease, all 25 showed immunofluorescence.Smears prepared from leucocytes of normal healthy persons, treated identically, gave no immunofluorescence. Further trials are being carried out to look for reverse transcriptase in cells of persons at various stages of remission.

REVERSE TRANSCRIPTASE ACTIVITY IN AN ORBITAL TUMOR ASSOCIATED TO ACUTE MYELOMONOCYTIC LEUKEMIA IN CHILDREN.

Chloroma-like ocular lesions in Turkish children with acute myelomonocytic leukemia (AMML) have been reported by Cavdar et al. (1971); these lesions account for approx. one-third of the cases suffering from AMML. The eye lesions consisted of orbital tumor, exophthalmos, proptosis, chemosis, corneal opacity, and swollen eye lids. The authors believe that the term chloroma is not suited to these orbital tumors, since a) the tumors were devoid of the characteristic green color, b) no periosteal or other bone changes were present, and c) no greyish color was observed in the bone marrow. For these reasons, the authors suggest the term granulo-cytic sarcoma (Cavdar et al., 1971).In most cases, the ocular lesions were noted before the diagnosis of leukemia; varying from 20 days to 8 months before the onset of leukemic disease.Viral probe carried out on one orbital tumor revealed the presence of a group-specific (GS-3) antigen, previously observed in murine cells, as an expression of type-c virus (Cavdar, Dr.A.O.:personal communication). This motivated us to look for the presence of reverse transcriptase activity in the orbital tumor associated to AMML.

Approximately 9.1g of the orbital tumor was combined with 90 ml of buffer containing 50 mM tris/HCl (pH 7.5), 1 mM dithiothreitol (DTT), 0.5 mM EDTA and 5 mM magnesium chloride; then homogenized for 5 min at low speed and 8 min at high speed in a Waring blendor (ice-water cooled). The suspension was filtered through a monolayer of nylon stocking then centrifuged at 900g and 10,000g to remove the nuclei and mitochondria. The resulting supernatant was layered on to a 25 % w/w saccharose cushion (in homogenizing buffer) and centrifuged at 171,000g for 2 hr. The microsomal pellet obtained was used to extract the reverse transcriptase activity. The methods employed in the isolation and purification of reverse transcriptase are essentially the same, as described in chart 1 (Fig. 1).

The phosphocellulose column adequately separated the RNA-directed DNA polymerase activity from the other DNA polymerase activities, as shown in Fig. 7. DNA polymerase assay of fractions, employing poly rA. oligo dT as template-primer, showed the peak enzyme activity eluted from the phosphocellulose column with 0.21 M KCl in buffer.

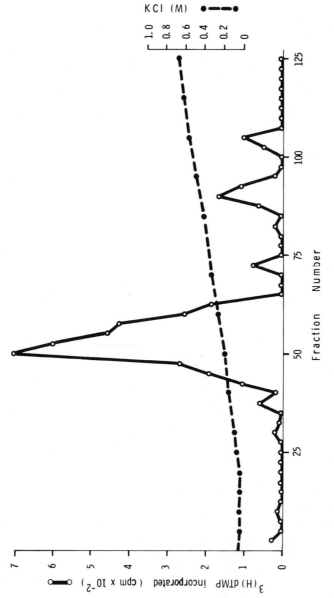

FIG. 7 Phosphocellulose chromatography of material eluted from DEAE-
cellulose (DE52) column with the 0.05 M-KCl wash.

*Fractions were assayed for DNA polymerase activity as described
in the experimental section, utilizing poly rA.oligo dT as template-
primer. Reverse transcriptase activity of the orbital tumor was eluted
at 0.21M KCl concentration.*

TABLE 5

DNA-POLYMERASE ACTIVITIES AT VARIOUS PURIFICATION STEPS

DNA polymerase assays were carried out at 30°C for 60 min in a reaction mixture of 0.05 ml, which contained: 50 mM Tris/HCl pH 7.8, 60 mM KCl, 0.4 mM MnCl₂, or 8 mM MgCl₂ and 1 mM DTT. The primer template conc. used was 50 ug/ml; other conditions are same as under materials and methods. Numbers in brackets give the endogenous incorporation.

SOURCE OF PROTEIN AND PROTEIN CONTENT	TEMPLATE-PRIMER: DIVALENT CATION: Activity and Purification	$(dT)_{12-18} \cdot (A)_n$ Mn++	Mg++	$(dG)_{12-18} \cdot (C)_n$ Mn++	Mg++	$(dT)_{10} \cdot (dA)_n$ Mn++	Mg++
Crude Tumor Homogenate (I)	Total[2]	9248.73	7339.43	2307.07	1398.83	11827.17	3145.97
6710 mg/90 ml	Specific[3]	1.38 (0.12)	1.09 (0.02)	0.35 (0.08)	0.21 (0.09)	1.76	0.47
	Purification fold	1.0	1.0	1.0	1.0	1.0	1.0
Disrupted Microsomal Pellet (II)	Total	1443.17	985.72	1248.91	1061.03	1328.34	272.48
38.0 mg/25 ml	Specific	37.98 (0.66)	25.94 (0.03)	32.87 (0.79)	27.92 (1.71)	34.56	7.17
	Purification fold	27.52	23.80	93.91	132.95	19.28	15.29
0.35 M KCl Eluate off DEAE 23 Cellulose (III)	Total	1122.46	465.24	281.49	883.58	892.64	213.0
15.84 mg/36 ml	Specific	70.86	29.37	17.77	55.78	56.35	13.45
	Purification fold	51.35	26.94	50.77	265.62	31.96	28.67
0.07 M KCl Eluate off DEAE 52 Cellulose (IV)	Total	573.84	204.36	255.43	80.28	264.03	57.22
0.525 mg/21 ml	Specific	1093.03	389.26	486.53	152.91	502.92	108.99
	Purification fold	792.05	357.12	1390.09	728.14	285.26	232.39
0.21 M KCl Eluate off Phospho-cellulose (V)	Total	38.38	6.46	4.69	1.56	0.01	<0.01
0.01 mg/2 ml	Specific	3838.07	646.16	469.16	156.38	1.14	<0.01
	Purification fold	2781.21	592.81	1340.46	744.67	0.64	<0.5

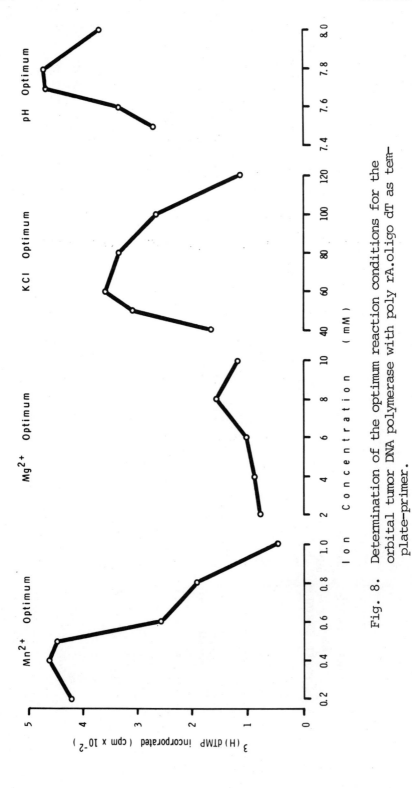

Fig. 8. Determination of the optimum reaction conditions for the
orbital tumor DNA polymerase with poly rA.oligo dT as template-primer.

*Reactions were performed under conditions described in Fig.7,
varying the ionic concentration, or pH.*

The activities of orbital tumor DNA polymerase at various steps of purification, using different template-primers are documented in Table 5.

The single peak of activity eluted from the phosphocellulose column at 0.21 M salt concentration(Fraction V, Table 5),represents a 1340-fold purification over the enzyme activity of the crude homogenate using poly rC. oligo dG as the template-primer, and 2781-fold purification using poly rA-oligo dT.

T A B L E 6

PRIMER-TEMPLATE ACTIVITIES OF THE ORBITAL TUMOR RNA-DEPENDENT DNA POLYMERASE

Assays were carried out for 60 min as described in Materials and Methods. The primer-template concentration used was 50 ug/ml; R(Mu)LV-70s RNA was used at a concentration of 20 ug per ml; and $(dT)_{12-18}$ at a concentration 20 ug/ml whre indicated. ^3H-dTTP was used as the labelled substrate for activated DNA, poly rA.oligo dT, poly dA.oligo dT, R(Mu)LV-70s RNA and oligo-dT. ^3HdGTP was used as the labelled substrate for $(dG)_{12-18}$, poly rC. oligo dG and poly rC(OMe). oligo dG. NT= not tested.

PRIMER-TEMPLATE	^{3}H- dNMP incorporated	
	(p moles/ mg protein / 60 minutes)	
divalent cation:	Mn^{2+}	Mg^{2+}
activated DNA	0. 31	0. 68
Poly rA.oligo dT	3476. 11	603. 07
Poly dA.oligo dT	1. 14	0. 01
Poly rC.oligo dG	461. 01	174. 92
Poly rC(OMe).oligo dG	53. 33	3. 95
Oligo dG	0. 1	NT
R(Mu)LV 70s RNA	138. 22	NT
R(Mu)LV 70s RNA+oligo dT	262. 61	NT
Oligo dT	0. 01	NT

The optimum reaction conditions for the orbital reverese transcriptase activity with poly rA. oligo dT as template-primer are shown
in Fig. 8. The Mn^{++} optimum for this reverse transcriptase is around
0.4 mM and that for Mg^{++} is 8 mM. The KCl optimum is 60 mM, and the
optimum pH of this enzyme is around 7.8.

As shown in Table 6 the purified reverse transcriptase from the
orbital tumor efficiently utilizes poly rA. oligo dT, poly rC.
oligo dG and poly rC(OMe). oligo dG as template primers; whereas, the
template primer poly dA. oligo dT is completely ineffective in this
system. These characteristics are similar to those reported for
reverse transcriptases purified from other mammalian RNA tumor viruses.
Furthermore, the data clearly indicate the failure of the purified
orbital reverse transcriptase to utilze oligo dG and oligo dT as an
initiator, concluding that this enzyme does not contain any terminal
deoxynucleotidyl transferase activity.The ability of the purified

T A B L E   7

PRELIMINARY RESULTS OF THE EFFECT OF VARIOUS TYPE-C VIRUS
DNA POLYMERASE ANTIBODIES ON THE REVERSE TRANSCRIPTASE OF
THE ORBITAL TUMOR

SOURCE OF DNA-POLYMERASE	SPECIFIC ANTI-REVERSE TRANSCRIPTASE (IgG) ADDED				
	IgG (ug)	Pre-immune IgG	anti-RLV RT IgG	anti-AMV RT IgG	anti-GaLV RT IgG
		^{3}H-dTMP incorporation (% of Enzyme Activity[a])				
SiSV- 1	8	93.4	91.2	94.5	17.4
	13	101	NT	NT	23.0
	32	101	79.0	NT	21.0
Orbital Tumor from AMML Patient	8	98.2	94.0	97.8	NT
	13	103	NT	NT	44.3
	32	114	93.2	NT	40.2

*Orbital tumor DNA polymerase (10 ul) was incubated with 10 ul of
non-immune rabbit sera IgG,or the indicated immune sera IgG at 4 °C
for 4 h, before assaying for the enzyme activity. For comaprison,
SiSV-1 reverse transcriptase was similarly challenged with immune and
non-immune sera. a) the % of ^{3}H-TMP incorporation expresses activity,
compared to that of enzyme without IgG. NT = not tested.*

enzyme to utilize 70s RNA from R(Mu)LV as template, and its stimulation by the primer oligo dT strengthen the belief that, the orbital reverse transcriptase is similar to the reverse transcriptases from known RNA tumor viruses.However, the final proof of its oncornaviral nature comes from the immunological studies, in which antibodies prepared against DNA polymerase from some RNA tumor viruses were tested for cross reaction towards the reverse transcriptase purified from the orbital tumor (Table 7)

As shown in Table 7, the DNA polymerases from SiSV-1 and the human orbital tumor are strongly inhibited by antibodies to gibbon-virus enzyme (GaLV-DNA polymerase). The cross reaction of SiSV-1 DNA polymerase with GaLV-DNA polymerase antibodies, used for comparative conclusions in our experiments, has been reported by Sarin and Gallo (1976). However, no cross reaction of the orbital enzyme was found with DNA polymerases from avian myeloblastosis virus (AMV), or Rauscher murine leukemia virus (RLV).

The immunological data reported in Table 7 are preliminary in the sense, that these studies require repetition. Due to very low amounts of the purified enzyme it was not possible to continue these studies further; however with the availability of more tumor material the immunological studies will be elaborated.

A C K N O W L E D G M E N T S

The authors wish to thank Dr. Robert C. Gallo (National Cancer Institute, MD, U.S.A.) for communicating unpublished results (prepublication manuscripts) to us, and for valuable discussions. We are grateful to Litton Bionetics, Kensington, MD., U.S.A., and to Dr. Jack Gruber (National Cancer Institute, MD, U.S.A.) for the gift of antisera against the DNA polymerases from RNA tumor viruses. We also thank Dr. H. Sonneborn (Biotest, Frankfurt) for his assistance in preparing antibodies against the splenic reverse transcriptase. We are indebted to Professor A.O.Cavdar, University of Ankara, for the availability of orbital tumor specimen.

This work was supported by the Stiftung Volkswagenwerk (grant No. 14 0305).

R E F E R E N C E S

1. ABRELL, J.W. & R.C. GALLO (1973): J. Virol. 12 , 431.
2. ALBERTS, B.M. & G. HERRICK (1971): Methods Enzymol. 21, 198.
3. BALTIMORE, D. & D. SMOLER (1971): Proc.Natl.Acad.Sci.U.S. 68,1507.
4. BHATTACHARYAA, J., M.XUMA, M. REITZ, P. SARIN & R.C. GALLO (1973) Biochem. Biophys. Res. Commun. 54, 324.

5. BOLLUM, F.J. (1960): J. Biol. Chem. 235, 2399.
6. CAVDAR,A.O., A. ARCASOY, S.GÖZDASOGLU & B.DEMIRAG (1971): The Lancet April 3, 1971, 680.
7. CHANDRA, P. & L.K. STEEL (1977): Biochem. J. 167, 513.
8. CHANG, L.M.S. (1973): J. Biol. Chem. 248, 3789.
9. FRIDLENDER, B., M. FRY, A. BOLDEN & A. WEISSBACH (1972): Proc. Natl.Acad.Sci.,U.S. 69, 452.
10. GALLO, R.C., R.G. SMITH, D.H. GILLESPIE and R.E. GALLAGHAR (1974) Advances in Biosci. 14, 547.
11. GALLO, R.C., R.E. GALLAGHER,N.R. MILLER, H. MONDAL, W.C. - SAXINGER, R.J. MAYER, R.G. SMITH & O.H. GILLESPIE (1975): Cold Spring Harbor Symp. Quant. Biol. 39, 933.
12. GALLO, R.C., W.C. SAXINGER, R.E. GALLAGHER,D.H. GILLESPIE, F.- RUSCETTI, M.S. REITZ, G.S. AULAKH and F. WONG-STAAL (1976): Cold Spring Harbor Symp. Quant. Biol. on "Origins of Human Cancer", Sept. 7-14, 1976, in press.
13. GRANDGENETT, D.P., G.F. GERARD & M. GREEN (1972): J. Virol. 10, 1136.
14. KAWAKAMI, T., S.D. HUFF, P.M. BUCKLEY,D.J. DUNGWORTH, S.P.- SNYDER and R.V. GILDEN (1972): Nature(New Biol) 235, 170.
15. LEWIS, B.J., J.W. ABRELL, R.G. SMITH & R.C. GALLO (1974): Biochim. Biophys. Acta 349, 148.
16. LOEB, L.A. (1974): Enzymes 10, 173.
17. MONDAL, H., R.E. GALLAGHER & R.C. GALLO (1975): Proc. Natl. Acad. Sci., U.S. 72, 1194.
18. OHNO, T., R.W. SWEET, R.HU, D. DEJAK & S. SPIEGELMAN (1977): Proc.Natl.Acad.Sci., U.S.74 , 764.
19. SARIN,P.S. & R.C. GALLO (1976): Biochim. Biophys. Acta 454,212.
20. SCHLABACH, A., B.FRIDLENDER, A. BOLDEN, & A. WEISSBACH (1971): Biochem.Biophys.Res.Commun. 44, 879.
21. SEDWICK,W., T. WANG & D. KORN (1972): J.Biol.Chem. 247, 5026.
22. SEDWICK,W., T. WANG & D. KORN (1972 a): J.Biol.Chem. 247, 7948.
23. SMITH,R.G. & R.C. GALLO (1972):Proc.Natl.Acad.Sci.,U.S. 69,2879.
24. SNYDER, S.P., D.L.DUNGWORTH, T.G.KAWAKAMI, E. CALLAWAY & D. LAU (1973): J. Natl. Cancer Inst. 51, 89.
25. SPIEGELMAN,S. (1976) in: Modern Trends in Human Leukemia II (Edts. R.Neth,R.C.Gallo,K.Mannweiler & W.C.Moloney),J.F.Lehmann Verlag. München, p. 391.
26. TEICH, N.M., R.WEISS, S.SALAHUDDIN, R.E.GALLAGHER, D.GILLESPIE & R.C. GALLO (1975): Nature (London) 256, 551.
27. THEILEN, G.H., D. GOULD, M. FOWLER & D.L. DUNGWORTH (1971): J. Natl. Cancer Inst. 47, 881.
28. TODARO, G.J. & R.C. GALLO (1973): Nature (London) 244, 206.
29. TRONICK,S., E. SCOLNICK & W. PARKS (1972):J.Virol. 10, 885.
30. WITKIN, S., T. OHNO & S. SPIEGELMAN (1975): Proc. Natl. Acad. Sci., U.S. 72, 4133.

IMMUNITY IN MAN AGAINST C-TYPE TUMOR VIRUS ANTIGENS:

A PROGRESS REPORT

Reinhard Kurth[1], Adolfine Huesgen[1] and Natalie M. Teich[2]

[1] Friedrich-Miescher-Laboratorium
Max Planck Gesellschaft
7400 Tübingen
West Germany

[2] Imperial Cancer Research Fund
Lincoln's Inn Fields
London WC2A 3PX
England

INTRODUCTION

The dogma that oncogenic type C retroviruses exist only in lower animals had to be abolished with the isolation of the simian sarcoma virus (SSV) / simian sarcoma associated virus (SSAV) complex from a fibrosarcoma of a woolly monkey (Wolfe et al., 1971). This discovery, as well as subsequent isolations of C-type viruses from other subhuman primates like baboons (baboon endogenous virus, BEV; Benveniste et al., 1974) and gibbons (gibbon ape leukemia virus, GALV; Kawakami et al., 1972) initiated yet another wave of attempts to demonstrate C-type viruses in man. Much evidence has accumulated for the presence of retrovirus particles, virus antigens, reverse transcriptase and viral nucleic acids in both normal and malignant human tissues (for references see Kurth and Mikschy, 1978). These initially positive results subsequently met with some scepticism when other laboratories reported negative results concerning tumor viral footprints in human cells (Charman et al., 1974; Sarma et al., 1974; Stephenson and Aaronson, 1976).

Another approach for the study of viral infection is to screen sera for the presence of anti-viral antibody which may indicate previous infection. In several species where C-type viruses have clearly been demonstrated naturally occurring antibodies are widespread among adult animals (Weiss and Biggs, 1972; Ihle et al.,

1974; Essex, 1975; Kawakami et al., 1973; Aoki et al., 1976).

We have used this approach to investigate human sera for the presence of IgG-antibodies reactive with antigens of BEV and the SSV(SSAV) complex. In initial experiments (Kurth et al., 1977) detergent-lysed, iodinated virus preparations were used as antigens in indirect radioimmunoprecipitation assays (RIPA) with human sera. These experiments suggested the presence of anti-viral antibodies in the majority of sera obtained from healthy blood donors.

In subsequent investigations, metabolically labeled virus antigen preparations (Kurth and Schmitt, 1977) as well as purified virus polypeptides (Kurth et al., 1978; Kurth and Mikschy, 1978) were employed and shown to react with antibodies in normal human sera.

Analogous to the situation in animals, it is the 70 000 daltons virus envelope glycoprotein (abbreviated gp70) which is predominantly recognized by human sera. In a few instances, two other major viral structural proteins of 28 000 daltons (p28) and 15 000 daltons (p15) are also precipitable by human antibodies.

In this communication, immunological parameters are described which influence the precipitation of the recently purified (Thiel et al., 1977) gp70 envelope glycoprotein of the SSV(SSAV) complex. We will also discuss experimental difficulties which may help to explain why these human antitumor virus antibodies were originally somewhat difficult to detect.

EXPERIMENTAL APPROACH AND ARTEFACTS

Radioimmunoprecipitation assays are presently the most sensitive immunological techniques for the detection of antigens in solution, as it is possible to detect as little as 0.01 ng protein antigen when such antigens are radioactively labeled with ^{125}iodine to specific activities of $> 10^8$ cpm/µg of protein. However, in our hands, labeling of purified virus antigens to such high specific activities usually resulted in a drastic loss of immunogenicity as judged by the reduced proportion that remains immunoprecipitable. Therefore we prefer to label purified virus polypeptides to specific radioactivities not higher than about 5×10^6 cpm/µg of protein.

Our version of the RIPA has been described previously (Kurth et al., 1977; Kurth and Schmitt, 1977). We used an indirect technique employing a second antiserum (e.g. goat anti-human IgG) for the cross-linking of virus antigen- human antibody complexes. The details for competition RIPA have also been described (Kurth et al., 1977; Kurth and Mikschy, 1978).

In all RIPA, normal goat sera as well as specific anti-gp70 SSV(SSAV) goat antisera were included as controls. Once positively reacting human sera had been found, one such serum was always included as additional positive control. Likewise, a non-reactive human sample was always included to monitor nonspecific background precipitation.

During the course of the RIPA studies, it became apparent that both the structural integrity of antibodies and, even more importantly, of the antigen molecules are of utmost importance to obtain successful antigen-antibody binding. Repeated freezing and thawing of antisera or IgG preparations leads to loss of titer. Purified virus antigens exhibit a similar thermolability. The labeling procedure, radiation destruction and serum proteases active during the incubation times in the RIPA represent additional hazards for the structure and immunogenicity of the viral antigens.

The gp70 virus glycoprotein of the SSV(SSAV) complex was purified (Thiel et al., 1977) and kindly made available by Drs. H.-J. Thiel and W. Schäfer, Max Planck-Institut für Virusforschung, Tübingen. Gp70 was labeled by the chloramine-T method (Kurth et al., 1975).

Immediately after labeling, virus polypeptides were protected with cold carrier protein (e.g. myoglobin) and separated from unbound Na ^{125}I by Sephadex G-25 column chromatography. Labeled antigen was stored in aliquots at -70°C and could be used for about four to six weeks without loss of immunogenicity. To reduce proteolytic cleavage during the RIPA, fresh phenylmethanesulfonyl fluoride (PMSF) was added to the antigen solution on the day of test (Kurth and Mikschy, 1978).

RESULTS AND DISCUSSION

Normal human sera (NHS) titrated against gp70 SSV(SSAV) fall into several categories (Fig. 1). About half of all sera tested do not react appreciably and titrate like NHS #40. The other serum samples show varying titers with the highest titer sera having 20% precipitation endpoints at dilutions between 1:1600 and 1:6400.

To underline the immunological nature of the precipitations pictured in Fig. 1, homologous competition RIPA were performed (Fig. 2). Competing unlabeled gp70 SSV(SSAV) is able to displace all labeled gp70 SSV(SSAV) when used in excess amounts. One could suspect from the relatively shallow slope of the curves when intermediate-titer sera are employed (e.g. NHS #37, NHS #38) that a number of antibody populations with different specifications take part in the precipitation reaction, an indication that a set of antigenic determinants on the molecule can be recognized by human sera.

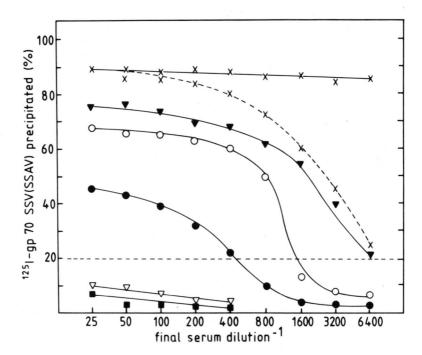

<u>Fig. 1:</u> RIPA curves of NHS and animal control sera titrated against
iodinated gp70 SSV(SSAV). 10 μl serum or 2-fold dilutions
thereof were used. Addition of antigen and anti-immunoglo-
bulin G antisera during the RIPA led to a final 25-fold dilution of the testsera. Input antigen: 4 μg. NHS 23: ▼ ;
NHS 37: ○ ; NHS 38: ● ;   NHS 40: ▽ ; normal goat serum: ■ ;
goat anti-SSV(SSAV) antiserum: x-x; additional 100-fold dilution of the goat antiserum: x---x.

        Another way to quantitate anti-viral titers in NHS is to deter-
mine their maximal precipitating activity under conditions of antigen excess (Table 1). Conversely, under conditions of antibody excess, it becomes clear that NHS are only able to precipitate a
characteristic percentage of the input antigen (Fig. 1, discussed
in detail by Kurth and Mikschy, 1978). At first we assumed that
this plateau effect was due to proteolytic cleavage of gp70 SSV(SSAV)
into its major degradation product gp 45 (Thiel et al., 1978). When
purified gp45 SSV(SSAV) became available through the courtesy of
Drs. H.-J. Thiel and W. Schäfer, its immunogenicity for NHS was
quickly noted (Kurth and Mikschy, 1978). Those human sera which react well with gp70 SSV(SSAV) also react well with gp45 SSV(SSAV)
(Table 2). Conversely, sera without anti-gp70 SSV(SSAV) activity
remain negative for gp45 SSV(SSAV).

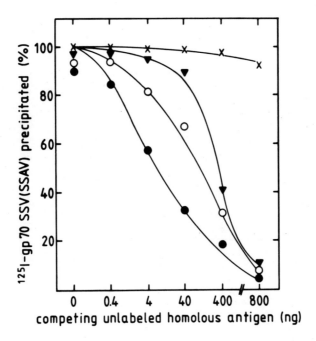

Fig. 2: Homologous RIPA competition assay. Unlabeled gp70 SSV(SSAV) competed with 4 μg iodinated gp70 SSV(SSAV). Symbols for sera as in Fig. 1

A plateau effect, as shown for gp70 SSV(SSAV) in Fig. 1, was again observed for gp45 SSV(SSAV). Such plateaus are characteristic when C-type virus antigens are recognized by the so-called inter-species-specific antigenic determinants (Thiel et al., 1978). These "interspec-determinants" are shared by C-type viruses originating from different species. The plateau effect seen here could there-fore best be explained by postulating that the human antibodies were originally induced by a virus immunologically related, but not identical, to SSV(SSAV).

At present, it cannot be ruled out that a cross-reacting non-viral antigen was responsible for the antibody induction. However, to our knowledge, antigens cross-reacting with C-type tumor viruses have not yet been described. When high and low titer NHS were tested against bacterial (e.g. BCG) as well as other viral antigens (va-rious adenovirus, influenza and poliovirus strains), the emerging patterns of reactivity were entirely different from the pattern seen against C-type viruses (R.K., H.-J. Gerth, P. Minden, unpublished data), somewhat eliminating the possibility that certain NHS from

"high responder" persons react strongly against all antigenic stimuli.

Table 1: Maximal amount of gp70 SSV(SSAV) viral antigen precipitable
         by high, intermediate and negative titer normal human sera

Serum	Serum Quantity and Dilution	Input Antigen	Precipitated Antigen
normal goat serum	10 µl (1:40)	32 ng	0.9 ng (2.8 %)
goat anti-SSV(SSAV)	10 µl (1:400)	"	30.1 ng (94 %)
NHS 23	10 µl (1:40)	"	17.6 ng (55 %)
NHS 24	"	"	6.1 ng (19 %)
NHS 29	"	"	5.8 ng (18 %)
NHS 26	"	"	2.0 ng (6.1 %)
NHS 33	"	"	0.6 ng (1.9 %)

Table 2: Maximal amount of gp45 SSV(SSAV) viral antigen precipitable
         by high, intermediate and negative titer normal human sera

Serum	Serum Quantity and Dilution	Input Antigen	Precipitated Antigen
normal goat serum	10 µl (1:40)	25.6 ng	0.6 ng (2.2 %)
goat anti-SSV(SSAV)	10 µl (1:400)	"	24.6 ng (96 %)
NHS 23	10 µl (1:40)	"	13.8 ng (54 %)
NHS 24	"	"	5.4 ng (21 %)
NHS 31	"	"	5.9 ng (23 %)
NHS 26	"	"	0.8 ng (3.0 %)

The question whether different sera recognize the same or different determinants on gp70 SSV(SSAV) was investigated by pooling

various NHS to test for a synergistic increase in maximal precipitating activity. These RIPA have to be performed under conditions
of antibody excess. As can be seen from Table 3, pooled NHS precipitate approximately as much as the highest serum in the group. The
absence of a synergistic increase in precipitating activity indicates that the NHS all recognize the same determinants on the antigen molecule. This would seem to represent another indirect piece
of evidence that the viral antigen is recognized via a limited subset of ("interspec"?) determinants, reducing the possibility that
non-viral antigens have induced many populations of antibodies specific for different determinants on the antigen.

Table 3: Maximal immunoprecipitation of gp70 SSV(SSAV) antigen
         (3.2 ng = 100 %) by individual and combined human sera

Serum	Quantity and Dilution	gp70 SSV(SSAV) precipitated (%)
normal goat serum	10 µl (1:40)	9.4
goat anti-SSV(SSAV)	1 µl (1:200)	98.5
NHS 4	10 µl (1:40)	54.2
NHS 23	"	97.6
NHS 4 + 23	2x5 µl (1:40)	98.4
NHS 24	10 µl (1:40)	50.5
NHS 29	"	41.0
NHS 30	"	32.3
NHS 31	"	56.0
NHS 24 + 29 + 30 + 31	4x2.5 µl (1:40)	50.9
NHS 21	10 µl (1:40)	13.4
NHS 26	"	9.1
NHS 32	"	10.8
NHS 33	"	12.6
NHS 21 + 26 + 32 + 33	4x2.5 µl (1:40)	9.7

For reasons unknown at present, the antibody titers against
C-type virus antigens are low even in those sera where they are
very easily demonstrable (e.g. NHS #23 and #37 in Fig. 1) in compa-

rison to titers frequently observed after infections by other viruses like, for example, influenza or polio. Even in the case of
two laboratory workers, where we have reason to suspect laboratory
exposure to SSV(SSAV), the titers as measured in Fig. 1 do not exceed 1:6400. C-type viremia has never been ovserved in man. There
are apparently non-immunological mechanisms that prevent massive
viral replication and/or dissemination in man, possibly limiting
the need for an excessive immune response. This assumption is supported by the finding that the complement systems in man and some
other higher animals can specifically lyse C-type viruses (Welsh
et al., 1975, 1976). In gibbon apes, it was recently shown that
this lytic activity can be present concomitantly with anti-viral
antibodies (Gallagher et al., 1978).

In mice, a non-immunoglobulin factor which specifically neutralizes xenotropic mouse C-type viruses has been partially characterized (Levy, 1974; Fischinger et al., 1976; Leong et al., 1977).
It remains to be seen whether an analogous factor, which would have
similar implications as discussed above for the complement-mediated
virolysis, also operates in man.

In the absence of epidemiological data supporting horizontal
C-type virus transmission in man, one could also speculate that the
anti-viral antibodies in man are the result of endogenous virus expression activated in certain cells. Moroni and Schuman (1977) as
well as Wecker et al. (1977) have shown recently that lymphocyte
stimulation in mice may lead to C-type virus production and gp70
expression on the lymphocyte plasma membrane. Such stimulation
could certainly explain the presence and relatively low titers of
the anti-viral antibodies.

There is another facet that should be brought to attention.
Very recent antibody affinity studies, again using gp70 SSV(SSAV) as
antigen, revealed the presence of both high and low affinity antibodies in NHS (F. Katz and R.K., unpublished data). High affinity
antibodies were demonstrable only in blood donors selected for their
relatively high titers. Low affinity antibodies were detected in
practically all NHS, even in those which score negative in RIPA
titrations. Surprisingly, these low affinity antibodies have also
been found in normal sera from goats and rabbits! They may be the
result of cross-reactions to non-viral antigens. Alternatively, the
hypothesis cannot be dismissed at present that practically all animal and human sera may contain a class of low affinity antibodies
due to constant exposure to endogenous or exogenous C-type viruses.

A physiological role for C-type viruses, particularly in differentiation and embryogenesis, has often been proposed (discussed,
for example, by Todaro, 1978) but remains to be defined. In man,
budding particles have been observed in placental trophoblasts
(Kalter et al., 1973; Imamura et al., 1976; Roter-Dirksen and Levy,

1977) and it is noteworthy that during pregnancy an increased, but transient anti-viral immunity can be observed (Hirsch et al., 1978; Thiry et al., 1978). It is tempting to speculate that the presence of C-type virus particles during embryogenesis may be due to a yet unknown viral function in the differentiation of developing cells. However, because of the present lack of more precise data it still remains to be elucidated whether C-type viruses possess more than occasional transforming functions in animals and possibly in man.

DIRECTION OF FUTURE WORK (OUTLOOK)

The epidemiological studies using human sera and C-type virus antigens primarily served two purposes. Firstly, it had to be elucidated whether sera containing anti-viral antibodies exist at all. We believe that such antibody positive sera have now clearly been demonstrated. Secondly, the immune reactivity in groups of patients with various malignant and autoimmune disorders is presently under intensive study. Consistent presence or absence of high affinity anti-viral antibodies may indicate viral involvement in the etiology of the disease. This, in turn, would trigger detailed immunological investigations to demonstrate viral footprints in the diseased tissues.

ACKNOWLEDGEMENTS

We are indebted to Drs. W. Schäfer and H.-J. Thiel for the kind provision of purified virus antigens. We also gratefully acknowledge the technical assistance of Mrs. U. Mikschy and Ch. Baradoy and thank Mrs. U. Netuschil for expert secretarial assistance. This work was supported by the Deutsche Forschungsgemeinschaft, grant No. Ku 330/3.

REFERENCES

1. AOKI, T., LIU, M., WALLING, M.J., BUSHAR, G.S., BRANDCHAFT, P.B., and KAWAKAMI, T.G. (1976): Science 191, 1180

2. BENVENISTE, R.E., LIEBER, M.M., LIVINGSTON, D.M., SHERR, C.J., TODARO, G.J., and KALTER, S.S. (1974): Nature 248, 17

3. CHARMAN, H.P., KIM, N., WHITE, M., and GILDEN, R.V. (1974): J. Natl. Cancer Inst. 52, 1409

4. ESSEX, M. (1975): Adv. Cancer Res. 21, 175

5. FISCHINGER, P.J., IHLE, J.N., BOLOGNESI, D.P., and SCHÄFER, W. (1976): Virology 71, 346

6. GALLAGHER, R.E., SCHRECKER, A.W., WALTER, C.A., and GALLO, R.C. (1978): J. Natl. Cancer Inst. 60, 677

7. HIRSCH, M.S., KELLY, A.P., CHAPIN, D.S., FULLER, T.C., BLACK, P.H., and KURTH, R. (1978): Science 199, 1337

8. IHLE, J.N., HANNA, M.G., Jr., ROBERSON, L.E., and KENNEY, F.T. (1974): J. Exp. Med. 139, 1568

9. IMAMURA, M., PHILLIPS, P.E., and MELLORS, R.C. (1976): Am. J. Path. 83, 383

10. KALTER, S.S., HELMKE, R.J., HEBERLING, R.L., PANIGEL, M., FOWLER, A.K., STRICKLAND, J.E., and HELLMAN, A. (1973): J. Natl. Cancer Inst. 50, 1081

11. KAWAKAMI, T., HUFF, S., BUCKLEY, P., DUNGWORTH, D., SNYDER, S., and GILDEN, R. (1972): Nature New Biol. 235, 170

12. KAWAKAMI, T.G., BUCKLEY, P.M., McDOWELL, T.S., and DE PAOLI, A. (1973): Nature New Biol. 246, 105

13. KURTH, R., FRIIS, R.R., WYKE, J.A., and BAUER, H. (1975): Virology 64, 400

14. KURTH, R., TEICH, N.M., WEISS, R., and OLIVER, R.T.D. (1977): Proc. Natl. Acad. Sci. U.S.A. 74, 1237

15. KURTH, R., and SCHMITT, C. (1977): Med. Microbiol. Immunol. 164, 167

16. KURTH, R., TEICH, N.M., and WEISS, R. (1978) in: Advances in Comperative Leukemia Research (eds.: P. Bentvelzen, J. Hilgers and D.S. Yohn), Elsevier-North Holland Biomedical Press, pp 41

17. KURTH, R., and MIKSCHY, U. (1978): Proc. Natl. Acad. Sci. U.S.A., in press

18. LEONG, J.C., KANE, J.P., OLESZKO, O., and LEVY, J.A. (1977): Proc. Natl. Acad. Sci. U.S.A. 74, 276

19. LEVY, J.A. (1974): Am. J. Clin. Path. 62, 258

20. MORONI, C., and SCHUMANN, G. (1977): Nature 269, 600

21. ROTER-DIRKSEN, E., and LEVY, J.A. (1977): J. Natl. Cancer Inst. 59, 1187

22. SARMA, P.S., SHARAR, A., WALTERS, V., and GARDNER, M. (1974): Proc. Soc. Exp. Biol. Med. 145, 560

23. STEPHENSON, J.R., and AARONSON, S.A. (1976): Proc. Natl. Acad. Sci. U.S.A. 73, 1725

24. THIEL, H.-J., BERGHOLZ, C., BEUG, H., DEINHARDT, F., SCHWARZ, H., and SCHÄFER, W. (1977): Z. Naturforsch. 32c, 884

25. THIEL, H.-J., BEUG, H., GRAF, T., SCHWARZ, H., SCHÄFER, W., BERGHOLZ, C., and DEINHARDT, F., Virology, in press

26. THIRY, L., SPRECKER-GOLDBERG, S., BOSSENS, M., and NEURAY, F. (1978): J. Natl. Cancer Inst. 60, 527

27. TODARO, G.J. (1978): Brit. J. Cancer 37, 130

28. WECKER, E., SCHIMPL, A., and HÜNIG, T. (1977): Nature 269, 598

29. WEISS, R.A., and BIGGS, P.M. (1972): J. Natl. Cancer Inst. 49, 1713

30. WELSH, R.M., Jr., COOPER, N.R., JENSEN, F.C., and OLDSTONE, M.B.A. (1975): Nature 257, 612

31. WELSH, R.M., Jr., JENSEN, F.C., COOPER, N.R., and OLDSTONE, M.B.A. (1976): Virology 74, 432

32. WOLFE, L.G., DEINHARDT, F., THEILEN, G.H., ROBIN, H., KAWAKAMI, T., and BUSTAD, L.K. (1971): J. Natl. Cancer Inst. 47, 1115

RNA TUMOR VIRUS-RELATED COMPONENTS IN INTRACISTERNAL A-TYPE

PARTICLES FROM MURINE AND HUMAN PLASMA CELL TUMORS

B.J. Weimann, J. Schmidt, and B. Takacs

Basel Institute for Immunology
487 Grenzacherstrasse 487
Postfach, 4005 Basel 5, Switzerland

Oncogenic viruses have been recognized as causative agents capable of inducing tumors in animals. Although most human tumors are not associated with viruses, cytoplasmic particles from some human malignant tissues have been observed at densities characteristic for C-type RNA tumor viruses carrying a RNA-dependent DNA polymerase and RNA. These particles as well as some virus isolates from human tissues were found to be related to the murine leukemia virus (MuLV) group, or to the gibbon ape leukemia virus (GaLV) and simian sarcoma virus (SSV) group as shown by common antigenic determinants or by nucleotide sequence homology. Since there is no conclusive evidence yet for the existence of B- or C-type RNA tumor viruses in humans, viral isolates from human tumors or their components are compared to primate RNA tumor viruses. Because of this lacking evidence, it is speculated that other particles, like intracisternal A-particles, carried by tumor cells, may be involved in the establishment of tumors. These intracisternal A-particles are present in many transformed cells, especially in murine plasma cell tumors (1). They have been occasionally found in normal cells during early embryonal stages (2), but it is not known whether they are involved in the differentiation of normal cells or whether they represent an early expression of oncogenic RNA viruses. Formed by budding at the membranes of the endoplasmic reticulum, they remain within the cisternae. They are regarded as RNA tumor viruses on the basis of their morphology and of their biochemical characteristics, notably their high molecular weight RNA and RNA-dependent DNA polymerase activities. Although their morphology and some of their biochemical characteristics suggest a relationship to oncogenic viruses, their biological significance is still unclear.

We have examined the possibility of whether intracisternal A-type particles from plasma cell tumors of either murine or human origin contain components which are also found in infectious C-type viruses. Our experimental systems were 1) the chemically induced mouse plasma cell tumors MPC 11 and MOPC 104E, each carrying intracisternal A-particles, and Abelson murine leukemia virus (A-MuLV) (3) and 2) a human lymphoblastoid cell line, designated PHD, established from the bone marrow of a male patient with Polycythemia vera (4), and simian sarcoma virus (SSV), isolated from a fibrosarcoma of a woolly monkey (5), a non-human primate. Experimentally, we tried 1) to detect RNA-dependent DNA polymerases (6,7) in intracisternal A-particles and 2) to inhibit their enzymatic activities by antisera directed against the DNA polymerases of either murine or primate RNA tumor viruses (8).

Electron micrographs on cross sections of fixed human cells revealed particles which resembled in structure and location the intracisternal A-particles of murine plasma cell tumors (1). As they bud into the cisternae of the endoplasmic reticulum, these particles consisted of two concentric shells surrounding a relatively electronlucent centre with an average diameter of 800 Å. They were never found at the outer cell membrane or in the extracellular space. C-type viruses could not be induced by either halogenated analogues of thymidine, 2-deoxy-D-glucose, testosterone or arginine deprivation.

Like the majority of other human cell lines derived from either normal or malignant lymphoid sources, the PHD cells produce and secrete immunoglobulins. Analysis of the radiolabelled biosynthetic product on 5-30% linear sucrose gradients showed a peak in the 19 S region. After SDS-polyacrylamide gel electrophoresis two defined bands were found coinciding with that of reference heavy (μ) and light chains of IgM molecules. Nearly all cells had cytoplasmic and surface IgM as shown by immunofluorescence. The cells expressed the Epstein-Barr nuclear antigen (EBNA).

To demonstrate a relationship between enzymatic activities associated with intracisternal A-particles and those of infectious C-type viruses, enzymes were partially purified by column chromatography on phosphocellulose and their enzymatic activities were then studied in the presence of antisera directed against the reverse transcriptases of C-type RNA tumor viruses. For this purpose, intracisternal A-particles were isolated from microsomal vesicles of mechanically disrupted cells by treating the postnuclear fraction with low concentrations of the nonionic detergent Non-

idet P40. After equilibrium density centrifugation of intracisternal A-type particles from either murine or human cells in linear
sucrose gradients, we consistently observed three peaks of DNA
polymerase activity on the template-primer $poly(rA) \cdot oligo(dT)$ at
approximate densities of 1.30, 1.24 and 1.20 - 1.22 g/cm^3. Electron micrographs revealed that murine A-particles banding at the
1.30 g/cm^3 density region had well preserved structures consisting
of two concentric membrane layers surrounding an electrontrans-
parent core (9). They were mainly found as single particles and
only a small proportion as aggregates. Deformed particles were
observed at the density of 1.24 g/cm^3, whereas defective particles
limited by only one membrane layer were found in the 1.20 - 1.22
g/cm^3 region. DNA polymerases associated with A-particles center-
ing around those densities were solubilized by detergent and sonic
treatment, and then separated by column chromatography on phosphocellulose. Each particle fraction was associated with three DNA
polymerases, which were termed DNA polymerase 1, 2 and 3, respectively. They eluted at salt concentrations of around 0.30 M, 0.45 M
and 0.65 M KCl. The relative amounts of individual DNA polymerases
from different A-particles varied considerably. DNA polymerase 1
transcribed $poly(rA).oligo(dT)$, $poly(rC) \cdot oligo(dG)$ and $poly(2'-0-$
$methylcytidylate) \cdot oligo(dG)$, $poly(rCm) \cdot oligo(dG)$, but was nearly
inactive on poly $d(A-T)$. DNA polymerase 3, however, utilized
effectively poly $d(A-T)$, but not $poly(rC) \cdot oligo(dG)$ or $poly(rCm) \cdot$-
$oligo(dG)$ as templates. The incorporation data obtained with the
three DNA polymerases on different templates are shown in Table 1.
In a cytoplasmic extract of the human cells, two DNA polymerases
were observed on $poly(rA) \cdot oligo(dT)$. They eluted around 0.35 M
and 0.48 M KCl.

Serological analysis on the enzymes of murine and human origin
was performed with antisera raised against Rauscher murine leukemia
virus (R-MuLV) reverse transcriptase or against simian sarcoma
virus (SSV) reverse transcriptase, respectively. If such antibodies inactivated the A-particle enzymes, it would indicate a certain similarity between them and the reverse transcriptase of C-type
RNA tumor viruses. The incorporation data obtained in the presence
of antiserum are expressed as the percentage of control experiments
performed without antiserum. Tests with goat anti-(R-MuLV reverse
transcriptase) on Friend and Abelson murine leukemia viruses gave
complete inhibition. Normal goat serum had no effect on the enzymes. In Table 2 we have listed the enzyme inactivation results
obtained on the three DNA polymerases of A-particles from the
murine plasmacytomas. DNA polymerase 1 was completely inactivated.

Table 1: Template activities of DNA polymerases from murine
intracisternal A-particles after chromatography on phosphocellulose

A-particles banding at density (g/cm^3)	DNA polymerase	Incorporation of deoxynucleotide monophosphate (pmol) on:		
		poly(rA)· oligo(dT)	poly(rC)· oligo(dG)	poly d(A-T)
1.30	1	19.0	1.20	0.4
	2	25.9	0.45	1.42
	3	29.5	0.1	4.4
1.24	1	23.3	0.32	0.7
	2	3.7	0.2	0.3
	3	7.1	<0.1	1.55
1.20-1.22	1	47.0	0.6	0.65
	2	2.8	<0.1	<0.1
	3	0.65	<0.1	0.3

The standard assays for each enzyme were performed on different
templates as described previously (9). Values for individual templates were expressed in pmol of incorporated deoxynucleotide monophosphates. Enzymes eluting from phosphocellulose at 0.30 M, 0.45 M
and 0.65 M KCl were termed DNA polymerase 1, 2 and 3, respectively.

The slope of the inhibition curve is like that of Abelson murine
leukemia virus reverse transcriptase. This enzyme seems to be a
true viral reverse transcriptase, corroborated by its inhibition
pattern and utilization of poly(2'-O-methylcytidylate)·oligo(dG)
as template. The second activity was only partly inhibited (15 -
30%), with no further reduction on increasing the concentration of
antiserum. It is likely, therefore, that this fraction contained
at least two polymerizing enzymes. No effect whatever was observed on the DNA polymerase 3. The lack of inhibition, the incorporation data obtained on poly(rA)·oligo(dT) and poly d(A-T),
and centrifugation data, suggest that this enzyme may be the cellular DNA polymerase γ. The DNA polymerase from human cells eluting
from phosphocellulose at 0.35 M KCl was assayed in the presence of
goat anti-(SSV reverse transcriptase) antiserum. Purified DNA polymerase from simian sarcoma virus was completely neutralized by the
antiserum. The human DNA polymerase could not directly be neutralized by the antiserum. However, we would note a serological relationship only when the relevant antibodies inactivate the active
site of the enzyme. Cross-reacting antibodies would not alter its
activity. To precipitate complexes of anti-(SSV reverse transcriptase) antibodies and of the human DNA polymerase, anti-sheep
immunoglobulins were added to the mixture. Using this procedure

about 20% of the human DNA polymerase activity could be removed
with the precipitate. The result showed that anti-(simian sarcoma
virus reverse transcriptase) antibodies bound to the human DNA
polymerase independent of the active site of the enzyme. It also
seems likely that at least two independent enzymatic entities
were present in that fraction, similar to those obtained on the
murine DNA polymerase 2.

Table 2: Inhibition of DNA polymerases from murine intracisternal
A-particles by anti-(Rauscher leukemia virus reverse transcriptase)
antiserum.

A-particles banding at density (g/cm^3)	DNA polymerase	Incorporation of ^{3}H dTMP control (cpm)	Incorporation in presence of 34 µg antiserum (cpm)	Inhibition %
	1	2600	110	95.0
1.30	2	2430	2185	10.0
	3	3580	3685	0
	1	1700	59	97.5
1.24	2	332	235	30.0
	3	644	735	0
	1	4035	359	98.0
1.20-1.22	2	--	--	--
	3	605	638	0

Molecular weight determinations of the viral (A-MuLV and SSV)
as well as the particle-associated DNA polymerases from murine and
human cells were done by SDS-polyacrylamide gel electrophoresis.
Radiolabelled and unlabelled DNA polymerases were precipitated by
the relevant antibodies and then bound to Sepharose-coupled protein
A of Staphylococcus aureus. Using this indirect precipitation
method, apparent molecular weights of 80,000 daltons were determined for the Abelson murine leukemia virus reverse transcriptase
and for the intracisternal A-particle associated enzyme from the
murine plasmacytoma MOPC 104E. The native form of the reverse
transcriptase of the subhuman primate simian sarcoma RNA tumor
virus was found to exist as a single polypeptide chain with an
apparent molecular weight of 85,000 daltons. Spontaneous degradation of the SSV DNA polymerase was observed, generating stable
polypeptides of 70,000, 45,000 and probably 78,000 daltons. All
these breakdown products still had most of the enzymatic properties
and shared the common antigenic determinants against which the
antiserum was raised. The native form was able to dimerize and

was found as high molecular weight form after centrifugation in
linear sucrose gradients, while the 70,000 dalton breakdown product lost the property to dimerize and was found as low molecular
weight form. It appears that a 15,000 dalton polypeptide chain
was cleaved from the 85,000 dalton chain. The newly generated
70,000 dalton enzyme is then unable to dimerize. After precipitation of the human DNA polymerase with anti-(simian sarcoma
virus reverse transcriptase) antiserum and radio-iodination of the
complexes, an apparent molecular weight also of 85,000 daltons was
found.

     In this report we describe some observations made on enzymatic
activities carried by intracisternal A-particles from plasma cell
tumors of murine and human origin. Both types of tumors lacking
the evidence for infectious C-type particles belong to the
B-lymphocyte lineage. Intracisternal A-particles were observed by
electron microscopy in these plasma cell neoplasias. We always
found a co-sedimentation of the enzymatic activities with isolated
A-particles as shown by incorporation of deoxymonophosphates into
polymer on synthetic templates and by electron microscopy. This
suggests a physical association of DNA polymerases with A-particles.
Viral DNA polymerases may be distinguished from the normal cellular
DNA polymerases on the basis of their physical properties, subcellular location, template specificities and their serological
differences. The DNA polymerases of A-particles satisfy the criteria for reverse transcriptases, such as transcription of specific
template-primers, presence of ribonuclease H and the inhibition by
antisera directed against viral DNA polymerases from C-type RNA
tumor viruses. In addition, their salt elution patterns from
resins, their optimum reaction conditions and their molecular
weights are very similar to those of viral DNA polymerases. Hybridization studies (J. Schmidt et al., unpublished observations) suggest that only parts of the genomes from intracisternal A-particles
and C-type viruses share sequence homology. Therefore, a precursor relationship of intracisternal A-particles to C-type viruses
seems to be unlikely. The DNA polymerases of the two types of
particles are, however, similar, as shown by their serological relationship. It may be that the intracisternal A-particles constitute a different kind of oncogenic particle sharing only the reverse transcriptases with C-type viruses. The results observed in
the human system show that viral information of a DNA (Epstein-Barr
virus) and of a RNA tumor virus (simian sarcoma virus related) are
expressed in these cells. It is not known whether the expression
of functions of two different viruses is required for human lymphocyte transformation. Interactions between Herpes and RNA tumor
viruses in the avian system and co-expression of the EBV genome

and RNA tumor virus related sequences in Burkitt's tumors are known
to occur (10,11).

References

1. Dalton, A.J., Potter, M., and Merwin, R.M. J. Nat. Cancer Inst.
    26, 1221-1267 (1961).
2. Wivel, N.A. and Smith, G.H. Int. J. Cancer 7, 167-175 (1971).
3. Abelson, H.T. and Rabstein, L.S. Cancer Res. 30, 2213-2222
    (1970).
4. Weimann, B.J., Kluge, N., Dube, S.K., von Ehrenstein, G.,
    Krieg, J.C., Kind, J. and Ostertag, W. J. Natl. Cancer Inst.
    55, 537-542 (1975).
5. Theilen, G.H., Goule, D., Fowler, M., and Dungworth, D.L.
    J. Natl. Cancer Inst. 47, 881-889 (1971).
6. Baltimore, D. Nature 226, 1209-1211 (1970).
7. Temin, H.M. and Mizutani, S. Nature 226, 1211-1213 (1970).
8. Todaro, G.J. and Gallo, R.C. Nature 224, 206-209 (1973).
9. Schmidt, J., Pragnell, I.B. and Weimann, B.J. Eur. J. Biochem.
    73, 493-497 (1977).
10. Peters, W.P., Kufe, D., Schlom, J., Frankel, J.W., Prickett,
    C.O., Groupé, V., Spiegelman, S. Proc. Nat. Acad. Sci. USA
    70, 3175-3178 (1973).
11. Kufe, D., Magrath. I.T., Ziegler, J.L. and Spiegelman, S.
    Proc. Nat. Acad. Sci. USA 70, 737-741 (1973).

MORPHOLOGY OF SOFT-AGAR COLONIES FROM NORMAL AND LEUKEMIC HUMAN BONE MARROW

R. NETH[1], B. HEINISCH[1], H. HELLWEGE[1],
G. MARSMANN[2] and H. BECKMANN[1]

[1]Molekularbiologisch-hämatologische Arbeitsgruppe und [2] Abteilung für Gerinnungsforschung
und Onkologie an der Universitätskinderklinik
2000 Hamburg, W. Germany

In vitro methods of bone marrow cells in semisolid media have been known since the beginning of this century (4,6). Maxinow and others showed more than 50 years ago, using plasmaclot cultures, that pluripotent lymphoid stem cells cna differentiate in vitro into eosinophils, mono-cytes and macrophages (Fig. 1a) dependent on a growth factor produced in the bone marrow.

Since about 1970 soft agar techniques for the study of granulopoietic differentiation (7) and plasmaclot techniques for the study of erythropoietic differentiation (9, 10) of human blood cells are available. Using these techniques, Maxinow's theory (6) about hemopoietic cell proliferation and differentiation could be confirmed.

Modern experimental hematologists use the nearly hundred-year-old classification of human blood cells sometimes rather uncritical for the characterization of blood cells grown in vitro. Simple quantitative evalua-tion of colony formation alone does not yield enough in-formation regarding differentiation patterns. Also it is not sufficient to base the classification of a cell as for example an eosinophil (Fig. 1c) or macrophage (Fig. 1d) solely on growth characteristics or insuffi-cient cytological methods like orcein staining (Fig. 1b). Rather the morphological characterization of human blood cells grown in vitro should be based on classical hematological techniques like the Pappenheim or Wright staining procedures.

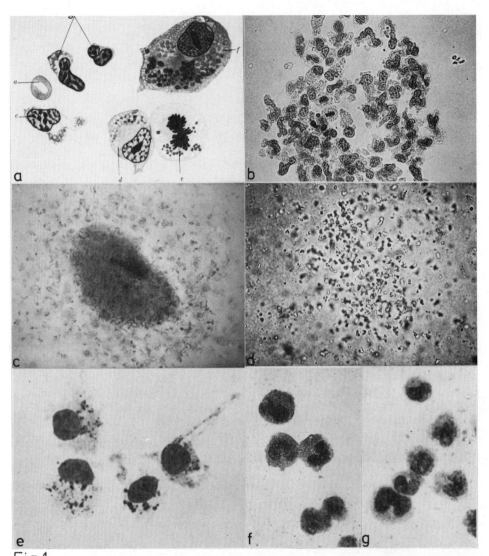

Fig.1

a) In vitro differentiation of lymphocytes (b) and monocytes (c) from rabbit blood (Awrorow and Timefejewsky
1914 cited in A. Maxinow (6) and H.Fisher (4). a. Erythrocyte, b) small lymphocyte and c) monocyte after 2 hours
of in vitro culture, d) and e) differentiated cells after
4 days and f) 7 days of in vitro culture. b) Orcein stained
colony, c) and d) soft agar colonies c) thick and d)
scattered, e-g)isolated cells from soft agar colonies,
e)macrophages, Pappenheim stain, f)eosinophils and g)
monocytes, peroxidasereaction, Giemsa stain.

The only systematic cytological studies of colony
formation in soft agar we are aware of have been done
by Shoham et al. (8) and by us (1, 2). In the present
investigation we demonstrate cytological, cytochemical
and immunocytochemical criteria from more than 1,000
colonies of normal and leukemic bone marrow grown in
soft agar.

MATERIAL AND METHODS

a. Source of material

Bone marrow was obtained by aspiration from the
ilias crest or sternum. For cytological, cytochemical
and immuncytochemical classification the usual criteria
were used (Fig. 4).

b. Cell Separation

For the separation of leukocytes the method of
Böyum (3) was used. The resulting buffy coat was suspended in culture medium. The nucleated cells were counted
with a hemocytometer. For the preparation of feeder
layer, granulocytes and monocytes were counted. The cell
layer was prepared by suspending two or three drops of
aspirated bone marrow into the culture medium, followed
by a hypertonic shock, repeated twice for lysis of erythrocytes, and by counting the number of mononucleated
bone marrow cells, omitting non-dividing cells like
metamyelocytes and polymorphs.

c. Culture Technique

Agar cultures were prepared using the double layer
agar technique of Pike and Robinson (7). McCoy's 5A medium containing 15 % fetal calf serum and supplemented
with amino acids and vitamins, was mixed in a 9:1 ratio
with boiled 5 % agar (Difco). After addition of the
appropriate number of leukocytes ($1.5-1.8 \times 10^6$), 1 ml
of this agar cell medium mixture was pipetted into 35 mm
plastic Petri Dishes (Falcon Plastics). These prepared
feeder layers were stored at 37° C in a humidified incu-
bator continuously flushed with 8 % CO_2. The washed bone
marrow cells were mixed with culture medium and boiled
3 % agar, in a ratio of 9:1; of this, 1 ml aliquots were
then pipetted onto the feeder layer. The final concentration of the cell layer was 1×10^5 mononucleated bone
marrow cells per ml. Following this preparation, no aggregates, clumps, or tissue fragments were found in bone
marrow suspensions or in agar. The dishes were incubated
for three weeks. During this time, at intervals of 12 to

14 days, the number of colonies was counted with an inverted microscope (Diavert) at 40x magnification. Only
those colonies containing 50 or more cells were counted.
For each experiment, at least four plates with and two
plates without feeder layer were examined; the counts
were expressed as the mean result of these plates. The
number of colonies in two plates never varied more than
10 % for bone marrow cells, and maximally 100 % for
peripheral blood leukocytes.

d. Source of Colony Stimulating Factor

A feeder layer of peripheral blood leukocytes was
used as source of colony stimulating factor (CSF). Since
the induction of proliferation of colonies depends on
the age of the feeder layer, the feeder layer was used
during the day of preparation or only few days later.
After seven days of incubation, the feeder layer had
lost about 50 % of its original stimulating activity
(1).

The number of granulocytes in the feeder layer was
not allowed to exceed 1×10^6 cells per ml. At this concentration of granulocytes the feeder layer contained
nearly $1-2 \times 10^5$ monocytes per ml.

e. Cytologic Analysis of Colonies

For cytologic analysis, colonies were picked out of
the agar under the inverted microscope with an angled
(ca. 110°) micro-hematocrit. They were put on slides
and incubated for 10 minutes in a humidified chamber
with a 1 % solution of agarase (Calbiochem., Los An-
geles). The colonies were prepared according to the
method of Testa and Lord (11). After incubation, the
agarase was drawn off carefully, and the colonies were
fixed according to the cytochemical reaction necessary
(10 % formalin alcohol for peroxidase reaction, 60 %
cold acetone for acid phosphatase reaction). Fixation
solution was dropped onto the slide. Then a coverslip
was placed on top of the drop. This in turn was covered
with a piece of filter paper and gently pressed. The
slide was frozen on dry ice for 10 minutes, the cover
slip was removed quickly, and the slide immediately
dried. The colony cells were stained with May-Grünwald-
Giemsa, respectively for peroxidase (12), or acid
phosphatase (8).

f. Demonstration of Immunoglobulins

To demonstrate immunoglobulin with plasma cells,
some colonies were fixed as described above, stained

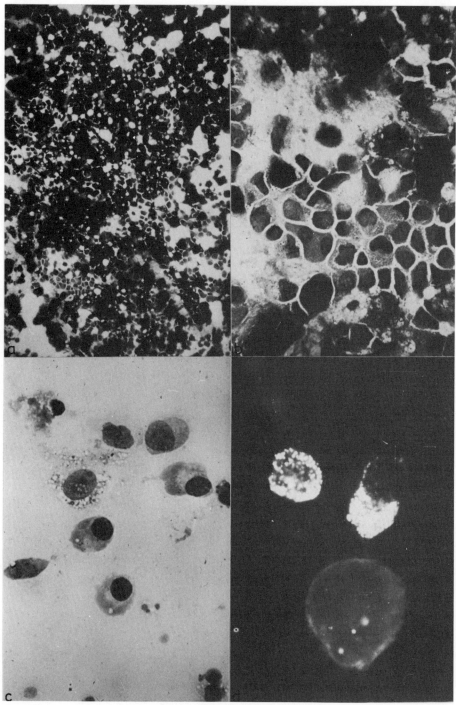

Fig. 2   See text RESULTS

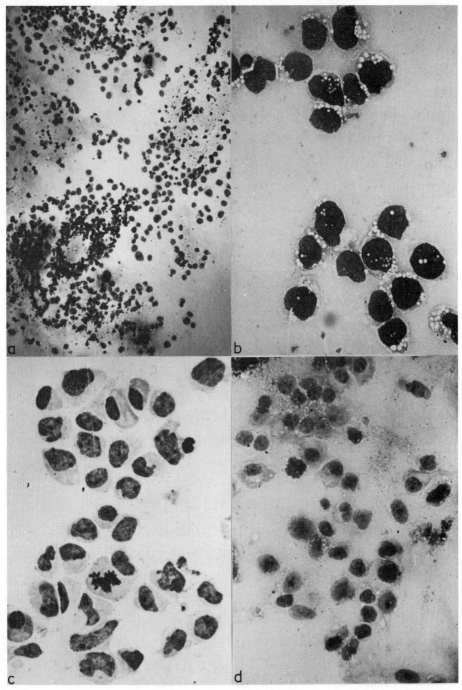

Fig.3   See text RESULTS

for 30 minutes with FITC conjugated anti-human immuno-globulins and then washed three times with PBS.

The colonies were investigated with a Leitz ortholux microscope equipped with an Opak-Fluor vertical illuminator.

RESULTS

A summary of the results is shown in Fig. 4. Beside the quantitative analysis of colony formation the cytological and cytochemical methods allow a classification of the cellular composition of these colonies. We found macrophages (Fig. 1e), always strong acid phosphatase positive (Fig. 2a and b), strong peroxydase positive eosinophils (Fig. 1f), and weak peroxydase positive monocytes (Fig. 1g). In dense (Fig. 1c) as well as in scattered (Fig. 1d) colonies, beside this in colonies from bone marrow of leukemic patients, we saw plasma cells (Fig. 2c) and blast cells (Fig. 3a- d).

Using immunofluorescence techniques we were able to demonstrate that these plasma cells produce immuno-globulins in vitro (Fig. 2d). Additional labelling was carried out with specific antisera against IgG, IgA, IgM, kappa and lambda chains (Fig. 5).

Diffusible factors, produced by the feeder layer, showed no effect on the proliferation of leukemic blast cells (Fig. 5) since blast cell colonies grow autonomously in the soft agar culture. In contrast, normal colonies grown without feeder layer were only very rarely found in the cases studied here.

DISCUSSION

The results described here (Fig. 1e-g, 2a,b, Fig. 4) show that under the culture conditions used, bone marrow cells mainly produced colonies consisting of monocytes and macrophages. In addition, pure eosinophil colonies and mixed colonies of monocytes and eosinophils were observed. Beside this in colonies derived from leukemic patients plasma cells (Fig. 2, Fig. 4) and blast cells (Fig. 3, Fig. 4) were observed. In the meantime more than 3000 bone marrow colonies from normal persons and leukemic patients have been investigated using the soft agar technique and the results described here have been confirmed. By this method in no case neutrophilic granulocytes have been observed in the colonies. In two cases we found plasma cells in bone marrow colonies from normal persons, however never

Cytology, Cytochemistry and Immunocytochemistry of Colony-Cells

| Cell Type of Colony | Cytology | | Cytochemistry | | Immunocytochemistry |
	Nucleus	Cytoplasm	Peroxydase	Acid Phosphatase	Fluorescence of Cytoplasm
neutrophil granulocyte	band or segmented	pink	positive	negative or faint positive	negative
eosinophil granulocyte	band or segmented	pink	positive	positive	negative
monocyte	oval, notched horseshoe	grayish-blue	negative faint positive	faint positive	negative
macrophage	round, excentrically placed	blue, grayish-blue, vacuolated	negative	strong positive	negative
plasma cell	round, excentrically placed	deep blue, halo near nucleus	negative	faint diffuse positive, positive granules	positive

Cytological Classification of Colonies (%)

diagnosis	number of patients	number of colonies analyzed	mon	mac	mon mac	eos	mon eos	mac eos	mon mac eos	mon mac eos neu	pc mon mac	pc mon mac eos	pc bc mon mac	bc mon mac
ALL untreated	21	164	70,5	8.	12	2	2	–	0,5	–	4	–	0,5	0,5
CR ALL	33	331	53	9	6	2	4,5	4	5	3	7	6	0,5	–
PR ALL	5	97	44	10	4	–	4	–	1	–	29	1	6	1
AML untreated	12	74	18,5	–	–	16,5	5	1	5	4	27	14	6,5	2,5
CR AML	5	76	64	5	2,5	2,5	6,5	.1	–	–	–	17	2,5	–
PR AML	7	21	58	4,5	4,5	–	–	–	–	–	9	24	–	–
CML remission	2	83	59	2,5	21	1	2,5	–	–	–	5	10	–	–
normal bone marrow	15	180	76	2,5	6	5,5	5	1	4	–	–	–	–	–
	n = 110	n = 1,026												

CR = complete remission, PR = partial remission, mon = monocyt, mac = macrophag, eos = eosinophil, neu = neutrophil, pc = plasma cells, bc = blast cells

Fig. 4

See Text.

Figs. 4 and 5 partly published in MODERN TRENDS
IN HUMAN LEUKEMIA II, 1976,
F. Lehmann-Verlag, München.

Dependence of Normal and Leukemic Colony Formation on CSF

| patient | diagnosis | number of colonies[1] / 1 x 10⁵ mononuclear bone marrow cells | | | |
| | | with feeder layer | | without feeder layer | |
		normal	pathologic	normal	pathologic
P.	ALL	1,3	0,3	∅	∅
D.	ALL				
	untreated	0,8	9	∅	14
	untreated	0,8	0,3	∅	∅
W.	AMML				
	untreated	∅	1	∅	2
O.	AMML				
	untreated	∅	0,4	∅	1
B.	ALL				
	PR	78	0,7	∅	∅
H.	AML				
	PR	96	1,8	∅	2
	CR	95	0,5	∅	0,3
Z.	AML				
	PR	7	1,5	∅	0,3
	PR	31	1	∅	1,5
	CR	55	1,2	2	0,5
D.	AML				
	PR	224	0,2	∅	0,3
K.	AMoL				
	PR	238	1,5	∅	1,3
H.	AMoL				
	PR	1,5	1,3	∅	2,5
W.	AML				
	CR	59	1	∅	1

[1] = mean of five plates
CR = complete remission – PR = partial remission

Demonstration of Immunoglobulins in Plasma Cells from Soft Agar Colonies

patient	diagnosis	anti-Ig	anti-IgG	anti-IgM	anti-IgA	anti-kappa	anti-lambda
D.	ALL						
	untreated	nt	+ (2)	nt	nt	+ (1)	+ (2)
B.	ALL partial						
	remission	+ (1)	+ (1)	nt	– (2)	+ (6)	+ (6)
Z.	AML partial						
	remission	nt	+ (3)	+ (1)	+ (3)	+ (3)	+ (3)
H.	AML partial						
	remission	+ (5)	– (2)	– (2)	nt	nt	nt
	complete						
	remission	nt	nt	– (1)	+ (1)	+ (1)	+ (1)
Wa.	AML comple-						
	te remission	+ (4)	nt	nt	nt	+ (1)	+ (1)
We.	AMML						
	untreated	+ (4)	+ (2)	– (1)	nt	nt	nt
O.	AMML						
	untreated	nt	nt	nt	nt	nt	+ (1)

demonstration of immunoglobulins using FITC coupled anti-human-immunoglobulin (goat), and anti-IgG, anti-IgM, anti-IgA (H-chain specific; rabbit), anti-kappa, anti-lambda (rabbit)
+ = positive immunofluorescence / / – = negative immunofluorescence / / nt = not tested / / ( ) = number of colonies studied

Fig.5   See Text

blast cells.

The diagnosis of hematological diseases and the experimental investigation of factors influencing proliferation and differentiation of normal and leukemic blood cells must be based not only on colony counting but also on a morphological classification of the cells. It is therefore desirable to have simple techniques, which allow both the quantitative and qualitative evaluation of colonies. In preliminary experiments we found that Axelrad's plasmaclot technique (9), originally introduced for erythropoietic cells, with a standardized placenta condition medium is a simple method meeting these requirements for granulopoietic cells as well.

Blood cells proliferated and differentiated in vitro should be classified according to the classical hematological nomenclature only after unequivocal identification by classical hematological techniques. If the morphological diagnosis in clinical hematology would be based on the methods and interpretations of some experimental hematologists, this would certainly be fatal for many patients.

REFERENCES

1. BECKMANN, H., H. SOLTAU, M. GARBRECHT, K. WINKLER (1974): Klin. Wschr. $\underline{52}$, 603.

2. BECKMANN, H., R. NETH, H. SOLTAU, J. RITTER, K. WINKLER, M. GARBRECHT, K. HAUSMANN & G.RUTTER (1976): in, Progress in Differentiation Research. 383, Elsevier/North Holland Biomedical Press B.V., Amsterdam.

3. BÖYUM, A. (1968): J. clin. Lab. Invest. (Suppl. 97) $\underline{21}$, 1.

4. FISHER, A. (1930): Gewebezüchtung, Verlag Rudolph Müller u. Steinicke, München.

5. LEDER, L.D. (1967): in,Der Blutmonocyt. Springer-Verlag, Berlin-Heidelberg-New York.

6. MAXINOW, A. (1927): Bindegewebe und blutbildende Gewebe, Handb. d. Mikr. Anat. (W.V. Mollendorf) Bd. 2, Julius Springer-Verl., Berlin.

7. ROBINSON, W.A., J.E. KURNICK & B.L. PIKE (1971): Blood $\underline{38}$, 500.

8. SHOHAM, D., E. BEN DAVID, L. ROZENSZAJN (1974):
         Blood 44, 221.

9. STEPHENSON, J.R., A.A. AXELRAD, D.L. McLEOD &
         M.M. STREEVE (1971): Proc. Natl. Acad. Sci.,
         U.S.A. 68, 1542.

10. TEPPERMAN, A.D., J.E. CURTIS & E.A. McCULLOCH (1974):
         Blood 44, 659.

11. TESTA, N.G. & B.J. LORD (1970): Blood 36, 586.

12. UNDRITZ, E. (1972). Hämatologische Tafeln Sandoz -
         II. Auflage, Sandoz 1972.

S E C T I O N III

The role of DNA tumor viruses in human cancer

Convenor

Dr. Fred RAPP
The Milton S. Hershey Medical Center
College of Medicine
Dep. of Microbiology
Hershey, Pennsylvania 17033

U.S.A.

IN SITU CYTOLOGICAL HYBRIDIZATION TO DETECT HERPES SIMPLEX VIRUS RNA IN HUMAN TISSUES

J.K. McDougall[1], D.A. Galloway[1] and C.M. Fenoglio[2]

[1]Cold Spring Harbor Laboratory, Cold Spring Harbor, New York 11724 and
[2]College of Physicians and Surgeons of Columbia University, New York, New York 10032.

Herpesvirus type 2 (HSV-2) has been regarded as a candidate oncogenic virus in humans for at least a decade (Rawls et al., 1968), yet it has not been possible to arrive at any definitive conclusions regarding the possible role of this virus in cervical cancer (Rawls et al., 1977). Apart from the obvious inability to satisfy Koch's postulates in a human situation, the results from molecular biological attempts to detect HSV-2 DNA in cervical tumors have, with one exception (Frenkel et al., 1972), proved negative (Zur Hausen et al., 1974; Pagano, 1975). Sero-epidemiological surveys continue to offer tantalizing clues suggesting an association between HSV-2 and cervical carcinoma (Rawls et al., 1969; Nahmias et al., 1970; Skinner et al., 1971; Sprecher-Goldberger et al., 1972; Adam et al., 1974; Kawana et al., 1974; Skinner et al., 1977) and it has been proposed (Aurelian et al., 1977) that a putative HSV-2-coded antigen is found frequently enough in cervical tumor biopsies to have diagnostic value.

One of the major problems encountered at the molecular level has been that the HSV-2 DNA probes used in various hybridization techniques are not sufficiently sensitive to allow negative results to be conclusive. By analogy with the results from other DNA viruses (e.g., SV40 and adenoviruses) it is necessary to exclude the presence of as small a region as 1-2% of the HSV-2 genome per cell, since an equivalent amount of a specific region of each of the smaller oncogenic viruses is capable of initiating and maintaining the transformed phenotype (Graham et al., 1974; Sambrook et al., 1974). As the "transforming" genes of HSV-2 have not to date been localized on the genome it has not been

possible to prepare a radioactive probe with equivalent sensitivity to that available for SV40 and adenovirus reassociation
kinetics experiments. The use of probes representing the entire
HSV-2 genome limits detection to a value well in excess of 1-2%
of the genome/diploid cell.

The examination of tumor or putative tumor tissue, as opposed
to transformed cell lines, is further complicated by a number of
factors, e.g., the tumor sample--especially in the case of
biopsied material--may be small in mass and consist of both
neoplastic and normal tissues. The extraction of DNA and RNA
from such samples results in a dilution of the nucleic acid
sequences from the neoplastic cells and thus increases the risk of
false negatives.

The in situ cytological hybridization technique (John et al.,
1969; Gall and Pardue, 1969) has been used to detect and localize
satellite DNA sequences (Corneo et al., 1970; Jones et al., 1972),
globin messenger RNA (Harrison et al., 1973) and virus DNA (Orth
et al., 1970; McDougall et al., 1972; Zur Hausen et al., 1972;
Wolf et al., 1973; Dunn et al., 1973; Watkins, 1973). One of the
most significant studies provided the first indication that
Epstein-Barr virus DNA could be detected in the epithelial cells
of nasopharyngeal carcinoma (Wolf et al., 1973). This technique
is therefore of potential value in the localization of viral DNA
to areas of tissue or particular cell types within a tumor. The
probability of there being sufficient viral DNA integrated to be
routinely detectable by the in situ method is very low since, in
most cells transformed by DNA viruses, only limited regions of the
viral genome persist and these are present in low copy number
(Sambrook et al., 1974; Frenkel and Leiden, 1978). The detection
of virus RNA using a radioactive DNA probe increases the probability of detection as the target sequences are an amplification of
the persisting viral DNA. One of the most attractive features of
the method is that cytological hybridization permits the study of
individual cells or sub-populations of cells for an evaluation of
their content of viral RNA transcripts. We have previously
examined HSV-2 transformed cells (Copple and McDougall, 1976),
using the in situ technique to detect virus mRNA in cloned populations of the 333-8-9 cell line (Duff and Rapp, 1971) and in
frozen sections of tumors induced in hamsters. The results from
these experimental tumors have encouraged us to develop the method
for wider use in screening frozen sections of human tissue for
evidence of viral sequences in situations where the virus may be
present either in latent form or associated with neoplastic cells.

IN SITU HYBRIDIZATION TO DETECT VIRUS-SPECIFIC RNA

Herpesvirus type 2 DNA, extracted from virions banded in
sucrose gradients or directly from infected cells as described by

Walboomers and Schegget (1976), was purified by centrifugation
in NaI equilibrium density gradients and labelled with ^{3}H using
the nick translation method (Maniatis et al., 1976). The specific
activity of the probe was approximately 10^7 cpm/ug. HSV-2
infected and transformed cells grown on glass slides and frozen
sections of tumors induced in hamsters by inoculation of the
transformed cells were fixed in absolute ethanol at -20^0C. The
slides were dried and 10 ul of denatured probe in 6xSSC, containing
$5x10^5$ cpm, was applied, covered with a glass coverslip and
incubated at 68^0C for 18 hours. After extensive washing in 2xSSC
at 4^0C the slides were dehydrated through an ethanol series, dried
and dipped in photographic emulsion. Results from these cytological hybridizations are shown in Figure 1.

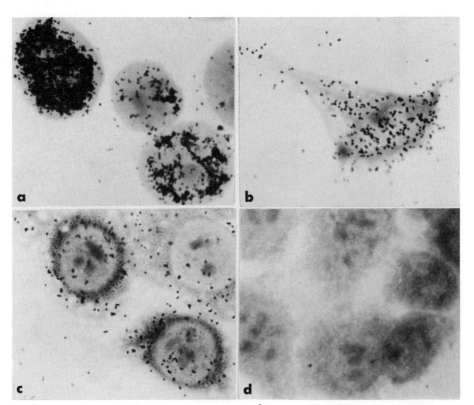

Figure 1. In situ hybridization of ^{3}H HSV-2 DNA to (a) HSV-2 infected BHK cell nuclei, denatured in 0.07N NaOH. Autoradiographic
grains are over areas of viral DNA synthesis; (b) HSV-2 infected
cell not denatured, grains indicate hybridization to viral RNA;
(c) HSV-2 transformed cells not denatured; (d) uninfected cells.

IN SITU DETECTION OF HSV RNA IN SENSORY GANGLIA

Persistence of Herpes simplex virus in nervous tissue has
been demonstrated experimentally in mice (Stevens and Cook, 1971;
Cook and Stevens, 1976) and rabbits (Stevens et al., 1972) and by
recovery of the virus from human sensory ganglia (Bastian et al.,
1972; Baringer, 1974). The evidence supporting HSV latency is
documented in a recent review by Stevens (1978).

One of the techniques used to demonstrate the presence of
HSV DNA in the neurons of sensory ganglia was the hybridization
in situ of radioactive viral-specific complementary RNA to sections
of ganglia (Stevens and Cook, 1974; Zur Hausen and Schulte-
Holthausen, 1975). The state of the virus when latent in the
neurons is unknown and could be in any form, from viral DNA
(integrated or as free molecules) to incomplete virions. In order
to establish whether any transcription of the latent HSV genome
could be detected in neurons we hybridized ^{3}H-HSV-2 DNA to frozen
sections of human sensory ganglia obtained at autopsy.

The preliminary results from these studies show that viral
specific RNA can be detected in some neurons (Figure 2). The
background level of grains over supporting cells is very low,
providing a high degree of confidence in the application of this
method for the detection of viral RNA in other situations where

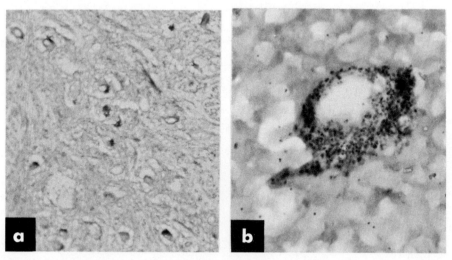

Figure 2. In situ hybridization to human sensory ganglia. (a) low
power of frozen section after hybridization with ^{3}H HSV-2 DNA.
(b) high power magnification of ganglion cell showing localization
of grains. Preparations not denatured, autoradiograph exposure
4 weeks.

persistence of the viral genome may not have been previously
established.

IN SITU DETECTION OF HSV RNA IN HUMAN CERVICAL TISSUE

Using the same virus DNA probe we have examined a series of
human cervical biopsies taken for pathological diagnosis. The
results from these cytological hybridizations indicate that HSV-2
RNA can be detected in areas of cells undergoing pre-malignant
changes (Figure 3), autoradiographic grains being most frequently
associated with neoplastic cells but are also in some sections
associated with macrophages and lymphoid cells in the areas of
abnormality. The nick-translated HSV-2 DNA probe does not
hybridize to normal cells or to human DNA bound to nitrocellulose
filters under conditions which detect $5x10^{-5}$ ug of contaminating human DNA in the probe. Hybridization of other viral
DNA probes to cervical sections has proven negative. The results
from this series of cervical biopsies are shown in Table 1,
negative tissues are from sections which do not contain any area
of abnormality which can be related by pathological examination
to malignant or pre-malignant changes.

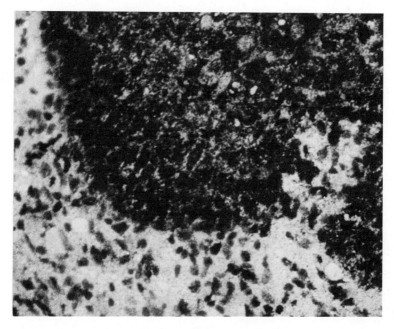

Figure 3. *In situ* hybridization to frozen section of human
cervical tissue. An area of intraepithelial neoplasia showing
autoradiographic grains localized in the abnormal epithelial cells
after hybridization with ^{3}H HSV-2 DNA. Section not denatured,
exposure 6 weeks.

TABLE 1
CERVICAL BIOPSIES (42 CASES)

Diagnosis	In situ hybridization with ^{3}H-HSV-2 DNA	
	HSV-2-RNA positive	HSV-2-RNA negative
CIN I-III	10	4
Squamous Metaplasia	2	2
Negative Diagnosis	1	23
Total	13	29

The results from in situ cytological hybridizations described here are at the least indicative of a significant presence of HSV-2 RNA in cervical tumor tissue. Infection of the human genital area with HSV-2 is common and is a recognized venereal disease (Kessler, 1977), consequently it is possible that we have detected viral RNA synthesized in virus replication. As HSV-2 can persist in ganglia there could be re-activation of latent virus with consequent replication in the area of neoplasia. It would be surprising if HSV-2 replication occurred preferentially in the neoplastic tissues when all cells are permissive and we have no evidence to suggest that these patients were undergoing acute infection at the time of biopsy or that infectious virus was present in the tissues. In situ hybridizations using restriction endonuclease derived fragments of HSV-2 DNA should identify the regions of the viral genome from which the observed RNA species are transcribed, these studies are now in progress.

REFERENCES

Adam, E., Kaufman, R.H., Melnick, J.L., Levy, A.H., and Rawls, W.E. (1974) Amer. J. Epidemiol. 98, 77.

Aurelian, L., Strnad, B.C., and Smith, M.F. (1977) Cancer 39, 1834.

Bastian, F.O., Rabson, A.S., Yee, C.L., and Tralka, T.S. (1972) Science 178, 306.

Baringer, J.R. (1974) N. Engl. J. Med. 291, 828.

Cook, M.L. and Stevens, J.G. (1976) J. Gen. Virol. 31, 75.

Copple, C.D. and McDougall, J.K. (1976) Int. J. Cancer 17, 501.

Corneo, G., Ginelli, E., and Polli, E. (1970) J. Mol. Biol. 48, 319.

Duff, R. and Rapp, F. (1971) J. Virol. 8, 469.

Dunn, A.R., Gallimore, P.H., Jones, K.W., and McDougall, J.K. (1973) Int. J. Cancer 11, 628.

Frenkel, N., Roizman, B., Cassai, E., and Nahmias, A. (1972) Proc. Nat. Acad. Sci. USA 69, 3784.

Frenkel, N. and Leiden, J. (1978) in "Integration and Excision of DNA Molecules", eds. P.H. Hofschneider and P. Starlinger, Springer-Verlag, Heidelberg. p. 71.

Gall, J.G. and Pardue, M.L. (1969) Proc. Nat. Acad. Sci. USA 63, 378.

Graham, F.L., Abrahams, P.J., Mulder, C., Heijneker, H.L., Warnaar, F.A., DeVries, F.A.J., Fiers, W., and Van der Eb, A.J. (1974) Cold Spring Harbor Symp. Quant. Biol. 39, 615.

Harrison, P.R., Conkie, D., Paul, J., and Jones, K.W. (1973) FEBS Letters 32, 109.

John, H.A., Birnsteil, M.L., and Jones, K.W. (1969) Nature 233, 528.

Jones, K.W., Prosser, J., Corneo, G., Ginelli, E., and Bobrow, M. (1972) in "Symp. Medica Hoechst. Modern Aspects of Cytogenetics", F.K. Schattauer, Verlag, Stuttgart.

Kawana, T., Yoshino, K., and Kassamatsu, T. (1974) Gann 65, 439.

Kessler, I. (1977) Cancer 39, 1912.

Maniatis, T., Kee, S.G., Efstratiadis, A., and Kafatos, F.C. (1976) Cell 8, 163.

McDougall, J.K., Dunn, A.R., and Jones, K.W. (1972) Nature 236, 346.

Nahmias, A.J., Josey, W.E., Naib, Z.M., Luce, C.F., and Duffey, A. (1970) Amer. J. Epidemiol. 91, 539.

Orth, G., Jeanteur, P., and Croissant, O. (1970) Proc. Nat. Acad. Sci. (Wash.) 68, 1876.

Pagano, J.S. (1975) J. Infect. Dis. 132, 209.

Rawls, W.E., Tompkins, W.A.F., Figueroa, M., and Melnick, J.L. (1968) Science 161, 1255.

Rawls, W.E., Tompkins, W.A.F., and Melnick, J.L. (1969) Amer. J. Epidemiol. 80, 547.

Rawls, W.E., Bacchetti, S., and Graham, F.L. (1977) in "Current Topics in Microbiology and Immunology", ed. W. Arber et al., Springer-Verlag, Heidelberg. p. 71.

Sambrook, J., Botchan, M., Gallimore, P.H., Ozanne, B., Pettersson, U., Williams, J., and Sharp, P.A. (1974) Cold Spring Harbor Symp. Quant. Biol. 39, 615.

Skinner, G.R.B., Thouless, M.E., and Jordan, J.A. (1971) J. Obst. Gynaecol. 78, 1031.

Skinner, G.R.B., Whitney, J.E., and Hartley, C. (1977) Archiv. Virol. 54, 211.

Sprecher-Goldberger, S., Thiry, L., Gould, I., Fassin, Y., and Gampel, C. (1972) Amer. J. Epidemiol. 97, 103.

Stevens, J.G. and Cook, M.L. (1971) Science 173, 843.

Stevens, J.G., Nesburn, A.B., and Cook, M.L. (1972) Nature N.B. 235, 216.

Stevens, J.G. (1978) in "Advances in Cancer Research", eds. G. Klein and S. Weinhouse, Academic Press, New York. p. 227.

Walboomers, J.M.M. and Schegget, J.T. (1976) Virology 74, 256.

Watkins, J.F. (1973) J. Gen. Virol. 21, 69.

Wolf, H., Zur Hausen, H., and Becker, V. (1973) Nature N.B. 244, 245.

Zur Hausen, H. and Schulte-Holthausen, H. (1972) in "Oncogenesis and Herpesviruses I", 1st Int. Symp. I.A.R.C., Lyon. p. 73.

Zur Hausen, H., Schulte-Holthausen, H., Wolf, H., Dorries, K., and Egger, H. (1974) Int. J. Cancer 13, 657.

Zur Hausen, H. and Schulte-Holthausen, H. (1975) in "Oncogenesis and Herpesviruses II", 2nd Int. Symp. I.A.R.C., Lyon. p. 117.

ANALYSIS OF EPSTEIN-BARR VIRUS FROM

HUMAN LYMPHOBLASTOID LINES

Harald zur Hausen and Karl-Otto Fresen

Institut für Virologie, Zentrum für Hygeine
Universität Freiburg
Hermann-Herder-Str. 11, 7800 Freiburg
Federal Republic of Germany

The Epstein-Barr virus (EBV) has been implicated as the possible etiological agent of two human tumors, Burkitt's lymphoma (BL) and nasopharyngeal carcinoma (NPC) (see review zur Hausen, 1975). Since it has also been identified as the causative virus of infectious mononucleosis, it is presently difficult to understand the reasons for its dual role in pathogenesis within the same host species.

There exists the possibility that besides differences in the host response to this viral infection different strains of EBV may be responsible for the development of specific clinical symptoms. The following tries to summarize recent experiments of our laboratory which provide support for the existence of EBV heterogeneities, even within individual cells of the same line. Two viral isolates were analyzed: EBV from the P3HR-1 line which originated from a BL tumor (Hinuma et al., 1967) and virus from the B95-8 line (Miller and Lipman, 1973) which was obtained from marmoset cells after transformation with EBV derived from a patient with infectious mononucleosis. Both viral isolates induce the EB virus-specific nuclear antigen (EBNA) upon infection of B-lymphocytes. P3HR-1 EBV moreover induces the early antigen complex EA (Henle et al. 1971) in EBV genome carrying and genome-negative lymphoblasts, but fails to immortalize human umbilical cord lymphoblasts. B95-8 virus in contrast efficiently induces transformation but does not induce EA.

Heterogeneity in EBNA Expression:

The establishment of human B lymphoma lines, devoid of
detectable EBV DNA sequences and negative for EBNA
(Klein et al., 1974) provided a reliable method for EBV
titration by determining EBNA induction. At the same
time it became possible to obtain EBNA-converted sublines of such cells (Clements et al., 1975, Fresen and
zur Hausen, 1976) and to study EBNA expression in cells
of their clones (Fresen et al., 1977).

Infection of BJA and Ramos cells, both derived
from EBV-negative BL, with EBV from P3HR-1 or B95-8
cells resulted in the gradual conversion of such cells
to EBNA expression after periods of 2 to 8 months of
continuous cultivation (Clements et al., 1975; Fresen
and zur Hausen, 1976). In contrast to cells converted
by the B95-8 virus, P3HR-1 virus converted BJA and Ramos
cells revealed a remarkable heterogeneity in EBNA expression. Besides nuclei exhibiting brilliant staining,
a substantial number of nuclei expressed a faint-granular EBNA pattern. Upon cloning it was possible to obtain sublines revealing either the faint-granular or
the brilliant pattern only (Fresen et al., 1977). This
indicated that differences in EBNA expression were due
to the infecting viral genomes rather than to mutational
changes of the cells, and the interpretation was supported by the observation that B95-8 virus-conversion of
the same cells led uniformly to the brilliant form of
EBNA expression.

Both types of P3HR-1 virus converted clones also
showed characteristic differences in the persistence
of EBNA expression. Whereas cells from clones revealing
the faint-granular pattern were uniformly EBNA-positive,
brilliantly EBNA-expressing clones always segregated
some EBNA-negative cells. This segregation was apparently due to the loss of EBV genomes since one EBNA-negative subclone was obtained which was devoid of detectable
EBV DNA. The segregation was observed for more than 1
year of continuous cultivation.

These data suggested that at least 2 different
populations of EBV molecules coexist in P3HR-1 cells;
one being responsible for the faint granular EBNA-ex-
pression with continuous persistence of the respective
genomes within the converted cells. The second one induces the brilliant EBNA pattern, but there is apparently a defect in this type of genome with regard to regulation of the persistence of viral DNA within the con-

verted cells. EB viral plasmid DNA has been demonstrated within such cells (Fresen et al., unpublished data),
and the continuous segregation of EBNA-negative cells
could result from an uneven distribution of replicated
viral plasmid DNA among daughter cells (Fresen et al.,
1977).

Complementation in EA Synthesis

The EA complex was originally discovered by the observation that certain sera reacted differently when tested against nonproducer cells of the Raji and 64-10
lines superinfected with P3HR-1 EBV as compared to VCA-
synthesizing cells of the P3HR-1 or EB3 lines (Henle
et al., 1970 b, 1971 a). By differential fixation at
least two subcomponents were discovered, the D- (diffuse)
component being methanol-ethanol resistant and the R-
(restricted) component which is not demonstrable after
alcohol fixation (Henle et al., 1971 a). Henle et al.
(1971 b, c, 1973) reported the observation that patients with BL frequently reveal antibody titers directed against the R-subtype of the EA complex whereas
antibodies in patients with nasopharyngeal carcinoma
and to some extent also in patients suffering from infectious mononucleosis predominantly react with the D-
subcomponent.

EA was classified as an early antigen on the basis
of the kinetics of its appearance (Henle et al., 1970)
and its inducibility in the presence of IUDR or ara-
binosine cytoside (Gergely and Klein, 1971 a, b). EA
is efficiently induced in a variety of lymphoblastoid
lines harbouring EBV genomes by superinfection with the
P3HR-1 virus isolate (Henle et al., 1970; Klein et al.,
1972; Diehl et al., 1972). EA is also induced after
treatment of Raji, NC-37 and some other lymphoblastoid
cells with IUDR (Hampar et al., 1972; Gerber, 1972;
Klein and Dombos, 1973). In Raji and NC-37 lines only
EA but not VCA-synthesizing cells are observed after
IUDR induction, whereas superinfection with the P3HR-1
virus results in a varying percentage of cells also revealing VCA synthesis.

Induction of EA was selected for a further investigation of the heterogeneity of P3HR-1 EBV (zur Hausen
and Fresen, 1977). By comparing EA induction in EBV-
converted BJA and Ramos cells as well as in cells of
their nonconverted parental lines after infection with

P3HR-1 EBV, it became obvious that the presence of EBV
genomes prior to infection enhanced EA induction considerably. Such lines revealed on average 14 times more
EA-synthesizing cells than the EBV genome-free parental
lines.

The analysis of the kinetics of EA induction after
infection with varying dilutions of P3HR-1 EBV provided
additional information (zur Hausen and Fresen, 1977).
In cells of EBV-genome-harbouring lines EA induction
followed the expected line for first order kinetics.
In contrast, in cells of EBV-negative lines EA was induced apparently according to second order kinetics.
These data argue strongly in favor of a complementation
model between resident viral genomes and the superin-
fecting EBV. They also indicate that two P3HR-1 EBV
genomes have to enter a BJA or Ramos cell before EA
synthesis is initiated.

These results seem to underline the concept of
intracellular heterogeneity of EBV from P3HR-1 cells.
They apparently also point to a biological interaction
between the heterogenous viral genome populations mani-
festing itself in EA induction. One could speculate on
a role of this interaction for the consistently high
spontaneous induction rate of P3HR-1 cells as observed
for more than a decade after their original establishment (Hinuma et al., 1967).

Partial Denaturation Mapping of EBV DNA

The partial denaturation pattern of EBV from B95-8 and
P3HR-1 cells has been analyzed (Delius and Bornkamm,
1978). A total of 32 molecules from B95-8 EBV showed
a homogenous and reproducible pattern of denaturation
loops. In marked contrast, DNA molecules obtained from
P3HR-1 EBV clearly revealed a heterogeneity in the denaturation pattern. At least two patterns could be dis-
cerned: besides 55 molecules fitting into one pattern,
20 molecules were analyzed which exhibited a very distinct denaturation pattern. The distribution of these
loops cannot be attributed to a simple structural rearrangement of identical genes.

Rescue of Transforming Viruses from Raji
and NC-37 Cells

Tanaka et al. (1976) observed a considerable induction

of viral DNA synthesis in Raji cells following superinfection with the P3HR-1 virus. The same authors also
noted virus particle production in these cells (personal communication) which was correlated with the demonstration of VCA in some of the superinfected cells.
Transforming virus was rescued at low titer (Nonoyama,
personal communication). We were able to confirm and
to extend these observations (Fresen et al., in preparation). Superinfection of both Raji or NC-37 cells
with non-transforming filtered virus concentrates from
P3HR-1 cells led to the recovery of transforming virus
from both types of culture for lymphoblastoid lines
of diploid cells karyologically distinct from Raji and
NC 37 cells were established from human umbilical cord
blood when this was in turn infected with preparations
of this recovered transforming virus. The yield of
transforming virus from superinfected Raji or NC 37
cells was low and visible growth of the infected cord
blood lymphocytes was not achieved before 4 to 6 weeks
following infection (Fresen et al., in preparation).

These results indicate that besides complementation in EA synthesis the non-transforming P3HR-1
virus apparently rescues transforming resident viruses
from Raji and NC 37 cells.

A "New" Antigen in Ramos Cells After Infection with B95-8 EBV

Infection of Ramos cells with B95-8 EBV resulted in
the induction of a nuclear antigen (Ram-ag) which was
demonstrated by indirect immunofluorescence (Fresen
et al., 1978). This antigen is distinct from EBNA,
for Ram-ag was present in a smaller percentage of cells
than EBNA and was also induced in Ramos cells already
EBNA-converted by B95-8 or P3HR-1 EBV. In addition,
absorption studies removed EBNA reactivity of sera
without affecting significantly the titers of Ram-ag
antibodies.

Antibodies to Ram-ag were found in the majority
of EBV-reactive individuals at varying titers. Sera
from patients with acute infectious mononucleosis regularly were devoid of detectable reactivity. This shows
some resemblance to the EBNA reactivity.

Ram-ag has only been induced in Ramos cells but
not in the EBV-negative BJA-B line. In addition, besides cell-specificity a remarkable virus-specificity

was noted for its induction: only EBV from B95-8 cells
and from another EBV-transformed marmoset line (Nyevu,
Miller et al., 1976) was able to induce this antigen in
Ramos cells, whereas P3HR-1 virus failed to do so (Fresen et al., 1978).

The induction of a specific antigen exclusivity by
B95-8 and Nyevu-virus preparations may point to a heterogeneity of these viruses as well. The specificity
of this induction for Ramos cells, however, points to
the additional role of a cellular factor. Further studies have to elucidate the nature of this antigen.

Conclusions

This study shows a remarkable heterogeneity of individual EB virus preparations. In addition, some biological interactions between the heterogenous virus molecules have been established: complementation in EA
synthesis and rescue of transforming EB viruses from
genome-carrying nonproducer cells after infection with
the non-transforming P3HR-1 isolate. It remains to be
established whether such interactions play also a role
in the pathogenesis of EBV-associated diseases.

Acknowledgements

We gratefully appreciate the skillfull technical assistance of Mrs. Gabriele Menzel and Mrs. Susanne Zabel.
This study has been supported by the Bundesministerium
für Forschung und Technologie (BCT 99) and by the Deutsche Forschungsgemeinschaft(Ha 449/12)

Literature

Clements, G. B., Klein, G., and Povey, S., 1975
        Production of an EBNA positive subline from an
        EBNA negative human lymphoma cell line without
        detectable EBV DNA by EBV infection.
                Int. J. Cancer, 16, 125-133

Delius, H., and Bornkamm, G. W.
        Heterogeneity of Epstein-Barr virus. III. Compari-
        son of a transforming and a non-transforming virus
        by partial denaturation mapping of their DNA.
                J. Virol. in press

Diehl, V., Wolf, H., Schulte-Holthausen, H., and zur
Hausen, H., 1972
    Re-exposure of human lymphoblastoid cell lines to
    Epstein-Barr virus.
        Int. J. Cancer, 1o, 641-651.

Fresen, K. O., and zur Hausen, H., 1976
    Establishment of EBNA-expressing cell lines by in-
    fection of Epstein-Barr virus (EBV) -genome-negative
    human lymphoma cells with different EBV strains.
        Int. J. Cancer, 17, 161-166.

Fresen, K. O., Merkt, B., Bornkamm, G. W., and zur Hausen, H., 1977
    Heterogeneity of Epstein-Barr virus originating
    from P3HR-I cells. I. Studies on EBNA induction.
        Int. J. Cancer, 19, 317-323.

Fresen, K. O., Cho, M. S. and zur Hausen, H., 1978
    Heterogeneity of Epstein-Barr virus. IV. Induction
    of a specific antigen by EBV from two transformed
    marmoset cell lines in Ramos cells.
        Submitted for publication

Gerber, P., 1972
    Activation of Epstein-Barr virus by 5-bromodeoxyuri-
    dine in virus free human cells.
        Proc. Nat. Acad. Sci. (Wash.), 69, 83-85.

Gergely, L., Klein, G., and Ernberg, I., 1971 a
    Appearance of Epstein-Barr virus-associated anti-
    gens in infected Raji cells.
        Virology, 45, 1o-21.

Gergely, L., Klein, G., and Ernberg, I., 1971 b.
    Host cell macromolecular synthesis in cells con-
    taining EBV-induced early antigens, studied by
    combined immunofluorescence and radioautography.
        Virology, 45, 22-29.

Hampar, B., Derge, J. G., Martos, L. M., and Walker, J.
L., 1972
    Synthesis of Epstein-Barr virus after activation
    of the viral genome in a virus negative human
    lymphoblastoid cell (Raji) made resistant to 5-brom-
    deoxyuridine.
        Proc. Nat. Acad. Sci. (Wash.), 69, 78-82.

Henle, W., Henle, G., Zajac, B., Pearson, G., Waubke,
R., and Scriba, M., 197o

Henle, G., Henle, W., and Klein, G., 1971 a
    Demonstration of two distinct components in the
    early antigen complex of Epstein-Barr virus infec-
    ted cells.
        Int. J. Cancer, 8, 272-282.

Henle, G., Henle, W., Klein, G., Gunvén, P., Clifford,
P., Morrow, R. H., and Ziegler, J. L., 1971 b.
    Antibodies to early Epstein-Barr virus-induced
    antigens in Burkitt's lymphoma.
        J. Nat. Cancer Inst., 46, 861-871.

Henle, W., Henle, G., Niederman, J. C., Klemola, E.,
and Halita, K., 1971 c.
    Antibodies to early antigens induced by Epstein-
    Barr virus in infectious mononucleosis.
        J. Infect. Dis., 124, 58-67.

Henle, W., Henle, G., Gunvén, P., Klein, G., Clifford,
P., and Singh, S., 1973
    Patterns of antibodies to Epstein-Barr virus-in-
    duced early antigens and Burkitt's lymphoma. Com-
    parison of dying patients with long-term survivors.
        J. Nat. Cancer Inst. 5o, 1163-1173.

Hinuma, Y., Konn, M., Yamaguchi, J., Wudarski, D. J.,
Blakeslee, J. R., and Grace, J. Y., 1967
    Immunofluorescence and Herpes-type virus particles
    in the P3HR-I Burkitt lymphoma cell line.
        J. Virol. 1, 1o45-1o51.

Klein, G., and Dombos, L., 1973
    Relationship between the sensitivity of EBV-carry-
    ing lymphoblastoid lines to superinfection and the
    inducibility of the resident viral genome.
        Inter. J. Cancer, 11, 327-337.

Klein, G., Dombos, L., and Gothoskar, B., 1972
    Sensitivity of Epstein-Barr virus (EBV) producer
    and non-producer human lymphoblastoid cell lines
    to superinfection with EB-virus.
        Int. J. Cancer, 1o, 44-57.

Klein, G., Lindahl, T., Jondal, M., Leibold, W., Ménézes,
J., Nilsson, K., and Sundstrom, Ch., 1974
    Continuous lymphoid cell lines with B-cell charac-
    teristics that lack the Epstein-Barr virus genome,
    derived from three lymphomas.
        Proc. Nat. Acad. Sci. 71, 3283-3286.

Miller, G., and Lipman, M., 1973
    Release of infectious Epstein-Barr virus by marmo-
    set leucocytes.
        Proc. Nat. Acad. Sci. USA 7o, 19o-194.

Miller, G., Coope, D., Wiederman, J., Pagano, J., 1976
    Biological properties and viral surface antigens
    of Burkitt's Lymphoma and Mononucleosis derived
    strain of Epstein-Barr Virus released from trans-
    formed marmoset cells.
        J. Virology, 18, 1o71-1o8o.

Tanaka, A., Miyagi, M., Yajima, Y., and Nonoyama, M.,
1976
    Improved Production of Epstein-Barr Virus DNA for
    Nucleic Acid Hybridization Studies.
        Virology 74, 81-85.

zur Hausen, H., 1975
    Oncogenic herpesviruses
        Biochim. Biophys. Acta, 417, 25-53.

zur Hausen, H., and Fresen, K.-O., 1977
    Heterogeneity of Epstein-Barr virus. II. Induction
    of early antigen (EA) by complementation.
        Virology 81, 138-143.

TRANSFORMATION OF MAMMALIAN CELLS BY HERPES SIMPLEX VIRUS

K. Munk, G. Darai[+], R.M. Flugel, J. Lombardo, and D. Komitowski

Inst. für Virusforsch., DKFZ
[+]Inst. für Med. Virol. d. Univ
6900 Heidelberg, FRG

A number of viruses of the herpesvirus group are proven to be oncogenic. These viruses induce tumours, mostly lymphoproliferative neoplasias either in natural hosts or in laboratory animals. Other viruses of this group, however, are only suspected to be oncogenic. Direct evidence for oncogenicity of these viruses either in natural hosts or by tumour development after experimental infection is still lacking. Herpes simplex virus (HSV) belongs to those viruses which are only suspected to be oncogenic.

So far, experiments to prove the oncogenicity of HSV by inducing tumours in the laboratory animal after infection with this virus have failed. It is therefore not possible to induce tumours in vivo. Thus, the proof for the oncogenic capacity of the HSV can only be given by testing the ability of the virus to neoplasticly transform cells in tissue culture. The malignancy of the in vitro transformed cells has to be demonstrated in experiments in which the transformed cells grow into tumours after transplantation into the isogeneic animal.

The suggestion that HSV might be oncogenic does not derive only from the well-known seroepidemiological studies, but also from the fact that HSV shares so many biological properties with those viruses of the herpesvirus group which are indeed oncogenic even under natural conditions. The stage of latency merits particular attention here. From the clinical appearance of the

recurrency of the herpes lesions, it is evident that HSV
is able to enter the productive and the non-productive
host-virus relation as well, where the productive infection is expressed in the acute herpes lesions and the
non-productive host-virus interaction takes place in the
latent phase during the interim time between the occurrence of the herpes lesions. Therefore, the properties
of the HSV as they are expressed in the latency phase in
human HSV infection resemble some properties of viruses
known to be oncogenic. We can conclude that a non-productive virus-host relationship is one of the prerequisites for the expression of oncogenic functions.

In the papovavirus-host cell system the phenomenon
of the non-permissive cells is known which gives support
to the induction of the cell transforming processes (1).
In the HSV host cell system, however, it is known that
under normal conditions all cells are permissive for HSV.
Thus, in all attempts to transform cells in vitro by HSV
it was first necessary to find and to work out conditions
under which the lytic functions of the HSV are inhibited.
The various methods by which this was achieved will be
discussed in detail later.

While generally discussing the cell transformation
experiments with HSV, one should first make a distinction between two different aims of these experiments. In
one type of experiments it was intended to alter the
cell only in one particular and distinguished property.
It was planned to demonstrate that a cell acquires a biochemical function lacking so far in these cells such as
synthesis of thymidine kinase after non-permissive infection with HSV. The thymidine kinase was proven to be
coded for by the viral DNA.

In the other type of transformation studies it was
the aim of the experiments to prove the oncogenic potential of HSV. In these experiments the conversion of a
normal cell into a tumour cell with all relevant properties have been achieved.

Table 1 gives an historical survey on these experiments. However, in the table are listed those experiments only by which a neoplastic cell transformation was
achieved.

In the further discussion of the experimental method
and details of the transforming experiments by HSV one
has to distinguish between two methodological principles.
As it was pointed out before, the prerequisite for all

TABLE 1

EXPERIMENTAL APPROACHES TO DEMONSTRATE
THE ONCOGENIC POTENTIAL OF HSV TYPE 1 AND 2

METHOD	CELLS	CONVERSION	TUMOUR	REFERENCES
UV-IRRADIATED VIRUS	HAMSTER EMBR. FIBROBLAST	+	+	DUFF + RAPP 1971 - 72
SUPRAOPTIMAL INCUBATION TEMPERATURE OF 42°C	HUMAN EMBR. CELLS	+	–	DARAI + MUNK 1973
	RAT EMBR. FIBROBLAST	+	+	DARAI + MUNK 1974
TEMPERATURE SENSITIVE VIRUS MUTANTS	RAT EMBR. FIBROBLAST	+	+	MACNAB 1974
	HAMSTER EMBR. FIBROBLAST	+	+	TAKAHASHI + YAMANISHI 1974
PHOTODYNAMIC INACTIVATED VIRUS	HAMSTER EMBR. FIBROBLAST	+	+	LI ET AL. 1975
PHOTODYNAMIC AND SUPRAOPTIMAL TEMPERATURE OF 42°C	HUMAN EMBR. FIBROBLAST	+	–	KUÇERA + GUSDON 1976
	RAT EMBR. FIBROBLAST	+	+	KUÇERA + GUSDON 1976
SUBOPTIMAL INCUBATION OF 20°C	RAT EMBR. FIBROBLAST	+	+	DARAI ET AL. 1977

TABLE 2

CELL TRANSFORMATION WITH ALTERED
HERPES SIMPLEX VIRUS

Method	Cells	Transformation in vitro	Out-Growth of Tumor in vivo
UV-Inactivation	Hamster	+	+
Temperature - Sensitive Mutants	Rat Hamster	+ +	+ +
Photodynamic Inactivation	Hamster	+	+
Inactivation by High Energy Radiation	Human Tupaia	+ +	ND ND

transformation experiments was the establishment of a
non-permissive or a non-productive virus host cell system.
Such conditions were obtained by the various laboratories
in two different ways. One group of investigators inhibited the lytic function of the HSV by altering the inoculated virus, whereas the other group of authors
changed the cell conditions from those of permissive to
those of non-permissive cells.

In the following two tables the transformation experiments are presented. In Table 2 those experiments
are listed in which the virus was altered mainly by artificial reduction of the viral gene functions, particular
those functions which determine cell lysis as a consequence.

Duff and Rapp have used in their first series of experiments ultra-violet light-irradiated HSV and have
transformed hamster embryo fibroblasts into malignant
cells (2). In the next series of experiments HSV was used
which was partially inactivated by photodynamic treatment
(3). In this method virus was treated with a heterocyclic
dye such as neutral red, proflavine or toluidine blue and
viral infectivity was subsequently inactivated with ordinary light.

In another type of experiments Macnab used temperature-sensitive (ts)-mutants of HSV and achieved neoplastic transformation of rat embryo cells with these ts-
mutants without UV-inactivation of the virus (4). She
prevented the replication of the virus after infection by
keeping the cultures infected with the ts-mutants at the
non-permissive temperature of 38°C for the initial period
of the experiment. Later, generally after 10 days, at
38°C the cultures were shifted back to an incubation
temperature of 37°C. The recognizable foci of transformed
cells began to appear after about 21 days of incubation.

In our laboratory cell transformation experiments
have recently been performed with HSV which was inactivated by high energy irradiation. We investigated the possible influence of high energy rays on the transforming
capacity of HSV. It was found that the total inactivation
of HSV which was necessary for cell transformation in vitro can be achieved by a dosis of 2×10^6 rad using gamma
rays and by 5×10^6 rad using beta rays - which were generated by a linear accelerator. Figure 1 shows the corresponding inactivation curve. Total inactivations of HSV by
deuterons generated by a cyclotron require an energy of
6×10^6 rads (Fig.2a+b).

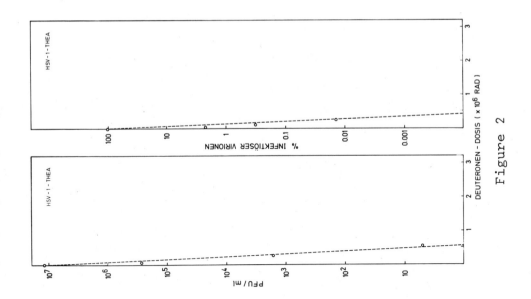

Figure 2

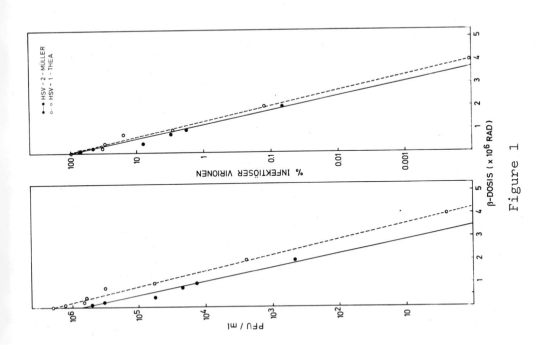

Figure 1

Human and tupaia embryonic fibroblasts were used
in order to transform these cells in tissue culture by
HSV the plaque forming ability of which had been completely inactivated by high energy rays. Preliminary results showed that inactivated HSV can transform these
mammalian cells in vitro. The transformed cells showed
all the properties characteristics for HSV-transformed
cells which were mentioned before. Experiments to prove
whether these cells are tumorigenic in vivo are in progress.

In the second type of experiments, in which the
host cell was changed to a non-permissive cell, a number of various methods have been applied (Table 3).

Garfinkle and McAuslan employed a continuous rodent
cell line which had been stably transformed by Rous-sar-
coma virus (5). This pre-transformed cell line was non-
permissive for HSV and additionally deficient in thymidine kinase synthesis. By HSV-infection of these cells,
the authors then induced the ability to synthesize thymidine kinase. It is known that this enzyme is coded for
by the persistant viral genome in these cells (6).

Another principally different technique to establish
a non-permissive host cell system which allows the application of wild-type HSV was initiated and performed in
our laboratory. As we will describe later, in further
detail, we used in one series of experiments the supraoptimal incubation temperature of 42°C for limited period
of incubation time and in the other series of experiments
we used the suboptimal incubation temperature of 20°C for
a certain period of time. The cells we used in these experiments were first human embryonic lung cells, later
rat embryo fibroblasts and recently tupaia embryonic
fibroblasts (7,8).

Kuçera and Gusdon performed experiments in which
the photo-dynamic inactivation of HSV and the incubation with the supraoptimal incubation temperature of
42°C were combined (9). These authors were successful in
transforming rat and human cells by these methods.

The characteristics of the HSV-transformed cells
are listed in Table 4.

Generally these can be defined as the parameters
for a successful cell transformation. In all experiments
mentioned so far, most of these parameters have been

TABLE 3

TRANSFORMATION OF NONPERMISSIVE CELLS
BY HERPES SIMPLEX VIRUS

Method	Cells	Transformation in vitro	Out-Growth of Tumor in vivo
RSV Pretransformed Cells	XC-Cells	+	−
Supraoptimal Incubation Temperature (42°)	Human	+	ND
	Rat	+	+
Suboptimal Incubation Temperature (20°)	Rat	+	+
Photodynamic Inactivation and Supraoptimal Incubation Temperature (42°)	Rat	+	+
	Human	+	ND

TABLE 4

CHARACTERISTICS OF THE HSV TRANSFORMED CELL

Characteristics
of the HSV Transformed Cell

Change in Morphology

Plating Efficiency

Growth in Soft Agar

Resistant to Re-Infection

Alteration of Karyotype

Stimulation of Cellular DNA

HSV-specific Antigen

Thymidine Kinase

Persistence of Viral DNA

Out-Growth of Tumor in vivo

described. The parameter for synthesis of thymidine kinase was only used in the thymidine kinase-deficient
host cell.

Our own cell transformation experiments are outlined in the next table (Fig.3) which describes the
standard protocols of the method to transform at either
the supraoptimal or at the suboptimal incubation temperature. These transformed cells diplayed properties
which are characteristic for HSV-transformed cells.

The questions of a possible interaction between herpesviruses and oncornaviruses during the HSV transformation process and their co-tumorigenicity is one of
the important aspects in the field of the oncogenic potential of herpesviruses. Type-C RNA viruses were activated in HSV-transformed cells (10) and these results
were confirmed by Hampar, Rapp and their co-workers (11).
Using different transformation methods HSV-transformed
rat cell clones which had been transformed at the non-
permissive temperature contained high levels of reverse
transkriptase activity.

Syncytia formation or giant cells typical for C-type
RNA particles with a small (6-8) number of nuclei was
also observed. These rat cells induced malignant tumours
in syngeneic animals. These results indicate that an activation of retroviruses could take place in cells transformed by HSV and is independent of the method of transformation. All these findings justify to consider the
hypothesis of a possible virus-virus co-tumorigenicity.

Since the first report of mammalian cells by HSV,
many efforts have been made to directly detect the genome of HSV in the transformed and tumour cells by nuclei acid hybridization. Minson et al. suggested that
the presence of HSV DNA in the 333-8-9 line of hamster
cells transformed by UV-irradiated HSV-2 is an unstable
characteristic of the cell line and that these sequences
may be lost at cell division (11). The possibility that
a small fragment of the HSV genome remained could not be
excluded. It is interesting in this context that Kraiselburd found five copies of fragment comprising only
23% of the total HSV genome by reassociation kinetics in
a cloned mouse L cell line which had been transformed by
HSV (13). In hamster cells which had been transformed
by HSV, Frenkel et al. found that the amount of HSV DNA
present in the cells varied in different transformed
cell lines and ranged from 8% to 32% (14). Our HSV-

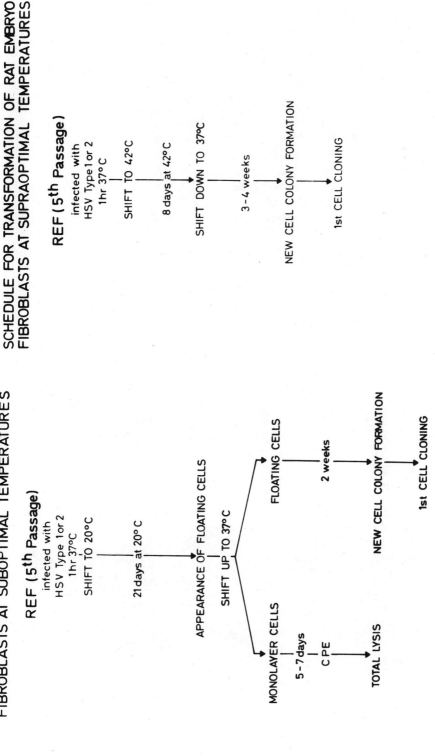

Figure 3

TABLE 5

RELATION OF THE SIZE OF THE LETHAL HSV DOSE TO THE AGE
OF INFECTED TUPAIAS

Age (days) Weight (g) *	Inoculated HSV	Route of application	PFU animal	Dead animals Number of animals
29 / 84	HSV-1 WAL	i.v.	2.5×10^2	4/4
35 / 107	HSV-1 WAL	i.p.	2.5×10^2	1/1
31 / 95	HSV-2 HG-52	i.p.	5.0×10^2	4/4
32 / 91	HSV-1 Thea	s.c.	1.0×10^3	2/2
31 / 81	HSV-2 Müller	s.c.	1.0×10^3	2/2
40 / 107	HSV-2 HG-52	i.p.	1.0×10^5	7/9
45 / 128	HSV-2 HG-52	i.p.	1.0×10^5	2/3
150 / 172	HSV-2 HG-52	i.p.	1.0×10^3	0/1
150 / 173	HSV-2 HG-52	i.p.	1.0×10^5	0/1

* AVERAGE VALUES

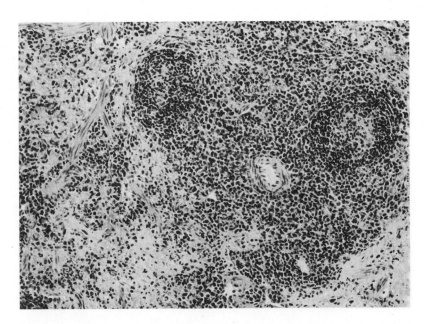

Histological picture of Tupaia spleen after HSV
infection.

transformed rat cell lines gave negative results at a
level of detection of one copy of 10% of the complete
HSV genome per 50 cells by DNA-DNA reassociation kinetics.
When the RNA-DNA hybridization technique was used, it
was found that less than 1% of the HSV genome per one
cell is present in the HSV-transformed rat cell (G. Fey,
unpublished).

Direct evidence for tumour induction in vivo by HSV
is missing. Most investigators attempted to induce tumours by HSV in rodents. These experiments failed, because first, the life-span of rodents is limited, and a
long-time observation therefore not possible. Second,
the high rate of induction of spontaneous tumours in these
animals make such experiments impossible. These experiments can only be approached and convincingly performed,
if an animal is available which meets the following requirements, namely a long life-span, a very low rate of
spontaneous tumour induction and is susceptible for HSV.
We found that the animal of choice is the tree shrew, also called tupaia. This primitive prosimian is highly susceptible for HSV and lives for 8 to 14 years. The rate
of spontaneous tumours to a study by Elliot et al. is under 0.1% (15). Our own observations confirm the results.
Since 1976 my laboratory has been involved in studying
the broad virological aspects of the tree shrew.

One of the projects was to study the pathogenesis
of HSV in tupaias. We found that juvenile tree shrews are
highly susceptible to HSV, type 1 and type 2 (Table 5).
The high susceptibility for HSV-2 ended, if the animal
reached the age of 60 to 70 days. In contrast, the susceptibility for HSV-1 remained unchanged for a longer
period of time. The animals which survived the HSV-infection were studied for recovery of latent virus which
was successful in 25%. The virus could be recovered from
the spinal cord of animals infected. All organs of the
infected animals were studied by histo-pathological investigations. A remarkable finding was that the spleen of
some animals which were sacrificed 6 months p.i. showed
pre-neoplastic cell formation, typical for the beginning
of malignant lymphomas (Fig.4). This would be a first
evidence for a possible induction of a neoplasia in vivo
by HSV.

These observations could lead us into right direction that using these special animals it will be possible
to throw light upon the unsolved problem of the in vivo
oncogenicity by HSV.

REFERENCES

1. Sambrook, J. (1972). Adv. Cancer Res. 16, 141-180.

2. Duff, R., and Rapp, F. (1971). J. Virol. 8, 469-477.

3. Rapp, F., Li, L.J., and Jerkofsky, M. (1973). Virology 55, 339-346.

4. Macnab, J.C.M. (1974). Virology 24, 143-1

5. Garfinkle, B., and McAuslan, B.R. (1974). Proc. nat. Acad. Sci. U.S.A. 71, 220-224.

6. Kit, S. (1976). Cell Biochem. 11, 161-182.

7. Darai, G., and Munk, K. (1973). Nature New Biol. 241, 268-269.

8. Darai, G., and Munk, K. (1976). Int. J. Cancer 18, 469-481.

9. Kučera, L.S., and Gusdon, J.P. (1976). J. Gen. Virol. 30, 257-261.

10. Flügel, R.M., Darai, G., Braun, R., and Munk, K. (1977). J. Gen. Virol. 36, 365-369.

11. Hampar, B., Aaronson, S.A., Derge, J.G., Chakrabarty, M., Showalter, S.D., and Dunn, C.J. (1976). Proc. nat. Acad. Sci. U.S.A. 33, 288-293.

12. Minson, A.C., Thouless, M.E., Eglin, R.P., and Darby, G. (1976). Int. J. Cancer 17, 493-500.

13. Kraiselburd, E., Gage, L.P., and Weissbach, A. (1976). J. mol. Biol. 97, 533-542.

14. Frenkel, N., Locker, H., Cox, B., Roizmann, B., and Rapp, F. (1976). Virol. 18, 885-893.

15. Elliot, O.S., Elliot, M.W., and Lisco, H. (1966). Nature 211, 1105.

THE ONCOGENIC PROPERTIES OF HUMAN CYTOMEGALOVIRUS

Fred Rapp and Barbara A. McCarthy

Department of Microbiology
The Pennsylvania State University College of Medicine
Hershey, Pennsylvania 17033 USA

Two herpesviruses, Marek's Disease virus and the Lucké virus, are known to cause malignant disease in their natural hosts, the chicken and frog, respectively. Two human herpesviruses, herpes simplex virus (HSV) and Epstein-Barr virus (EBV), are now routinely associated with certain malignancies in humans (51). A third human herpesvirus, cytomegalovirus (CMV), is found in many tissues and body secretions. It causes congenital disease and represents a feared secondary consequence to patients on immunosuppressive therapy. Its role in human neoplasia is not known, although it has been associated with tumors of the genitourinary tract and with Kaposi's sarcoma. The virus can stimulate host DNA synthesis and can transform rodent and human cells in culture. The transformed cells are morphologically altered, contain virus antigens and virus-specific nucleic acids, and are malignant when transplanted to an appropriate host. Cell lines from the tumors have been established and partially characterized. These observations strongly suggest that CMV is an oncogenic agent (Table 1) with the potential to cause neoplasia in humans. A background on CMV, its history, its role in clinical disease, the expression of antibody, and the characteristics of its DNA will be presented briefly before the oncogenic properties of this virus are discussed.

HISTORY OF THE DISCOVERY OF CMV

The first description of the clinical condition now recognized as cytomegalic inclusion disease occurred in 1904 when Jesionek and Kiolemenoglou (34) reported the presence of protozoan-like cells in the kidneys, liver, and lungs of a premature

Table 1

Evidence for Causal Role of Viruses in Carcinogenesis

Epidemiological evidence:	Association of virus with tumors in nature.
	Reduced incidence with vaccine.
Biological evidence:	Infectious virus in tumor cells.
	Tumor induction in vivo.
	Transformation of cells in vitro.
Biochemical evidence:	Virus nucleic acids in tumor cells.
Immunological evidence:	Virus-specific antigens in tumor cells.
	Antibodies to virus antigens in patients.
	Antibodies prognostic.

---

infant. Subsequent reports identified similar giant cells with Goodpasture and Talbot in 1921 (24), suggesting the use of the term cytomegalia because of the size of the cells. In the same year, Lipschütz (39) observed that the intranuclear inclusions were similar to those seen in herpetic lesions and suggested that the inclusion disease was due to a virus. Today, we know that congenital cytomegalic inclusion disease is the result of a human CMV infection which is, most probably, acquired in utero from the asymptomatically infected mother (26,42,65,67). As early as 1932, the characteristic cytomegalic inclusion bodies were detected in salivary glands from 12% of the autopsy material examined (13). In 1952, the clinical manifestation referred to as salivary gland virus disease, was detectable by inclusion bodies in typical cells in the urinary sediment (14). This discovery paved the way for three simultaneous, but independent, isolations of CMV: in 1956, Dr. Margaret G. Smith isolated CMV from the submaxillary salivary gland tissue of a dead infant (60) and in the same year, Dr. Wallace Rowe and his coworkers isolated the virus from human adenoidal tissue, hence the name AD169 (54) for this isolate. Weller et al. (69) also successfully isolated the agent from liver biopsy material and this isolate, known as the Davis strain, was the first CMV recovered from a living patient. The name, cytomegalovirus, now commonly used in place of "salivary gland virus" or the "viruses of cytomegalic inclusion disease", was suggested by Weller and his colleagues in 1960 (68).

CLINICAL DISEASE DUE TO CMV

Each year in the United States, more than 3,000 infants are born seriously retarded as a result of congenital CMV infection (40). In addition to mental retardation, these children may also suffer from other birth defects due to CMV infection, namely blindness and deafness. Approximately one percent of all infants are born infected with CMV and 10% of these infants will suffer from one or more of the following diseases: cytomegalic inclusion disease, enlarged spleen and liver, hepatitis, blood abnormalities, and microcephaly. One of the most dreaded diseases of infancy is cytomegalic inclusion disease with clinical manifestations that include: jaundice, petechiae, chorioretinitis, microcephaly, central nervous system disease (including seizures, spastic diplegia, deafness and microphthalmia), hepatosplenomegaly, pneumonia, mental and psychomotor retardation, diarrhea, cerebral calcifications, chronic gastroenteritis, thrombocytopenia and prematurity (42). Follow-up studies on children with nonfatal cases of cytomegalic inclusion disease demonstrate that many of these patients go on to acquire unusual sequelae as they mature (42). Only rarely has cytomegalic inclusion disease been encountered in adults (70).

A study by Dr. James B. Hanshaw, in which 8,600 newborns were screened for evidence of CMV infection, yielded a virus recovery of approximately 0.6% (51.6) as reviewed by Marx (40). Those children with infections at birth had lower intelligence quotient scores than control children. Congenital CMV infections may result from: 1) primary infection of the mother during pregnancy; 2) reactivation of a latent virus carried by the woman; 3) localized cervical CMV infecting the fetus; or 4) venereally acquired infections. Since acquisition of congenital CMV infections may result from one of the modes of transmission mentioned above, it is necessary to consider the possibility that these viruses may be, and, in fact, probably are transmitted sexually. Cytomegaloviruses are known to cause cervicitis, urethritis and intrauterine infections which are asymptomatic (12). Such CMV infections of the female genital tract are common during pregnancy and may be the source of neonatal infections (45). It is now known that maternal humoral immunity may not protect the fetus against congenital CMV infection (61). Lang and Kummer in 1972 (37) reported the case of a 23-year-old male recovering from CMV mononucleosis. They followed this case closely and determined that CMV was replicating in the genital tract and that a high titer of CMV persisted in the semen for weeks, although the patient was asymptomatic. In a later study (38), these same investigators detected CMV in the semen of six individuals, thus establishing the presence and persistence of CMV in semen and indicating that sexual transmission might be involved in the spread of some CMV infections. In a recent

study, Chretien et al. (4) noted the development of CMV mononucleosis in two men after sexual contact with a woman who had
had a similar but medically unverified illness several months
before. CMV was cultured from the woman's urine and cervix. A
new sexual contact of one of the men was also found to have
evidence of recent CMV infection. The roommates of the first
woman did not develop the disease and serologic tests failed to
demonstrate the development of a CMV infection. Thus, a CMV
mononucleosis syndrome may result from the acquisition of CMV by
venereal infection. Although several clinicians thought that the
etiology of Paul-Bunnell-positive and Paul-Bunnell-negative
mononucleosis were different, it was not until 1965 that the CMV
infectious mononucleosis syndrome was first described by Klemola
and Kääriäinen (36). They observed that complement-fixing
antibodies to CMV rise in patients with clinically diagnosed
infectious mononucleosis without a positive heterophil agglutination test. No significant rise of the complement-fixing antibody
titer to CMV was demonstrated in a single case among those suffering from infectious mononucleosis with a positive heterophil
agglutination test. A significant rise in the neutralizing
antibody titer to CMV has also been detected in all patients with
the heterophil-negative mononucleosis-like syndrome.

        CMV infection is also a grave concern to transplant surgeons
and the recipients of donor blood and organs. Three sources of
risk exist for these patients: 1) the blood donor; 2) the transplanted organ; and 3) reactivation of the patient's own latent
CMV infection. There are other factors to be considered: a
second stimulation of CMV by foreign white cells, drugs, and the
stress of surgery (11). It is known that a number of blood
donors experience prolonged viremia (6). If blood from such a
person is transfused into a susceptible patient, a whole range of
disease manifestations may be observed from subclinical infection
to the post-transfusion syndrome (28,50). A study by Monif
et al. (44) suggests that blood may be a vehicle for infectious
CMV particles and that exclusion of seropositive donors should be
initiated to reduce the chance of CMV infection. The transplanted kidney is also a source of CMV infection and a prospective study by Ho et al. (29) reported a significant correlation
between the development of CMV infection and the seropositivity
of the donor, particularly when the recipient was seronegative.
Another report (59) details two patterns of CMV infection in
renal transplant recipients. A benign form exists in which fever
and leukopenia occur within 6 months post-transplant with renal
biopsy evidence of rejection and brisk antibody responses to CMV.
The lethal form is also accompanied by fever and leukopenia
within 6 months post-transplant, but progresses through a typical
four-week course of prostration, orthostatic hypotension, and
mild hypoxemia, progressing to severe pulmonary and hepatic
dysfunction, muscle wasting, central nervous system depression

and death. The antibody responses to CMV are minimal in the
lethal form and renal biopsy does not show rejection. Upon
autopsy, CMV is found in the lungs, liver, kidneys, gastrointestinal tract, and brain. It is possible to control the lethal
syndrome; however, successful management depends largely on rapid
clinical recognition and immediate reduction of immunosuppressive
therapy. The first report of CMV-induced vasculitis producing
skin ulcerations in a renal transplant patient reaffirms the
potential dangers of this ubiquitous virus (43). Clinicians
should be aware of the possible occurrence of skin ulceration due
to CMV. Bone marrow transplantation has also been associated
with the activation of CMV and its associated diseases (53).

We have discussed several conditions that are associated
with CMV reactivation: pregnancy, organ transplantation, transfusion, and malignancy. These conditions share two common features: 1) the body is in a state of varying degrees of immunosuppression, and 2) the presence of foreign antigens. The antibody status of the patient to CMV will determine whether clinical
illness will follow reactivation of the virus.

A final clinical manifestation that was recently linked to
CMV infection is the Guillain-Barré Syndrome (58). Of ten
patients studied, nine had a prior CMV infection as detected by
virus-specific IgM present in high titers in the serum, and five
yielded CMV from the urine. The etiology of Guillain-Barré
Syndrome is not clear and the possible involvement of CMV as the
causative agent is still highly speculative. Although CMV is
known to cause encephalitis, chronic CMV encephalitis leading to
death in newborns is rare and encephalitis in adults usually has
a benign outcome (3). Successful treatment of CMV encephalitis
in immunologically normal adults has been accomplished with
vidarabine (48). A double encephalitis caused by HSV and CMV has
been reported in an adult but this double infection seems to be
unique (71).

Since CMV is known to cause a broad spectrum of clinical
diseases in humans (Table 2), studies have been conducted to
investigate the formation and expression of antibodies in acutely-
infected and in latently-infected, but healthy individuals.
Complement-fixing and neutralizing antibodies have been detected
in the serum of CMV-infected infants and their mothers (41,46).
In addition, virus antigen has been detected in CMV-infected
cells by fluorescein-labeled antibody (66). Congenital CMV
infections will result in the production of IgM and elevations in
IgM levels are useful in detecting intrauterine infections due to
CMV. Fluorescent antibody techniques have been used to determine
the early IgM antibody response in adults with CMV infections.
In 1966, Hanshaw suggested that a complement-fixing antibody
titer greater than 1:8 in a young infant usually results from an

Table 2

Diseases Due to Human Cytomegalovirus

| Disease | |
Confirmed Etiology	Associated Etiology
Cytomegalic Inclusion Disease	Prostatic Cancer
Congenital defects	Kaposi's Sarcoma
Abortion	Cervical Cancer
Mononucleosis-like syndrome	Guillain-Barré Syndrome
Interstitial Pnemonia	Bladder Cancer
Microcephaly	
Blood abnormalities	
Hepatitis	

active infection rather than from passive transfer of antibody from the mother (25). In older individuals acquiring CMV infection for the first time, the rise in antibody, as in other virus infections, is usually over a three-week course. A report by The et al. (63) established that CMV early antigen and late antigen differed with regard to distribution and antigenic specificity. Sera collected before the onset of CMV infection did not have antibodies to either late or early antigen, thus supporting the idea that the infection was primary. The patients then developed antibodies to the late antigen which reached a peak in the acute phase of disease and remained at high levels. The antibodies to early antigen showed a late rise as well as an early decrease. The CMV-induced antibodies to early antigen were found only in acutely infected patients but not in healthy donors or in patients with other herpesvirus infections. Thus, the presence of antibodies to early antigen may be helpful in diagnosing recent and acute CMV infections. In another study by Dr. Laszlo Geder (15), nuclear antigens were induced by CMV as early as three hours post-infection when the anti-complement immunofluorescence (ACIF) test was used. The staining pattern and early appearance of the nuclear antigen is similar to the EBV nuclear antigen. This work was confirmed by Giraldo et al. (21) who also determined that there is no cross-reactivity between

early antigens of CMV, HSV and EBV. The and colleagues (62)
investigated the presence of antibodies against CMV-induced early
antigens in the sera of immunosuppressed renal-allograft recipients. Of fifteen recipients, eight seroconverted from 47 to 137
days post-transplantation; five with CMV antibodies at the time
of transplantation showed rises in the antibody response to CMV
early antigen, and two recipients remained seronegative until
four years after transplantation. These data support this group's
early results that antibodies to CMV early antigen reflect an
active virus proliferation in the host and that antibodies against
CMV late antigen are present in latent infection (63). In a
separate study, CMV was isolated from cervical secretions of
patients at a venereal disease clinic (64). Patients whose
cervical secretions were reactive for IgG and secretory IgA
antibodies, demonstrated antibody to the early antigen. It is
not yet clear whether the presence of secretory IgA antibody is
associated with the recent acquisition of a CMV infection and
whether the secretory IgA antibody functions in a protective
fashion in genital CMV infections.

CMV DNA

     Since 1973, several laboratories have concentrated their
efforts on the characterization of human CMV DNA. Huang et al.
(32) reported in 1973 that the density of CMV DNA as determined
by analytical ultracentrifugation was 1.716 g/cm^3 and that the
molecular weight of CMV DNA is approximately 10^8. A recent
report by Kilpatrick and Huang (35) provides additional information on the human CMV genome. Contour length measurements of CMV
DNA indicate that more than one size class of virus DNA is
encapsidated. There is apparently a class averaging 100 x 10^6
daltons as well as a less abundant class of larger CMV DNA
molecules averaging 150-155 x 10^6 daltons. The alignment of the
partial denaturation maps of both class molecules reveals six
unique zones contained in a length equal to the longest class.
Five of these zones are linked in a specific sequence and maintain the same relative orientation. These features indicate the
absence of major inversions within these zones. The sixth zone
may occur at either end of the five zone series but never at both
ends. DNA-DNA reassociation kinetics have been used with the S1
enzyme differential digestion technique to determine homology of
human CMV DNA to EBV, HSV types 1 and 2 (HSV-1 and HSV-2), and
simian and murine CMV DNA (33). No relatedness, or less than 5%
detectable homology, exists. Human CMV can stimulate the synthesis of host cell DNA and RNA (55). This important discovery by
St. Jeor et al. (55) provided the groundwork for the study by
Huang in which a human CMV-induced DNA polymerase was detected
(30). Further experiments by Huang using nucleic acid hybridization demonstrated the specific inhibition of human CMV DNA

synthesis in virus-infected human fibroblasts by phosphonoacetic acid (31). When the drug was removed the inhibition was reversible and virus DNA synthesis resumed. Albrecht et al. (1) reported the induction of cellular DNA synthesis and increased mitotic activity in hamster embryo fibroblast cells which were abortively infected with human CMV. However, DeMarchi and Kaplan (5) found that activation of cellular DNA synthesis is apparently not essential for virus DNA or virus antigen synthesis. St. Jeor and Weisser (56) report the persistence of CMV in human lymphoblasts and peripheral leukocyte cultures. Unpublished experiments by St. Jeor and Walboomers indicated that CMV induces higher levels of cellular thymidine kinase instead of coding for its own thymidine kinase. This work was extended by Závada et al. (72) in 1976 when they reported that the AD169 strain of human CMV did not induce a viral thymidine kinase and by Estes and Huang (10) who also reported that strains AD169 and Towne did not induce a virus-specific thymidine kinase. Further characterization of the human CMV-stimulated thymidine kinase enzymes demonstrated that they are of cellular origin.

TRANSFORMING AND ONCOGENIC POTENTIAL OF CMV

It is well known that CMV, like many other herpesviruses, has the propensity to infect an individual and produce overt disease or subclinical infection. CMV is also capable of entering a latent state after residing for long periods of time in individuals who are asymptomatic. Latency is one characteristic that has brought CMV under much suspicion for a possible role in the development of malignancy. It is known that human CMV can induce oncogenic transformation of hamster embryo fibroblast cells (2) and can stimulate the synthesis of host cell DNA and RNA (55). These properties are commonly associated with oncogenic herpesviruses as demonstrated by the initial studies of Duff and Rapp in 1971 (7) and 1973 (8). In 1975 (52), Rapp et al. reported that cells from human prostate tissue which apparently had been infected in vivo with CMV grew in vitro to passage levels higher than those usually attained by normal cells (Figs. 1 and 2). Virus was not rescuable after several passages, although CMV-specific antigens and nucleic acids could be detected. At the time, it was not clear whether the cells were transformed by CMV or whether they were chronically infected and released virus at levels too low for detection. As a result, additional studies were initiated to examine the transforming ability of the Mj virus isolate. Geder et al. (18) were able to demonstrate that CMV-Mj-infected human embryo lung cells can establish long-term persistent infection and that occasional cell transformants can arise in the cultures. These resulting cell transformants contain CMV-specific membrane and intracellular antigens and share common antigens with CMV-transformed hamster

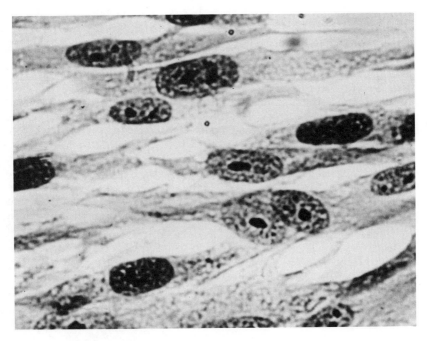

Figure 1.   Normal human embryo fibroblast cells.

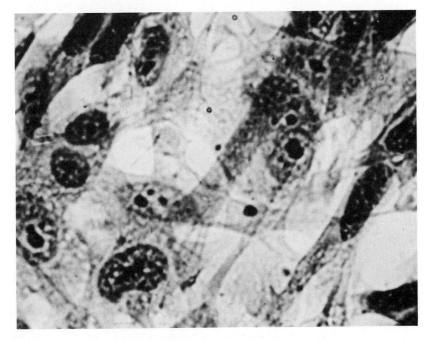

Figure 2.   Human embryo fibroblasts transformed by cytomegalovirus.

cells. The cells were also able to induce nondifferentiated
tumors when injected into weanling athymic nude mice. A cell
line, CMV-Mj-HEL-2 was subsequently established from the in vitro
transformation of HEL cells by CMV. The transformed cells ceased
to demonstrate contact-inhibition, grew in soft agarose, and
possessed easily detectable CMV-antigenic markers at early
in vitro passages. This line proved to be oncogenic when inoculated into athymic nude mice (17). After an average latent
period of 19 days, 62% of the animals developed tumors (Fig. 3).
The tumor cells were poorly differentiated but may have been of
epithelial origin. Uninfected HEL cells and latently infected
human prostatic fibroblasts were nononcogenic in the nude mouse.
CMV-related intracellular and membrane antigens were detected by
indirect immunofluorescence and ACIF techniques in cells cultured
in vitro from the tumors. During prolonged in vitro cultivation,
diverse alterations in oncogenicity, CMV-related antigenicity,
karyotypic markers, resistance to superinfection with herpesviruses, and induction of immune response were observed. The
oncogenicity of the transformed cells was inversely proportional
to the rate of expression of virus-related antigens in the cell
population (16). A new herpesvirus has been recovered from one
of the transformed cell lines (Geder, Figueroa and Rapp,

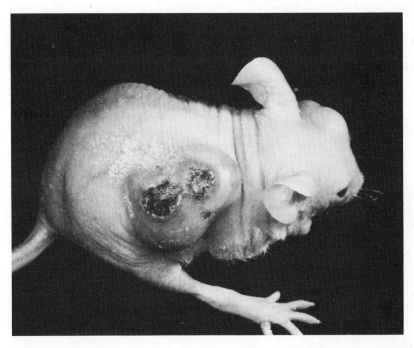

Figure 3. Athymic nude mouse with tumor induced by cytomegalo-
virus-transformed cells.

unpublished observations). This new herpesvirus (Fig. 4) has
biological and biochemical properties resembling CMV and HSV.
Base sequence homology between this new virus DNA and HSV-2 DNA
has been detected, although the density and the restriction
enzyme patterns of the virus DNA do not resemble CMV or HSV DNA
(Hyman, Oakes, Iltis, Dawson and Rapp, unpublished observations).

This laboratory is also involved in studying the etiology of
prostate cancer and the possible involvement of CMV in the initiation of this malignant condition (Fig. 5). In a preliminary
study by Geder et al. (20), prostate cell cultures were screened
for herpesvirus-specific markers. Sera from prostatic cancer
patients were shown to react two times more frequently in immunofluorescence tests with the cytoplasmic membrane of CMV-transformed human cells than the sera of a control group. These
observations suggest the presence of CMV markers in some prostatic cancer cell lines and establish the in vitro transformation
of human cells by a human prostatic CMV isolate. In another
study by Sanford et al. (57), it was reported that two cell lines
derived from tissue from human prostatic carcinoma survived more
than 20 passages in vitro and demonstrated CMV-specific membrane
antigens. Significant humoral antibody titers against CMV and
cell-mediated lymphocytotoxicity against these transformed cells
were demonstrated in patients with urinary tract tumors. Geder
and Rapp (19) demonstrated that intranuclear CMV-related antigens
can be detected in CMV-transformed human cells by the ACIF test.
Staining of the nuclei of CMV-transformed cells by ACIF correlated with the presence in the sera of CMV antibodies against

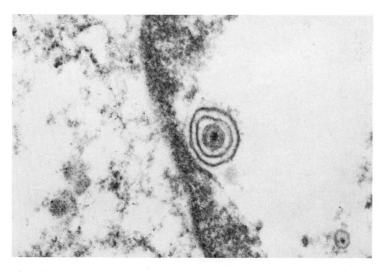

Figure 4. New herpesvirus resembling cytomegalovirus and herpes
simplex virus isolated from transformed cell lines.

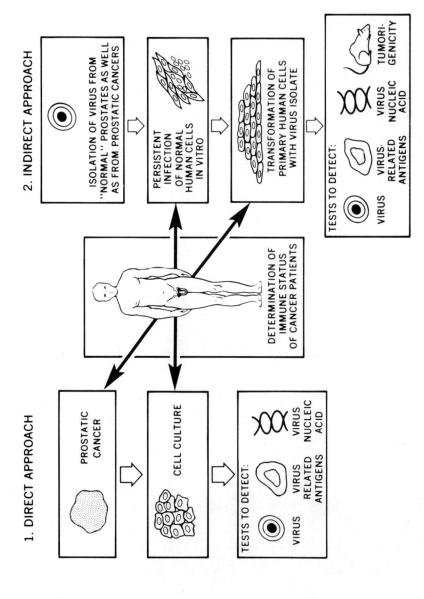

Figure 5. Approach to study the etiology of prostatic cancer.

late-phase intracellular and early intranuclear antigens of CMV-
infected cells. Immune sera from patients with prostatic cancer
or those individuals in the convalescent phase of an acute CMV
infection who had a CMV antibody titer greater than 1:64, demonstrated nuclear reactivity. A relationship seems to exist between the early nuclear antigens of CMV-infected cells (15) and
the nuclear antigens of transformed cells.

Cytomegalovirus has also been associated with cervical
cancer and Kaposi's sarcoma, although the evidence to support a
role for CMV in these diseases has been meager. Antibodies to
CMV have been detected more often in sera of women with atypia
than in sera of women with other cervical disorders or in sera of
healthy controls (47). CMV has also been detected in the cervix
during the last trimester of pregnancy more often than HSV-2.
In 1975, Giraldo et al. (22) analyzed sera from patients with
Kaposi's sarcoma. The sera were examined for antibody titers to
CMV, EBV, HSV-1 and HSV-2 using indirect hemagglutination,
complement-fixation, virus neutralization, and indirect immunofluorescence techniques. All Kaposi's sarcoma sera contained CMV
neutralizing antibodies. Patients in regressive stages of the
disease showed significantly elevated anti-CMV titers by indirect
hemagglutination. However, patients in progressive stages of the
disease did not show a serologic association with CMV. There was
no significant association with antibodies to EBV, HSV-1 or
HSV-2 among regressors or progressors. Glaser et al. (23) characterized a herpes-like virus (K9V) isolated from a cell culture
derived from a tumor biopsy specimen from a patient with Kaposi's
sarcoma. The presence of CMV-type antigens in K9V-infected human
fibroblasts was detected by immunofluorescence and complement-
fixation assays. The density of the K9V DNA was consistent with
the density of CMV DNA. Peculiarities noticed in K9V, are similar
to characteristics observed in the Mj strain of CMV which transforms human fibroblasts. The virus was more cell-associated in
human fibroblasts than other laboratory strains, spread of cytopathology was slow, and total regression of cytopathology was
common when persistent infection was established. It is possible
that the K9V strain of CMV may play a role in the etiology of
Kaposi's sarcoma.

CONTROL OF INFECTION DUE TO CMV

Scientists have been searching for safe, effective therapies
to control congenital infection due to CMV. Elek and Stern (9)
suggested that adolescent girls be inoculated with a live strain
of CMV so that the incidence of primary CMV infection during
pregnancy could be reduced. In studies with volunteers, they
found that subcutaneous inoculation was capable of stimulating
neutralizing and complement-fixing antibody production without

serious side effects. A weighing of the pros and cons concerning a CMV vaccine was discussed by Hanshaw (27). He considered the long-term safety, effectiveness, need, benefits, and cost of such a vaccine. Plotkin et al. (49) reported the results of clinical trials in which male volunteers were immunized with the Towne strain of human CMV. The volunteers were inoculated subcutaneously with the virus and this induced seroconversion in all seronegative volunteers and a booster antibody response in some previously seropositive individuals. Many more tests need to be conducted before the safety and efficacy of a CMV vaccine can be determined.

CONCLUSIONS

1.   CMV is ubiquitous in the human population and is found in many organs and secretions.

2.   Spread of the virus is broad, involving respiratory, intrauterine, and venereal routes.

3.   The virus often causes persistent and latent infections and is most readily reactivated by immunosuppression.

4.   CMV stimulates host cell DNA synthesis and can transform human cells in culture to malignancy.

5.   Although the role of the virus in a variety of human illnesses is well documented, its role in cancer is still speculative.

ACKNOWLEDGMENTS

This work was supported by contract #NO1-CP-5-3516 within the Virus Cancer Program of the National Cancer Institute and by grants CA 18450 and CA 16365 awarded by the National Cancer Institute, National Institutes of Health.

REFERENCES

1. Albrecht, T., Nachtigal, M., St. Jeor, S. C. and Rapp, F. Induction of cellular DNA synthesis and increased mitotic activity in Syrian hamster embryo cells abortively infected with human cytomegalovirus. J. Gen. Virol. 30: 167-177, 1976.

2. Albrecht, T. and Rapp, F. Malignant transformation of
    hamster embryo fibroblasts following exposure to ultra-
    violet-irradiated human cytomegalovirus. Virology 55:
    53-61, 1973.

3. Brown, P. Viral Encephalitis. In Current Diagnosis, Fifth
    Edition, H. F. Conn and R. B. Conn, eds. W. B. Sanders
    and Co., Philadelphia, pp. 126-136, 1977.

4. Chretien, J. H., McGinnis, C. G. and Muller, A. Venereal
    causes of cytomegalovirus mononucleosis. J.A.M.A. 238:
    1644-1645, 1977.

5. DeMarchi, J. M. and Kaplan, A. S. Replication of human
    cytomegalovirus DNA: Lack of dependence on cell DNA
    synthesis. J. Virol. 18: 1063-1070, 1976.

6. Diosi, P., Moldovan, E. and Tomescu, N. Latent cytomegalo-
    virus infection in blood donors. Brit. Med. J. 4: 660-
    662, 1969.

7. Duff, R. and Rapp, F. Properties of hamster embryo fibro-
    blasts transformed in vitro after exposure to ultra-
    violet-irradiated herpes simplex virus type 2. J.
    Virol. 8: 469-477, 1971.

8. Duff, R. and Rapp, F. Oncogenic transformation of hamster
    embryo cells after exposure to inactivated herpes
    simplex virus type 1. J. Virol. 12: 209-217, 1973.

9. Elek, S. D. and Stern, H. Development of a vaccine against
    mental retardation caused by cytomegalovirus infection
    in utero. The Lancet, January 5, 1974, 1-5.

10. Estes, J. E. and Huang, E.-S. Stimulation of cellular
    thymidine kinases by human cytomegalovirus. J. Virol.
    24: 13-21, 1977.

11. Evans, A. S. Symposium on cytomegalovirus infections:
    Opening remarks. Yale J. Biol. Med. 49: 3-4, 1976.

12. Evans, T. N. Sexually transmissible diseases. Am. J.
    Obstet. Gynecol. 125: 116-133, 1976.

13. Farber, S. and Wolbach, S. B. Intranuclear and cytoplasmic
    inclusions ("protozoan-like bodies") in salivary glands
    and other organs of infants. Am. J. Path. 8: 123-126,
    1932.

14. Fetterman, G. H. New laboratory aid in clinical diagnosis
     of inclusion disease of infancy. Am. J. Clin. Path.
     22: 424-425, 1952.

15. Geder, L. Evidence for early nuclear antigens in cyto-
     megalovirus-infected cells. J. Gen. Virol. 32: 315-
     319, 1976.

16. Geder, L., Laychock, A., Gorodecki, J. and Rapp, F. Altera-
     tions in biological properties of different lines of
     cytomegalovirus-transformed human embryo lung cells
     following in vitro cultivation. In Oncogenesis and
     Herpesviruses. Proceedings of the Symposium on Onco-
     genesis and Herpesviruses (eds. G. de Thé, W. Henle and
     F. Rapp), International Agency for Research on Cancer,
     Lyon, France, 1978, in press.

17. Geder, L., Kreider, J. and Rapp, F. Human cells transformed
     in vitro by human cytomegalovirus: Tumorigenicity in
     athymic nude mice. J. Natl. Cancer Inst. 58: 1003-
     1009, 1977.

18. Geder, L., Lausch, R. N., O'Neill, F. J. and Rapp, F.
     Oncogenic transformation of human embryo lung cells by
     human cytomegalovirus. Science 192: 1134-1137, 1976.

19. Geder, L. and Rapp, F. Evidence for nuclear antigens in
     cytomegalovirus-transformed human cells. Nature 265:
     184-186, 1977.

20. Geder, L., Sanford, E. J., Rohner, T. J. and Rapp, F.
     Cytomegalovirus and cancer of the prostate: In vitro
     transformation of human cells. Cancer Treatment Re-
     ports 61: 139-146, 1977.

21. Giraldo, G., Beth, E., Hammerling, U., Tarro, G. and
     Kourilsky, F. M. Detection of early antigens in nuclei
     of cells infected with cytomegalovirus or herpes simplex
     virus type 1 and 2 by anti-complement immunofluorescence,
     and use of a blocking assay to demonstrate their specifi-
     city. Int. J. Cancer 19: 107-116, 1977.

22. Giraldo, G., Beth, E., Kourilsky, F. M., Henle, W., Henle,
     G., Miké, V., Huraux, J. M., Andersen, H. K., Gharbi,
     M. R., Kyalwazi, S. K. and Puissant, A. Antibody
     patterns to herpesviruses in Kaposi's sarcoma: Sero-
     logical association of European Kaposi's sarcoma with
     cytomegalovirus. Int. J. Cancer 15: 839-848, 1975.

23. Glaser, R., Geder, L., St. Jeor, S., Michelson-Fiske, S. and
     Haguenau, F. Partial characterization of a herpes-type
     virus (K9V) derived from Kaposi's sarcoma. J. Natl.
     Cancer Inst. 59: 55-59, 1977.

24. Goodpasture, E. W. and Talbot, F. B. Concerning the nature
     of protozoan-like cells in certain lesions of infancy.
     Am. J. Dis. Child. 21: 415-425, 1921.

25. Hanshaw, J. B. Congenital and acquired cytomegalovirus
     infection. The Pediatric Clinics of North America 13:
     279-293, 1966.

26. Hanshaw, J. B. Congenital cytomegalovirus infection: A
     fifteen year perspective. J. Infect. Dis. 123: 555-
     561, 1971.

27. Hanshaw, J. B. A cytomegalovirus vaccine? Am. J. Dis.
     Child. 128: 141-142, 1974.

28. Henson, D. Cytomegalovirus inclusion disease following
     multiple blood transfusions. J.A.M.A. 199: 278-280,
     1967.

29. Ho, M. Suwansirikul, S., Dowling, J. N., Youngblood, L. A.
     and Armstrong, J. A. The transplanted kidney as a
     source of cytomegalovirus infection. New Engl. J. Med.
     293: 1109-1112, 1975.

30. Huang, E.-S. Human cytomegalovirus. III. Virus-induced
     DNA polymerase. J. Virol. 16: 298-310, 1975.

31. Huang, E.-S. Human cytomegalovirus. IV. Specific inhibi-
     tion of virus-induced DNA polymerase activity and viral
     DNA replication by phosphonoacetic acid. J. Virol. 16:
     1560-1565, 1975.

32. Huang, E.-S., Chen, S.-T. and Pagano, J. S. Human cyto-
     megalovirus. I. Purification and characterization of
     viral DNA. J. Virol. 12: 1473-1481, 1973.

33. Huang, E.-S. and Pagano, J. S. Human cytomegalovirus. II.
     Lack of relatedness to DNA of herpes simplex I and II,
     Epstein-Barr virus, and nonhuman strains of cytomegalo-
     virus. J. Virol. 13: 642-645, 1974.

34. Jesionek, A. and Kiolemenoglou, B. Ueber einen Befund von
     protozoënartigen Gebilden in den Organen eines heredi-
     tärluetischen Fötus. München Med. Wochenschr. 51:
     1905-1907, 1904.

35. Kilpatrick, B. A. and Huang, E.-S. Human cytomegalovirus
     genome: Partial denaturation map and organization of
     genome sequences. J. Virol. 24: 261-276, 1977.

36. Klemola, E. and Kääriäinen, L. Cytomegalovirus as a possi-
     ble cause of a disease resembling infectious mononu-
     cleosis. Brit. Med. J. 2: 1099-1102, 1965.

37. Lang, D. J. and Kummer, J. F. Demonstration of cytomegalo-
     virus in semen. New Engl. J. Med. 287: 756-758, 1972.

38. Lang, D. J. and Kummer, J. F. Cytomegalovirus in semen:
     Observations in selected populations. J. Infect. Dis.
     132: 472-473, 1975.

39. Lipschütz, B. Untersuchungen über die Aetiologie der Krank-
     heiten der Herpesgruppe (Herpes zoster, Herpes geni-
     talis, Herpes febrilis). Arch. f. Dermat. u. Syph.
     136: 428-482, 1921.

40. Marx, J. L. Cytomegalovirus: A major cause of birth de-
     fects. Science 190: 1184-1186, 1975.

41. McAllister, R. M., Straw, R. M., Filbert, J. E. and Goodheart,
     C. R. Human cytomegalovirus. Cytochemical observa-
     tions of intracellular lesion development correlated
     with viral synthesis and release. Virology 19: 521-
     531, 1963.

42. Medearis, D. N., Jr. Observations concerning human cyto-
     megalovirus infection and disease. Bull. Johns Hopk.
     Hosp. 114: 181-211, 1964.

43. Minars, N., Silverman, J. F., Escobar, M. R. and Martinez,
     A. J. Fatal cytomegalic inclusion disease. Arch.
     Dermatol. 113: 1569-1571, 1977.

44. Monif, R. G., Daicoff, G. I. and Flory, L. L. Blood as a
     potential vehicle for the cytomegaloviruses. Am. J.
     Obstet. Gynecol. 126: 445-448, 1976.

45. Montgomery, R., Youngblood, L. and Medearis, D. N., Jr.
     Recovery of cytomegalovirus from the cervix in preg-
     nancy. Pediatrics 49: 524-531, 1972.

46. Numazaki, Y., Yano, N., Morizuka, T., Takal, S. and Ishida,
     N. Primary infection with human cytomegalovirus:
     Viral isolation from healthy infants and pregnant
     women. Am. J. Epidemiol. 91: 410-417, 1970.

47. Pacsa, A. S., Kummerländer, L., Pejtsik, B. and Pali, K. Herpesvirus antibodies and antigens in patients with cervical anaplasia and in controls. J. Natl. Cancer Inst. 55: 775-781, 1975.

48. Phillips, C. A., Fanning, W. L., Gump, D. W. and Phillips, C. F. Cytomegalovirus encephalitis in immunologically normal adults, successful treatment with vidarabine. J.A.M.A. 238: 2299-2300, 1977.

49. Plotkin, S. A., Farquhar, J. and Hornberger, E. Clinical trials of immunization with the Towne 125 strain of human cytomegalovirus. J. Infect. Dis. 134: 470-475, 1976.

50. Prince, A. M., Szmuness, W., Million, S. J. and David, D. S. A serologic study of cytomegalovirus infections associated with blood transfusion. N. Engl. J. Med. 284: 1125-1131, 1971.

51. Rapp, F. Question: Do herpesviruses cause cancer? Answer: Of course they do! J. Natl. Cancer Inst. 50: 825-832, 1973.

52. Rapp, F., Geder, L., Murasko, D., Lausch, R., Ladda, R., Huang, E. and Webber, M. Long-term persistence of cytomegalovirus genome in cultured human cells of prostatic origin. J. Virol. 16: 982-990, 1975.

53. Rinaldo, C. R., Hirsch, M. S. and Black, P. H. Activation of latent viruses following bone marrow transplantation. Transplantation Proceedings 8: 669-672, 1976.

54. Rowe, W. P., Hartley, J. W., Waterman, S., Turner, H. C. and Huebner, R. J. Cytopathic agent resembling human salivary gland virus recovered from tissue cultures of human adenoids. Proc. Soc. Exp. Biol. Med. 92: 418-424, 1956.

55. St. Jeor, S. C., Albrecht, T. B., Funk, F. D. and Rapp, F. Stimulation of cellular DNA synthesis by human cytomegalovirus. J. Virol. 13: 353-362, 1974.

56. St. Jeor, S. and Weisser, A. Persistence of cytomegalovirus in human lymphoblasts and peripheral leukocyte cultures. Infect. Immun. 15: 402-409, 1977.

57. Sanford, E. J., Geder, L., Laychock, A., Rohner, Jr., T. J.
     and Rapp, F. Evidence for the association of cyto-
     megalovirus with carcinoma of the prostate. J. Urology
     118: 789-792, 1977.

58. Schmitz, H. and Enders, G. Cytomegalovirus as a frequent
     cause of Guillain-Barré syndrome. J. Med. Virol. 1:
     21-27, 1977.

59. Simmons, R. L., Matas, A. J., Ratazi, L. C., Balfour, H. H.,
     Hoivard, R. J. and Najarian, J. S. Clinical char-
     acteristics of the lethal cytomegalovirus infection
     following renal transplantation. Surgery 82: 537-546,
     1977.

60. Smith, M. G. Propagation in tissue cultures of cytopatho-
     genic virus from human salivary gland virus (SGV)
     disease. Proc. Soc. Exp. Biol. Med. 92: 424-430,
     1956.

61. Stagno, S., Reynolds, D. W., Huang, E.-S., Thames, S. D.,
     Smith, R. J. and Alford, C. A., Jr. Congenital cyto-
     megalovirus infection. Occurrence in an immune popula-
     tion. New Engl. J. Med. 296: 1254-1258, 1977.

62. The, T. H., Andersen, H. K., Spencer, E. S. and Klein, G.
     Antibodies against cytomegalovirus-induced early anti-
     gens (CMV-EA) in immunosuppressed renal-allograft
     recipients. Clin. Exp. Immunol. 28: 502-505, 1977.

63. The, T. H., Klein, G. and Langenhuysen, M. M. A. C. Anti-
     body reactions to virus-specific early antigens (EA) in
     patients with cytomegalovirus (CMV) infection. Clin.
     Exp. Immunol. 16: 1-12, 1974.

64. Waner, J. L., Hopkins, D. R., Weller, T. H. and Allred, E.
     N. Cervical excretion of cytomegalovirus: Correlation
     with secretory and humoral antibody. J. Infect. Dis.
     136: 805-809, 1977.

65. Weller, T. H. Cytomegaloviruses: The difficult years. J.
     Infect. Dis. 122: 532-539, 1970.

66. Weller, T. H. The cytomegaloviruses: Ubiquitous agents
     with protean clinical manifestations. I. New Engl. J.
     Med. 285: 203-214, 1971.

67. Weller, T. H. and Hanshaw, J. B. Virologic and clinical
     observations on cytomegalic inclusion disease. N.
     Engl. J. Med. 266: 1233-1244, 1962.

68. Weller, T. H., Hanshaw, J. B. and Scott, D. E. Serologic
        differentiation of viruses responsible for cytomegalic
        inclusion disease. Virology 12: 130-132, 1960.

69. Weller, T. H., Macaulay, J. C., Craig, J. M. and Wirth, P.
        Isolation of intranuclear inclusion producing agents
        from infants with illnesses resembling cytomegalic
        inclusion disease. Proc. Soc. Exp. Biol. Med. 94: 4-
        12, 1957.

70. Wong, T.-W. and Warner, N. E. Cytomegalic inclusion disease
        in adults. Arch. Path. 74: 403-422, 1962.

71. Yanagisaiva, N., Toyokura, Y. and Shiraki, H. Double
        encephalitis with herpes simplex virus and cytomegalo-
        virus in an adult. Acta Neuropath. 33: 153-164, 1975.

72. Závada, V., Erban, V., Rezácová, D. and Vonka, V. Thymidine-
        kinase in cytomegalovirus infected cells. Arch. Virol.
        52: 333-339, 1976.

EPIDEMIOLOGICAL EVIDENCE IMPLICATING THE EPSTEIN-BARR VIRUS

IN BURKITT'S LYMPHOMA AND NASOPHARYNGEAL CARCINOMA ETIOLOGY

Guy de-Thé[1]

International Agency for Research on Cancer

Lyon, France

INTRODUCTION

Epidemiologists and experimental cell biologists differ profoundly in their approach to try and uncover the origin of human cancers. Neither group appears to be close to understanding the origin of human tumours. The time has come when scientists of different backgrounds and visions should come together in a multidisciplinary attempt to determine the specific causes and to try to control them.

The study of the Epstein-Barr virus (EBV) and of its role in human oncogenesis was privileged with such an integrated approach and today EBV is the first virus for which epidemiological evidence has been obtained for its playing a role in cancer causation in man.

Let us first ask how the epidemiological characteristics of EBV compare with those of Burkitt's lymphoma (BL) or of nasopharyngeal carcinoma (NPC), then present the case of the Burkitt's lymphoma prospective study and discuss the prospects for nasopharyngeal carcinoma. Finally, we shall see how intervention represents the final step in proving causation.

---

1 At present on sabbatical leave at the Department of the Regius Professor of Medicine - ICRF - Cancer epidemiology Unit - Oxford - England.

1. HOW DO THE EPIDEMIOLOGICAL CHARACTERISTICS OF EBV
COMPARE WITH THOSE OF BURKITT'S LYMPHOMA (BL) OR
OF NASOPHARYNGEAL CARCINOMA (NPC)?

There is, at first glance, an unresolvable contradiction between
the ubiquitous spread of EBV infection throughout the world and the
restrictive geographical distribution of the associated diseases:
infectious mononucleosis in the temperate climates and high socio-
economic groups; Burkitt's lymphoma in the Equatorial belt of
Africa; nasopharyngeal carcinoma in South-East Asia. But let us
take a closer look.

1.1 The Age-Specific Prevalence of EBV Infection Depends
Upon Socio-Economic Development

Henle et al. (1969) first stressed the role of socio-economic
classes in the age-specific prevalence of EBV infection, as measured
by antibodies to EBV structural antigens (VCA, or virion capsid
antigens). He observed dramatic differences in the proportion of
individuals having VCA antibodies in the first two decades of life
between inhabitants of the "slums" in US towns and those living in
high class areas. Children aged 5-7 years were found to be infected at 60% in the first group versus 20% in the high social groups.
The mode of transmission of EBV infection is not well-known, but
saliva is considered to be the main vector, since it contains
"transforming" EBV (as tested by the immortalization test on cord
blood lymphocytes) (Chang & Golden, 1971). Bad hygienic conditions
and possibly overcrowding (Hinuma et al., 1969) facilitate the
transmission of EBV, possibly by saliva contaminated objects, or
food. The proportion of healthy carriers varies greatly between
areas: Gerber et al. in 1976 found transforming EBV in the saliva
of 10% of healthy Americans and in 50% of Equatorial Africans.
Unfortunately, no data are available on this proportion in NPC-
susceptible groups in South-East Asia.

In order to have comparative data from areas which vary greatly
in the frequency of EBV-associated diseases, we studied representative samples of the general population in Singapore, Hong Kong
and Uganda. As seen in Fig. 1, significant differences were observed in both the age-specific prevalence of EBV infection and the
immune response to viral antigens, between areas with a high incidence of NPC or BL (Singapore and Uganda). Could the fact that
by three years of age, practically all children in Uganda are infected by EBV, be relevant to BL prevalence in this part of the
world?

Two alternatives can be proposed:

a) Since only one child out of 1,000 will ever develop a BL

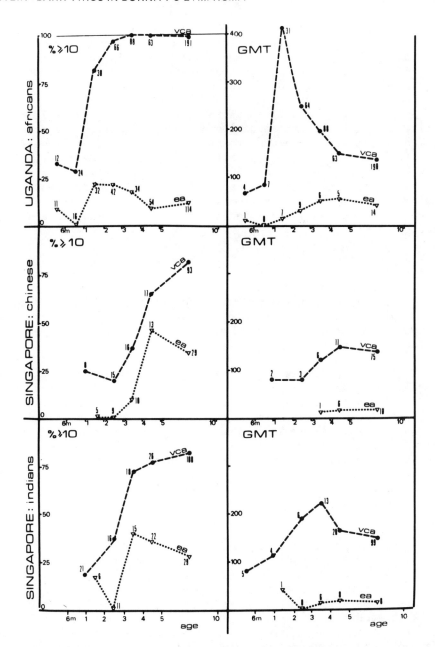

Figure 1: Prevalence (curves at left) and geometric mean titres
(GMT of positive sera curves at right) of antibodies to VCA and EA
in representative samples of three populations: Ugandans (at high
risk for BL), Chinese Singaporeans (at high risk for NPC) and
Indian Singaporeans (at no risk for BL or NPC). (The numbers of
sera for each point of the curves are noted). Reproduced with
permission from Lancet.

tumour, one could suppose that BL candidates are the very few who have escaped early primary EBV infection. Delayed infection would, under extreme conditions, induce a "malignant" infectious mononucleosis. If this were the case, BL candidates should lack EBV antibodies when bled prior to the incubation period.

b)   An opposite alternative has been proposed (de-Thé, 1977), namely, that the extreme situation of early infection observed in tropical areas may be related to BL development. If this were the case, the BL candidates would be recruited in the cohort of children infected very early in life. How early is difficult to determine, since we do not know if transplacental infection could occur in equatorial areas, in association with congenital malaria, for example, or if primary EBV infection could occur under maternal antibodies.

These are important questions which could only be answered by studying the natural history of EBV infection during the first years of life in areas where BL occurs. The critical importance of age of infection in experimental viral oncology is well established (Gross, 1970) and in certain viral diseases the age of primary infection, by poliovirus,   for example, is known to be the determining factor for paralytic poliomyelitis.

     The oncogenic potential of EBV in man is obviously expressed under extreme circumstances, one of these possibly being the early age of primary infection. The socio-economic development which will take place in Equatorial Africa should be accompanied by changes in perinatal hygiene habits, which in turn will affect EBV transmission and, if our hypothesis is correct, BL incidence. The long term interest in socio-economic changes taking place in areas of high BL incidence, such as the West Nile District of Uganda, or the North Mara District of Tanzania, should permit the following of natural events and prove, or disprove, the proposed hypothesis.

1.2   Burkitt's Lymphoma Appears to be Related to Environmental Biological Factors

     The historical Burkitt's safari in 1958-59 (Burkitt, 1962) still represents the most original epidemiological study in recent medical history and still holds true. Burkitt found that this lymphoma was restricted to areas where the average temperature was at least $60^{o}F$ and the yearly rainfall at least 30 inches. In the equatorial belt of Africa, the tumour is not seen above 5,000 feet (Burkitt, 1962). An association with hyper- or holoendemic malaria was proposed in the early 1960's (Dalldorf et al., 1964) and in fact was found to be very strong in the North Mara District of Tanzania (Fig. 2). Only a small cliff of a few hundred feet limits the plateau, but is sufficient to separate the BL-free plateau (as

observed for the last 10 years) from the high BL incidence lowlands.
In order to investigate malaria as a causal factor for BL development, the IARC, with the Tanzanian Government, has established a
malaria intervention project in the North Mara District, where
chloroquine tablets are given twice a month to all children aged 0
to 10 years. The decline in BL incidence in the treated population,
as compared to a neighbouring, untreated population, will establish
the role of malaria (IARC Annual Report, 1977). If, however, the
BL incidence does not drop significantly, one will be entitled to
suspect the role of the anopheles as the vector of another oncogenic
agent. How hyper- or holoendemic malaria would act in BL development is a matter of speculation. O'Connor (1970) has proposed that

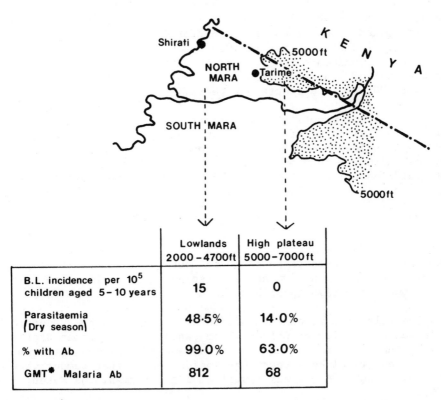

	Lowlands 2000 – 4700ft	High plateau 5000 – 7000 ft
B.L. incidence per 10^5 children aged 5 – 10 years	15	0
Parasitaemia (Dry season)	48.5%	14.0%
% with Ab	99.0%	63.0%
GMT* Malaria Ab	812	68

*Geometric mean titres

Figure 2: Frequency of Burkitt's lymphoma and malaria in North Mara
District, Tanzania.

heavy malaria burden, in aggressing the reticulo-endothelial and immune systems, would increase the pool of "target cells" for EBV transformation.   One could also suggest that congenital malaria which exists in hyper- or holoendemic malaria areas would allow transplacental EBV infection to take place, which would lead to still-born infants, but in mild cases could create favourable conditions for later development of BL.   These hypotheses, however, hardly explain certain epidemiological characteristics of BL, such as the space-time clustering and the seasonal variations observed in Uganda (Williams et al., 1974, 1978).   It appears as if there were a precipitating or triggering event very close (a few weeks) to the clinical onset of the disease, the nature of which is unknown.

1.3   Nasopharyngeal Carcinoma Is Linked to Genetic Factors and Also to Environmental Factors

Figure 3 gives the geographical distribution of NPC and one can see two geographical regions of interest: Cantonese Chinese and also mixed populations of South-East Asia are at very high risk for NPC (Incidence ⩾ 20 per 100,000 inhabitants per year).   An intermediate incidence area covers the Northern part of East Africa and a number of countries around the Mediterranean (incidence 1.5 to 9 per 100,000 inhabitants per year).

The role of genetic factors in NPC development is suggested by epidemiological data indicating that South-East Asian populations with high incidence of NPC are all genetically related to Cantonese Chinese, although they have very different cultural patterns. Familial clustering of NPC cases has been described (Ho, 1967, 1972). Blood genetic markers have been sought in NPC patients and Simons et al. (1975) have described a specific HLA profile associated with high NPC risk: this consists of the haplotype A2-BSIN2 (the SIN2 antigen being observed only in mongoloid populations).   The existance of an NPC disease susceptibility gene (DSG) has been postulated and is believed to be close to, but outside, the HLA region and might represent an immune response gene controlling the response to a common infection (possibly the EBV).

The role of environmental factors is suggested by the decrease in incidence in migrant Chinese from Canton to the United States, but, at the same time, even after two generations, the American Chinese have retained a very high incidence for that tumour when compared to white Americans (Buell, 1973;   Fraumeni and Mason, 1974).

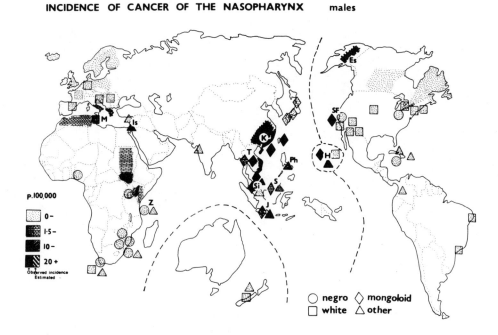

INCIDENCE OF CANCER OF THE NASOPHARYNX   males

Figure 3: World Distribution of NPC

One can recognize four levels of incidence:

(a)   The highest (20 per 10^5) being in the southern province of Kwantung in the People's Republic of China and in Cantonese immigrants in South-East Asia (SEA)

(b)   The next highest (10-20 per 10^5) being in Cantonese immigrants outside SEA: e.g., in the US (Hawaii and San Francisco)

(c)   Intermediate incidence (1.5-9 per 10^5) surrounds the Mediterranean and the Rift Valley in East Africa

(d)   Low incidence (≥1.5) covers the rest of the world.

Geometric figures refer to Cancer Registries, whereas shaded areas refer to estimated incidence from relative frequency data.

(Map kindly prepared by Ms Paula Cook, Department of the Regius Professor of Medicine, University of Oxford, United Kingdom).

Key: ES = Eskimos, H = Hawaii, Is = Israel, J = Java, K = Province of Kwantung in the People's Republic of China, M = Malta, Ph = Philippines, S = Sumatra, SF = San Francisco.

2. PROSPECTIVE STUDIES TO TEST SPECIFIC
HYPOTHESES REGARDING CAUSATION

Circumstantial evidence for a causal role of EBV in the development of BL and NPC has accumulated through experimental studies,
but direct evidence can only be provided by epidemiological studies
aimed at revealing the pre-tumour events and the EBV profile of
the candidates for the development of Burkitt's lymphoma. The
final epidemiological evidence will, indeed, be given by a direct
intervention against the causative virus.

We conducted a long term, prospective, sero-epidemiological
survey in Uganda between 1968 and 1978, which was successful in
establishing the EBV profile associated with the high risk of
development of Burkitt's lymphoma. This study involved 42,000
children aged 0-8 years, who were visited, interviewed, registered,
bled once and then carefully followed up in order to uncover all
the Burkitt's lymphoma cases arising within that cohort. The study,
which took place in the West Nile District of Uganda, has now yielded 14 BL cases for whom we have pre-BL sera (de Thé et al., in
press; IARC Annual Report, 1977). The pre-BL sera (collected at
time intervals ranging from 7-54 months prior to the clinical diagnosis of BL) and the post-BL sera were tested for EBV reactivities
together with a number of controls of the same age, sex and locality. Whereas no differences were observed between future cases and
controls for EBNA and EA reactivities, significantly higher VCA
titres were observed in the pre-BL sera when compared to different
matched controls. The VCA/GMT for pre-BL sera was 425 versus 125
for controls. These differences were found to be significant at
the p = 0.01 level. Thus one can calculate an increased risk of
developing BL in children having VCA titres of 2 or more dilutions
above the mean for the general population standardized for age,
sex and locality and this was found to be 30 times higher than that
for the general population.

A remarkable and unexpected stability of VCA titres was observed at tumour onset. This stability of VCA titres in years prior
to BL development indicated that high VCA titres previously observed in BL patients were, in fact, present long before the clinical
onset of the disease. Antibodies to EA developed in 8 of the 14
cases after clinical diagnosis, 7 of these having antibodies
directed against the R component.

The pre- and post-BL sera, as well as their controls, were
also tested for antibodies to herpes simplex virus, cytomegalovirus
and measles virus at the Center for Disease Control, Atlanta,
Georgia, USA (Dr P. Feorino). No significant differences were observed in antibody levels between cases and controls, except that
measles antibody titres were lower in pre-BL sera than in controls,
this being on the border line of significance. Malaria parasite

counts at the time of the main bleeding showed no difference between pre-BL and controls, but at the time of disease onset, the
BL patients had significantly fewer parasites than the controls,
probably due to anti-malarial drugs having been taken prior to
presentation at the hospital for BL diagnosis.

The above results strongly support a causal role for EBV infection in the development of Burkitt's lymphoma. The high VCA
titres are believed to be the marker of a long-standing EBV infection, linked either to infection very early in life, or to an abnormal host response to an otherwise normal EBV primary infection.
I have proposed that very early infection in life, possibly in the
pre- or post-natal period, might be one of the critical events
leading to BL development (de-Thé, 1977). The results of the
prospective study are compatible with such a hypothesis.

Among the 14 BL cases for whom we had collected sera prior to
disease onset, 10 had profiles as described above, that is, high
VCA titres long before tumour development. However, there were
four cases who did not fall into that category, three with atypical
characteristics (de-Thé et al., in press).

It appears that there are two types of lymphoma in tropical
regions: EBV-associated and EBV-free lymphomas. The "EBV-associated" lymphomas would have high VCA titres a long time prior to
tumour onset and exhibit EBV markers in the tumour cells. In
contrast, the "EBV-free" lymphomas would have, prior to and after
tumour onset, VCA titres similar to those of the general population
and tumour cells would lack detectable EBV markers. Whereas the
EBV-free lymphomas form the majority of childhood B-cell lymphomas
in temperate climates, they appear to be the exception in tropical
areas; their etiology is completely unknown. The EBV-associated
lymphoma would represent the disease described by Burkitt in
tropical regions.

In conclusion, the present results of this long term prospective study, which is being pursued in Uganda, together with the
experimental data showing the in vitro transforming and in vivo
oncogenic potential of EBV in New World primates, strongly support
a causal association between this virus and Burkitt's tumour. It should
be inferred, however, that the oncogenic potential of EBV in man
is realized under severe environmental conditions and that co-
factors are necessary (malaria being one of them).

3. PROSPECTS FOR NASOPHARYNGEAL CARCINOMA (NPC) STUDIES

The association between EBV and NPC rests upon data similar to
that associating the virus to BL, namely, the regular presence of
viral fingerprints at the epithelial tumour cell level (both are

betrayed by the presence of EBV genomes and the EBV-specific nuclear antigen) and by a strong immune response (both humoral- and
cell-mediated) of NPC patients to a series of EBV-specific antigens.
(For reviews see de Thé and Lenoir, 1977; Klein, 1975; Proceedings
of the Kyoto Symposium, 1978). However, proof of the causal nature
of the association between this virus and NPC is still a matter of
debate. This virus is a natural host of the oropharynx and there
is always a possibility that the viral infection takes place in
the epithelial tumour cells, secondary to transformation into
carcinoma. Henderson et al. (1976, 1977) favour such a hypothesis,
based on the fact that a few tumours arising in the oropharyngeal
area have elevated VCA titres. This not our view point, since,
when we compared nasopharyngeal carcinoma patients originating from
different geographical areas, we did in fact observe differences
up to three-fold between different groups of NPC patients, but
always a similar ratio of the GMT of NPC versus other tumours,
when compared within each area, varying from six to 20-fold from
VCA to EA respectively (de Thé et al., 1978).

However, as in the case of Burkitt's lymphoma a prospective
study could help to enlighten the relationship between EBV and NPC
by determining the EBV profile prior to the development of the
tumour. If candidates for NPC had an EBV profile different from
that of the general population, either a long time prior to tumour
development, or even at relatively short periods prior to clinical
onset of the disease (let us say six months to a year), this would
reinforce the association with the virus and permit the identification of the cohort at highest risk. Future etiological studies
could be carried out and eventually a vaccine could be tried on
this highest risk group.

Furthermore, a short term prospective study would allow the
establishment of whether IgA antibodies to both VCA and EA, which
have been found in the serum and saliva of NPC patients (Henle and
Henle,1976; Ho et al., 1977; Desgranges et al., 1977), are already
present at the pre-clinical stage of the disease. If this were
the case, then early detection of the tumour in mass surveys in
high incidence areas, such as the People's Republic of China,
could be envisaged. This would lead to better control of the
disease by early treatment. From the methodological point of
view, this prospective study would only require a follow up of,
say, 5,000 male Cantonese Chinese aged 45-54 years, as they should
yield around 25 cases over a period of 5 years. Dr Ho, in Hong
Kong, is carrying out a prospective follow up of family members of
NPC patients, who represent a high risk group for the tumour, and
hopes to collect sera prior to the development of some tumours in
that context. However, the difficulty here is that the expected
number of cases is not well established and the ideal situation
would be to follow up a group of Cantonese males irrespective of
their relationship to an NPC case. It is of interest to note here

that the EBV serology, and more specifically the antibody directed
against early antigen (EA) both in the IgG class and in the IgA
class, appears to be a very useful tool for clinicians in establishing NPC in low incidence areas, for evaluating the prognosis
of the tumour and for monitoring the treatment. Clinically oriented
studies are being implemented in this context and this certainly
represents a very important spin-off of the EBV studies carried out
over the last few years.

4. INTERVENTION AS THE FINAL STEP IN PROVING CAUSATION

The ultimate aim of epidemiology is to prevent a disease by
intervention against putative causal factors. Such an intervention,
if successful, would provide the final evidence for causation,
which sometimes may not be obtainable otherwise. In the case of
EBV and human malignancies, intervention can take place either
against co-factors, such as malaria, or against the EBV.

4.1 Intervention Against Malaria to Prevent BL

The relation which seems to exist between holo- or hyperendemic
malaria and high incidence of Burkitt's lymphoma provides a unique
opportunity for intervention, since an anti-malaria project, if
ineffectual for preventing Burkitt's lymphoma, would nevertheless
save a large number of lives (up to 20% of children in Equatorial
Africa die of malaria before 5 years of age). The IARC has recently implemented a project in the North Mara District, where
chloroquine tablets are distributed to all children aged 0-10 years.
The incidence of Burkitt's lymphoma has been followed up since 1970
in that area and any dramatic change in this incidence will be attributed to the intervention scheme. If the incidence decreases
dramatically (within two years or so), this will support the view
that malaria acts as a promoter close to clinical onset of BL.
However, if congenital malaria were to represent a critical factor
(possibly responsiblefor congenital EBV infection), or if malaria
would act very early in life, one may not observe a decline in
BL incidence before 5-6 years from now. During that period, socio-
economic changes will take place in Tanzania and it will be very
difficult to interpret the results and to assess the specific role
of the intervention scheme or the cultural changes.

4.2 Intervention Against the Virus - Is It Timely
To Discuss an EBV Vaccine?

In the naturally occurring lympho-proliferative Marek's disease
of chickens, vaccination with attentuated virus or with live apatho-
genic turkey herpesvirus, has been very successful (Purchase, 1976).

The question was recently posed by Epstein: why not develop an EBV
vaccine to bring the final proof of the causal relationship between
this virus and human malignancies? (Epstein, 1976). Technically,
an EBV vaccine is not in sight, but the successful utilisation of
a membrane vesicule preparation of herpesvirus saimiri (HVS) transformed cells in preventing lymphomas induced by this virus in non-
human primates (Pearson and Scott, 1977) should form the experimental basis for developing similar research programmes in the field
of EBV. The logical steps for assessing the value of an EBV vaccine
would be first to try it in preventing infectious mononucleosis in
temperate climates and socio-economically developed countries and
later on to prevent human malignancies, such as BL and NPC.
Concerning Burkitt's lymphoma, it might be difficult to convince
the Public Health authorities of the practical value of an EBV
vaccination, when anti-malaria intervention can be as successful
and much more profitable from their point of view. In contrast,
if certain antigenic preparations were found to have a prognostic
value in CMI tests for NPC patients, vaccination in the highest
risk group, as characterized by the proposed prospective study (see
above), might be readily acceptable in areas where this tumour is
endemic and represents the most common ENT malignancy in males.
However, it is obvious that the development of a vaccine and its
assessment in man will require the development of an experimental
model in non-human primates.

    In conclusion, the development of any malignant tumour repre-
sents a multifactorial process and the question for the epidemio-
logist is not to determine whether the Epstein-Barr virus is the
sole cause of BL and/or NPC, but to determine whether the virus is
involved in the causation of the disease and whether it is a factor
against which intervention is feasible. The conquest of human
malignancies will only come about by further integrating multidisciplinary approaches where the epidemiologists will have to work
hand in hand with laboratory scientists.

                              REFERENCES

Burkitt, D. A "tumour safari" in East and Central Africa. Brit.
    J. Cancer, 16:379-386, 1962.

Buell, P. Race and place in the etiology of nasopharyngeal cancer:
    a study based on California death certificates. Int. J. Cancer,
    11:268-272, 1973.

Chang, R.S. and Golden, H.D. Transformation of human leukocytes
    by throat washing from infectious mononucleosis patients.
    Nature (London), 234:359-360, 1971.

Dalldorf, G., Linsell, C.A., Barnhart, F.E. and Martyn, R. An epidemiological approach to the lymphomas of African children and Burkitt's sarcoma of the jaws. Perp. Biol. Med., 7:435-449, 1964.

Desgranges, C., de-Thé, G., Ho, J.H.C. and Ellouz, R. Neutralizing EBV-specific IgA in throat washings of nasopharyngeal carcinoma (NPC) patients. Int. J. Cancer, 19:627-633, 1977.

de-Thé, G. Is Burkitt's lymphoma related to perinatal infection by Epstein-Barr virus? Lancet, i:335-338, 1977.

de-Thé, G., Lavoué, M.F. and Muenz, L. Differences in EBV antibody titres of patients with nasopharyngeal carcinoma originating from high, intermediate and low incidence areas. In: Proceedings of an International Symposium on Etiology and Control of Nasopharyngeal Carcinoma. IARC Scientific Publication, International Agency for Research on Cancer, Lyon, France, 1978.

de-Thé, G., Geser, A., Day, N.E., Tukei, P.M., Williams, E.H., Beri, D.P., Dean, A., Bornkamm, G.W., Feorino, P. and Henle, W. Epidemiological evidence for the causation of Burkitt's lymphoma by the Epstein-Barr virus - Results of the Ugandan prospective study. Nature, in press.

de-Thé, G. and Lenoir, G. Comparative diagnosis of Epstein-Barr virus related diseases: Infectious mononucleosis, Burkitt's lymphoma and nasopharyngeal carcinoma. In: Kurstak, E. ed., Comparative Diagnosis of Viral Diseases. New York, Academic Press, 1977.

Epstein, M.A. Implications for a vaccine for the prevention of Epstein-Barr virus infection: ethical and logistic considerations. Cancer Res., 36:711-714, 1976.

Fraumeni, J.F. Jr. and Mason, T.J. Cancer mortality among Chinese Americans, 1950-69. J. Natl. Cancer Inst., 52:659-665, 1974.

Gerber, P., Nkrumah, F.K., Pritchett, R. and Keiff, E. Comparative studies of Epstein-Barr virus strains from Ghana and the United States. Int. J. Cancer, 17:71-81, 1976.

Gross, L. Oncogenic viruses. Pergamon Press, Oxford, 1970.

Henderson, B.E., Louie, E.W., Jing, J.S. et al. Risk factors associated with nasopharyngeal carcinoma. N. Engl. J. Med., 295:1101-1106, 1976.

Henderson, B.E., Louie, E.W., Jing, J.S. and Alena, B. Epstein-
    Barr virus and nasopharyngeal carcinoma: is there an etiologic
    relationship? J. Natl. Cancer Inst., 59:1393-1395, 1977.

Henle, G., Henle, W., Clifford, F., Diehl, V., Kafuko, G.W., Kirya,
    E.G., Klein, G., Morrow, R.H., Munube, G.M.R., Pike, M.C., Tukei,
    P.M. and Ziegler, J.L. Antibodies to EB virus in Burkitt's
    lymphoma and control groups. J. Natl. Cancer Inst., 43:1147-
    1157, 1969.

Henle, G. and Henle, W. Epstein-Barr virus specific IgA serum
    antibodies as an outstanding feature of nasopharyngeal carcinoma.
    Int. J. Cancer, 17:1-7, 1976.

Hinuma, Y., Ohta-Hatuno, R. and Suto, T. High incidence of Japanese
    infants with antibody to a herpes-type virus associated with
    cultured Burkitt's lymphoma cells. Jap. J. Microbiol., 13:309-
    311, 1969.

Ho, J.H.C. Nasopharyngeal carcinoma in Hong Kong. In: Muir, C.S.
    and Shanmugaratnam, K. eds., Cancer of the Nasopharynx. UICC
    Monograph Series, Vol.1, Munksgaard, Copenhagen, 1967. pp.58-63.

Ho, J.H.C. Nasopharyngeal carcinoma (NPC). In: Advances in Cancer
    Research, Klein, G., Weinhouse, S. and Haddow, A. eds., Academic
    Press, New York, London. pp.57-92, 1972.

Ho, H.C., Ng, M.H. and Kwan, H.C. IgA antibodies to Epstein-Barr
    virus capsid antigens in saliva of nasopharyngeal carcinoma
    patients. Br. J. Cancer, 35:888-890, 1977.

International Agency for Research on Cancer, Annual Report 1977,
    Lyon, France.

Klein, G. The Epstein-Barr virus and neoplasia. N. Engl. J. Med.
    293:1353, 1975.

O'Connor, G.T. Persistent immunologic stimulation as a factor in
    oncogenesis with special reference to Burkitt's tumour. Am. J.
    Med., 48:279-285, 1970.

Pearson, G. and Scott, R.E. Isolation of virus free herpesvirus
    saimiri antigen - positive plasma membrane vesicles. Proc. Natl.
    Acad. Sci. USA, 75:2546, 1977.

Proceedings of the Kyoto International Symposium on Etiology and
    Control of Nasopharyngeal Carcinoma. de-Thé, G. and Ito, Y. eds.
    IARC Scientific Publications No. 20, 1978.

Purchase, H.G. Prevention of Marek's disease: a review. Cancer
    Res., 36:696-700, 1976.

Simons, M.J., Day, N.E., Wee, G.B., Chan, S.H., Shanmugaratnam, K. and de-Thé, G. Immunogenetic aspects of nasopharyngeal carcinoma (NPC). III. HL-A type as a genetic marker of NPC predisposition to test the hypothesis that EBV is an aetiologic factor in NPC In: de-Thé, G., Epstein, M.A. and zur Hausen, H. eds., Oncogenesis and Herpesviruses II. IARC Scientific Publications No.11, Vol. 2, International Agency for Research on Cancer, Lyon, France, 1975. pp.249-258.

Williams, E.H., Day, N.E. and Geser, A.G. Seasonal variation in onset of Burkitt's lymphoma in the West Nile District of Uganda. Lancet, ii:19-22, 1974.

Williams, E.H., Smith, P.G., Day, N.E., Geser, A., Ellice, J. and Tukei, P. Space-time clustering of Burkitt's lymphoma in the West Nile District of Uganda, 1960-75. Brit. J. Cancer, 37:109-122, 1978.

INTERFERENCE BY DEFECTIVES OF BK VIRUS

J. van der Noordaa, C.J.A. Sol, A. van Strien and C.Walig

Laboratorium voor de Gezondheidsleer
Universiteit van Amsterdam
Mauritskade 57
Amsterdam

INTRODUCTION

The synthesis of defective interfering particles after high multiplicity infection has been reported for a wide variety of viruses and it has been suggested that defective interfering particles may play a role in establishing persistent infections (1). In view of the persistence of the human papovavirus BK (2) in its natural host we have analysed the interfering properties of a class of variants of BK virus (BKV). The variants were prepared by serial undiluted passage of BKV in primary human embryonic cells and were subsequently studied by isolation and characterization of their DNA. isolation and characterization of their DNA.

MATERIALS AND METHODS

Cell cultures and media

Primary human embryonic cells were obtained from 6 - 12 week old gestation products and were cultured in Eagle's basal medium supplemented with 10% calf serum and antibiotics (100 u. penicillin/ml and 100 µ g streptomycin/ml). Cultures of primary rat kidney cells were derived from the kidneys of 5 day old Wistar rats.

Virus, assay and serial passage

BK virus (strain Gardner) was obtained from Dr. Takemoto
(N.I.H. Bethesda, U.S.A.). Non-defective stock virus was prepared
by low multiplicity infection (0.001 pfu/ml) of confluent cultures
of primary human embryonic cells.
The virus was harvested after 14 - 21 days when about 75% of the
cells showed cytopathological lesions and was titrated on monolayer
cultures of primary human embryonic cells in 5 cm Falcon petri dishes.
A 0.9% agar overlay was added one day after inoculation and after 24
days the plaques were stained by neutral red (0.01% in final agar
overlay). The titre of the crude lysate used as stock virus was
5×10^6 pfu/ml.
Stock virus was tested for the presence of defectives by agarose gel
electrophoresis of 1 µg of the viral DNA which permits the detection
of 10 nanograms of discretely migrating contaminating DNA(3).
For the preparation of serial passage virus roller bottle cultures
of primary human embryonic cells were infected at a m.o.i. of 5;
therefore 10 ml of non-defective stock virus was added to 10^7 cells
in 60 ml of medium. When nearly all cells showed cytopathological
lesions cultures were frozen and each of the succeeding cultures
was inoculated with 4 ml of the preceding culture.

Extraction, purification and electrophoresis of viral DNA

For extraction of the viral DNA the infected cells were
detached from the glass by freezing-thawing and cells and virus were
sedimented for 2 hours at 25.000 rev/min at 4° C in a SW 27.1 rotor
(Beckmann). The viral DNA was extracted from the pellet by the Hirt
procedure (4) and was further purified by equilibrium centrifugation
in caesium chloride containing ethidium bromide (5).
The ethidium bromide was removed by isoamyl alcohol extraction and
subsequent dialysis against 10mM-tris HCL, 1mM NA-EDTA, PH 7.5.
The viral DNA was analysed by electrophoresis through 1.5% agarose
containing ethidium bromide (6). Hind III digestion products were
analysed by electrophoresis through a horizontal slab gel (12 x 12 x
0.5 cm) of 2.5% agarose at 8v/cm gel.

Electron microscopy of viral DNA

For length measurements of normal and variant BKV DNA the
aqueous method of Davis et al. (7) was used. The DNA had been
converted from the closed circular form to the open circular form
by the method described by Greenfield et al.(8). Open circular
PM_2DNA was added to the spreading solution as length marker. The mol.
wt of PM_2 DNA (6.37×10^6 dalton) has previously been determined (3).
Heteroduplexes were prepared and spread for electron microscopy
by a modification of the RNA spreading procedure of Robberson et al.
(9): 5 µl of a mixture of Eco RI cleaved normal and variant BKV DNA

(100 µg/ml in 10 mM tris pH 7.6) was added to 40 µl of 80% (v.v.)
formamide, 4M urea. This mixture was kept at 53°C for 30 seconds to
denature the DNA. After cooling to 20°C, 5 µl of 0.2 M NaCl, 1 µl
of open circular PM_2DNA (200 µg/ml in 10 mM tris pH 7.6) and 2.5 µl
cytochrome-c (1 mg/ml in 20 mM tris, 2 mM E.D.T.A. pH 8.5) were
added and the DNA was allowed to renature for 1 hr. The DNA was then
spread on a hypophase of double distilled water and after 10 min.
the DNA was picked up on carbon coated copper grids which then were
shadowed with Pt at an angle of 9° while rotating.
The grids were examined in a Philips EM-300 electron microscope at
60 kV. Micrographs were taken at a magnification of 15000 on Kodak
Eastman 5302 film. The negatives were enlarged 8 times and the DNA
molecules were measured with a Hewlett Packard model 10 calculator
and a digitizer model 9864A.

Infectivity, T antigen and transformation assay of viral DNA

The infectivity of viral DNA was tested in primary
human embryonic kidney cells after treatment with DEAE-dextran
(10,11). Monolayer cultures in 5 cm Falcon petri dishes were
washed twice with phosphate buffered saline.
The cells were incubated for 30 min. at room temperature with 1 ml
PBS containing 500 µg of DEAE-dextran (Pharmacia)..
After removal of the DEAE-dextran the viral DNA was added in 0.2 ml
samples. After 15 min. the cells were washed with PBS and the medium
was supplied. An agar overlay (0.9%) was added the next day and
plaques were counted after 24 days.
The transforming ability of the viral DNA was investigated by
employing the Ca phosphate method (11, 12).
The DNA was diluted in hepes buffer (PH 7.05), calcium chloride
was added to a final concentration of 125 mM and calf thymus DNA
was added as carrier. This mixture was kept at room temperature
for 30 minutes and then 0.5 ml of the diluted DNA was added to
subconfluent cultures of primary rat kidney cells in 5 cm Falcon
petri dishes. The final concentrations of BKV DNA were 0.5 and
1.0 µg of DNA per dish in the presence of 5 µg of calf thymus
DNA per dish.
After 4 weeks cultures were fixed and stained with Giemsa and the
number of transformed foci were counted. Control cultures were
mock infected with and without calf thymus DNA.
The indirect immunofluorescence test for detection of tumour and
viral antigens was employed.
The BKV anti T serum was obtained from BKV tumour bearing hamsters
(11) and the anti-hamster conjugate was purchased from Nordic.
For assay of T-antigen coverslip cultures of BSC-1 cells were
pretreated for 30 minutes with 100 µg of DEAE-dextran and then
infected with 25-100 nanogram of viral DNA. After 24 hours
the cultures were fixed and stained.

For V (viral) antigen cells were treated in the same way and stained
after 4 days with a hyper immune rabbit anti BKV serum (neutralizing
titre ±512), followed by anti rabbit conjugate (Nordic).

Replication assay of viral DNA

Semiconfuent BSC-1 cells in 25 cm^2 Falcon bottles
were infected with normal or variant BKV DNA as described before.
At 24 h. after infection medium was removed and replaced by 2 ml
medium without calfserum and supplemented with 10 µ C_i of methyl ^{3}H
thymidine (24 Ci/mmol) per ml. At 48 h after infection viral DNA
was extracted by the Hirt procedure (4). The lysis buffer contained
a known amount of ^{14}C labeled SV40 DNA that had previously been
digested with endonucleases Hind II + III which allowed determination
of the recovery of viral DNA. The Hirt supernatant was twice extracted with phenol, once extracted with chlorophorm-isoamyl alcohol
(24:1 v.v.) and the DNA was concentrated by ethanol precipitation.
The precipitate was dried and then dissolved in 50 µl 10 mM Tris pH
7,6, 5% sucrose (w.v.).
5 µl samples were removed to determine the recovery of ^{14}C DNA.
Then samples containing nearly equal amounts of ^{14}C labeled DNA
fragments were subjected to agarose (1,5%) slab gel electrophoresis
for 18 hours at 1 V/cm gel.
Subsequently the DNA was transferred to a nitro-cellulose sheet by
the blotting procedure (13). Prior to the transfer of the DNA the
gel was irradiated with X-ray (60,000 rad from a 100 kV source) to
introduce nicks in covalently closed circular DNA which improved
detection. After blotting the nitrocellulose sheet was washed in
0,3 M NaCl 0.03 M Nacitrate (pH 7.0), air dried and briefly immersed
in a 10% (w.v.) solution of PPO in toluene and then air-dried.
The nitrocellulose sheet was placed for 24 h at -70°C on Royal
X-omat röntgenfilm (14).

Restriction endonucleases

The enzymes Hind II+ dIII, Eco R I and Pst I were
prepared according to the procedure described (15).
Incubation mixtures were for Hind II + d III; 6,6 mM tris pH 7,5,
6,6 mM $MgCl_2$, 6,6 mM 2 mercapto-ethanol, 50 mM NaCl, for Eco R I;
90 mM tris pH 7,9, 10 mM $MgCl_2$, for Pst I; 6,6 mM tris pH 7,6,
6,6 mM $MgCl_2$, 6,6 mM 2-mercapto ethanol.
With 1 µl of each enzyme preparation a complete digest of 1µ g BKV
DNA, dissolved in 20-200 µl, was obtained within 1 h incubation at
37°C.

RESULTS

After 10 serial passages the viral titre of the passages 1,5 and 10
was determined and was respectively 5.5 x 10^5, 1.0 x 10^5 and 2.10^{+4}
pfu/ml.

The viral DNA from each passage was analysed by agarose gel electrophoresis. As early as after one passage a band of viral DNA which
migrated slightly more rapidly than normal genome length DNA could
be observed in the electropherogram.
The relative amount of faster migrating DNA increased during the
following passages and in the fifth passage a third species with
an intermediate mobility band was visible, which had disapppeared
at passage 10. At that stage only one band of faster moving DNA
could be distinguished while only a small amount of normal DNA had
remained. The DNA from passage 10 was chosen for further study.
Because of the close proximity of the 2 bands separate isolation
of the variant DNA from the gel was difficult and an additional step
was necessary to separate the variant from normal DNA. Therefore
the total viral DNA from passage 10 was treated with various restriction endonucleases and the variant DNA appeared resistant to the
Providencia Stuarti (Pst) I restriction enzyme, while the normal
genome length DNA was converted to the linear form.
This difference in cleavage by the Pst enzyme enabled us to separate
the form I variant DNA from the form III normal BKV DNA by equilibrium centrifugation in CsCl-EthBr.
The length of the variant DNA measured by electronmicroscopy was
93% of parental BKV DNA (Table 1). Further examination of denatured
and renatured Eco RI linears of variant DNA revealed no heteroduplex
structures indicating genetic homogeneity of the DNA.
Heteroduplex analysis with Eco RI cleaved normal and variant BKV DNA
showed two configurations of heteroduplexes (fig. 1). Both configurations contained two single strand regions; the larger one was at
the same location in both types and the smaller one in two different
locations. Length measurements showed that the large single strand
region represented a segment of the BKV DNA which reflected the
genetic deletion in the variant DNA.
The short single strand region originates from the variant DNA in
the heteroduplex; the two different locations of this single strand
regions in the two types of heteroduplexes are separated by DNA with
a length that equals the length of the single strand which is
consistent with the presence of a repeated sequence in the variant
DNA. The heteroduplex analysis permitted the construction of a
physical map of the variant DNA (shown in figure 2). Based on the
absence of the Pst I site of the variant DNA (situated at .31 on
the physical map of BKV DNA, to be published) the genetic deletion
starts at .28 clockwise from the Eco RI cleavage site and extends
to .53. The loss in length of 25% by this genetic deletion is
partly compensated by a repeat of the DNA segment located between
.53 and .71 on the physical map of parental BK DNA. The positions
of the Hind III cleavage sites on BKV parental DNA are slightly
different from those published (17) and might be due to a different
gel system used in analysing the cleavage product.
According to the physical map digestion of the variant DNA with Hind
III showed the formation of parental A and C fragments, the fragment

Table 1. Length and molecular weight of normal and variant BKV DNA
determined by comparative length measurements with PM_2 marker DNA

Type of DNA	relative length		molecular weight (megadalton)
BKV normal	100	$(84)^a$	3.22 $\pm$ 0.11
PM_2		(77)	6.37 $\pm$ 0.16
BKV variant	93.2 $\pm$ 0.8	(107)	3.00 $\pm$ 0.12
PM_2		(111)	6.37 $\pm$ 0.14

[a] number of molecules measured

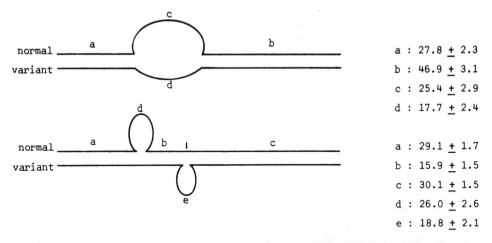

a : 27.8 $\pm$ 2.3
b : 46.9 $\pm$ 3.1
c : 25.4 $\pm$ 2.9
d : 17.7 $\pm$ 2.4

a : 29.1 $\pm$ 1.7
b : 15.9 $\pm$ 1.5
c : 30.1 $\pm$ 1.5
d : 26.0 $\pm$ 2.6
e : 18.8 $\pm$ 2.1

Fig. 1. Schemes of two representative heteroduplex molecules formed
by hybridization of Eco RI cleaved normal and variant BKV DNA. For
each type of heteroduplex the results of length measurements of
respectively 72 and 46 molecules are shown. The figures represent
the percentage of length of the parental genome.

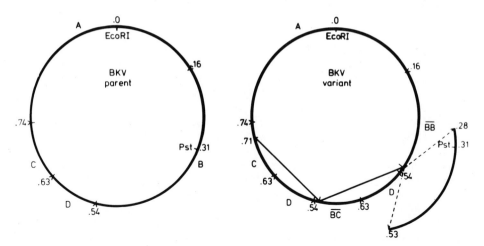

Fig. 2. Physical map of the genome of BKV deletion variant compared to BKV parent genome; ➤, Hin d III cleavage sites. The deleted region is indicated by the wedge-shaped extension from the circle and the repeated region by the chords.

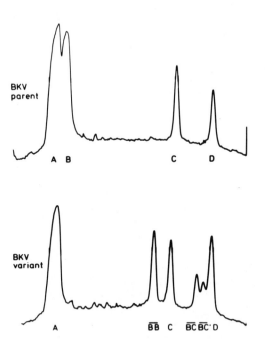

Fig. 3. Hin d III digests of BKV parent and variant genomes. Scanning of slab gels after electrophoresis.

D in bimolar amount and two new fragments (fig.3). One new fragment
(BB) composed of two parts of the parental B fragment is slightly
larger than the parental C fragment and the second new fragment (BC)
has a size intermediate between C and D. However as shown in fig.3
instead of the one new fragment with a mobility between that of
fragment C and D two fragments are present in less than unimolar
amount which indicates that the variant DNA consists of two
populations with an estimated size difference of 20 base pairs in
the BC fragment. The biological activity of this variant DNA was
compared to that of the normal BKV DNA by determining the infectivity, T-antigen inducing and transforming ability. The results of
3 replicate experiments are summarized in table 2. The infectivity
was very low and was probably due to contaminating normal DNA.
The variant DNA did not induce T-antigen and no transformation of
primary rat kidney cells could be established. The variant DNA
could not induce V-antigen.
The ability of variant DNA to interfere with the infectivity of
normal DNA was tested by coinfection of cells with respective DNA's
(table 3). A 10 to 100 fold excess of variant DNA resulted in a
strong reduction of the number of plaques by normal DNA and coinfection with equal amounts of variant and normal DNA still gave
rise to a 10 fold reduction in infectivity of normal DNA.
The results of the replication assay of viral DNA are shown in fig.4.
Variant DNA is not able to autonomous replication while coinfection
with normal DNA results in replication of the variant DNA which
markedly interferes with the replication of normal DNA.

DISCUSSION

Serial passage of undiluted BK virus in primary
human embryonic cells resulted in a decreasing yield of infectious
virus. Analysis of the viral DNA after 10 passages revealed the
presence of smaller size classes of DNA. It was noted that variant
DNA was already present after one passage and that during further
passage most of the viral DNA of genome length was replaced by a
size class of DNA which measured 93% of the size parental DNA.
Further analysis of this new size class of viral DNA showed a
genetic deletion of 25% which in length was partly compensated for
by a direct repeat of a 18% segment (.53 - .71).
The deletion contained the recognition site for the Pst restriction
enzyme of the BKV genome; linear wild type BKV DNA prepared by
digestion with the Pst I enzyme is also unable to induce T antigen
and transformation (manuscript in preparation). The genetic
homogeneity of the deletion mutant DNA was shown by heteroduplex
analysis which did only show heteroduplex molecules as mentioned
before. However from restriction enzymes analysis it appeared that
the deletion mutant DNA consisted of two populations with a size
difference of 20 base pairs, which had remained unnoticed by
heteroduplex analysis.

Table 2. Infectivity, induction of T-antigen and transformation efficiency of normal and variant BKV DNA

Experiment number	Infectivity (pfu/µg)		Induction of T-antigen (pos.nuclei/µg)		Efficiency of transformation (foci/µg)	
	normal	variant	normal	variant	normal	variant
I	6.0×10^{4a}	1.0×10^1	2.3×10^{3b}	< 20	16^c	0
II	4.0×10^4	0.25×10^1	4.5×10^3	< 20	13	0
III	NT^d	NT	4.5×10^3	< 20	7	0

[a] Average number of plaques in 4 dishes.
[b] Average number of T-ag pos. nuclei on 2 coverslips.
[c] Average number of foci in 4 dishes.
[d] Not tested.

Table 3. Infectivity of normal BKV DNA after co-infection with variant BKV DNA

Co-infection	Infectivity (pfu/µg)
normal DNA + variant DNA	4.0×10^{3a}
	1.2×10^4
	4.0×10^4
normal DNA + Phi x 174 DNA [b]	4.0×10^5
normal DNA	5.0×10^5

[a] 2.0×10^{-3} µg of normal DNA with respectively 2.0×10^{-1}, 2.0×10^{-2}, 2.0×10^{-3} µg of variant DNA.
[b] 2.0×10^{-3} µg of normal DNA with 2.0×10^{-1} µg Phi x 174 DNA.

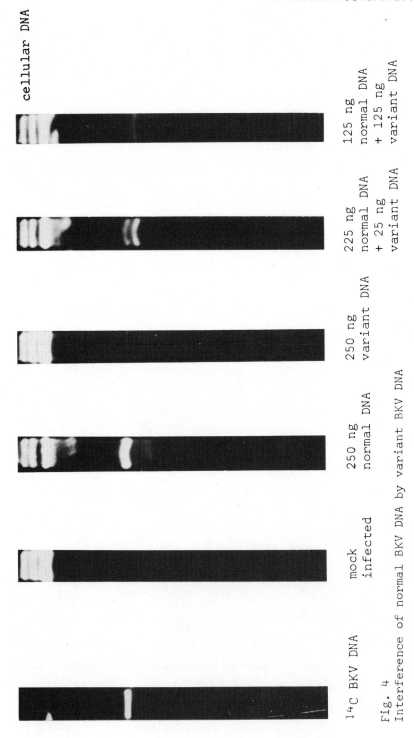

Fig. 4
Interference of normal BKV DNA by variant BKV DNA

Fig. 4. Interference of normal BKV DNA by variant BKV DNA.

Table 4. Properties of deletion
mutant BKV-DNA

Induction of T-antigen	-
Transformation of rat cells	-
Viral DNA replication	-
Induction of V-antigen	-
Plaque formation	-
Interference with plaque formation by wt BKV-DNA	+

The results of our studies of the biological activity of the variant
DNA are summarized in table 4. The variant DNA was unable to
induce T antigen, to transform rat cells, to replicate itself,
to induce viral antigen and to give rise to plaques.
The only biological activity which could be detected was interference with viral DNA replication and the production of wild type
virus.
Our findings on interference agree with those of Scott et al.
(16) who described a SV 40 deletion mutant whose only biological
property consisted of interference with wild type virus by inhibition of the replication of wild type DNA.
These authors suggested that the interference may be due to competition for a limiting initiation factor (e.g. gene A product)
which interacts with the initiation site for DNA replication and
may therefore be related with the number of initiation sites.
Because of the duplication in the variant BKV DNA the presence
of two initiation sites for DNA replication seems likely and
therefore the mechanism by which the variant BKV DNA interferes
may be as suggested by Scott et al. (16).
The mechanism of persistence of BKV in its natural host might be
explained by assuming that variants which effectively interfere
with the production of wild type virus also are generated in vivo.
Since the defectives depend on non-defective virus for replication
but then replicate to excess and interfere with the non defective
virus cyclic production of normal and defective virus may ensue.

SUMMARY

Serial undiluted passage of wild type BKV in primary
human embryonic cells resulted in the formation of a variant with a
genetic deletion of 25%. The variant DNA was unable to express
early functions like T - antigen induction and transformation.
The variant DNA could only replicate in the presence of normal helper
DNA and strongly interfered with the replication of normal DNA.

Acknowledgements

We wish to thank Ineke Zwaan for her skilled assistance
in preparing the figures and tables.

REFERENCES

1. Huang, A.S. and Baltimore, D. (1970)
   Defective viral particles and viral disease processes.
   Nature 226, 325-328.

2. Gardner,S.D., Field, A.M., Coleman, D.V. and Hulme, B. (1971)
   New human papovavirus (BK) isolated from urine after renal
   transplantation.
   The lancet i, 1253-1257.

3. Sol, C.J.A., Walig, C., ter Schegget, J., Van der Noordaa. J.(1975)
   Analysis of defective SV 40 by agarose geleleotrophoresis.
   J. gen. Virol. 28.285-297.

4. Hirt, B. (1967)
   Selective extraction of polyoma DNA from infected mouse cell
   cultures.
   Jrl of molecular Biology 26. 365-369.

5. Radloff, R., Bauer, W. and Vinograd, J. (1967)
   A dye-buoyant-density method for the detection and isolation of
   closed circular duplex DNA; the closed circular DNA in HeLa cells.
   Proc. National Acad. Sciences U.S.A. 57, 1514-1521.

6. Aay,C and Borst, P. (1972)
   The gel electrophoresis of DNA.
   Biochem. et Biophys. Acta 269.192-200.

7. Davis, R.W., Simon, M. and Davidson, N. (1971)
   Methods in Enzymology 21., 413-428.

8. Greenfield, L., Simpson, L. and Kaplan, D. (1975)
   Conversion of closed circular DNA molecules to single-nicked
   molecules by digestion with DNA-ase I in the presence of ethidium
   bromide.
   Biochem. Biophys. Acta 407, 365-375.

9. Robberson, D.L., Aloni, Y., Attardi, G. and Davidson, N.(1971)
   Expression of the mitochondrial genome in HeLa cells. VI. Size
   determination of mitochondrial ribosomal RNA by electron
   microscopy.
   Jrl of molecular Biology 60, 473-484.

10.McCutchan, J.H. and Pagano, J.S. (1968)
   Enhancement of the infectivity of simian virus 40 deoxy-
   ribonucleic acid with diethylaminoethyl dextran.
   Jrl national Cancer Inst. 41, 351-357.

11. Noordaa, J. van der (1976)
    Infectivity, oncogenicity and transforming ability of BK virus
    and BK virus DNA.
    Jrl gen. Virol. 30, 371-373.

12. Abrahams, P.J. and van der Eb, A.J. (1975)
    In vitro transformation of rat and mouse cells by DNA from
    simian virus 40.
    Jrl of Virology 16, 206-209.

13. Southern, E.M. (1975)
    Detection of specific sequences among DNA fragments separated
    by gel electrophoresis.
    Jrl molecular Biology 98, 503-517.

14. Laskey, R.A. and Mills, D. (1975)
    Quantative film detection of ^{3}H and ^{14}C in polyacrylamide gels
    by fluorography.
    European Jrl of Biochemistry 56, 335-341.

15. Crawford, L.V. and Robbins, A.K. (1976)
    The cleavage of polyoma virus DNA by restriction enzymes Kpn I
    and Pst I.
    Jrl gen. Virology 31, 315-322.

16. Howley, P.M., Mullarkey, M.F., Takemoto, K.K. and Martin, M.A.
    (1975).
    Characterization of human papovavirus BK DNA.
    Jrl Virology 15, 173-181.

17. Scott, W.A., Brockman, W.W. and D. Nathans (1976)
    Biological activities of deletion mutants of simian virus 40.
    Virology 75, 319-334.

THE ROLE OF HOST-VIRUS INTERACTION FOR THE DEVELOPMENT

OF HERPESVIRUS INDUCED MALIGNANCIES OF NEW WORLD PRIMATES

Hans Wolf and Gary J. Bayliss

Max von Pettenkofer-Institut, University of München

Pettenkoferstraße 9a, D-8000 München 2

THE ROLE OF THE HOST ORGANISM FOR THE ONCOGENIC EXPRESSION OF
LYMPHOTROPIC HERPESVIRUSES

Considerable knowledge has been accumulated on the biology of Herpesvirus saimiri (HVS) and Herpesvirus ateles (HVA). Hunt et al
1970 and Wolfe et al 1971 showed that HVS and HVA induce tumors in
white lipped cotton topped and common marmosets with very high
efficiency. The same was shown for owl monkeys (Hunt et al 1970,
Ablashi et al 1971,Cicmanec et al 1974). However, there have been
no reports on the occurence of HVS or HVA induced malignancy in the
natural host, the squirrel monkey Saimiri sciureus or the spider
monkeys Ateles geoffroyi and fusciceps respectively. At the present
time, we do not know the reasons for the differential behaviour of
these viruses in the natural host and the experimental host.
This relationship was studied in some detail by using HVS as the
tumorinducing agent and squirrel monkeys, owl monkeys and marmosets
as experimental hosts (Klein et al 1973). They found that there was
a correlation between the time at which antibodies developed against
the viral antigens and the titers of those antibodies on the on hand
and the development of tumors on the other hand. Rapid immunresponse
as observed in the natural host, seemed to protect the animal from
the development of clinical disease with or without tumor development. Conversly in marmosets antibodies developed late and positive
virus isolation from peripheral lymphocytes sometimes preceeded the
development of the generally low titers of antibodies. Owl monkeys
had an intermediate behaviour as far as antibody response was concerned and also with respect to the rather delayed development of tumors.
The interpretation of these findings was that a competent immune-
system is required for effective defense against tumor development.

315

.However, this is not necessarily so, it could also be that the
reason is the relatedness or nonrelatedness of cellular and viral
DNA. The natural host, for example, could be deprived by a probably
phylogenetic loss of the right anchor sites for insertion of viral
DNA in certain control genes. Alternatively, the host might have
been selected as a strong suppressor of the oncogenic manifestation
of HVS. In favour of this hypothesis one might consider the fact
that there is no squirrel monkey cell-line transformed by Herpesvirus
saimiri although one can isolate HVS from the circulating lymphocytes
of squirrel monkeys. Some virus excretion is observed from the oropharynx and cagemates, even if they belong to a different species,
may be infected. Barahona (Barahona et al 1975) reported that an owl
monkey, caged with a squirrel monkey, developed a neoplasia which
was successfully linked to an infection with HVS. At the present
time we do not know whether these observations are due to a smoul-
dering infection or to real latency. The parallel to Epstein Barr
Virus and Herpes simplex virus might suggest the latter. From all the
experimental hosts which are susceptible to tumor induction by HVS,
virus carrying suspension cell-lines could be isolated after infection. It has been shown that these cells carry T-cell charactcristics
(Wallen et al 1973). Returning to the role of the immune system there
have been reports on tumor prevention by killed vaccines (Laufs and
Steincke, 1975) and by live attenuated strains (Schaffer et al 1975).
Subcellular DNA free components were used for immunization (Pearson
and Scott, 1977). The latter animals were not challenged with live
virus. However, at least the experiments using virus vaccines would
probably support a theory based on the evolutionary selection of
squirrel monkeys with immune systems competent for tumor prevention.
This would imply that squirrel monkeys acquired during their phylo-
genesis the ability to respond to an infection with HVS, whereas marmosets and owl monkeys did not. In this context it would be interesting to know how fetal or suckling squirrel monkeys behave upon exposure to HVS when they are not protected by maternal antibodies.

The problems with Herpesvirus vaccines, especially with their possible application to humans, are twofold: (i) It was shown that HVS
DNA alone can be oncogenic in marmosets (Fleckenstein et al 1976).
(ii) The Herpesvirus saimiri marmoset system is not comparable to
the interaction of EBV of man because there is already an immune
competence as shown by rapid and high levels of antibody production.
The appearance of a tumor is a very rare event. In the Herpesvirus
saimiri marmoset monkey system vaccination might merely shift an incompetent system to a competent one. Tumors might still develop in
the challenged animals as well as in the natural host in similar frequency as BL in man and still not be observed with the number of animals studied and observation times available.
The DNA of HVS and HVA isolates has been characterized (Fleckenstein et al 1978). As of now there are 2 clearly distinct strains
of HVA known with 2.4% mismatching base pairs, and based on restriction enzyme analysis, 3 strains of HVS. No differences in biological behaviour have been linked to these genetic variations.

PROPERTIES OF POTENTIAL DNA TUMOR VIRUSES

So far we have been concerned with primates of the Americas and their T—cell tropic herpes viruses HVS and HVA. Most interestingly, in contrast, the lymphotropic herpesviruses of old world primates are all B—cell tropic. This tropism to certain cell types appears to be virus specified because, from marmosets with HVA induced disease, cell-lines with T—cell markers are obtained whereas in-fection with EBV leads to the production of cell-lines with B-cell characteristics. The best known of the B-cell tropic viruses of old world primates is the Epstein-Barr-Virus of man, though we know that at least Chimpanzees (Landon et al 1969), Baboons (Falk et al 1976, Lapin et al 1976) and Orang-utans (Rasheed et al 1977) are hosts to similar viruses. Even with Epstein-Barr-Virus we do not yet have detailed knowledge of the events involved in the in-duction of neoplastic transformation.

Although the association of Herpes simplex virus to human cancer still has to be studied further (see McDougall et al these pro-ceedings) it is at least a virus with the ability for latency be-sides its lytic expression and as such an interesting and well studied system and model. One of the prerequisites of at least a DNA containing tumor virus is the ability to undergo latency un-less viral genes persist in a fragmented form only, as it was ob-served in experimental Adenovirus systems (Gallimore et al 1974). In order to approach the basis of latency it is of considerable interest to know and to define first the regulatory events during the full expression of the viral genome which is present in the lytic cycle of virus regulation.

Regulation of Late Viral Proteins in Cells Lytically Infected with Herpes simplex Virus

In the case of HSV it has been shown (Honess and Roizmann, 1975) that there are 3 major classes of proteins. α-proteins are first made and switch on the synthesis of ß-proteins, the latter switch off the pro-duction of α-proteins, γ-proteins are made last. Our interest in this study will focus on the regulation of the synthesis of late proteins. Amongst these is the majority of structural proteins of the virus. Proteins of that group are strictly associated with the lytic cycle, their appearance is always followed by cell death though proteins appearing earlier in the lytic cycle seem to be sufficient for that effect (Honess and Roizmann, 1975).

Because of the time of appearance of γ-proteins the initiation of their synthesis may be linked only to the preceding synthesis of ß-proteins or it may be linked as well to the replication of viral DNA. The experiments described in the following were designed to give an answer whether there is a separate mechanism to switch on the synthesis of late proteins or whether the detectability of late proteins only after the replication of viral DNA has merely quanti-

tative causes. This means simply that 10.000 viral genomes can transcribe more m-RNA and make it available for translation into proteins
than one or few parental viral DNA molecules. The apparent regulation would then be only a question of the sensitivity of detection.
The results were as follows:

The amount of γ-polypeptides made in HSV-1 infected cells was dependent on the multiplicity of infection when inhibitors of DNA
synthesis like Hydroxyurea or Phosphoneacetate were present.

Figure 1 shows for HSV-1 at a multiplicity of 1 in the presence of
Phosphonoacetate, that the synthesis of host proteins is only poorly
shut down and that most polypeptides are either not made or made in
significantly reduced amounts.

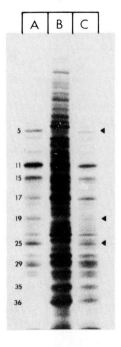

Fig.1: The autoradiogramm shows polypeptides separated on 9% Acrylamide gels. The proteins were synthesized in Hep-2 cells infected
with 1 pfu of HSV-1 (F-strain) per cell. The cultures were labelled
from 13.5 to 14 hrs post infection with a mixture of L(U-14C)leucine,
L(U-14C)isoleucine and L(U-14C) valine (NEN 300 mCi/ml) at a concentration of 2 µCi/ml and harvested immediately after labelling.
A modification of the procedures for labelling, collection, electrophoresis, autoradiography and quantitation of polypeptides of Honess and Roizmann (1975) was used. Details will be published elsewhere (Wolf and Roizmann,in prep.). A: infected cells without drug
B:cells were infected and maintained in the presence of 100 µg of
phosphonoacetate per ml of medium. C:cells were treated as in B,
5 hrs post infection the drug was washed out.

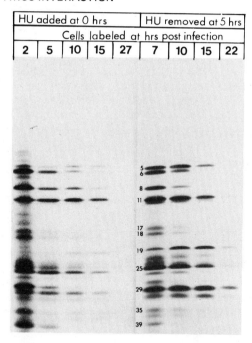

HU added at 0 hrs					HU removed at 5 hrs			
Cells labeled at hrs post infection								
2	5	10	15	27	7	10	15	22

Fig.2: The autoradiogram shows polypeptides of Hep-2 cells infected with 500 pfu of HSV-1 (F) per cell in the presence of 4 mg/ml
of hydroxyurea. The samples were pulse labelled for 30 minutes with
C^{14} amino acids at time points shown in the heading of the figure
and harvested as described in fig.1.

Figure 2 shows in a comparison of Hydroxyurea (HU) containing and
reversed cultures when the inhibitors were washed away 5 hours
post infection that, with a multiplicity of 500, γ-proteins, examp-
lified by proteins 5,19 or 25, are synthesized in only slightly
reduced amounts as compared to the uninhibited infection. It has
been shown, however, (Honess and Watson, 1977) that high concentrations of PAA (500 µl/ml) have a drastic effect on the synthesis
of γ-proteins.
Figure 3 shows that the results in HSV-2 infected cells were basically similar with the remarkable exception that some polypeptides
especially number 9 and 10 are hardly detectable at all multiplicities tested when the inhibitors of DNA synthesis including PAA
at the relatively low dose of 100 µg/ml were present.
In a second set of experiments we looked for the functional half-
life of viral messenger RNA. Several hours after the infection
Actinomycin D or Cordicepin was added to the cultures in order to
block the transcription and the processing of viral messenger RNA
respectively. At various time points thereafter the cultures were
pulse labelled for 15 to 30 minutes with C^{14} amino-acids. Figure
4 shows a set of those samples 17 hours after the infection, that
is 5 hours after the addition of the inhibitors (for B). The figure shows also the desitometric measurement of such autoradio-

grams. Proteins like No.19 are missing in the Actinomycin D treated
samples. Others are reduced and only a few are barely influenced at
this rather late time point. The quantitative analysis of the den-
sitometric scans (Wolf and Roizman,in prep.) shows, that there are
several kinetic classes of proteins. For HSV type 1 proteins No. 5,
15,19,25 decline rapidly whereas polypeptides No.23,27,29 are very
stable. Proteins like No.6,8,24 follows intermediate kinetics.

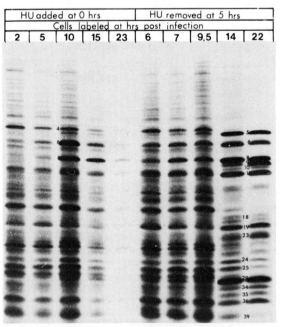

Fig.3: The autoradiogram shows polypeptides of Hep-2 cells infected with 500 pfu of HSV-2 (G) per cell in the presence of 4 mg/ml
of hydroxyurea. The samples were pulse labelled for 30 minutes with
C^{14} amino acids at timepoints shown in the heading of the figure
and harvested as described in fig.1.

Figure 5 shows in a comparison of the data of the two sets of experiments that these proteins whose messenger RNA's have a very
short functional half-life, are the same as those which are not
synthesized at low multiplicities of infection when the replication
of viral DNA is blocked.
From these and other data not shown here we can draw the following
conclusions: (i) Because many γ-messenger RNA's have a short functional half-life the synthesis of γ-polypeptides is especially dependent on the supplementation of polyribosomal RNA with fresh
messenger RNA. (ii) The amount of viral DNA available for transcription influences the synthesis of γ-polypeptides. (iii) The synthesis
of some γ-polypeptides (type 2) seems to be strongly dependent on
active replication. The functional half-life of α and β messenger
RNA is considerably longer, therefore the synthesis of the corresponding proteins is less dependent on the multiplication of the

template viral DNA. The inhibition of the appearance of late proteins in virus transformed cells might be caused by the inhibition of replication of viral DNA without requiring additional mechanisms.

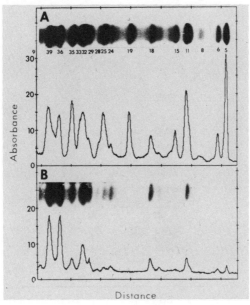

Fig.4: Scans of the autoradiogram shown on top of the trace of Hep-2 cells infected with 50 pfu HSV-1 (F) per cell.
A:untreated infected cells,B:cells treated with Actinomycin D (4 μg/ml) from 12 hrs post infection. The cultures were labelled for 15 minutes at 16.5 hrs post infection and harvested as described in fig.1.

Regulation of Protein Synthesis in EBV infected Raji Cells

In case of the Epstein-Barr-Virus it has been shown (Bayliss and Nonoyama,1978) that superinfection of the Epstein-Barr-Virus genome carrying Raji cells with EBV derived from P3 HR1 cells leads to similar effects as are known for HSV. The synthesis of host macromolecules is effectively shut down and viral proteins are induced with different patterns of synthesis.Besides that, viral DNA is made and it was shown that the cycle is a complete lytic one because progeny virus of such a superinfection differs from the infecting virus in its ability to transform cord blood cells (Nonoyama and Yajima, 1976).
Figure 6 shows protein patterns obtained by pulse labelling Cycloheximide treated superinfected Raji cells 12 hours post infection
It can be seen that there is a sequence in the appearance of these proteins. Table I lists them in the order of their appearance. When Phosphonoacetate, as an inhibitor of viral DNA replication, is added at the time of infection the pattern of synthesis of late viral proteins shows remarkable changes.

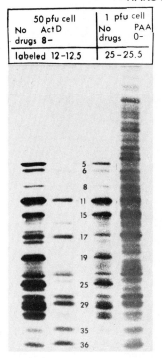

Fig.5: The autoradiogram shows polypeptides from Hep-2 cells infected with HSV-1 (F). Samples were prepared as described in fig.1.
Slot 1: untreated cells infected with 50 pfu/cell.Slot 2: cells infected with 50 pfu/cell, treated with Actinomycin D (4 µg/ml) from
5 hrs post infection. Slot 3: untreated cells infected with 1 pfu
per cell, slot 4: cells infected with 1 pfu/cell in the presence of
phosphonoacetate and maintained with the drug. Samples of slot 1
and 2 were harvested 12 hrs post infection and those for slot 3 and
4 at 17 hrs post infection.

Figure 7 shows this for several time points of labelling. Proteins
of molecular weights around 140,130,80 and 40 thousand are not
synthesized in the presence of phosphonoacetate or made in greatly
reduced amounts.Because of the difficulty of the system we have
as yet no data on the possible effects of very high multiplicities
of infections on the pattern of protein synthesis. So we do not
know whether we have a system comparable to HSV type I or type II
infected cells. In the previous section it was shown that HSV type
I late viral proteins were made without replication of viral DNA
when the multiplicity of infection is high enough. In HSV tpye 2
in contrast protein 9 and 10 are only made following the synthesis
of viral progeny DNA.

Table I summarized the available data on EBV induced proteins and
gives a tentative grouping based on our observations. The protein
with a molecular weight of 85,000 is the only one protein thus far
observed to be synthesized immediately after superinfection in
addition to the viral protein or proteins anyhow present in the

EBV genome carrying Raji cells. Its synthesis is required for the synthesis of the group II and III proteins which followed from cyclo-heximide experiments (fig.6). The distinction of group II and III was mainly based on their dependence on the replication of viral DNA at the multiplicity tested and on their time of appearance.

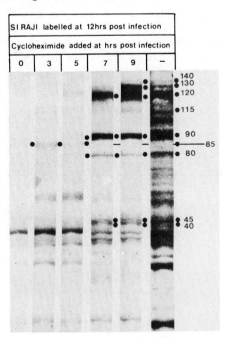

Fig.6: The effect of Cycloheximide (CH) on the synthesis of pro-teins in SI Raji cells. 6×10^7 Raji cells were mixed with virus prepared from 40 times the number of P3 HR1 cells in 3 ml. The sam-ple was divided into 6 portions. To the first 50 µg/ml CH was added. After 1 hour MEM was added to the cells (sample 0 was made 50 1g/ml with respect to CH) to give a cell density of 10^6/ml and the cul-tures returned to 37°C. At 3h, 5h, 7h and 9h CH was added to the respective cultures. At 12h the drug was removed by washing 4 times. The washed cells together with an untreated infected sample (-) were resuspended in methionine free MEM (containing 10 µCi ^{35}C methionine/ml at 2×10^6 cells per ml and incubated at 37°C for 30 minutes. After the pulse the cells were washed with PBS, resuspen-ded in 10% glycerol and sonicated, samples were assayed for pro-tein and TCA precipitable ^{35}S. After denaturation and reduction by heating to 100°C in 2% SDS,0. 2% 2-mercaptoethanol 50 µl samples containing 50 µg protein were applied to polyacrylamide slab gels (7-15% gradient of acrylamide). Virus induced polypeptides are indicated by a small dot placed to the right of the profile.

Figure 8 gives a flow chart of the data derived from the previous table including additional observations which are published and

discussed elsewhere (Bayliss and Nonoyama, 1978). Raji cells which
carry the EBV genome in a repressed state express at least one
virus specified protein-EBNA, however, further expression of the
viral genome appears to be blocked by a host cell factor (RSF)
(Glaser and Nonoyama, 1974). Superinfection of these cells at high
multiplicities leads to the synthesis of 3 groups of protein, the
synthesis of groups I and II appears to be unrelated to the synthesis of viral DNA, however, the synthesis of the third group was
inhibited by treatment of infected cells with inhibitors of viral
DNA replication. Although host DNA synthesis is effectively inhibited in the infected cultures only a small number (up to 30%) of

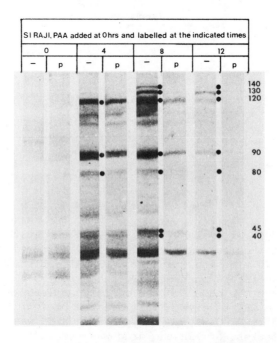

Fig.7: Effect of PAA on the Synthesis of SI Raji Cell Specific
Proteins: 4x10[7] Raji cells were mixed with virus prepared from 40
times the number of HR1 cells in 2 ml, 100 µg/ml PAA was added.
After 1 hour at room temperature MEM containing 100 µg/ml PAA was
added to give a final cell concentration of 10[6] cells/ml. The cells
were divided into 4 portions and placed at 37°C. At 0,4,8 and 12 h
PI the cells were pelleted and resuspended in methionine free MEM
containing 100 µg/ml PAA and 10 µCi/ml ^{35}S methionine at a concentration of 2x10[6] cells/ml. After a 30 min pulse at 37°C the cells
were proceeded as described in the legend to fig 6. (P) signifies
that the samples were prepared as described above. (-) signifies
that the samples were prepared as above except that the PAA was
omitted. Virus induced polypeptides are indicated by a dot placed
between the (P) and (-) profiles for any particular time point.

the cells actually synthesize VCA and even fewer (up to 10%) contain virus particles (Yajima and Nonoyama, 1976, Seigneurin et al 1977) indicating that most of the cells in the infected cultures are abortively infected.

PROTEIN MW x 10⁻³	TIME OF SYNTHESIS						CONTROL GROUP	DNA SYNTHESIS REQUIRED
	0	3	5	7	9	12		
140							III	+
130							III	+
120							II	−
115							III	+
90							II	−
85							I	−
80							II	−
45							III	+
40							III	+

Table I: Summarizing the properties of EBV induced proteins.

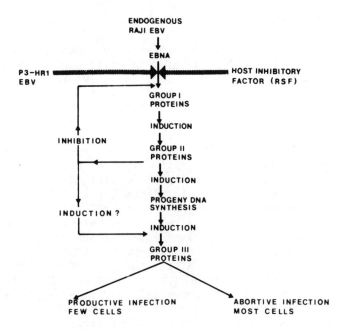

Fig.8: Flow chart of the appearance of virus induced proteins in EBV superinfected Raji cells.

SUGGESTED MODEL FOR VIRUS-HOST-INTERACTION

The scheme presented in figure 9 shows proposed steps of interaction in a cell infected with a virus like EBV or HVS or any other
tumor virus and shall also serve to sum up our observations.

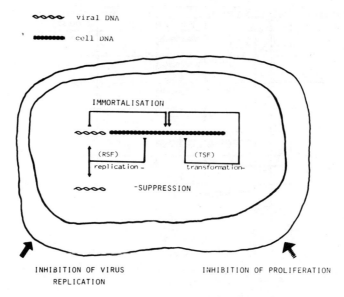

Fig.9: Model for tumor-virus - Host interaction. The explanation
follows from the text.

Virus present in a cell in a low number of genomes may express
only a certain portion of its genetic material. This follows from
the experiments with HSV shown in fig.5 and also to some exted from
the experiments with EBV in Raji cells shown in fig.7. We do not
know whether the limitted expression of the endogenous EBV in Raji
cells is caused by the same mechanism. At least in the latter case
one might speculate that this is due to some action of the host.
This interaction is labelled RSF (replication suppressing factor).
The viral genomes induce cell proliferation by means of an acti-
vator of cellular genes for continued cellular division or by in-
activating a cellular repressor for those genes. Alternatively
the viral genomes may induce the neoplastic transformation only
after integration in the right site of the host genome acting like
a transposon. However, as discussed earlier, the example of HVS
in squirrel monkey cells might be interpreted in that way that a
cellular property or product inhibits that transformation event.
This interaction is labelled TSF (Transformation suppressing
factor)and could be active in potential cancer cells. This additional step, which is not necessarily only a one step mechanism
itsself, leaves also room for the action of carcinogens or other
effects known to promote carcinogenesis. The observation that can-

cer development follows multihit-kincetis (for review see: Peto 1977)
is complimentary to such a model.
In addition this model allows for the action of apparently very
effective transforming agents like EBV. When the integration site
of viral genes causing neoplastic transformation is located at
the locus of TSV synthesis and inactivate this gene, transformation
could occur without further action.

This model is based on observations in several herpesvirus-natural
host-experimental host systems and is not a present testable. How
ever, this should change as the techniques for investigating host
cell response to virus infection improve.

Acknowledgements: Part of the work (with HSV) was done in the laboratory of Dr. Roizman, University of Chicago during a fellowship of
H.W. supported by DFG (Wo 227/1), part was done in collaboration
with M.Nonoyama at Rush Presbyterian St.Lukes Medical School Chicago
during a NATO-fellowship (B/RF-4620) of G.J.B.

Literature:
Ablashi,D.V.,Loeb,W.F.,Valerio,M.G.,Adamson,R.H.,Armstrong,G.R.,
     Bennet,D.G.,Heine,U.: Malignant lymphoma with lymphocytic
     leukemia induced in owl monkeys by Herpesvirus saimiri. J.
     nat.Cancer Inst. 47, 837-855 (1971).

Barahona,H.,Melendez,L.V.,Hunt,R.D.,Forbes,M.,Fraser,C.E.O.,Da-
     niel,M.D.: Experimental horizonal transmission of herpesvirus
     saimiri from squirrel monkeys to an owl monkey. J.Infect.Dis.
     132, 694-697 (1975).

Bayliss,G.J.,Nonoyama,M.: Mechanisms of infection with Epstein-Barr
     Virus. III The synthesis of proteins in superinfected Raji cells.
     Virology, in press (1978).

Cicmanec,J.L.,Loeb,W.F.,Valerio,M.G.: Lymphoma in owl monkeys (Ao-
     ties trivigatus) inoculated with Herpesvirus saimiri: clinical,
     haematological and pathologic findings. J.med.Primatology 3, 8-
     17 (1974(

Falk,L.,Deinhardt,F.,Nonoyama,M.,Wolfe,L.G.,Bergholz,C.,Lapin,B.,
     Yakoleva,L.,Agrba,V.,Henle,G.,Henle,W.: Properties of a baboon
     lymphotropic herpesvirus related to Epstein-Barr virus. Int.J.
     Cancer, 18, 798-807 (1976)

Fleckenstein,B.,Bornkamm,G.W.,Werner,F.-J.: The role of Herpesvirus
     saimiri genomes in oncogenic transformation of primate cells.
     Bibl.Haematol.(Basel) 43, 308-312 (1976).

Fleckenstein,B.,Bornkamm,G.W.,Mulder,C.,Werner,F.-J.,Daniel,M.D.,

Falk,L.A.,Delius,H.: Herpesvirus ateles DNA and its homology with
    Herpesvirus saimiri nucleic acid. J. Virol. 25, 361-373 (1978).

Gallimore,P.H.,Dharp,P.A.,Scambrook,J.: Viral DNA in transformed cells
    II. A study of the sequences of Adenovirus 2 DNA in nine lines
    of transformed rat cells using specific fragments of the viral
    genome. J. Mol. Biol. 89, 41-72 (1974).

Glaser,R.,Nonoyama,M.: Host cell regulation and induction of EBV. J.
    Virol. 14, 174-176 (1974).

Honess,R.W.,Roizman,B.: Regulation of Herpesvirus macromolecular
    synthesis: Sequential transition of polypeptide synthesis
    requires functional viral polypeptides. Proc.Nat.Acad.Sci.
    USA 72, 1276-1280 (1975).

Honess,R.W.,Watson,D.H.: Herpes simplex virus resistance and sensi-
    tivity to phosphonoacetic acid. J. Virol., 21, 584-600 (1977).

Hunt,R.D.,Melendez,L.V.,King,N.W.,Gilmore,C.E.,Daniel,M.D.,Wiliam-
    son,M.E.,Jones,T.C.: Morphology of a disease with features
    of malignant lymphoma in marmosets and owl monkeys inoculated
    with Herpesvirus saimiri. J.nat.Cancer Inst. 44, 447-465 (1970).

Klein,G.,Pearson,G.,Rabson,A.,Ablashi,D.V.,Falk,L.,Wolfe,L.,Dein-
    hardt,F.,Rabin,H.: Antibody reactions to Herpesvirus saimiri
    (HVS) induced early and late antigens (EA and LA) in HVS in-
    fected squirrel marmoset and owl monkeys. Int. J. Cancer 12,
    270-289 (1973).

Landon,J.C.,Ellis,L.B.,Zeve,V.H.,Fabrizio,D.P.: Herpes type virus
    in cultured leukocytes from chimpanzees. J.nat.Cancer Inst.
    40. 181-192 (1968).

Lapin,B.A.: Epidemiology of leukemia among baboons of Sukhumi monkey
    colony. Bibl. Haematol. 43, 212-215 (1976).

Laufs,R.,Steincke,H.: Vaccination of non-human primates against
    malignant lymphoma. Nature, 253, 71-72 (1975).

Pearson,G.R.,Scott,R.E.: Isolation of virus-free Herpesvirus sai-
    miri antigenpositive plasma membrane vesicles. Proc.nat.
    Acad.Sci. USA 74, 2546-2550 (1977).

Peto,R.: Epidemiology, multistage models, and short-term mutagenicity
    tests. in: Origins of Human Cancer: Cold Spring Harbor Conferen-
    ces on cell proliferation, Vol.4, Hiatt, Watson,Winsten eds.
    Cold Spring Harbor Laboratory (1977).

Rasheed,S.,Rongey,R.W.,Bruszweski,J.,Nelson-Rees,W.A.,Rabin,H.,
    Neubauer,R.H.,Esra,G.,Gardner,M.B.: Establishment of a cell-
    line with associated Epstein-Barr virus from a leukemia or-
    ganutan. Science, 198, 407-409 (1977).

Seigneurin.J.-M.,Vuillaume,M.,Lenoir,G., deThê,G.: Replication of
    Epstein-Barr virus: Ultrastructural and immunfluorescent stu-
    dies of P3 HR1 -superinfected Raji cells. J. Virol. 24, 836-845
    (1977).

Schaffer,P.A.,Falk,L.A.,Deinhardt.F.: Attenuation of Herpesvirus
    saimiri for marmosets after successive passage in cell culture
    at 39°C. J.nat.Cancer Inst. 55, 1243-1246 (1975).

Wallen,W.C.,Neubauer,R.H.,Rabin,H.,Cicmanec,J.L.: Nonimmune rosette
    formation by lymphoma and leukemia cells from Herpesvirus sai-
    miri infected owl monkeys. J.nat.Cancer Inst. 51, 967-975 (1973).

Wolf,H.,Roizman,B.: The regulation of γ(structural) polypeptide-
    synthesis in Herpes simplex virus (HSV) 1 and 2 infected cells.
    Oncogenesis and Herpesviruses III. Henle,W. and Rapp.F. (eds.).
    Switzerland, IARC Scientific Publications, in press (1978).

Wolfe,L.G.,Falk,L.A.,Deinhardt,F.: Oncogenicity of Herpesvirus sai-
    miri in marmoset monkeys. J.nat.Cancer Inst. 47, 1145-1162 (1971).

Yajima,J.,Nonoyama,M.: Mechanisms of infection with Epstein-Barr
    virus I: Viral DNA replication and formation of noninfectious
    virus particles in superinfected Raji cells. J.Virol. 19, 187-
    194 (1976).

SECTION IV

Immunological control mechanism of neoplasia

Convenor

Dr. George KLEIN

Dep. of Tumor Biology

Karolinska Institutet

104 01 Stockholm 60

Sweden

HOST RESPONSES TO SPONTANEOUS RAT TUMOURS

R. W. Baldwin, M. J. Embleton and M. V. Pimm

Cancer Research Campaign Laboratories

University of Nottingham, Nottingham, U.K.

INTRODUCTION

In recent years it has become widely accepted that many types
of experimental animal tumour exhibit neoantigens capable of
eliciting rejection responses. These tumour rejection antigens
have been identified in tests showing that tumour transplanted into
syngeneic hosts pre-immunized in a variety of ways, but often with
attenuated tumour cells, is rejected. In some instances, also,
these tumour immune rejection responses have been demonstrated in
tumour-bearing animals by showing that whilst the primary tumour
may be outside host control, a concomitant challenge with cells of
the same tumour can be rejected (Vaage, 1971; 1974). This evidence
has been used to reinforce the view that properly designed immunotherapy can be effective in the treatment of small amounts of tumour
such as pulmonary metastatic deposits following, or concurrent with,
conventional therapy of the primary tumour (Hersh et al., 1977;
Baldwin and Pimm, 1978).

These propositions have been developed to a considerable extent
from studies with selected animal tumours induced either by chemical
carcinogens or oncogenic viruses. It is important to recognise,
however, that the expression of tumour cell surface products which
function as rejection antigens is not an obligatory response to
neoplastic transformation. For example, whilst tumour specific
rejection antigens have been identified upon sarcomas induced by
chemical carcinogens (e.g. 3-methylcholanthrene, MCA) in several
species, a proportion of the tumours will lack this type of neoantigen (Bartlett, 1972; Prehn, 1975). Similarly, hepatic and
mammary tumours induced in rats by N-2-fluorenylacetamide only
infrequently express tumour specific antigens at levels capable of

333

inducing significant levels of immunity against transplanted tumour
cells (Baldwin and Embleton, 1969a; 1971).

Against this background knowledge with tumours induced with
extrinsic agents, it was pointed out very early in the development
of contemporary tumour immunology that naturally occurring tumours
may not be immunogenic as defined by tumour rejection tests. Since
these spontaneous tumours arise with low frequency within inbred
populations of animals, relatively few studies of their immuno-
genicities have been reported, but in early studies it was
established that spontaneous murine sarcomas were not immunogenic
in comparison with MCA-induced sarcomas (Prehn and Main, 1957);
the criterion for immunity in these studies being the capacity to
reject tumour grafts. This point was further evaluated in a series
of studies with spontaneous rat mammary carcinomas and sarcomas
(Baldwin and Embleton, 1969b; 1974), which again established that
a significant proportion of the tumours did not exhibit tumour
rejection antigens. In several instances it was possible to use
challenge inocula as low as 10^2 tumour cells so that in practical
terms these tumours were non-immunogenic.

There is still far too little evidence available to make valid
judgements upon the relative merits of spontaneous or experimentally-
induced tumours as models for human disease (Baldwin, 1976a; Weiss,
1977). Nevertheless, it is perhaps more realistic to evaluate
tumours of low immunogenicity such as those induced by chronic low
dose carcinogen treatment or arising without deliberate inducement.
In order to put these points into perspective, the role of host
factors in controlling growth of transplanted tumours has been
examined using spontaneous rat mammary carcinomas and sarcomas.
These have been studied firstly for tumour specific immune responses
and secondly for the capacity to manipulate non-specific responses
in controlling tumour growth.

IMMUNOGENICITY OF SPONTANEOUS TUMOURS

In this discussion spontaneous tumours will be defined as
those arising without deliberate inducement and with low incidence,
for which no aetiological agent is known. The study of immunogenicity of these tumours has of necessity to be carried out by
transplantation studies in syngeneic animals and the most appropriate
means of evaluation is by challenge-protection experiments. For
these reasons we will exclude the following:-

a. Murine mammary tumours and leukaemias, which are known to
    have a viral aetiology;
b. Other tumours of high incidence (>10% of adult animals);
c. Tumours in outbred populations;
d. Tumours arising from injection of cultured cells, spontaneously

transformed in vitro.

With these exclusions, there is a paucity of such studies
reported in the literature, possibly owing to the rarity in which
spontaneous tumours are found in laboratory animals, few of which
are likely to live to an advanced age.

The earliest report on the immunogenicity of spontaneous
tumours was by Prehn and Main (1957) where it was clearly shown
that fibrosarcomas induced by MCA were capable of inducing a tumor
rejection response in mice immunized by amputation of a limb bearing
a growing transplanted tumour. These mice rejected trocar grafts
of the immunizing tumour, which grew in controls. When seven
spontaneous fibrosarcomas were tested by the same methods, however,
no immunity could be detected and it was concluded that they were
deficient in tumour specific rejection antigens (TSRA) of the type
expressed by MCA-induced tumours (Table 1). It was possible in
these studies that weak rejection responses were induced but were
overcome by trocar graft challenges. Thus Hammond et al. (1967)
using a similar method of immunization, gave low doses of tumour
cells in suspension for challenge and by this means were able to
demonstrate weak immune responses against three spontaneous fibrosarcomas and two myoepitheliomas in mice. Administration of sub-
threshold doses of cells also afforded protection against subsequent
challenge with cell doses which produced tumours in control mice.
Immunization with irradiated cells was unsuccessful suggesting that
the antigens involved were radiosensitive. A similar radio-
sensitivity was also indicated with a spontaneous rat leukaemia,
against which no immunity to challenge with as few as 100 cells
could be induced with cells attenuated by X-irradiation (5,000 R),
nitrogen mustard, iodoacetate of glutaraldehyde (Wrathmell and
Alexander, 1976). However, immunization with leukaemia cells
treated with low doses of mitomycin C (5 mg/10^7 cells/ml) significantly retarded growth of challenge inocula, although at higher
doses of mitomycin C immunogenicity was abolished. In a report
by Vasa-Thomas et al. (1977) three lymphoma lines were established
in inbred hamsters, and all three were found to induce tumour rejection responses against 10^3 to 10^4 lymphoma cells following immunization with cells inactivated by 5,000 R X-irradiation.

The studies referred to above involved few tumours or a limited
number of tumour types, but Hewitt et al. (1976) published results
of a long-term study in which 27 tumours of various types comprising
leukaemias, carcinomas and sarcomas were examined. Not all of the
experiments described were specifically designed to demonstrate
tumour immunity, but nevertheless they could be expected to yield
evidence for any immune responses that may have been evoked as a
result of tumour transplantation. No such evidence was obtained,
and in attempts to specifically immunize mice against seven tumours

TABLE 1

Immunogenicity of Spontaneous Tumours

Authors	Tumour Type	Species	No. of Tumours	Immunogenicity
Prehn, R. T., and Main, J. M. (1957)	Fibrosarcoma	Mouse	7	−
Hammond, W. G., Fisher, J. G., and Rolley, R. T. (1967)	Fibrosarcoma	Mouse	3	+
	Myoepithelioma	Mouse	2	+
Wrathmell, A. B., and Alexander, P. (1976)	Leukaemia	Rat	1	+−
Hewitt, H. B., Blake, E. R., and Walder, A. S. (1976)	Sarcomas	Mouse	10	−
	Carcincmas	Mouse	10	−
	Leukaemia	Mouse	5	−
	Endothelioma	Mouse	2	−
Vasa-Thomas, K. A., Ambrose, K. R., Bellomy, B. R., and Coggin, J. H. (1977)	Lymphoma	Hamster	3	+

with irradiated cells, this treatment resulted in enhanced tumour growth rather than resistance to challenge. The authors concluded that spontaneous animal tumours lacked any neoantigens capable of evoking transplantation resistance, and presented their findings as a critique in which they dismissed the relevance of previous studies by other workers involving immune responses to virus-induced or chemically-induced tumours.

Immunological studies with spontaneous rat tumours have been carried out in our laboratory for more than a decade and have so far included 20 tumours of different types (Table 2), but our findings are less negative than those of Hewitt et al. (1976). The earliest report (Baldwin, 1966) showed that rats immunized against a spontaneous squamous cell carcinoma by ligation of a sub-cutaneously growing tumour graft were able to reject a subcutaneous inoculum of as many as $5x10^6$ cells which grew in all controls. In spite of resistance to subcutaneous challenge, however, the treated rats often succumbed eventually to lung metastases. Treatment with irradiated (15,000 R) tumour cells did not confer resistance against this tumour, and neither method of immunization was effective against a second tumour, a reticulum cell sarcoma.

A series of nine mammary carcinomas arising in the same WAB/Not rat strain was also studied (Baldwin and Embleton, 1969b). With six of these tumours, no immunity could be detected following treatment with irradiated tumour or surgical excision of subcutaneously growing tumour grafts. One tumour (Sp4) was consistently immunogenic so that immunity could be induced against inocula of at least $2x10^4$ cells, representing a 20-fold higher cell dose than that growing in controls (Table 2). Two other tumours were weakly immunogenic, immunized rats rejecting only 10^3 cells which was the threshold dose for growth in normal rats. More recent experiments have shown that spontaneous rat sarcomas have a similar frequency of immunogenicity. Thus, of nine sarcomas so far studied, one was weakly immunogenic, two were more strongly immunogenic and six were deficient in detectable tumour rejection antigens. Other spontaneous tumours examined in our laboratory include three nephroblastomas and a chemodectoma, all of which were apparently non-immunogenic (Table 2).

It was shown by Hammond et al. (1967) that weak immunity detected against spontaneous murine fibrosarcomas or myoepitheliomas was specific for the immunizing tumour, and Baldwin and Embleton (1969b) showed that there was no antigenic cross-reactivity between three immunogenic rat mammary tumours. Similarly, induction of immunity to a spontaneous rat fibrosarcoma did not result in resistance against either of two cross-challenge spontaneous sarcomas (Embleton and Middle, in preparation). This indicates that the antigens detected on spontaneous tumours by in vivo transplantation methods are individually specific like those of

TABLE 2

Rejection Responses to Transplanted Subcutaneous Tumours in Preimmunized Syngeneic WAB/Not Rats

Tumour	Site of Origin	Tumour Type	Min. Cell Inoculum Growing in Controls	Max. Cell Inoculum Rejected by Immunized[1] Rats	Immunogenicity Index[2]
Sp1	Skin	Squamous ca.	10^3	10^5	100
Sp2	Subcutaneous	Sarcoma	10^5	$<10^5$	0
Sp7	Subcutaneous	Sarcoma	5×10^4	5×10^6	100
Sp20	Subcutaneous	Sarcoma	2×10^5	$<2 \times 10^5$	0
Sp24	Subcutaneous	Sarcoma	10^3	10^3	1
Sp25	Subcutaneous	Sarcoma	5×10^4	$<5 \times 10^4$	0
Sp41	Subcutaneous	Sarcoma	5×10^4	2×10^5	4
Sp3	Breast	Carcinoma	10^3	10^3	1
Sp4	Breast	Carcinoma	10^3	10^5	100
Sp6	Breast	Carcinoma	10^3	$<10^3$	0
Sp9	Breast	Carcinoma	10^3	$<10^3$	0
Sp11	Breast	Carcinoma	10^2	$<10^2$	0
Sp14	Breast	Carcinoma	10^4	$<10^4$	0
Sp15	Breast	Carcinoma	10^3	10^3	1
Sp21	Breast	Carcinoma	5×10^4	$<5 \times 10^4$	0
Sp22	Breast	Carcinoma	10^3	$<10^3$	0
Sp45	Kidney	Nephroblastoma	10^6	$<10^6$	0
Sp63	Kidney	Nephroblastoma	5×10^4	$<5 \times 10^4$	0
Sp78B	Kidney	Nephroblastoma	10^4	$<10^4$	0
Sp71	Skin	Chemodectoma	5×10^5	$<5 \times 10^5$	0

[1] Rats were immunised by implantation of irradiated (15,000 R) tumour or by excision of growing tumour.

[2] Ratio of cell growth inocula rejected by immune rats to minimum inoculum growing in controls.

chemically-induced tumours. In the case of rat mammary carcinomas, it was further shown that antibody reacting against a consistently immunogenic tumour (Sp4) was specific only for this tumour as judged by membrane immunofluorescence studies (Baldwin and Embleton, 1970). However, later studies indicated that in vitro tests for cell-mediated cytotoxicity in tumour-bearing rats detected cross-reacting antigens in rat mammary carcinomas and these were identified as embryonic antigens re-expressed on the malignant cells.

The overall conclusion concerning the immunogenicity of spontaneous tumours in inbred animals is that the frequency of immunogenic tumours is less than is commonly observed with chemically-induced or virus-induced tumours, and even where immune responses are detected, they are often extremely weak in terms of the maximum number of tumour cells rejected by immunized animals and especially when compared to the minimum challenge inoculum required to produce progressive tumour growth in normal hosts. However, it is incorrect to assume that all spontaneous tumours are non-antigenic, since evidence from various groups shows that rejection antigens are demonstrable on a proportion of such tumours when appropriate methods are used for their detection.

Immune Responses to Modified Spontaneous Tumour Cells

Although only a minority of spontaneous rat tumours express detectable rejection antigens, almost all the examples tested express embryonic antigens demonstrated by in vitro reactions with serum or lymphoid cells from multiparous rats (Baldwin and Embleton, 1974; Baldwin and Vose, 1974). These do not function as transplantation antigens in conventional immunization procedures, and it has been suggested that this may be due to their mobility and consequent shedding from the cell surface (Price and Baldwin, 1977). Accordingly, attempts have been made to induce immunity to some of these tumours by pretreating syngeneic hosts with fixed cells which are incapable of shedding cell surface components, in the expectation that the stabilized antigens may be more immunogenic. Formalinized cells of nine different spontaneous tumours have been tested for immunogenicity compared with intact cells as shown in Table 3. In most cases cells from tumours of weak or moderate immunogenicity were rendered non-immunogenic after fixation but there were two examples in which immune responses were observed. The first was sarcoma Sp7 which normally is moderately immunogenic. In one experiment using high numbers of formalinized Sp7 cells, immunity to challenge with 10^5 tumour cells was achieved although in a subsequent experiment with lower numbers of cells no immunity to challenge with 2×10^4 tumour cells was detectable. However, in this experiment it was nevertheless possible to demonstrate antibody with specificity for Sp7 cells in the serum of treated rats using a membrane immunofluorescence test. Another positive

TABLE 3

Immune Responses to Formalin Treated Spontaneous Rat Tumour Cells

Tumour	Tumour Type	Challenge Cell Dose	Tumour Challenge Growth		Serum[1] Antibody
			Treated Rats	Control Rats	
Sp1	Squamous ca.	10^3	5/5	3/4	–
Sp4	Mammary ca.	2×10^4	5/5	5/5	–
Sp15	Mammary ca.	2×10^3	5/5	4/4	–
Sp22	Mammary ca.	5×10^3	5/5	3/4	–
Sp7[2]	Fibrosarcoma (a)	10^5	0/4	4/4	NT
Sp7	Fibrosarcoma (b)	2×10^4	5/5	4/4	+
Sp41	Fibrosarcoma	5×10^4	3/5	4/5	–
Sp63	Nephroblastoma	10^5	3/5	4/4	–
Sp66	Nephroblastoma	10^6	5/5	3/4	NT
Sp71	Chemodectoma	10^5	4/4	4/4	

[1] Antibody detected in serum of treated rats by membrane immunofluorescence. NT = not tested.

[2] Two experiments performed independently; formalinized cells were used at a two-fold higher inoculum in experiment (a) than in (b).

example was mammary tumour Sp22 which is non-immunogenic by the
usual criteria. The administration of formalinized Sp22 cells
induced significant retardation of tumour growth after challenge,
although complete protection was not achieved (Figure 1). The
remaining tumours were completely negative, even with examples
which are immunogenic in an untreated form. This is in agreement
with studies by Price et al. (1978) who showed that glutaraldehyde
fixation of cells of immunogenic chemically-induced tumours
rendered them non-immunogenic, although in this case it was
possible to demonstrate intact antigens on the surface of the fixed
cells. For example, treatment of radiation attenuated (15,000 R)
rat hepatoma D23 cells with glutaraldehyde at a concentration as

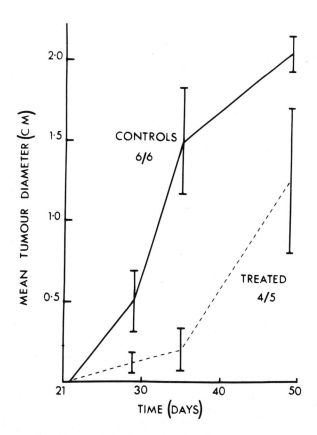

Figure 1. Immunization with formalinized mammary carcinoma Sp22
cells. Rats were injected three times with mammary carcinoma Sp22
cells treated with 10% formal saline (10^6 cells per injection) at
weekly intervals. One week after the last inoculum they were
challenged subcutaneously with 1×10^3 Sp22 cells.

low as 0·001% rendered them incapable of initiating tumour immunity
in normal rats (Price et al., 1978). Nevertheless, these
glutaraldehyde treated tumour cells still expressed the D23 specific
antigen as detected by reaction with syngeneic tumour immune serum
in membrane immunofluorescence or complement dependent cytotoxicity
tests. It has not been established conclusively that the serologically defined tumour specific antigen is identical with that
initiating tumour rejection responses even though it exhibited the
same individual specificity and this could explain the discrepancy
in these findings. A similar loss of immunogenicity following cell
treatment with glutaraldehyde has been reported, however, in other
studies on the cell mediated response to murine alloantigens
(Bubbers and Henney, 1975) and trinitrophenyl-modified cells
(Forman, 1977). This suggests that whilst glutaraldehyde treatment
stabilizes cell surface antigens, treatment may render them
incapable of initiating immune responses, perhaps because they are
now too firmly fixed as a consequence of cross-linking treatment.
This could result, for example if release of tumour antigen from
the cell surface and processing by macrophages is required in the
initiation of a tumour immune response (Brunda and Raffel, 1977).

   Alternative approaches have been proposed for increasing the
immunogenicity of weak or non-immunogenic tumours through chemical
modification of tumour cell surface proteins. In general these
approaches have not been greatly effective so that, for example,
modification of murine tumour cells by introduction of chemically
distinct groups did not markedly increase the immunogenic potential
of the tumour (Staab and Anderer, 1977). As already indicated,
however, simple chemical modification of cell surface components
may not be sufficient if by so doing the treatment severely alters
cell membrane turnover (Price and Baldwin, 1977). Another approach
for stimulating cell mediated immunity to weak tumour associated
antigens has been reported by Lachmann and Sikora (1978). In this
case, PPD was coupled to concanavalin A by glutaraldehyde treatment
and this complex allowed to bind to murine MCA-induced sarcoma cells.
These PPD-linked tumour cells were then shown to produce an enhanced
tumour rejection response in BCG-sensitized mice and it was
concluded that the effect was provided by antigenic help from PPD
provoking strong T cell responses. This procedure has not yet been
evaluated in other tumour systems but it does have the advantage of
adding T dependent antigens to the tumour cell surface whilst the
use of concanavalin A as carrier minimizes cell surface damage.

   In addition to chemically modifying existing cell surface
antigens it is also possible to introduce new receptors by a variety
of means. Most attention so far has been given to methods whereby
virus infection of tumour cells results in the expression of viral
antigens, these cells then being used to induce immunity against
non-infected tumour cells. This approach has proved effective with
a number of tumour systems (Kuzumaki et al., 1978; Kobayashi et al.,

1977) but has the inherent disadvantage that viral material has to be introduced. A completely different approach to modifying the antigenicity of weakly immunogenic spontaneous rat tumours has been initiated using mammary carcinoma Sp22 as an example. Cells of this tumour were treated in culture with MCA in the presence of irradiated rat embryo feeder cells to provide conditions for metabolic activation of the carcinogen. By this treatment, it was hoped to induce antigenic changes of the type observed in chemically transformed murine embryo or prostate cells (Mondal et al., 1970; Embleton and Heidelberger, 1972; 1975). A total of 18 MCA-treated tumour Sp22 clones were isolated and grown in vivo. Initially these cells were tested for loss of alloantigen by comparison of their capacity to absorb antibody from KX/Not anti WAB/Not) alloantiserum with that of parent (untreated) Sp22 cells this being taken as evidence of carcinogen-induced changes (Haywood and McKhann, 1971). Three clones demonstrated some loss of allo-antigen by this assay and these are being evaluated for immunogenicity.

NON-SPECIFIC IMMUNITY

Responses initiated when bacterial agents such as bacillus Calmette Guérin (BCG) or C. parvum (CP) are administered so as to localize in tumour deposits have been shown to control or even suppress tumour growth (Baldwin, 1978; Baldwin and Pimm, 1978; Scott, 1974; Scott and Milas, 1978) and so these approaches have been evaluated against a series of spontaneous rat tumours including sarcomas and mammary carcinomas. In the initial screening system designed to identify active bacterial preparations, the growth of tumour cells injected in admixture with these agents into normal syngeneic rats has been determined. As summarized in Table 4 injection of BCG (Glaxo percutaneous vaccine) in admixture with cells derived from both sarcomas and mammary carcinomas suppressed growth of subcutaneous tumours. The tumour challenge inocula rejected by this treatment ranged from 10^3 to 2×10^6 tumour cells and in some instances was greater than that in pre-immunized rats (Table 4). For example, the maximum tumour cell challenge rejected in pre-immunization tests with mammary carcinoma Sp4 was 10^5 cells, whereas when injected in contact with BCG up to 5×10^5 tumour cells was controlled. Similar responses were obtained using other BCG preparations such as the Trudeau Pasteur strain (TMC 1011) and the Pasteur immunotherapy reagent Pasteur F (Table 5). Tumour inhibition was also induced in some cases with the methanol extraction residue of BCG (MER), but the most pronounced and consistent response was obtained using a heat killed, preservative free, C. parvum preparation (Wellcome CN 6134). This is further emphasized by the tests with mammary carcinoma Sp15 in which injection of 1×10^5 tumour cells cannot be completely controlled by any of the preparations (Fig. 2), but nevertheless C. parvum

TABLE 4

BCG Contact Suppression of Subcutaneously Transplanted Tumours
of Spontaneous Origin

Tumour	Mixed Subcutaneous Inoculum		Tumour Takes in:	
	Tumour Cells	BCG µg Dry Wt.*	Test	Controls
Sarcoma: Sp7	$2x10^5$	70	0/5	3/5
	$5x10^5$	350	0/4	3/4
Sp24	$2x10^4$	70	0/15	10/15
	$1x10^5$	70	6/19	19/20
	$2x10^5$	70	9/15	15/15
	$5x10^5$	70	5/5	5/5
Sp41	$2x10^5$	175	0/5	5/5
	$5x10^5$	70	5/10	10/10
	$1x10^6$	70	10/15	15/15
	$2x10^6$	70	4/9	11/11
	$5x10^6$	70	3/5	4/4
Mammary Ca.: Sp4	$1x10^4$	35	0/10	10/11
	$5x10^4$	35	3/15	15/16
	$5x10^5$	300	0/6	5/5
Sp15	$1x10^3$	350	1/7	5/5
	$2x10^3$	175	5/5	5/5
	$5x10^4$	70	10/10	10/10
Sp22	$1x10^3$	175	10/10	10/10
	$2x10^3$	175	5/5	5/5

* Glaxo percutaneous vaccine

TABLE 5

Adjuvant Contact Suppression : Spontaneous Rat Tumours

Tumour/ Cell Dose	Tumour Incidence from Cells in Admixture with:					
	BCG Glaxo (200µg)	BCG TMC 1011 (80µg)	BCG Pasteur F (160µg)	MER (100µg)	C.parvum CN 6134 (100µg)	Control
Mammary Ca.:						
Sp4/$5x10^5$	0/6	0/6	0/6	0/6	0/6	6/6
Sp15/$1x10^5$	6/6	6/6	6/6	6/6	6/6	6/6
Sp22/$1x10^5$	6/6	6/6	6/6	5/6	6/6	6/6
Sarcoma:						
Sp7/$2x10^5$	–	5/6	–	4/6	0/6	5/5
Sp24/$5x10^5$	2/6	3/6	4/5	4/5	0/5	5/5

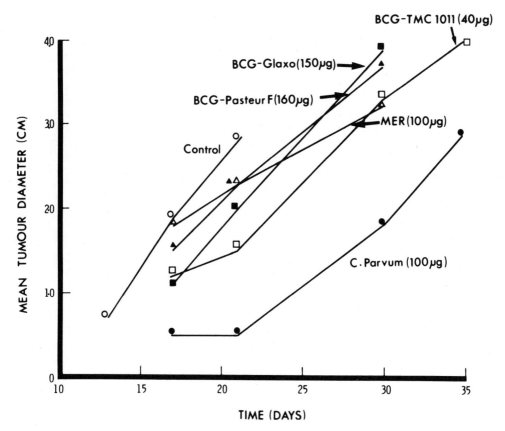

Figure 2.   Adjuvant contact suppression of spontaneous rat mammary carcinoma Sp15.

(CN 6134) was much more effective than any of the other agents in suppressing tumour development.

The mechanism of rejection of transplanted tumours established from spontaneous mammary carcinomas and sarcomas following contact of tumour cells with bacterial preparations has not yet been adequately defined, although the host factors involved in this type of response have been examined with a number of chemically-induced tumours.   BCG shows no direct cytotoxicity when cultured with tumour cells indicating that its local in vivo tumour suppressive action depends upon host responses.   However, adjuvant contact suppression can be demonstrated in immunosuppressed hosts and there is evidence that T lymphocytes are not necessarily involved.   This is illustrated by tests with the MCA-induced rat sarcoma Mc7 showing that suppression of growth of transplanted tumour cells injected in admixture with BCG (Glaxo) was effective in rats immunosuppressed by 450 R whole body irradiation (Pimm and Baldwin, 1976a).   Also

xenografted rat tumours including sarcoma Mc7 were rejected by
contact with BCG or C. parvum in athymic mice (Pimm and Baldwin,
1975; 1976b; Pimm et al., 1978). Similar effects have been
reported with experimentally-induced osteogenic sarcomas, tumour
growth being suppressed when tumour cells were injected in
admixture with BCG into rats deprived of T lymphocytes by adult
thymectomy, whole body irradiation and bone marrow reconstitution
(Moore et al., 1976). It is also relevant that in the rat sarcoma
Mc7 studies, 450 R whole body irradiation totally abrogated the
generation of systemic tumour specific immunity in animals rejecting
tumour cells admixed with BCG. Intact rats rejecting tumour cell-
BCG vaccines were also able to reject a simultaneous challenge with
tumour cells at a contralateral subcutaneous site. Tumour
challenges grew out in immunosuppressed rats, however, even though
they successfully rejected the mixed inoculum of tumour cells and
BCG. Similarly suppression of rat tumour cells injected in
admixture with BCG or C. parvum into athymic mice did not render
the treated mice resistant to a subsequent challenge with the same
tumour (Pimm and Baldwin, 1975).

The above studies indicate that T lymphocyte responses to
tumour specific antigens on rat tumours are not obligatory in the
suppressive effects initiated by BCG or C. parvum contact with
tumour cells. But there is evidence, albeit still inconclusive,
to suggest that immunogenic tumours are more susceptible than non-
immunogenic tumours to this type of growth suppression. For example,
with the immunogenic mammary carcinoma Sp4, BCG contact treatment
prevents growth of 5×10^5 tumour cells this being 500 times greater
than the minimum inoculum for tumour growth (Table 4). With two
other mammary carcinomas Sp15 and Sp22 showing little immunogenicity,
the ratio of the minimum tumour inoculum to challenge suppressed by
BCG contact is no greater than that needed for growth in untreated
controls. This pattern of BCG contact responses is reflected in
the susceptibility of these tumours to intralesional therapy when
developing in mammary pad tissue (Greager and Baldwin, 1978). This
correlation is by no means clear cut, however, and as illustrated
in Table 4 both immunogenic and non-immunogenic sarcomas showed
comparable susceptibilities to suppression by BCG contact with
tumour cells.

While T lymphocytes do not appear to be essential for BCG
contact suppression of growth of transplanted tumours, phagocytic
cells have been strongly implicated as an essential effector cell.
Systemic administration of fine particulate silica, reported to be
preferentially toxic for macrophages, has been shown to abrogate
the suppressive properties of BCG injected intralesionally into
subcutaneously developing MCA-induced rat sarcomas (Chassoux and
Salomon, 1975). Also this treatment abrogates the rejection
response induced when cells from rat sarcomas or hepatomas are
injected in admixture with BCG into either intact rats or athymic

mice (Hopper et al., 1976; Moore and Nisbet, 1978). The requirement
for macrophages in BCG contact suppression of these rat tumours is
further emphasized by studies showing that addition of paraffin oil-
induced peritoneal exudate cells from normal rats to a mixed
inoculum of rat hepatoma D23 cells and BCG facilitated the rejection
response allowing control of up to 20 times the inoculum normally
suppressed (Pimm et al., 1978; Hopper and Pimm, 1978). Removal of
glass adherent phagocytic cells, leaving only lymphocytes and polymorphs, abrogated the augmenting effect of the peritoneal exudate
cell preparations. Similar analyses have not yet been carried out
with the spontaneously arising mammary carcinomas and sarcomas, but
it has been shown that there is a marked correlation between the
extent of macrophage infiltration into these tumours and their
susceptibility to BCG contact mediated suppression of tumour growth
(Baldwin, 1976b).

The current status of these studies does not identify
unequivocally the host mediated events involved in tumour growth
suppression by contact with bacterial preparations. Macrophage
localization at the tumour deposit is clearly required, but this
in itself is not sufficient since an additional stimulus such as
that provided by BCG is required. This may simply reflect the
involvement of activated macrophages, but it cannot be excluded
that other host cells are required. It would seem that T lymphocyte
responses are not obligatory, however, although these may enhance
rejection of immunogenic tumours and also lead to the development
of systemic tumour immunity. The role, if any, of other lymphocyte
populations is still unresolved but the involvement of normal killer
cells may be suspected since they are known to be stimulated by BCG
(Herberman and Holden, 1978) and C. parvum (Oehler et al., 1978).
Furthermore it has been established that natural cell mediated
cytotoxicity in rats is sharply diminished by treatment with silica
in doses (50 mg/rat intraperitoneally) which had no effect on
proliferative responses of host lymphocytes to concanavalin A
(Oehler and Herberman, 1978). This dose of silica is comparable
to that used to show a requirement for phagocytic cells in BCG or
C. parvum mediated contact suppression of growth of rat tumours
(Hopper et al., 1976). Therefore if it is argued that macrophages
are required to maintain a high level of NK cell activity (Oehler
and Herberman, 1978) these cells may be involved in the local
tumour rejection response initiated following infiltration of
bacterial adjuvants into tumor deposits. It is important to
recognise, however, that tumour growth is suppressed when BCG or
C. parvum are injected so as to contact with tumour cells whereas
these agents have little or no effect when injected intraperitoneally
although this latter treatment stimulates NK cell activity. This
would suggest that local effects involving activated macrophages
are particularly important in adjuvant contact suppression of
tumour growth.

Even though a more precise characterization of the effector cells involved in BCG contact suppression of tumour growth is required, there are several approaches deemed to be of merit in attempting to improve responses to spontaneous tumours. Of these, the most obvious is the development of procedures which will increase macrophage accumulation at tumour deposits. This may be brought about, for example, by general stimulation of the reticuloendothelial system following systemic treatment with agents such as C. parvum. Alternatively specific localization of macrophages in tumour deposits may be increased through more effective agents than BCG. This approach is emphasized by the superior response of several rat tumours to contact with C. parvum and to a lesser extent MER when compared to BCG preparations (Willmott et al., 1978). A factor here which so far has received little attention is the effect of tumour products which adversely affect macrophage chemotaxis in vivo as well as in vitro (Pike and Snyderman, 1976; James, 1977). This is currently being evaluated with the spontaneous rat tumours to determine whether their low degree of macrophage infiltration compared to carcinogen-induced tumours such as MCA-induced sarcomas (Baldwin, 1976b) is due to inherent factors in the tumours and if so to evaluate whether their effects can be reversed.

IMMUNOTHERAPY OF SPONTANEOUS RAT TUMOURS

One of the objectives in studying specific and non-specific immune responses to spontaneous rat tumours has been to evaluate their potential for immunotherapy since these tumours may be appropriate models for human cancer. Considering first active specific immunotherapy, screening studies with a range of immunogenic carcinogen-induced rat tumours, e.g. MCA-induced sarcomas have established that immunostimulation with vaccines containing tumour cells admixed with either BCG or C. parvum can suppress tumours developing at distant sites (Baldwin and Pimm, 1973; Pimm and Baldwin, 1977). Even with these strongly immunogenic tumours, however, only small amounts of tumour can be suppressed and therapy is often unsuccessful if delayed for more than a few days after the initial implantation of tumour cells (Baldwin and Pimm, 1973). It follows, therefore, that these procedures will have only limited potential with the spontaneous rat sarcomas and mammary carcinomas, since these are much less immunogenic than the chemically-induced tumours. This has been confirmed in a series of studies using vaccines containing viable or radiation attenuated tumour cells admixed with BCG Glaxo percutaneous preparation, since it was only possible to consistently suppress growth of one mammary carcinoma (Sp4) when tumour cells were injected into a contralateral site (Pimm and Baldwin, 1978). Tests with two other mammary carcinomas and three sarcomas indicated that this type of therapy was totally ineffective, even when the challenge inoculum contained as few as 10^3 tumour cells. Significantly enhanced therapeutic responses

have not been obtained using other bacterial adjuvants such as
C. parvum in the immunizing vaccine (Willmott et al., 1978). Also
alternative sources of tumour antigen such as isolated membrane
preparations or solubilized fractions including 3M KCl or papain
extracts or serum-derived tumour antigen are unlikely to increase
the specific tumour immune response. This is illustrated by
studies showing that isolated membrane fractions from mammary
carcinoma Sp4 were not as effective as intact tumour cells for
inducing tumour specific immunity (Baldwin and Embleton, 1970).
With these spontaneous tumours, therefore, none of the existing
procedures are likely to lead to the development of effective
specific immunotherapy of established tumour deposits.

The non-specific effects mediated by infiltration of tumour
deposits with bacterial preparations appears to be more promising,
but these approaches are limited by the situations in which they
can be considered realistic. Of these, one of the most successful
systems so far developed has been for the treatment of rat mammary
carcinomas developing following injection of tumour cells into
mammary pad tissue (Greager and Baldwin, 1978). This can be
exemplified by considering treatment of mammary pad implants of the
spontaneous mammary carcinoma Sp4 (Fig. 3). In untreated rats, a
mammary pad challenge with 10 Sp4 cells produces progressively

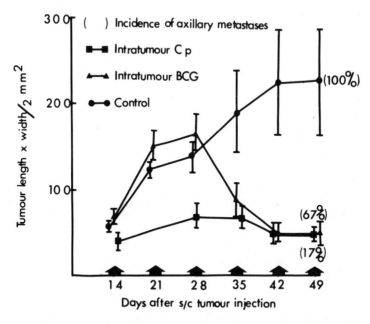

Figure 3. Influence of multiple intratumour injections of BCG
(Glaxo) or C. parvum (Wellcome CN 6134) on the growth and spread of
rat mammary carcinoma Sp4.

growing tumours which metastasize to the regional lymph nodes and
subsequently to more distant sites, especially lung. Intralesional
treatment with BCG (Glaxo percutaneous vaccine) 15 days after
tumour implantation initially had no effect on tumour growth, but
after three consecutive weekly treatments, growth of the mammary
tumour was controlled. Even so, 2/3rd of the rats developed regional
lymph node metastases. A more pronounced therapeutic effect was
obtained following intralesional injection of C. parvum (Wellcome
CN 6134) so that the primary mammary tumour implant did not
significantly grow and none of the rats developed regional lymph
node metastases (Fig. 3). In contrast to the effective responses
to mammary carcinoma Sp4, intralesional injection of either BCG or
C. parvum into two other spontaneous mammary carcinomas Sp15 and
Sp22 was essentially ineffective (Greager and Baldwin, 1978). This
is consistent with the response of these tumours to suppression
when tumour cells are injected in admixture with either BCG or
C. parvum (Table 4) which appears to be related to the inherent low
levels of macrophage accumulation in these tumours (Baldwin, 1976b).

CONCLUSIONS

These investigations on spontaneous rat sarcomas and mammary
carcinomas support the widely held view that spontaneous tumours
in general have limited immunogenic potential. They are not
entirely devoid of tumour specific antigens, however, whilst most
also express foetal antigens. This emphasizes that procedures
designed to increase the recognition of weak tumour antigens may
make these tumours more generally susceptible to active specific
immunotherapy.

Many of these tumours can be controlled by non-specific
effects mediated by activation of tumour infiltrating macrophages.
This approach perhaps has the greatest potential for therapy and
suggests that more well defined agents than viable or dead
bacterial suspensions should be sought. There are now several subcellular fractions of BCG showing tumour suppressive activity
including the methanol extraction residue of BCG as well as BCG
cell wall preparations (reviewed in Baldwin and Pimm, 1978). These
products are still too crude, however, and the aim should be to
introduce more well defined products such as cord factor isolated
from cell walls of mycobacteria and synthetic trehalose esters
e.g. trehalose-6-6'-mycolate (Lederer, 1976). Also products such
as N-acetyl-muramyl-L-alenyl-D-isoglutamine which represents the
minimum structure duplicating the adjuvant activity of the myco-
bacterial component of Freund's adjuvant (Audibert et al., 1976)
are of obvious interest. Whether the effects mediated by contact
with bacterial preparations requires recognition of tumour
associated antigens is still not resolved. Undoubtedly rejection
of non-immunogenic tumours can be induced when tumour cells are

injected in admixture with these agents. This is not reflected, however, in their sensitivity to intralesional therapy where there appears to be a correlation between tumour antigen expression and susceptibility to therapy (Greager and Baldwin, 1978). These findings again emphasize that introduction of new antigenic determinants may render tumour cells more susceptible to host control.

ACKNOWLEDGEMENTS

These studies are supported by a departmental grant from the Cancer Research Campaign, England, and by contracts NO1-CB-64042 and NO1-CB-64009 with the Tumor Immunology Program, National Cancer Institute, National Institutes of Health, U.S.A.

REFERENCES

Audibert, F., Chedid, L., Lefrancier, P. and Choay, J. (1976). Cell. Immunol. 21, 243.

Baldwin, R. W. (1966). Int. J. Cancer 1, 257.

Baldwin, R. W. (1976a). Cancer Immunol. Immunother. 1, 197.

Baldwin, R. W. (1976b). Transplant. Rev. 28, 62.

Baldwin, R. W. (1978). Develop. Biol. Standard. 38, 3.

Baldwin, R. W. and Embleton, M. J. (1969a). Int. J. Cancer 4, 47.

Baldwin, R. W. and Embleton, M. J. (1969b). Int. J. Cancer 4, 430.

Baldwin, R. W. and Embleton, M. J. (1970). Int. J. Cancer 6, 373.

Baldwin, R. W. and Embleton, M. J. (1971). Israel J. Med. Sci. 7, 144.

Baldwin, R. W. and Embleton, M. J. (1974). Int. J. Cancer 13, 433.

Baldwin, R. W. and Pimm, M. V. (1973). Br. J. Cancer 28, 281.

Baldwin, R. W. and Pimm, M. V. (1978). Adv. Cancer Res., in press.

Baldwin, R. W. and Vose, B. M. (1974). Br. J. Cancer 30, 209.

Bartlett, G. (1972). J. nat. Cancer Inst. 49, 493.

Brunda, M. J. and Raffel, S. (1977). Cancer Res. 37, 1838.

Bubbers, J. E. and Henney, C. (1975). J. Immunol. 114, 1126.

Chassoux, D. and Salamon, J.-C. (1975). Int. J. Cancer 16, 515.

Embleton, M. J. and Heidelberger, C. (1972). Int. J. Cancer 9, 8.

Embleton, M. J. and Heidelberger, C. (1975). Cancer Res. 35, 2049.

Forman, J. (1977). J. Immunol. 118, 1755.

Greager, J. A. and Baldwin, R. W. (1978). Cancer Res. 38, 69.

Hammond, W. G., Fisher, J. C. and Rolley, R. J. (1967). Surgery 62, 124.

Haywood, G. R. and McKhann, C. F. (1971). J. exp. Med. 133, 1171.

Herberman, R. B. and Holden, H. T. (1978). Adv. Cancer Res. 27, in press.

Hersh, E. M., Gutterman, J. U. and Mavligit, G. M. (1977). Ann. Rev. Med. 28, 489.

Hewitt, H. B., Blake, E. R. and Walder, A. S. (1976). Br. J. Cancer 33, 241.

Hopper, D. G. and Pimm, M. V. (1978). In The Macrophage and Cancer, eds. K. James, B. McBride and A. Stuart. pp. 182-187. Edinburgh.

Hopper, D. G., Pimm, M. V. and Baldwin, R. W. (1976). Cancer Immunol. Immunother. 1, 143.

James, K. (1977). In The Macrophage and Cancer, eds. K. James, B. McBride and A. Stuart. pp. 225-246. Edinburgh.

Kobayashi, N., Kodama, T. and Gotohda, E. (1977). Xenogenization of Tumor Cells. Hokkaido Univ. Med. Lib. Series, Vol. 9.

Kuzumaki, N., Fenyö, E. M., Giovanella, B. C. and Klein, G. (1978). Int. J. Cancer 21, 62.

Lachmann, P. J. and Sikora, K. (1978). Nature (Lond.) 271, 463.

Lederer, E. (1976). Chemistry and Physics of Lipids 16, 91.

Mondal, S., Iype, P. T., Griesbach, L. M. and Heidelberger, C. (1970). Cancer Res. 30, 1593.

Moore, M., Lawrence, N. and Nisbet, N. W. (1976). Biomedicine 24, 26.

Moore, M. and Nisbet, N. W. (1978). Develop. Biol. Standard. 38, 233.

Oehler, J. R. and Herberman, R. B. (1978). Int. J. Cancer 21, 221.

Oehler, J. R., Lindsay, L. R., Nunn, M. E., Holden, H. T. and Herberman, R. B. (1978). Int. J. Cancer 21, 210.

Pike, M. C. and Snyderman, R. (1976). J. Immunol. 117, 1243.

Pimm, M. V. and Baldwin, R. W. (1975). Nature (Lond.) 254, 77.

Pimm, M. V. and Baldwin, R. W. (1976a). Br. J. Cancer 34, 199.

Pimm, M. V. and Baldwin, R. W. (1976b). Br. J. Cancer 34, 453.

Pimm, M. V. and Baldwin, R. W. (1977). Int. J. Cancer 20, 923.

Pimm, M. V. and Baldwin, R. W. (1978). Unpublished findings.

Pimm, M. V., Hopper, D. G. and Baldwin, R. W. (1978). Develop. Biol. Standard. 38, 349.

Prehn, R. T. (1975). J. nat. Cancer Inst. 55, 189.

Prehn, R. T. and Main, J. M. (1957). J. nat. Cancer Inst. 18, 769.

Price, M. R. and Baldwin, R. W. (1977). Cell Surface Rev. 3, 423.

Price, M. R., Dennick, R. G., Robins, R. A. and Baldwin, R. W. (1978). Unpublished findings.

Scott, M. T. (1974). Semin. in Oncol. 1, 367.

Scott, M. T. and Milas, L. (1978). Adv. Cancer Res. 27, in press.

Staab, H.-J. and Anderer, F. A. (1977). Br. J. Cancer 35, 395.

Vaage, J. (1971). Cancer Res. 31, 1655.

Vaage, J. (1974). Cancer Res. 34, 2979.

Vasa-Thomas, K. A., Ambrose, K. R., Bellomy, B. B. and Coggin, J. H. (1977). J. nat. Cancer Inst. 58, 1287.

Weiss, D. W. (1977). Cancer Immunol. Immunother. 2, 11.

Willmott, N., Pimm, M. V. and Baldwin, R. W. (1978). Develop. Biol. Standard. 38, 39.

Wrathmell, A. B. and Alexander, P. (1976). Br. J. Cancer 33, 181.

IN SITU EXPRESSIONS OF HUMORAL IMMUNITY WITHIN A POLYOMA-VIRUS-INDUCED TUMOR

Maya Ran, Margalith Yaakubowicz and Isaac P. Witz

Department of Microbiology, The George S. Wise Center
for Life Sciences, Tel Aviv University, Tel Aviv,
Israel

INTRODUCTION

It is becoming increasingly clear that the assessment of
tumor immunity of cancer patients and tumor-bearing animals does
not, always, reflect the clinical status of the tumor-bearer and
that discrepancies are often evidenced between in vitro assays and
in vivo reality (1-5). It is equally clear that an accurate and
precise evaluation of the relations between the immune system of
the host and the tumor is an essential prerequisite for a rational
approach to improve the effective immune response against the tumor.

At present the assessment of host-tumor immune relations is
focused mainly on the systemic expressions of tumor immunity.
Thus, many investigators perform in vitro assays which measure the
anti-tumor reactivity of lymphocytes, macrophages or antibodies
originating from sites distant to the tumor: the circulation or
lymphoid organs of tumor bearers.

There is no reason to assume that the systemic expression of
tumor immunity is equal to that in the tumor site. Certain immuno-
cytes or antibodies expressing efficient anti-tumor reactivity
under laboratory conditions may be unable to reach the tumor site
due to various reasons such as inadequate vascularization, or to a
lack of the correct signals directing their homing to the site.
Other components may encounter no difficulty in reaching the tumor
site, or may even be attracted to it. Such a hypothetical imbalance in situ may bring about a completely different in vivo outcome than that suggested by assays utilizing effectors originating
from sites distant to the tumor.

Furthermore, the influence of the tumor's microenvironment on the expression of tumor immunity is neglected by most tumor immunologists. This is disturbing in view of the realization that the tumor site may contain a high concentration of specific (antigen; antibody; antigen-antibody complexes) and non-specific immunosuppressive substances (6 - 7) which may exert a significant influence on the local expressions of tumor immunity.

Recently, however, we are witnessing an encouraging trend in that the interest in local tumor immunity is extended and its importance in host-tumor interrelationship is considered more seriously. Thus, more studies are devoted to the presence, characterization and functions of cellular and humoral immune components residing in malignant tissues (6,8-14).

The work summarized below is mainly focused on humoral tumor immunity as expressed within the tumor tissue itself. Based on results in several laboratories, including ours, it has become clear that humoral immune components, i.e., immunoglobulins and complement, may be present within animal and human tumors (6). This basic finding lends itself to further investigations along the following lines:

1) The identity of the cells in the tumor to which Ig molecules are associated. Conceivably they could be tumor cells, or, alternatively, infiltrating host cells, such as Fc receptor-bearing lymphocytes, or macrophages. Are Ig-synthesizing B cells involved? It is not unlikely that some or even all of these alternatives could coexist.

2) The nature of binding of tumor-associated Ig to tumor-derived cells. Is it possible to identify among such Ig molecules antitumor antibodies directed against tumor-associated antigens? Are some of the tumor-associated Ig molecules serologically unrelated to tumor antigens? In this case, are they bound to tumor cells, to host cells, or to both? Also, in this case, the possible alternatives are not mutually exclusive.

3) The last, and probably the most important question concerns the biological role, if any, played by tumor-associated Ig in tumor growth, propagation and spread. It is important to emphasize that tumor-associated Ig molecules could be involved in tumor-host relationship even though they may not be antitumor antibody and although the tumor-derived Ig-associated cell may not be a tumor cell.

In choosing model systems to approach these questions one must employ tumors which usually evoke humoral immune responses. It thus appeared reasonable to use syngeneic virally-induced murine tumors where a significant amount of background information exists

concerning in vivo recognition of tumor antigens as inducers of
rejection and of other expressions of cellular and humoral immunity.
Polyoma-virus-induced sarcomas in mice seemed to be suitable models.

THE SEYF-a SYSTEM

SEYF-a is an ascites polyoma-virus-induced murine tumor
(15 - 16). It is at present at its 350th transplant generation
in syngeneic A.BY (H-2^b) mice. Studies on the immunogenicity of,
and the transplantation resistance to this and other polyoma-virus-
induced tumors were performed by Sjögren (15-16).

With the aid of an assay measuring complement-dependent cytotoxicity (CdL) we analyzed the antigenic specifications on the
membrane of SEYF-a cells by antibodies present in artificially
raised syngeneic or semi-syngeneic antisera (17). The approach
used in this study was to assay the capacity to mediate CdL to a
panel of target cells of unabsorbed antisera and antisera that
underwent fractional and sequential absorptions with different
tumor cells. The presence of several separate antigenic specificities on in vivo propagated SEYF-a cells became apparent. The
cells expressed a membrane antigen shared by other allogeneic polyoma-virus-induced murine sarcomas, but not by a considerable
number of non-polyoma-virus induced murine tumors (Witz et al., in
preparation). At least five additional separate membrane antigens
could be identified. Two of these were present on MuLV-induced
lymphoma cells, the first on Moloney-virus-induced YAC cells
(H-2^a) and the second on Gross-virus-induced GHA cells (H-2^k).
A third antigen was detected on EL-4 cells (H-2^b) and a fourth on
the ELD tumor cells (which are transplantable over the H-2 barrier). At least one (and possibly two) additional specificity/ties
was/were present on two cultured methylcholanthrene-induced H-2^b
sarcomas.

A.BY mice bearing sygeneic SEYF-a tumors develop circulating
anti-tumor antibodies mediating CdL of SEYF-a cells (18). It was
thus of interest to compare the specificity pattern of the hyperimmune artificially-produced anti-SEYF-a antibodies with that of
the circulating antibodies present in tumor bearers. In a study
which is essentially completed (Ran, Lee, Witz and G. Klein, in
preparation), it is evident that sera drawn from tumor-bearers have
a restricted specificity compared to the hyperimmune antisera. In
particular, sera drawn from mice shortly after inoculation (10-12
days) react with only 2 of the above mentioned antigenic specificities. Sera drawn later on from tumor-bearers react, however, with
more specificities than early sera. These findings show that the
entire antibody repertory that can be evoked in response to an
antigenic tumor such as SEYF-a appears gradually and may not be
expressed at all during the life span of the tumor-bearer. It is
thus possible that one could estimate the "biological age" of

certain tumors by the serological reactivity spectrum of the serum
of the tumor-bearer.

On account of the facts that the SEYF-a tumor evokes a
humoral immune response directed against several tumor-associated
antigens and in addition is relatively well characterized from a
serological point of view, we felt that it is a convenient system
in approaching some of the questions summarized above. We recognize however, the possibility that SEYF-a, being a serially transplanted tumor may have undergone alterations during its in vivo
passages. We draw our conclusions with a certain amount of caution
realizing that they may not always be generally applicable.
None the less the SEYF-a system has proved itself more than once
as capable of paving the way to previously unattempted approaches
to tumor serology. We hope to illustrate such approaches below.

THE NATURE OF INTERACTIONS BETWEN IN VIVO
PROPAGATING SEYF-a CELLS AND SEYF-a BOUND Ig

Ran et al. supplied for the first time direct and conclusive
evidence that the circulating cytotoxic anti-tumor antibodies
present in SEYF-a-bearing mice find their way to the tumor cells
in vivo (18). Tumor localized antibodies mediated complement-
dependent lysis of tumor cells, either after addition of exogeneous
complement to freshly harvested cells or after elution by low pH
buffers, when added with complement to indicator cells. The in vivo
coating of different types of tumor cells by tumor antibodies was
later also confirmed by other investigators (6). The SEYF-a bound
antibodies belonged to the IgG2a subclass (19) and their reactivity
pattern was found to be more restricted (i.e., they reacted with
less specificities) than the corresponding sera of tumor-bearing
mice   (Ran et al. in preparation).

In spite of the direct evidence that tumor antibodies localize
in vivo on SEYF-a cells the possibility should still be considered
that antibodies unrelated to any of the SEYF-a antigens may be
bound by cells lodging in the tumor. This possibility was supported
by our previous findings on TA-3/St cells, a non-lymphoid murine
tumor (20). It was demonstrated that tumor -derived cells originating in mice which were preimmunized with BSA or Ovalbumin, were
coated with anti BSA or Ovalbumin antibodies. These antibodies are
clearly serologically unrelated to tumor cell antigens. However,
the binding of the unrelated antibodies was shown to be mostly
limited to tumor-infiltrating Fc-receptor positive host cells.   In
a subsequent study (21), we demonstrated that the Fc-receptor
activity (assayed by immune-complex fixation) expressed by SEYF-a
cell populations was due to both infiltrating macrophages as well
as to tumor cells per se. The experimental evidence for the

presence of Fc-receptors on <u>in vivo</u> propagating SEYF-a tumor cells
was as follows: 1) The fixation of the immune complex by the
tumor-cell population could be inhibited by preincubating the cells
with syngeneic anti-SEYF-a antisera which did not react with normal
lymphocytes. 2) Depletion of phagocytes from the tumor cell
population, thus enriching for tumor cells, increased the inhibition
of complex fixation by the syngeneic anti-tumor antiserum. 3)
F(ab')2fragments of the syngeneic anti-tumor antibodies could also
inhibit immune-complex fixation. This indicated that the inhibition
of immune-complex fixation by the anti-tumor antibodies was not due
to the formation of "third-party" complexes composed of tumor cells
and the corresponding antibodies.

It is interesting to note that Fc receptors are probably
expressed only on <u>in vivo</u> propagating SEYF-a cells, but not on
cultured cells (22). The reasons for this discrepancy are unknown.

TIME ASSOCIATED CHANGES IN SOME OF THE PROPERTIES
OF SEYF-a ANTIBODIES

A.BY mice inoculated intraperitoneally with 2×10^6 SEYF-a
cells survive for over a month (35 ± 13 days). These tumor-bearers
can thus be conveniently studied for time-associated alterations in
patterns of host reactivity. We have investigated some parameters
of humoral anti-SEYF-a immunity, focusing on tumor-bound immunoglobulins, as a function of time after tumor inoculation.

Cytotoxic anti-tumor antibody are first demonstrable in the
serum of tumor bearers about 7-10 days after tumor inoculation.
Serum titers reach peak levels about two weeks later and stay high
until the death of the animals (18). Experiments performed by
Moav and Witz (19) indicated that the cytotoxic activity of the
anti-tumor antibodies is associated with the IgG2a population of
immunoglobulin. This conclusion was reached on the basis of the
finding that depletion of IgG2a molecules from cytotoxic serum
preparations completely abolished the cytotoxic activity from these
preparations. The fact that cytotoxic antibodies belonged exclusively
to the IgG2a subclass enabled us to calculate the specific cytotoxic
activity of serum and other Ig fractions. We defined specific cytotoxic activity as number of cytotoxic units (one cytotoxic unit=
the smallest amount of IgG (in µgr) causing a cytotoxicity index of
0.5 to SEYF-a cells) per unit of IgG2a (one unit of IgG2a = the
minimal amount of IgG (in µgr) giving a visible precipitation line
with a standard antiserum directed against IgG2a). We found that
the specific cytotoxic activity of serum drawn at late stages of
SEYF-a growth (26-35 days after inoculation) was 5-10 higher than
that of serum drawn at earlier stages, i.e. 16-20 days after tumor
inoculation. This increase is expected and it merely shows that

with tumor development there is an increase in the proportion of antitumor antibodies in the total circulating IgG2a.

Binding-affinity of anti-tumor antibodies to the corresponding cells is a very important factor if a comprehensive evaluation of the immunobiology of tumors is to be attained. This important parameter is however overlooked by most tumor serologist. Moav et al (23) determined the binding constants of Ig preparations orig- inating from SEYF-a-bearer serum to SEYF-a cells. They found that IgG preparations from such sera contain at least two distinct populations of molecules which differ from one another with respect to their binding constants to the tumor cells. One population is characterized by a high binding constant to SEYF-a cells, while the second population reveals a much lower binding constant to these cells. Normal mouse IgG preparations also bind to tumor cells - however, their binding constant is low.

Soluble antigens extracted from the corresponding SEYF-a cells were able to inhibit specifically the binding of IgG molecules with the high binding constants to the SEYF-a cells. Antigens extracted from non-related tissues did not affect the binding patterns of IgG to the SEYF-a cells. Moreover, IgG prepared from SEYF-a-bearing mice exhibited a high binding constant only when interacted with the corresponding SEYF-a cells, but not when inter- acted with non-corresponding ones. These results suggest that the IgG fraction with the high binding constant is composed mainly of antibodies to surface antigens of tumor cells.

No differences were found in the binding patterns of IgG isol- ated from tumor-bearer serum drawn at different intervals after tumor inoculation (19).

The ascitic fluid, being the immediate surrounding of the tumor cells was also assayed for the presence of anti-tumor antibodies. No antibodies could be detected in ascitic fluid up to at least 2 weeks after tumor inoculation. This observation was rather surp- rising in view of the fact that at the time where antibodies activity was not measurable in the ascitic fluid, anti-tumor anti- bodies were detectable both in the circulation as well as on the tumor cells bathing in the fluid (see below). Moreover, anti tumor antibodies coating tumor cells are in a dynamic equilibrium with the surrounding of the cells (6). They are transferred to the cells via the ascitic fluid but they do not stay fixed on the cells. A certain proportion is internalized while another is shed into the fluid. One explanation for the absence of free entibody in the ascitic fluid, while present in the serum and coating the ascites cells, is the presence of excess tumor antigen. This was found to be the case. Table 1 shows that ascitic fluid collected early after inoculation inhibited CdL of SEYF-a

TABLE 1

The ability of ascitic fluid to inhibit
or augment CdL of SEYF-a cells

Inhibitor (ascitic fluid collected at indicated post-inoculation day)	C.I mediated by anti-SEYF-a antibody without inhibitor[a]	C.I in the presence of indicated inhibitor dilution		
		1:4	1:8	1:16
	0.45			
12[b]		0.00	0.08	0.11
14[b]		0.03	0.15	0.21
19		0.20	0.20	0.21
21		0.34	0.31	0.34
25[c]		0.89	0.78	0.87

a)   A preparation of serum containing anti SEYF-a antibodies was assayed at a dilution causing a cytotoxicity index (C.I) of 0.45.

b)   The early ascitic fluids significantly inhibited CdL.

c)   The late ascitic fluid significantly augmented CdL.

---

cells mediated by anti-SEYF-a antibodies. The inhibition by the fluid could only be demonstrated when the inhibitor was added to the target-cell-antibody mixture. No inhibition occured at the target cell level. This finding supports the possibility that tumor antigen was responsible for the inhibition. The inhibitory activity progressively decreased until 3 weeks after tumor inoculation. At about that time, free antibodies appeared in the fluid. This was indicated by the fact that addition of ascitic fluid considerably augmented the cytotoxicity above the antiserum baseline. At that time the free antigen in the fluid was probably neutralized by excessive amounts of antibodies.

The most striking alteration in the properties of antitumor antibodies as a function time after tumor inoculation occured in the tumor-bound Ig population. As mentioned above the presence of an antibody coat on in vivo propagated SEYF-a cells was indicated by 2 separate tests. The one was the sensitivity of in vivo growing but not of cultured SEYF-a cells to exogenous complement (18). We functionally designate this antibody population as cell

bound. The second type of test revealing the presence of an antibody coat on SEYF-a cells was the presence of antibodies in low
pH eluates of such cells. Antibodies capable of mediating CdL of
indicator SEYF-a cells, were present in eluates of in vivo propagated but not of cultured cells. These antibodies are functionally
designated as elutable antibodies.

     Both cell-bound, as well as elutable antibodies appear on SEYF-a
at about the same time as they appear in the circulation. At about
two weeks after tumor inoculation the ascites SEYF-a cells are
highly sensitive to lysis by exogenous complement and relatively
high titers of antibodies can be eluted from such cells. IgG
eluted at that time is characterized by 2 features which clearly
differentiate it from IgG isolated from tumor-bearer serum (19).
1) The specific cytotoxic activity of eluate IgG was 25 - 100
times higher than that of serum IgG. 2). Eluate IgG contained a
homogeneous population of antibodies with a high binding constant
to the cells whereas serum IgG contained at least 2 major IgG
populations. One population had a high-binding constant to the
cells and another population had a low binding-constant. These
results indicate 1) a selective adsorption of relatively pure
anti-tumor antibodies onto the tumor cells at that time. 2) A
correlation between the exclusive presence of antibodies with a
high binding constant and a high specific cytotoxic activity.

     As the time after tumor inoculation progressed beyond 2 weeks,
cell bound anti SEYF-a antibodies either remained at plateau levels
or even decreased. In contrast, the titers of elutable antibodies
increased with time. This discrepency is not fully understood but
indirect evidence (24) suggests that immune complexes progressively
accumulating in the vicinity of the tumor were fixed by Fc receptors
expressed on the SEYF-a cells. These SEYF-a bound immune-complexes
were obviously unable to activate the added exogeneous complement.
By treating these complex-coated cell populations with the low pH
eluting buffer, a certain proportion of the immune complexes became
disocciated and the released antibody was then able to mediate CdL
of the indicator cells.

     Although the titers of the elutable anti SEYF-a antibody
increased with time after tumor implantation the specific cytotoxic
activity of the eluted antibodies decreased considerably (19). For
example, during the period from 15-20 days after inoculation to 25-
30 days after inoculation, the specific cytotoxic activity of the
eluate IgG decreased about 3 fold and was only 2-3 times higher than
that of serum IgG (19). This indicates the gradual accumulation at
the surface of old tumor cells either of IgG2a molecules with no
cytotoxic activity or of molecules with the capacity to inhibit
such an activity by competing against cytotoxic molecules for
antigenic determinants. Simultaneously the binding patterns of

eluted IgG preparations also changed with propagation time of the
tumors. IgG molecules eluted from old SEYF-a cells were heterogeneous with respect to their binding patterns to tumor cells. Such
preparations contained IgG molecules with high-binding constants to
SEYF-a cells as well as those with low binding-constants, in contrast to IgG eluted from young cells which contained exclusively the
former IgG molecule population.

It would be of obvious interest and importance to find out if
and how the progressive alterations in the expressions of in-situ
humoral tumor immunity described above contribute to the fact that
SEYF-a cells are able to escape tumor rejection mechanisms.

LYMPHOCYTOTOXIC ANTIBODIES IN SEYF-a ELUATES

A relationship between non-lymphoid malignancy and autoimmunity is indicated from the reports on the occurance of autoantibodies
in cancer patients (25-29).

There are several conceivable ways by which autoimmunity may
be connected with the development of malignancies. A non cause-
effect relationship may exist between autoimmunity and an increased
susceptibility towards malignancy if a central, not yet defined,
lesion occurs in the immunity system. Such a hypothetical lesion
may manifest itself in seemingly independent pathological phenomena
such as autoimmunity and cancer, which may be different expression of
the same fundamental misfunction. It is however, not unlikely that
a relationship between autoimmunity and malignancy is direct and
causative. It is conceivable, for example, that oncogenic viruses
or chemical carcinogens, by modifying the membrane of the transformed
cell, may bring about an autoimmune reactivity directed against
altered self-determinants (30).

These hypotheses are amenable to experimentation and we felt
that the SEYF-a system could be utilized in attempts to answer some
of the relevant questions.

In testing the activity spectrum of circulating antibodies in
SEYF-a bearers and of antibodies eluted from SEYF-a cells (Ran, Witz
and Klein in preparation) we found that eluates of SEYF-a cells
containing cytotoxic anti-SEYF-a antibodies mediated also complement-
dependent cytotoxicity of normal lymph-node cells, splenocytes,
thymocytes and to some degree also of bone-marrow cells (31).
Table 2 compares the sensitivity of thymocytes from various mouse
strains. The fact that AKR cells were essentially as sensitive as
C3H cells indicate that Thy 1 is not involved as target antigen for
the lymphocytotoxic antibodies in SEYF-a eluates. In view of the
high sensitivity of C57Bl/6 lymphocytes to these antibodies it may
be concluded that G_{IX} antigen is also not involved since the C57Bl/6

TABLE 2

The sensitivity of thymocytes from various strains to
CdL mediated by low pH eluates of SEYF-a cells

Origin of thymocytes	average cytotoxicity index [a] ± standard deviation mediated by SEYF-a eluates at indicated dilution		
	1:2	1:4	1:8
A.BY	0.28±0.06	0.16±0.05	0.11±0.09
C57B1/6	0.34±0.04	0.22±0.05	0.11±0.03
C3H	0.34±0.11	0.16±0.05	0.12±0.03
BALB/C	0.32±0.11	0.14±0.06	0.06±0.05
AKR	0.26±0.04	0.10±0.01	0.04±0.01

a)   Five different eluates were used in 5 different experiments.

mice are G_{IX} - negative (32).

The lymphocytotoxic antibodies in eluates belonged to the IgG
class and it seems that they were not carried into the tumor by
tumor-seeking lymphocytes or macrophages but localized on the tumor
cells themselves.

Sera of SEYF-a bearers also mediated a certain degree of CdL but
the pattern of cytotoxicity was different from that exhibited by
tumor eluates. In the serum the titer of lymphocytotoxic antibodies
was found to be lower than the titer of anti-SEYF-a antibodies.
Eluates, on the other hand exhibited similar titers towards both
target cells. Moreover, the eluates had a higher specific cytotoxic
activity than the serum. The results of CdL assays performed with
these materials at equal protein concentrations, showed that
whereas the eluates were cytotoxic at certain, low protein concentrations, serum was completely inactive at the same or even higher
concentrations. These results may indicate that tumor cells selectively absorbed lymphocytotoxic antibodies from the serum. Other
explanations are however, also possible.

The mechanism by which anti-lymphocyte antibodies are induced and
localize in SEYF-a tumors (possibly even on the tumor cells per se)
is unknown. This could be due to a cross reactivity between a tumor
associated antigen and a lymphocyte autoantigen, re-expression of T-

cell antigens on sarcoma cells (33), or to the formation of
antibodies directed against a tumor-localized T-cell product.
A possible mechanism explaining induction of such autoantibodies
(but not their in vivo localization within tumors) implies an
abnormal activation of anti-self B-cells by virus modified anti-
self T-cells (34); or by altered H-2 determinants on SEYF-a cells,
in a mechanism similar to TNP - self or TNP - tumor modification
(35-36).

A further insight into this phenomenon becomes a necessity in
view of preliminary unpublished results showing that thymocytotoxic
antibodies can also be eluted from another non-lymphoid tumor.

THE ASSOCIATION BETWEEN TUMOR
RESISTANCE AND ANTI-TUMOR ANTIBODIES

Sjögren (16) studied the mechanism of transplantation
resistance to polyoma-virus induced tumors, including SEYF-a, and
concluded that the resistance was due to cellular immunity.
Without underrating the importance and significance of cell-
mediated reactions, tumor-host relations cannot be correctly evaluated and completely understood without taking humoral reactions
into full consideration.

Although we realized that in vivo there is a complex interplay
between humoral and cell mediated immunity and that it may be very
difficult to separate between them, we made initial attempts to
analize if humoral immunity plays a role in the resistance to SEYF-a
as it seems to do in other tumor systems (37-42).Below is a
description of preliminary experiments dealing with this subject.

High Antibody Titers in Tumor-Bearers Whose Survival
was Prolonged by Early Removal of Their Tumor

Observational data collected for a period of one year indicated
that removal of the ascitic fluid from SEYF-a bearers prolonged significantly the survival of about 25% of the treated mice and caused
the complete cure of another 25%. The regressor mice were resistant
to a rechallenge of SEYF-a cells. In view of these data we carried
out experiments employing both male and female SEYF-a bearers from
which the ascites was removed at weekly intervals. It was seen
that removing the SEYF-a ascites at 2 weeks, and in males also at
3 weeks after inoculation but not later, or earlier than 2 weeks,
caused a statistically significant prolongation in the survival time
of these mice (in females from 3 2.6±12.0 days to 67.4±48.0 days
and in males from 46.4±13.5 days to 95.7±42.0 days when removed 2
weeks after inoculation and to 68.8±31.0 when removed 3 weeks after
inoculation).

TABLE 3

Antibody titers in the serum of long-term survivors

Sex	Ascites removed (weeks after inoculation)	Effect on Survival	Serum drawn (weeks after inoculation) and % of survivors at that time	$C.I_{50}$ Titer[a]
Females	2	Significant prolongation	6- (80%)	1:16
"	3	No effect	6- (20%)	<1:2
"	untreated		5-[b] (20%)	<1:2
Males	2	Signifcant prolongation	9- (60%)	1:64
"	3	" "	9- (40%)	1:32
"	untreated		7-[c] (40%)	1:4

a) $C.i_{50}$ titers = serum dilution causing a cytotoxicity index of 0.5

b) None of the untreated mice survived until 6 weeks after inoculation.

c) None of the untreated mice survived until 9 weeks after inoculation.

We compared the anti-SEYF-a antibody titers in control mice; in mice where the treatment was ineffective and in mice whose survival was prolonged by the treatment. The results summarized in Table 3, show that long term survivors had a higher antibody than control mice or mice whose survival was not prolonged by removal of their ascites. In some of the long-term survivors high antibody titers persisted up to 2-3 months after tumor inoculation.

Rejection of Tumor Cells by Regressor Mice Accompanied by a High Titer of Cytotoxic Antibodies

A group of 8 mice whose tumor completely regressed were re-challenged intraperitoneally with 2×10^6 SEYF-a cells which is a lethal dose to otherwise untreated mice. Mice were bled at weekly intervals and their serum was tested for its capacity to mediate CdL of indicator SEYF-a cells. The rechallenged mice became swollen during the first week after inoculation but the tumor regressed completely within two weeks. Thirty normal mice injected with the same inoculum died within 35 days. The rejection of the tumor by regressor mice was accompanied by a secondary humoral anti-tumor response (table 4). Antibodies appeared earlier and in higher titers in the rechallenged regressors than in tumor-bearing mice.

TABLE 4

Antibody titers in the serum of SEYF-a
bearers and in rechallenged regressors

Weeks after inoculation or rechallenge	Tumor Bearers	Rechallenged regressors
1	<1:2	1:256
2	1:16	1:512
3	1:32	1:512

a) C.I$_{50}$ titer = serum dilution causing a cytotoxicity index of 0.5.

The results summarized in the above 2 sections show that relatively high titers of anti-SEYF-a antibodies are associated with a state of resistance to SEYF-a tumors.

The Effect of Passively Administered SEYF-a Antibodies on SEYF-a Growth In Vivo

The results presented in the section on"Time associated changes in some of the properties of SEYF-a antibodies" suggested that excess tumor antigen is present in ascitic fluids of SEYF-a-bearers during the early stage (2-3 weeks) of tumor development (see also table 1). On account of this fact and the observations presented above namely that resistance to SEYF-a tumors is associated with relatively high titers of SEYF-a antibodies in the resistant mice, we tested the possibility that a passive administration of antibodies at an early stage of tumor growth might prove beneficial to the tumor-bearer.

A high titer tumor eluate (eluted from SEYF-a cells

propagated in vivo for 31 days and having a $C.I_{50}$ titer of 1:64),
was mixed with a lethal dose of 2×10^{6} tumor cells. The mixture
was injected i.m into (A.BY x C57Bl) F_1 hybrids. Hybrids rather
than syngeneic A.BY were chosen in order to overcome the relative
deficiency in some complement components (especially C'5. G. Dorval,
personal communication). The tumor diameter measured at weekly
intervals in these mice was significantly smaller than that of
tumors grown from cells mixed with low titer eluate (eluted from
11 days-old cells and causing a C.I. of 0.5 when undiluted). In
another experiment SEYF-a cells were incubated either with high
titer serum drawn from rechallenged regressors one week after
challenge, or with normal serum or again with eluates. The incubation mixtures were inoculated into (A.BY x C57Bl) F_1 hybrids.
The tumors which developed from cells incubated with regressor
serum or with high-titer eluates were found to be significantly
smaller than tumors which grew from cells incubated with normal
A.BY serum or with low-titer eluates. The results of both experiments are summarized in table 5. No significant differences between
the survival time of the various mouse groups was detected, however.

These preliminary results support the possibility that a
passive administration of anti SEYF-a antibodies at early stages of
tumor growth (when tumor antigen is in excess in the vicinity of the
tumor) may improve the condition of SEYF-a bearers. Optimal conditions for treatment will obviously have to be worked out.

CONCLUDING REMARKS

The prevailing dogma in tumor immunology states that whereas
cellular immunity mediated by T cells plays the major role in host
defence against antigenic tumors (e.g. 2) humoral immunity, on the
other hand, antagonizes the beneficial expressions of cellular immunity. Although the first part of the dogma is probably correct,
at least in most cases of antigenic malignancies there exists,
really, no solid information to confirm or negate its latter part
(43).

On the basis of quite a few studies from other laboratories
(37-42; 44-47) and in view of the results presented in this paper
it seems that the generally held opinion that humoral immune factors
are less likely to protect than to interfere with immune protection
may have been drawn too readily. A re-assessment of the role of
systemic and especially of local humoral immunity in protection
against tumor growth,or its facilitation,seems to be most timely.

TABLE 5

The in-vivo effect of anti-SEYF-a antibodies on tumor size

Average tumor diameter[a] in mm ± standard deviation

Experiment	Untreated	Low-titer eluate	High-titer eluate	Normal A.BY Serum	Serum of rechallenged regressors
1	16.6±6.0	12.6±5.0 [b]	5.9±6.7 [b]	NT	NT
2	NT	20.7±2.2 [c]	17.0±2.2 [c]	20.8±1.6 [d]	16.7±1.2 [d]

a) Measured on the 35th post inoculation day. Differences between the groups remained significant up to 7 weeks after inoculation.

b) Statistically significant differences (p<0.02-Students T test) between the tumor size in the mice treated with high or with low titer eluate.

c) Statistically significant differences (p<0.01-Students T test) between the tumor size in the mice treated with high or low titer eluate.

d) Statistically significant differences(p<0.01-Students T test) between the tumor size in the mice treated with serum from normal or from rechallenged regressors.

ACKNOWLEDGEMENTS

The efforts of Ms. Debora Edelman and Ms. Noa Leibowitch in establishing and maintaining our local A.BY colony are highly appreciated.

This investigation was supported by Grant Number I R01 CA20088-01 awarded by the National Cancer Institute DHEW and by a Behr-Lehmsdorff grant awarded by the Isreal Cancer Association.

REFERENCES

1. Takasugi, M., Mickey, M.R and Terasaki, P.I. Cancer Res. 33: 2898, 1973.
2. Herberman, R.B. Adv. Cancer Res. 19: 207, 1974.
3. Heppner, G., Henry, F., Stolbach, L., Cummings, F., McDonough, E. and Calabresi, P. Cancer Res. 35: 1931, 1975.
4. Bean, M.A., Bloom, B.R., Herberman, R.B., Old, L.J., Oettgen, H.F. Klein, G. and Terry, W.D. Cancer Res.35: 2902,1975.
5. Glaser, M., Lavrin, D.H. and Herberman, R.B. J. Immunal.116: 1507, 1976.
6. Witz, I.P. Adv. Cancer. Res. 25:95,1977.
7. Kamo, I. and Friedman, H. Adv. Cancer. Res. 25:271, 1977.
8. Evans, R. Transplantation 14: 468,1972.
9. Van Loveren H. and Den Otter, W. J. Nat. Cancer. Inst. 53: 1057,1974.
10. Haskill, J.S., Yamamura, Y. and Radov, L. Int. J. Cancer 16: 798, 1975.
11. Jondal, M., Svedmyr,E., Klein E. and Singh, S. Nature (London) 255: 405, 1975.
12. Kerbel, R.S. and Pross, H.F. Int. J.Cancer 18: 432, 1976.
13. Russell, S.W., Gillespie, G.Y., Hansen,C.B. and Cochrane,C.G. Int. J.Cancer 18: 331, 1976.
14. Moore, K and Moore, M. Int, J. Cancer 19:803, 1977.
15. Sjögren, H.A. J. Nat. Cancer Inst. 32:361, 1964.
16. Sjogren, H.A. J. Nat. Cancer Inst. 32:375, 1964.
17. Witz,I.P., Lee, N. and Klein,G. Int. J. Cancer, 18:243, 1976.
18. Ran, M., Klein, G. and Witz, I.P. Int. J. Cancer 17:90, 1976.
19. Moav, N. and Witz, I.P. J. Immunol. Meth. 1978, in press
20. Braslawsky, G.R., Yaackubowicz, M., Frensdorff, A. and Witz,I. P. J. Immunol. 116: 1571,1976.
21. Braslawsky, G.R., Serban, D. and Witz, I.P. Europ. J. Immunol. 6: 579, 1976.
22. Tracey, D.E., Pross, H.F., Jondal, M. and Witz, I.P. Int. J. Cancer, 15: 918, 1975.
23. Moav, N. Hochberg, Y., Cohen, G. and Witz, I.P. J. Immunol. Meth. 1978, in press.
24. Braslawsky, G.R., Ran, M. and Witz, I.P. Int. J.Cancer 18:116, 1976.
25. Yasuda-Yasaki, Y., and Yoshida, T.O. Scand. J. Immunol. 21: 357, 1975.
26. Forbes, A.P., Lake, J.R. and Bloch, K. Clin. Exp. Immunol.26: 426, 1976.
27. Wasserman, J., Glass, U. and Blomgren, H. Clin. Exp. Immunol. 19: 417, 1975.
28. Shirai, T., Miata, M., Nakase, A. and Itoh, T. Clin.Exp.Immunol. 26: 118, 1976.
29. Shiku, H., Takahashi, T., Resnick, L.A., Oettgen, H.F. and Old, L.J. J. Exp. Med. 145: 784, 1977.

30. Oth, D., Meyer, G. and Berebbi, M. Folia Biol. 23: 1, 1977
31. Ran, M. Yaakubowicz, M. and Witz, I.P. J. Nat. Cancer Inst. 1978, in press.
32. Klein, J. In: Biology of the Mouse Histocompatibility - 2 complex, Springer-Verlag, New York, 1975, pp. 279.
33. De Leo, A.B., Shiku, H., Takahashi, T., John, M. and Old, L.J. J. Exp. Med. 146: 720, 1977.
34. Bretcher, P. Cell. Immunol. 6: 1, 1973.
35. Shearer, G.M., Rehn, T.C. and Carbarino, C.A. J. Exp. Med. 141: 1348, 1975.
36. Galili, N., Noar, D., Asjö, B. and Klein, G. Eur.J. Immunol. 6: 473, 1976.
37. Fefer, A. Cancer Res. 29: 2177, 1969.
38. Essex, M., Klein, G., Snyder, S.P. and Harrold, J.B. Nature 233: 195, 1971.
39. Pearson, G.R., Redman, L.W. and Bass, L.R. Cancer Res. 33: 171, 1973.
40. Cantrell, J. L., Killion, J.J. and Kollmorgen, G.M. Cancer. Res. 36: 3051, 1976.
41. Haskill, J.S. and Fett, J.W. J. Immunol. 117: 1992, 1976.
42. O'Neill, G. J. Europ. J. Cancer 12: 749, 1976.
43. Currie, G.A. Bioch. Biophys. Acta-Cancer Rev. 458: 135, 1976.
44. Shin, H.S., Pasternack, G.R. Economou, J.S., Johnson, R.J. and Hayden, M.L. Science, 194: 327, 1976.
45. Shin, H.S., Economou, J.S., Pasternack, G.R., Johnson, R.J. and Hayden, M.L. J. Exp. Med. 144: 1274, 1976.
46. Byfield, J.E., Zerubavel, R. and Fankalsrud, E.W. Nature, 264: 783, 1976.
47. Reif, A.E., Robinson, C.M. and Smith, P.J. Ann. N.Y. Acad. Sci. 277: 647, 1976.

NATURAL KILLER AND TUMOR RECOGNIZING LYMPHOCYTE ACTIVITY IN MAN

Eva Klein, Farkas Vánky, Bernt M. Vose
and Markus Fopp

Department of Tumor Biology
Karolinska Institute and Radiumhemmet
Karolinska Hospital, S-104 01, Stockholm, Sweden

The concept that patients with solid tumors develop
an immunological response against their own tumor cells
is supported by results obtained with various immunological assays. These results are interpreted with caution
however and the issue is far from being proven decisively.
The lack of correlation with the clinical course of the
disease and the marginal, if any, effect of various form
of immunotherapy are obvious reasons for doubt the relevance of seemingly tumor specific results in vitro.

However, even in such experimental tumor system
where transplantation tests clearly demonstrate a host
response, the immune parameters detected in vitro do not
always reflect the in vivo events (13).

One of the important inconsistencies often mentioned,
is the in vitro cross reactivity of chemically induced
tumors, also with embryo cells, and their individual anti-
geneticity in rejection tests (8). Among in vitro cell
mediated immune reactions cytotoxicity is used most frequently.

Initially lymphocytotoxicity studies in both experimental systems and in patients with different tumor types,
were interpreted to show tumor specific selective reactivities (20). However frequent cytotoxicity obtained
with lymphocytes of healthy donors and untreated animals
led to the recognition that the capacity to attack certain tumor cell lines is a regularly occurring, not a
disease related phenomenon.

The discovery initiated intensive studies in several laboratories motivated mainly for two reasons: (1)
Characterization of a new cytotoxic phenomenon and (2)
In order to achieve a test condition which could be used
for tumor immunity studies, revealing disease related
effects, it is necessary to characterize and perhaps
eliminate this effect.

At present in vitro cytotoxicity tests aimed to
demonstrate disease related selective recognition are
preformed with the awareness that at least three known
effector mechanisms exist in which lymphocytes partici-
pate.   1.   T cells equipped with antigen recognizing
receptors (12).   2.   ADCC-antibody dependent cytotoxicity;   Cells affect targets which have been selected out
by the recognition of antibodies (26).   3.   NK - natural
killing - cells destruct on seemingly indiscriminative
basis by unknown mechanism (30).

Natural Killing

The NK effect is a general, in experimental animals,
age-related phenomenon (21,23).   Because of the lack of
knowledge about its initiation it was designated with the
attribute "natural" - natural killer - though it is not
excluded that it might be generated by classical immunization.   The nature of surface structure recognized by
the NK cells is still unknown.

There is a considerable interest presently in the
NK effect of the animal systems since one of the important questions is the in vivo relevance of the phenomenon.
Transplantation tests with a lymphoma line showed that
the repection of small inocula by semisyngeneic mice
paralleled the in vitro reactivity of the strain (24).

When an in vitro carried NK sensitive lymphoma line,
YAC-1, was retransplanted and propagated in mice its sensitivity declined (10).   This experiment and the rule
that cultured lines are highly sensitive would indicate
that this type of host response is extremely efficient
and only such cells can be established for longer time
in the host which lack the sensitivity to this mechanism.
Consequently, the NK system may represent a potent sur-
veillence mechanism.   While sensitivity is not an obligatory feature of tumor derived cell lines it may be
assumed that if during oncogenesis malignant cells with
sensitivity to the NK cell arise, these are eliminated.

Indicative for the role of NK cells in immune surveillance is the low incidence of naturally occurring
tumors in nude mice (35), expected to be unprotected
since they lack T cell mediated and T cell dependent
mechanisms considered to be crucial in graft rejection.
Spleen cells of nude mice have efficient NK activity
when tested in vitro (21,23). Arguments which do not
support the importance of NK mechanism in elimination
of the nascent tumor cells: 1. There is no correlation
between the NK efficiency and sensitivity to Moloney
virus induced leukemogenesis when different strains are
compared. Admittedly, leukemogenesis is the outcome of
several factors, some unrelated to immune response. 2.
MSV induced sarcomas regress in A mice as regularly as
in other strains but in this strain, in contrast to CBA
or CBA x C57 Bl F_1 mice, no cytotoxic activity was seen
when spleens or tumor infiltrating lymphocytes were
tested against the YAC-1 cells - one of the most sensitive NK targets (11). 3. Mice infected with Moloney
leukemia virus (a measure which leads to leukemia development) did not differ in spleen cell exerted cytotoxic
activity (anti-YAC-1)when tested in parallel with uninfected age matched controls (25). 4. Mice which carry
methylcholanthrene pellets and thus will develop sarcomas
were shown not to have any change in spleen NK efficiency
when compared with age matched controls (2). Such mice
were reported to have decreased numbers of antibody producing cells in the spleen (33).

The active lymphocytes are not the mature T or B
cells and in contrast to T cell mediated killing the
effect is not histocompatibility restricted (9,23). In
man the activity of a certain lymphocyte subset is correlated to the enrichement in Fc positive cells. The
activity of the SRBC rosetting T population is relatively
weak for which Fc positive cells are responsible. When
these are eliminated (about 10%) the T cells have no
effect (4).

The so called "null" fraction, i.e. the population
of nonadherent to nylon wool and depleted of SRBC rosetting cells is the most active on a per cell basis (3,22).
This represents about 10% of the total lymphocyte population. It is a highly heterogeneous population, rich in
Fc positive cells (about 50%) and the markers for B and T
cells are not clearly differentiated. About half of the
cells develop SIg when kept in culture (31). Some cells
have receptors for EBV, a property of B cells and coupled
to the C_3 receptors (16). Interestingly however, while
EBV receptors were detectable by virus absorption, the

early event of EBV infection, appearance of a specific
nuclear antigen (EBNA) was not induced. Thus the virus
could not infect the cells indicating that they are not
fully differentiated B cells. About half of the cells
have low avid SRBC receptors, they can be resetted when
either they or the erythrocytes are treated with neuraminidase (1,4). C_3 receptor carrying cells can also be
detected, a low proportion with the conventionalal EAC'
resetting technique and more when sheep cells are used as
EAC' indicators (6) supposedly detecting cells which carry both low avid E and C_3 receptors.

The human "null" subset is thus made up of cells
which are not fully differentiated yet, and some carry
surface markers which characterize both T and B cells.
Some of the lymphoblastoid lines are representative for
such cells in that they cannot be differentiated by B or
T markers. They are probably fixed in the degree of differentiation of the clone which was the origin of the
malignant transformation.

As mentioned above, the NK activity of the "null"
fraction is stronger than that of the total lymphocyte
population. After elimination of rosettes formed with
neuraminidase treated SRBC i.e. T cells with low avid E
receptors, the residual cells were still highly efficient.
Also after elimination of Fc receptor positive cells, the
residual cells were strongly active. Thus on the basis of
lymphocyte markers, it was not possible to subdivide the
"null" subset into populations with and without cytotoxicity (4).

It is conceivable that more than one lymphocyte type
can exert the effect and they may even act in collaboration. Peter et al.(27) supposed that one subset produces
soluble factors upon contact with the target and another
is induced by the factor(s) to exert the killing. Similarly, Takasugi et al. (37) and Troye et al.(39)assume the
collaboration of antibody producing cells, the killing
effect being at least in part ADCC. The effector cells
would either carry cytophyllic antibodies on their surface
and/or a small number of admixed antibody producing cells
contribute during the in vitro incubation. This assump-
ion is suggested by the fact that the subsets active in
NK thus far were shown to be efficient in ADCC systems
also. Even the organ distribution of the two types of
effect overlapped.

Another possibility is that cells do not operate on
the basis of a conventional antigen recognition. During

certain stages of differentiation or activation, thymus
dependent lymphocytes may acquire cytotoxic potential.
Cytotoxicity would be manifested against target cells
toward which the lymphocytes carrying recognition receptors. The efficiency of killing would be determined by
the target cell depending on its inherent sensitivity.
This assumption is strengthened by the finding that thymocytes and activated T cells recognize and attach to cells
of the same species (18). This recognition may be an important factor also in cytotoxicity of mitogen activiated
T lymphocytes which act preferentially on cells of their
own species (32).

        NK activity was found to be relatively decreased in
the spleen of tumor bearing animals (murine sarcoma virus
and methylcholanthrene-induced tumors and nude mice carrying grafts from human lymphoblastoid cell lines) (11) and
in the blood of tumor patients (29). In our series 47% of
cancer patients (the majority with lung carcinoma) failed
to exert cytotoxicity towards the highly NK sensitive K562
cell line while all the healthy donors tested in parallel
had strong reactivity (41).

        The composition of the blood lymphocyte population
did not differ with regard to the proportion of E rosetting and Fc receptor-bearing cells. Only rarely was activity exhibited by lymph node cells and tumor infiltrating
lymphocytes although cells with Fcreceptor were present in
both preparations. Tumor infiltrating lymphocyte preparations had in fact a high proportion (22%) EA rosettes.
Tumor infiltrating lymphocytes and lymph node cells had
good reactivity in other functional tests (PHA and MLC
assays).

        Even with lympho node preparations enriched for the
non-T and non-B cells, little evidence of cytotoxcity was
noted. Since cells bearing the Fc receptor were present
it seems that the expression of this does not per se en-
gender the lymphocytes with NK activity.

Reactivity of patients with their own tumor cells

        Since specific cellular recognition resides in the T
cell population and mature T cells have no NK effect -
either in man or mice and rats - detection of disease related cytotoxicity on cell lines is expected to be possible by using characterized lymphocyte subsets. The T cell
mediated effects can be investigated either directly or
after in vitro sensitization, achieved in culture when the
effector population is exposed to antigen carrying cells
for several days (17).

A new aspect of the T system has recently evoked considerable interest when it was discovered that effectors directed against virally or chemically altered cells have to share the histocompatibility antigens of the target in order to kill (15). The present view is that this restriction is not absolute and can be overridden to some extent especially in long term cytotoxic assays.

In view of this restriction it is questionable whether established cell lines can be used as prototype targets. Consequently it is likely that in search for tumor specific reactivities the experiments have to be performed in autologous systems. However, at least in one human disease - infectious mononucleosis - T cell mediated cytotoxicity was demonstrated in short term assay on allogeneic target cells (7,36). On the other hand experiments with breast cancer patients using similar lymphocyte subsets failed to reveal selective cytotoxicity towards breast cancer derived lines (5).

In an effort to eliminate at least some of the factors which hamper interpretation of results with cell lines two tests have been designed in our laboratory for measuring cell-mediated anti-tumor recognition in man, the autoogous tumor stimulation, ATS, and autologous lymphocyte cytotoxicity, ALC. In both tests, tumor cells separated from biopsy specimens were allowed to react with autologous lymphocytes.

We considered that the advantage of using biopsy cells is that the antigen source is not subjected to the modification and selective conditions of tissue culture. The disadvantages are the variability of the quality, the quantitative limitation and the laboriousity of tumor cell separation.

The autologous tumor stimulation (ATS)-test, registers DNA synthesis of lymphocytes following 6-day cultivation with mitomycin-treated biopsy cells (40). At least part of the responding cells belongs to the T subset. Lymphocytes attached to the tumor cells during the early period of co-cultivation were shown to rosett with SRBC. Moreover when prefractioned populations were used, the T-enriched fraction reacted while the T-depleted fractions did not.

In our initial series ATS was obtained in 30% of 197 patients with solid tumors (the majority with lung carcinomas or osteosarcomas). Improvement of the test conditions by using exclusively tumor cell enriched populations

of good viability as stimulators, the incubation of tumor
cells prior to the test (this step was introduced to allow
resynthesis of putative cell surface antigens if reomved
by the procedure of prepatation of tumor cell enriched
suspensions) and the use of T cell enriched responder population has given considerably increased positive cases
(60%). Thus the majority of patients seem to recognise
immunologically their own tumor cells. In table 1 results
of two experiments are given which indicate that the
lymphocytes are stimulated for DNA synthesis when confronted with autologous tumor cells and only exceptionally when
confronted with allogeneic. In 36 tested combinations
only 2 biopsies stimulated allogeneic lymphocytes.

Table 1

Autologous and Allogeneic Tumor Stimulation Given in
Reactivity Index, Which is Positive if > 4

Experiment 1

Responder patient	Stimulator Tumor Cells				
	a	b	c	d	e
a	5.7	1.4	0.7	8.7	1.0
b	3.7	30.6	1.4	8.0	0.7
c	1.4	2.4	7.8	13.0	0.5
d	2.2	1.0	0.5	1.3	-
e	-	-	-	-	0.9
Healthy Donor	-	2.8	0.8	-	-

Diagnosis: a, undiff. mesench.; b, sq. cell ca.; c and
d, adenocarcinoma; e, glioma

Experiment 2

	a	b	c	d
a	8.8	2.8	3.8	1.1
b	0.8	24.5	1.9	1.1
c	1.3	2.7	0.9	1.3

Diagnosis: a and b, glioma; c, adenoca. pulm.

Reactivity index: The ratio between the isotope uptake
in the test sample and that of the control sample.

The autologous lymphocytotoxicity (ALC) test was worked out recently (42). Short term ^{51}Cr-release micro-test was used to register the killing of biopsy cells.

In the experiments performed until present lympho-cytes were cytotoxic for autologous tumors in 16/29 cases. The specificity was investigated by criss cross tests. The results of 3 experiments are given in Table 2. In 1 and 2 the selective autologous effect is clear but in the third experiment the selectivity is only marginal. The ALC positive lymphocytes reacted with allogeneic tumor cells only in 4/52 combinations. Lymphocytes from healthy donors were negative in 13 experiments.

Table 2

Cytotoxicity of blood lymphocytes[x] against autologous and allogeneic biopsy cells

Exp.	Effector cells from Patient	Target Cells, % specific Cr51 release		
		1012	1008	
1	1012 osteosarcoma	24	0	
	1008 - " -	7	80	
		1008	1010[xx]	2274
2	1008 - " -	82	15	0
	2274 kidney cancer	2	0	24
		779	778	
3	779 glioma	24	16	
	778 - " -	14	3	
	780 - " -	12	3	
	Healthy blood donor	10		

[x]T cell enriched population obtained by passage through nylon column; effector: target 50:1; 4 hrs. assay.

[xx]Osteosarcoma

ALC positivity required blastogenesis. The opposite was not true i.e. not all cases with blastogenesis had cytotoxic activity (Table 3).

Table 3

Correlation between blastogenesis and cytotoxicity.

		1^O ALC	2^O ALC
ATS	+	9/29 (31%)	12/20 (60%)
	−	1/13 (8%)	0/7

The reactivities registered in autologous combinations, the effect of cocultivation leading to blastogenesis and the generation of cytotoxicity with maintained
autologous reactivity strongly suggest genuine tumor
specificities. Because biopsy cells are only exceptionally affected by NK cells such effect does not disturb the
experiments. It has to be emphasized that the cocultiva-
tions were performed in human serum. This is of major
importance because cultivation of lymphocytes in fetal
calf serum is known to generate non-discriminative cytotoxicity.

Comparison of our results with the earlier extensive
material on human tumors shows an important difference
because the latter indicated tissue specific tumor specificity. With various tumor types using short term cultured cells as targets cross reactivities between tumors
originating in the same tissue were reported (20). These
studies may have been devoid of NK effects because the
target cells were cultured only during a short time.
Apart from technical factors (48^h microcytotoxicity or
colony inhibition in the experiments of the Hellströms
and short term Cr^{51} release test in our series) the nature
of target cells is the main difference.

The preferential if not absolute autologous reactivity may be indicative for individual antigens or reflects
the influence of histocompatibility on T cell mediated
cytotoxicity. The earlier cross reactivities, indicating
tissue related specificities may be reconciled with the
duration of the cytotoxic test. In animal tumor systems
with strong antigenicity long term tests have overridden
the histocompatibility restriction, however there was
still a stronger effect if the effector and target cells
were histocompatible (38).

Acknowledgements

The work upon which this publication is based was
performed pursuant to Contract NO1-CB-64023 and NO1-CB-
74144 with the Division of Cancer Biology and Diagnosis,
National Cancer Institute, Department of Health, Education
and Welfare. Grants have also been received from the
Swedish Cancer Society. B.M.V. was supported by grants
from the Cancer Research Campaign of Great Britain; F.V.
by the Stanley Thomas Johnson Foundation, Bern, Switzerland; and M.F. by the Schweizerische Akademie der Mediz-
inischen Wissenschaften.

References

1. Abo, T., Yamaguchi, T., Shimizu, F. and Kumagia, K.:
   J. Immunol. 1976, 117: 1781.
2. Argov, S. and Klein, E., to be published.
3. Bakács, T., Gergely, P., Cornain, S. and Klein, E.:
   Int. J. Cancer 1977, 19: 441.
4. Bakács, T., Gergely, P. and Klein, E.: Cellular
   Immunol. 1977, 32: 317.
5. Bakács, T., Klein, E. and Ljungström, K.G.: Cancer
   Letters 1978, 4: 191.
6. Bakács, T., Klein, E., Yefenof, E., Gergely, P. and
   Steinitz, M.: Z. Immun.-Forsch. 1978. 154: 121.
7. Bakács, T., Svedmyr, E., Klein, E., Rombo, L. and
   Weiland, D.: Cancer Letters 1978, 4: 185.
8. Baldwin, R.W., Glaves, D. and Vose, B.M.: Int. J.
   Cancer 1974, 13: 135.
9. Becker, S., Fenyö, E.M. and Klein, E.: Europ. J.
   Immunol. 1976, 6: 882.
10. Becker, S., Kiessling, R. and Klein, G., to be publ.
11. Becker, S. and Klein, E.: Europ. J. Immunol. 1976,
    6: 892.
12. Cerottini, J.C. and Brunner, K.T.: Adv. in Immunol.
    1974, 18: 67, New York, Academic Press.
13. Cornain, S. and Klein, E.: Z. Immun.-Forsch. 1978,
    154: 101.
14. De Vries, J.E., Cornain, S. and Rümke, P.: Int. J.
    Cancer 1974, 14: 427.
15. Doherty, P.C., Blanden, R.V. and Zinkernagel, R.M.:
    Transpl. Rev. 1976, 29: 28.
16. Einhorn, L., Steinitz, M., Yefenof, E., Bakács, T.
    and Klein, G.: Cell. Immunol. 1978, 35: 43.
17. Engers, H.D. and MacDonald, H.R.: Contemp. Topics in
    Immuno-Biology. Plenum press, N.Y., 1976, 5: 145.
18. Galili, V., Galili, N., Vánky, F. and Klein, E.:
    Proc. Nat. Acad. Sci., in press.

19. Gatien, J.C., Schneeberger, E.E. et al.: Eur. J. Immunol. 1975, 5: 312.
20. Hellström, K.E. and Hellström, I.: Adv. Cancer Res. 1969, 12: 167.
21. Herberman, R.B., Nunn, M.F. and Lavrin, D.H.: Int. J. Cancer 1975, 16: 230.
22. Hersey, P., Edwards, A., Edwards, J., Adams, E., Milton, G.W. and Nelson, D.S.: Int. J. Cancer 1975 16: 173.
23. Kiessling, R., Klein, E. and Wigzell, H.: Eur. J. Immunol. 1975, 5: 230.
24. Kiessling, R., Petrányi, G., Klein, G. and Wigzell, H.: Int. J. Cancer 1975, 15: 933.
25. Klein, G. and Åsjö, B.: to be published.
26. MacLennan, I.C.M.: 1976. In: Clinical Tumor Immunology. Ed. J. Wybran and M. Staguet. Pergamon Press, Oxford, P. 47.
27. Peter, H.H., Eife, R.F. and Kalden, J.R.: J. Immunol. 1976, 116: 342.
28. Plata, F., McDonald, H.R. and Engers, H.D.: J. Immunology 1976, 117: 52.
29. Pross, H.F. and Baines, M.G.: Int. J. Cancer 1976, 18: 593.
30. Pross, H.F. and Baines, M.G.: Cancer Immunol. Immunotherap. 1977, 3: 75.
31. Schlossman, S.F. and Chess, L.: 1975. In: Clinical evaluation of immune function in man. Grune and Stratton Inc., p. 65.
32. Stejskal, V.: Scand. J. Immunol. 1976, 5: 479.
33. Stjernswärd, J.: J. Natl. Cancer Inst. 1965, 35: 885.
34. Stein, H. and Möller-Hermelink, H.K.: Brit. J. Haem. 1977, 36: 225.
35. Stutman, O.: Science 1974, 183: 534.
36. Svedmyr, E. and Jondal, M.: Proc. Natl. Acad. Sci. 1975, 72: 1622.
37. Takasugi, M., Koide, D., Akira, D. and Ramseyer, A.: Int. J. Cancer 1977, 19: 291.
38. Ting, C.-C. and Law, L.W.: J. Immunol. 1977, 117:1259.
39. Troye, M., Perlmann, P., Pape, G.R. Spiegelberg, H.L., Näslund, I. and Gidlöf, A.: J. Immunol. 1977, 119: 1061.
40. Vánky, F. and Stjernswärd j.: 1976. In vitro methods in cell mediated and tumor immunity. II. Eds. B. Bloom and J.R. David. Academic Press Inc., N.Y. 597.
41. Vose, B., Vánky, F., Argov, S. and Klein, E.: Eur. J. Immunol. 1977, 7: 753.
42. Vose, B., Vánky, F. and Klein, E. Int J. Cancer 1977, 20: 512.
43. Vose, B.M. and Moore, M.: Int. J. Cancer 1977, 19: 34.
44. Vose, B., Vánky, F., Fopp, M. and Klein, E.: Int. J. Cancer 1978, 21: 588.

CELL-MEDIATED IMMUNITY TO ROUS SARCOMAS IN JAPANESE QUAILS

M. Hayami, J. Ignjatovic, B. Gleischer,
H. Rübsamen, J. Stehfen-Gervinus, and
H. Bauer

Institut für Virologie
Justus-Liebig-Universität Giessen
63 Giessen, FRG

1. Introduction

The avian C-type tumor viruses offer several advantages for the study of tumor immunology. First, defined tumor virus strains are available: sarcoma viruses (ASV), able to transform embryonic fibroblasts in vitro, as well as transformation-defective leukosis viruses (ALV) which only replicate in fibroblasts without transforming them [1]. The group of avian RNA tumor viruses is subdivided into several subgroups, based on differences in the envelope glycoprotein gp85, which defines the virus host range as well as susceptibility to interference and neutralization [2] and shows subgroup-specific and group-specific antigenic determinants [3].

Secondly, most of these viruses replicate independently from any helper virus, leading to cell transformation by monoclonal virus strains. Furthermore, the unique possibility exists in the avian system to manipulate the immune functions of the natural host by eliminating selectively bursa-derived or thymus-dependent immune reactions.

The Rous sarcoma virus (RSV)-system in Japanese quails (JQ) is particularly useful, since these animals have never been shown to express endogenous viral genes [4], which might interfere with the identification of tumor antigens. In addition, with an appropriate virus dose it is possible to induce reproducibly tumors that grow transiently and then regress spontaneously or

385

tumors that grow progressively and kill the host.

2. Cell-mediated cytotoxicity (CMC) in the RSV-quail system

In regressor animals tumors appear 7 - 10 days after virus inoculation, reach peak size after 14 - 20 days and then quickly regress. It has been proposed, that the regression is mainly due to cell-mediated immune reactions [5], since in thymectomized quails regression very rarely occurs, whereas bursectomy does not affect recovery from the tumor [6].

It has been shown that spleen cells from JQ which have recovered from an ASV-induced tumor exert a strong cytotoxic effect in a microcytotoxicity assay against autochthonous or allogeneic RSV-transformed cultured QEC. Peak cytotoxicity is found shortly after tumor regression, while at maximum tumor size no immunity is detectable [7]. Spleen cells from an animal with progressively growing tumor do not show any cytotoxicity in vitro, but even are able to suppress the cytotoxic activity of spleen cells from regressor animals [8]. In addition, serum effects, such as blocking of the cytotoxicity of immune spleen cells or arming of normal spleen cells have been shown at different stages of tumor growth or regression [9,10,11]. Sera taken from JQ after tumor regression confered in most cases cytotoxic activity to normal spleen cells, whereas serum taken during tumor growth was able to block the cytotoxic reaction [9,10]. In addition, an early cytotoxicity inducing factor has been described to be found in the sera of JQ shortly after inoculation of the virus but before visible tumor growth [7,11].

3. Demonstration of tumor-associated antigens by cross-reactivity in vitro

In all these investigations, however, no attention has been paid to the nature of the antigens serving as target in the anti-tumor immune reactions in vivo and in vitro. Recently in this laboratory several studies have been performed to identify tumor-associated antigens on RSV-transformed quail cells using immune spleen cells in a 18-hr visual microcytotoxicity assay [12, 13].

The following cell populations were used as target cells in this cytotoxic reaction: a) Quail embryo cells (QEC) infected in vitro by ASV and ALV of various subgroups, b) an established quail cell line, designated

R(-):Q, consisting of QEC transformed by the Bryan high titer strain of RSV, BH(RSV), [14], which is a deletion mutant for the viral envelope glycoproteins [14], and c) an established quail cell line, designated MC3-5:Q, derived from a tumor induced in vivo by means of 3-methylcholanthrene (MC) [12]. Effector cells were taken from animals, which had recovered from a tumor induced by ASV of subgroup A or C or the BH(RSV) or from quails after repeated injections of ALV of subgroup A or C, as described in detail [12].

Table I

Cytotoxicity against transformed and untransformed quail cells

effector cells from JQ infected with

Target cells	ASV-A	ASV-C	BH(RSV)	ALV-A	ALV-C
ASV-A-transformed	+	+	+	+	−
ASV-C-transformed	+	+	+	−	+
R(-):Q	+	+	+	−	−
MC3-5:Q	+	+	NT	−	−
ALV-A-infected	+	−	−	+	−
ALV-C-infected	−	+	NT	−	+
normal QEC (low passage)	+	NT	NT	NT	NT
normal QEC (high passage)	−	−	−	−	−

+: significant cytotoxicity; −: cytotoxicity not significant; NT: not tested

Table I summarizes the results of these experiments. Spleen cells from ALV-infected JQ are able to destroy QEC infected in vitro with ALV or ASV of the same subgroup only. Spleen cells, however, from quails immunized with ASV or the Bryan strain of RSV are highly cytotoxic to QEC transformed by ASV of the same as well as of other subgroups, whereas the destruction of ALV-infected QEC is subgroup-specific. R(-):Q cells and the chemically transformed MC3-5:Q cells are destroyed to a similar extent as are ASV-transformed cells. Since

the R(-):Q and MC3-5:Q do not express viral structural
proteins on their surface, the CMC is presumably directed against antigens associated with the transformed
state of these cells. A weak, but significant cytotoxic
effect was obtained with uninfected primary QEC but not
with QEC after several passages.

4. Identification of several target antigens

It has been shown that the system described here it
is possible to block the cytotoxic activity by pre-
treatment of the effector cells with extracts from
various target cells [13,16]. The CMC can be blocked
completely by extracts of those cells that induced the
immune response in vivo as well as by extracts of the
respective in vitro target cells. Extracts from ALV-
infected, untransformed cells block only partially the
ASV-induced CMC against ASV-transformed cells and show
no blocking on R(-):Q or MC3-5:Q. Extracts from the
latter, which do not express any structural virus proteins on their surface, block only partially the CMC
against ASV-transformed targets. This partial blocking
observed is a qualitative effect, since with increasing
antigen concentration in the incubation mixture the
blocking remains partial, whereas mixing of extracts
which show only partial blocking each may yield a total
blocking [16].

Table II summarizes in a chess-board pattern the
blocking by various extracts of an SV-C-induced CMC
against various target cells.

Table II

Blocking capacity of various extracts on various target
cells [a]

| target cell | extracts from QEC transformed by infected with | | | | | |
	ASV-A	ASV-C	BH(RSV)	MC	ALV-A	ALV-C
ASV-A-transformed	T	T	P	P	P	P
ASV-C-transformed		T	P	P	P	P
R(-):Q	T	T	T	P	-	-
MC3-5:Q	T	T	T	T	-	-
ALV-C-infected	-	T	-	-	-	T

a): effector cells: ASV-C-induced; T: total blocking;
P: partial blocking; -: no blocking

Since extracts from MC3-5:Q block only partially the CMC against R(-):Q whereas R(-):Q extracts block completely against MC3-5:Q, the cells transformed by the defective sarcoma virus seem to express at least one antigen in addition to those expressed on the chemically transformed MC3-5:Q. These and experiments with mixtures of extracts which have been described in detail recently [16], were interpreted as shown in Table III.

Table III

Distribution of tumor-associated antigens on transformed and untransformed quail cells

Antigen	ASV- transf.	BH(RSV) transf.	ALV- infected	MC- transf.
s-gp85, subgroup-specific determinant of gp85	+	-	+	-
g-gp85, group-specific determinant of gp85	+	-	-	-
TSSA, non virion structural protein	+	+	-	-
EAg, embryonic antigen(s)	+	+	-	+

Four different target antigens could be distinguished: two of these are determinants of the viral envelope glycoprotein, a group-specific determinant, g-gp85, exposed on transformed cells only, and a subgroup-specific one, found on ALV-infected as well as on ASV-transformed QEC. As with g-gp85, two further antigens are expressed on the surface of transformed cells only, one, EAg, probably of embryonic origin and shared by ASV- and chemically transformed cells, and an antigen tentatively called transformation-specific surface antigen (TSSA), which is found only on virally transformed cells, but is not a viral structural protein.

Experiments with QEC transformed by temperature sensitive (ts) mutants of RSV indicate that the embryonic antigen disappears at the nonpermissive temperature as does the transformed phenotype. Since extracts from

these cells, prepared at 42° C, still block on R(-):Q,
ts ASV-transformed QEC still seem to contain the TSSA
at the nonpermissive temperature [17], though the localization is not known. Since the defect in ts mutants
of RSV has been assumed to be due to a point mutation
in the src gene [18], it has been speculated that the
TSSA may be the src gene product, which, though not
functioning, is still immunologically detectable at
the nonpermissive temperature [17].

5. Role of in vitro detected antigens for in vivo-pro-
    tection

To test which of the in vitro detectable target
antigens might act as transplantation antigen in vivo,
quails were injected with soluble extracts prepared
from the in vitro target cells with detergents and
enriched in glycoproteins by affinity chromatography
on lens culinaris lectin columns [17,19]. The results
obtained indicate, that immunizing with any of the
transformation-associated antigens described here may
protect against RSV challenge.

Surprisingly the effect of immunization was strongly
dependent on the route of antigen application: while
intravenous (i.v.) injection lead to immunity to a subsequent challenge with ASV, as measured by a decreased
growth rate and incidence of tumors, after intramuscular (i.m.) injection enhancement of tumor growth was
observed. This phenomenon could be explained at least
in part by the finding of suppressor cells in the
spleens of i.m. immunized quails. Using the in vitro-
CMC it was found, that spleen cells from i.v. injected
quails exerted a strong cytotoxic effect against target cells carrying the antigens used for immunization,
whereas spleen cells from i.m. immunized animals not
only were not cytotoxic, but even were able to suppress
the cytotoxic activity of the former. In addition,
blocking activity could be detected in the sera of i.m.
immunized quails and arming in the sera of i.v. injected animals [19]. These findings indicate that i.m.
immunization may lead to a complex derangement of the
immune function which may be comparable to events
taking place in a tumor-bearing host.

6. Conclusion

The system described above allows the reproducible
induction of antigenic tumors in vivo in combination

with a cell-mediated cytotoxicity assay for the detection of tumor immunity in vitro.

In addition, it is possible to distinguish and identify tumor-associated antigens by their capacity to block the cytotoxic reaction. Since, furthermore, tumor immunity or enhancement can be induced alternatively by experimental manipulation the RSV-system seems to be a unique model for the study of tumor immunology. This system should help to define the various components in the interaction of the host's immune system with the tumor cell finally giving a better understanding of the complex host-tumor relationship.

References

1. Bauer, H. (1974). Adv. Cancer Res. 20, 275-340

2. Vogt, P.K., Ishizaki, R., Duff, R. (1967). In: "Subviral Carcinogenesis" (Y. Ito, ed.) Aichi Center, Nagoya, Japan, 297-310

3. Rohrschneider, L.R., Bauer, H., Bolognesi, D.P. (1975). Virology 67, 234-241

4. Vogt, P.K., Friis, R.R. (1971). Virology 43, 223-234

5. Yamanouchi, K., Hayami, M., Fukuda, A., Kohune, F. (1968). Jap. J. med. Sci. Biol. 21, 393-404

6. Yamanouchi, K., Hayami, M., Miyakura, S., Fukuda, A.,Kohune, F. (1971). Jap. J. med. Sci. Biol. 24, 1-8

7. Hayami, M., Ito, M., Yoshikawa, Y., Yamanouchi, K. (1976). Jap. J. med. Sci. Biol. 29, 11 - 24

8. Hayami, M., Hellström, I., Hellström, K.E., Yamanouchi, K. (1972). Int. J. Cancer 10, 507 - 517

9. Hayami, M., Hellström, I., Hellström, K. E. (1973). Int. J. Cancer 12, 667 - 688

10. Hayami, M., Hellström, I., Hellström, K. E., Lannin, D. R. (1974). Int. J. Cancer 13, 43 - 53

11. Yoshikawa, Y., Yamanouchi, K., Fukuda, A., Hayami, M. (1976). Int. J. Cancer 17, 525 - 532

12. Hayami, M., Ignjatovic, J., Bauer, H. (1977). Int. J. Cancer 20, 729 - 737

13. Bauer, H., Ignjatovic, J., Rübsamen, H., Hayami, M. (1977). Med. Microbiol. Immunol. <u>164</u>, 197 - 205

14. Friis, R. R. (1972). Virology <u>50,</u> 701 - 712

15. Halpern, M., Bolognesi, D.P., Friis, R. R. (1976). J. Virol. <u>18,</u> 504 - 510

16. Ignjatovic, J., Rübsamen, H., Hayami, M., Bauer, H. (1978). J. Immunol., in press

17. Bauer, H., Hayami, M., Ignjatovic, J., Rübsamen, H., Graf, T., Friis, R. R. (1977). "Three days on Avian RNA Tumor Viruses" Pavia, Italy (S. Barlatti, C. de Guili, eds.), in press

18. Bernstein, A., MacCormick, R., Martin, G.S. (1976). Virology <u>70,</u> 206 - 209

19. Bauer, H., Hayami, M., Stehfen-Gervinus, J., in preparation

This work was supported by the SFB 47 of the Deutsche Forschungsgemeinschaft.

Dedicated to the Memory of James William McGinnis, Jr.

A SINGLE GENETIC LOCUS DETERMINES THE EFFICACY OF SERUM THERAPY AGAINST MURINE ADENOCARCINOMA 755a

Gary J. Roloson, Cecily A. Chambers, Darrow E. Haagensen, Jr., Ronald C. Montelaro and Dani P. Bolognesi

Duke University Medical Center, Department of Surgery Durham, North Carolina, U.S.A. 27710

INTRODUCTION

We have recently described a unique model system for immuno-therapy where immunological management of a highly lethal tumor, the ascites form of the Adenocarcinoma 755 (AD755a), could be carried out reproducibly and with remarkable efficiency (1). Some of the basic featues of this model are summarized in Table 1. The studies to be described in this report will concern themselves primarily with a more in depth analysis of the phenomenon of strain variation in relation to the protective capacity of the serum, and were done in an effort to gain some insight into the mechanism by which the serum mediates its powerful effect.

Preparation of Hyperimmune Anti-AD755a Antiserum

AD755a was uniformly lethal in B6 mice after intraperitoneal (ip) inoculation of as few as 50 cells per mouse (Table 1). In contrast, when AD755a cells were injected subcutaneously (sc) into B6 mice in a dose range between $1x10^5$ and $5x10^5$ cells, a transient nodule appeared that was resorbed completely by week 2-3 after injection. Mice that had rejected AD755a cells inoculated sc were resistant to a later ip challenge with these cells. On this basis, B6 mice were hyperimmunized against the AD755a cells by an initial sc inoculation of 10^4 AD755a cells followed by sc inoculations 2-3 weeks later of $1x10^5$ and $5x10^5$ cells respectively. Subsequently, increasing doses of AD755a cells from $1x10^4$ to $1x10^6$ were given ip over a period of seven weeks. After four additional ip inoculations with $1x10^6$ cells, serum was taken. Animals were boosted and bled monthly thereafter.

Table 1

CHARACTERISTICS OF AD755a TUMOR SYSTEM

AD755a is a "universal" tumor and is lethal in all mouse strains tested. Inoculation of fewer than 50 cells intraperitoneally gives 100% lethality and fewer than ten cells results in approximately 80% lethality. The tumor grows equally well in all strains tested.

Immunization in "syngeneic" C57Bl/6J mice by subcutaneous inoculation of AD755a provides protection against an intraperitoneal challenge of $>10^4 LD_{100}$ and this protection persists for greater than 90 days.

Serum or immune cells from mice hyperimmunized by multiple intraperitoneal injections after an initial subcutaneous immunization can transfer protection to a normal animal. Hyperimmune serum can transfer protection against 1×10^5 AD755a cells in quantities of 5-10 μl depending on the serum pool.

Preliminary study of the protective factor(s) shows it is contained in the IgG fraction. It has an effective half-life in vivo of greater than 4.5 days and less than 9.0 days.

Studies in several mouse strains have revealed that protective capacity of the serum is strain dependent.

Normal B6 mice were inoculated ip with various volumes of the immune sera at the same time that they were challenged with AD755a cells. Protection against 10^5 tumor cells was obtained with as little as 5-10 µl of B6 anti-AD755a serum. Subsequent experiments demonstrated that similar titration end points could also be obtained after sc or intravenous injection of the serum; this indicated that the serum and tumor cells did not need to be administered together for successful passive immunotherapy to be achieved. Finally, serum administered as late as 3 days after tumor inoculation was also protective, although larger quantities were required.

Protective Capacity of Immune Serum in Various Mouse Strains

Titration of B6 anti-AD755a immune serum against AD755a tumor cells given ip to other strains of mice revealed a significant strain specificity of the immune protective capacity (Table 2).

The results emphasize the variation observed earlier (1) where only a few strains were tested. The mice are arbitrarily subdivided into three groups based on their titration end point (see legend of Table 2).   All standard C57Bl strains, as well as strains 129/J, CBA/J and A/J, were protected by low quantities of serum (10 µl) including strains congenic at H-2 (*) and Fv-2 (**).

At the opposite end of the spectrum were mouse strains which were not protected by at least ten (AKR) or more than 30 times (BALB/cJ) the quantity of serum used to protect C57Bl/6J. Both $Fv-1^n$ (NIH) and $Fv-1^b$ (BALB) mice were members of this group, indicating no relationship to the Fv-1 gene. A variety of strains, however, could be protected by intermediate quantities of serum (group II).

Some conclusions can be drawn from this analysis which indicate that protection did not seem to correlate with the H-2 type or with two well-known viral markers. Moreover, the variations observed cannot be explained by a difference in growth rate of the tumor since at the dosage given (10^5 tumor cells), the tumor was uniformly lethal within very nearly the same time period after administration in all strains tested.

Genetic Analysis of the AD755a System

The strain variation observed could be due to a number of factors including several immunological and virological parameters. Since some of the loci controlling these factors are known, a genetic analysis of the system might provide some clues as to the significance of this variation, and even illuminate the nature of the mechanism of protection itself. Using C57Bl/6J (B6)(protected [P] at 10 µl) and BALB/cJ (C)(not protected [-] at 300 µl) mice, we

Table 2

STRAIN ANALYSIS FOR PROTECTION AGAINST THE AD755a TUMOR

Mouse Strain	Minimum Protective Volume (µl)	
C57B1/6J	10	
C57B1/6J (male)	10	
C57B1/6By	10	
*B6.C-H-2^d/By	10	
**B6.C-H-7^b/By	10	
C57B1/10J	10	
*B10.A/SgSn	10	
*B10-H-2^a-H-7^{b}Wts	10	I
B10.129(21M)/SnJ	10	
*B10.D2/nSn	10	
C57B1/KsJ	10	
129/J	10	
CBA/J	10	
A/J	10	
*B10.Br/SgSn	35	
C3H/HeJ	35	
C3H/HeJ (male)	35	
*C3H.SW/Sn	50	
DBA/2J	50	
SJL/J	50	
C58/J	50+	II
RF/J	50+	
NZB/BINJ	50+	
STU	50+	
P/J	75	
SEC/1ReJ	75	

Table 2 (cont'd)

Mouse Strain	Minimum Protective Volume (µl)	
DBA/1J	>75	
NIH/Sw	>75	
NIH/Sw (Nu/Nu)	>75	
PL/J	>75	
RII/2J	>75	III
SM/J	>75	
BUB/BnJ	>75	
BALB/c By	>75	
AKR	>100	
BALB/cJ	>300	
BALB/cJ (male)	>300	

(1)   Unless indicated, females were tested

(2)   Same serum pool used in all strains tested

(3)   Strains titrated at 0, 10, 20, 35, 50, 75 or
      100 and 300 µl where indicated. Four mice
      tested at each level.

*H-2 congenics

**Fv-2 congenics

carried out classical mating crosses (F_1, F_2, F_1 backcrosses) to establish the number of genes involved in the phenomenon and their penetrance (dominant or recessive).

F_1 Generation

Both F_1 breeding combinations, (C x B6) and the reverse (B6 x C) indicated that an intermediate quantity of serum (~75 μl) was required for protection of the F_1 hybrids and that there was no sex-linked effect (Table 3). The fact that these animals could be protected excludes the presence of a single dominant locus from BALB/cJ mice which blocks protection.

F_2 and F_1 Backcross Progeny Testing

The results of the second generation cross (C x B6) F_2 involving 313 mice, where protection was assayed at 15 μl of serum, are shown in Table 4. Since 22.4%, or one quarter of the mice resembled the B6 parent, this strongly suggests that a single locus is involved in the process. Studies to determine the percentage resembling the BALB/cJ parent confirm this notion (see Table 6). The observed values for the individual F_1 backcross generations are also in close agreement with the expected values for a single operative locus. A diagrammatic representation of the various crosses is presented in Figure 1.

Linkage Studies to Determine the Position of the Locus Controlling Protection

During the course of these experiments, we noticed that certain alleles controlling coat color might be linked to the protection locus. In crosses between BALB/cJ and C57Bl/6J mice, multiple genes located on separate chromosomes determine coat color (2). The a locus confers the agouti characteristic which is represented by hair with a visible yellow banding. The locus is dominant except in albino mice where melanin is not produced. The C57Bl/6J parents are black mice, homozygous nonagouti (aa), while BALB/cJ mice are white (no melanin) but homozygous at agouti for the wild-type allele (AA). In a cross between these two strains, one typically observes the following ratio in the F_2 generation: 9 agouti: 3 nonagouti: 4 albino.

Analysis of the (C X B6) F_2 generation at the 15 μl protection end point in relation to coat color yields the results outlined in Table 5. Assuming no linkage with any color marker, one would have expected that the percentage of mice protected in each category would be the same as the overall percentage protected (~25%). On the other hand, a close linkage to agouti should result in no pro-

Table 3

PROTECTION OF PARENTAL AND F_1 MICE BY IMMUNE SERUM

Mouse Strain	Minimum Quantity of Protective Serum
C57Bl/6 ⟶ Parental	15 µl
BALB/cJ ⟶	>300 µl
(B6 x C) F_1	75 µl
(C x B6) F_1	75 µl

Table 4

PROTECTION OF F_2 AND F_1 BACKCROSS (BC) PROGENY

By 15 µl OF IMMUNE SERUM

Cross	Number Of Mice	Percent Protected	Percent Expected For One Locus
(C x B6) F_2	313	22.4	25.0
(B6 x F_1) BC	50	42.0	50.0
(F_1 x C) BC	52	0	0

Table 5

LINKAGE OF IMMUNE PROTECTIVE CAPACITY

WITH COAT COLOR (15 µl) : F_2 GENERATION

	Total	Agouti	Nonagouti	Albino
Number of Mice (F_2)	313	175	49	89
Number of Mice Protected by 15 µl	70	25	28	17
Percent	22.4	14.3	57	19
% Expected (no linkage)	25	25	25	25
% Expected (linkage to agouti)	25	0	100	25

Parental Type	P|	|P P|	|- -|	|P -|	|-	TOTALS (% Protected)	
F_2	a|	|a a|	|A A|	|a A|	|A	Agouti	Nonagouti
Color	Nonagouti	Agouti	Agouti	Agouti			
Protected by 15 µl	+	−	−	−		0	100

TRANSMISSION OF LOCI INVOLVED IN PROTECTION AND THEIR
LINKED ALLELES TO F_1, F_2 AND BACKCROSS PROGENY

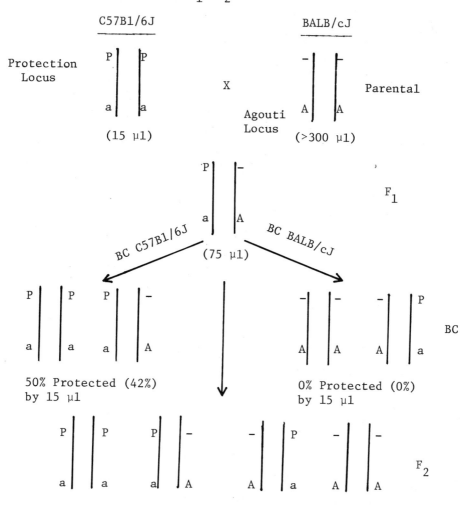

Fig. 1. Diagrammatic representation of genetic crosses between
C57B1/6J and BALB/cJ mice and their offspring demonstrating the
putative relationship between loci associated with protection
and that of the agouti coat color.

tection for agouti mice since these would resemble the BALB/cJ
parent; and complete protection of nonagouti animals (like B6
parents). The observed percentages represent significant deviations from either idealized situation.

Genetic Analysis of Protection Using 100 µl of Serum

Assessment of the protective capacity of 100 µl of serum was
chosen since this quantity of serum could protect all F_1 hybrid
mice in addition to animals behaving like parental B6. This quantity of serum, however, would not be able to protect mice resembling
parental BALB/cJ (see also Fig. 1). The results of this study are
presented in Table 6, and they support the contention of a one locus
phenomenon since 31.4% of the mice (in comparison to an idealized
25%) are not protected and thereby resemble the BALB/cJ parents.
Note that only 51 mice have been studied thus far such that the
numbers are expected to deviate slightly from ideal values.

This study is also useful for a linkage analysis to the agouti
locus. In this case the values observed correspond nearly exactly
with the expected values for linkage to agouti (for both the agouti
and nonagouti groups). Pertinent to the studies presented in Tables
5 and 6, albino mice cannot be adequately evaluated since both agouti
and nonagouti markers cannot be scored; but nevertheless, the values
obtained are in general conformity with the expected ones.

At first hand it would appear that there is a discrepancy between the results of Tables 5 and 6 with regard to actual values
relative to those expected. However, we have not thus far considered the phenomenon of recombination in these crosses and its effect
on the percentages observed. This point is illustrated in Figure 2
where an idealized comparison of the parental and recombinant types
in the F_2 generation with regard to protection and coat color employing both levels of antiserum (15 and 100 µl) is presented. This
analysis illustrates that whereas the recombinants can be scored using coat color as a marker when the 15 µl quantity is employed (e.g.
agouti mice which can be protected or a nonagouti mouse not protected
by 15 µl), none of the recombinants can be individualized when protection with 100 µl of serum is assessed (percentages with regard to
coat color are the same as parental type F_2).

This information explains at least in part the discrepancy between Tables 5 and 6 and suggests that the deviations from the expected values demonstrating linkage to agouti are due to the presence of recombinants which can be scored in the 15 µl but not the
100 µl analyses. Note also that the expected frequency of scoring
recombinants in the nonagouti category is 100% while only 33% can
be identified in the agouti category (Fig. 2). On this basis using
the data of Table 5, one can estimate a recombination frequency of

Table 6

LINKAGE OF IMMUNE PROTECTIVE CAPACITY

WITH COAT COLOR (100 µl) : F_2 GENERATION

	Total	Agouti	Nonagouti	Albino
Number of Mice (F_2)	51	23	4	24
Number of Mice Protected by 100 µl	35	15	4	16
Percent	68.6	65.2	100	66.6
% Expected (no linkage)	75	75	75	75
% Expected (linkage to agouti)	75	66.6	100	75

Parental Type	P	P	P	–	–	P	–	–		TOTALS
F_2	a	a	a	A	A	a	A	A		(% Protected)
Color	Nonagouti		Agouti		Agouti		Agouti		Agouti	Nonagouti
Protected by 100 µl	+		+		+		–		66.6	100

Fig. 2. Parental and expected recombinant F_2 genotypes involving the protection and agouti loci.

about 43% using either the nonagouti values directly (100-57%) or a corrected value for the agouti precentage (3x14.3%, since only one third of the recombinants are being scored). This tentatively places the allele associated with protection about 43 map units from the agouti locus. Since the agouti locus has been mapped, our function is located in chromosome 2, linkage group V (Fig. 3). Our preliminary data employing recombinant inbred strains suggests that the function maps toward the centromere from agouti (unpublished observations).

In summary, the genetic data support the conclusions drawn from the strain specificity that the protection function does not depend on H-2 (linkage group IX), or viral markers Fv-2 (linkage group II), Fv-1 (linkage group VIII) and Akv-1 (linkage group I). These conclusions are important for evaluating other parameters of this system which are to follow.

The Specificity of Protection is Dictated by Virus Associated Antigens

The mechanism by which AD755a tumor challenge is rejected and the identity of the antigens involved in the induction of immune transfer capacity remain to be defined. Possibly relevant to these questions were the observations of Brandes and Groth (3) that virus particles were present in both the solid and ascites form of Adeno-carcinoma 755. We have recently demonstrated that this agent, termed ADV (Adenocarcinoma-755a virus) is a type-C virus closely related to the Friend and Rauscher murine leukemia agents (4). Moreover, the B6 anti-AD755a serum could neutralize ADV and viruses of the FMR (Friend-Moloney-Rauscher) group, possessed a high antibody titer in radioimmunoassays with the major glycoprotein of Friend virus (gp71) and effectively lysed AD755a tumor cells or murine cells infected with Friend virus.

Indeed protection by this antiserum seems to correlate with an antigen associated with FMR viruses. Some of this information is summarized in Table 7. We have observed complete cross protection with universal tumors which likewise express FMR antigen, but none with tumors expressing unrelated viral antigens or no known viral antigens. Of considerable interest is that introduction of FMR viral antigens on a non virus-producing (NP) tumor (the Harvey sarcoma virus-induced C57Bl sarcoma [C57Bl (MSV HA)]) now renders this tumor ([C57Bl (MSV HA) FLV]) susceptible to rejection by an AD755a immune mouse.

Moreover, it has been possible to immunize mice with intact or disrupted Friend virus against challenge with AD755a. The viral specificity extends even to this parameter since AKR virus was not able to immunize against the tumor (Table 7).

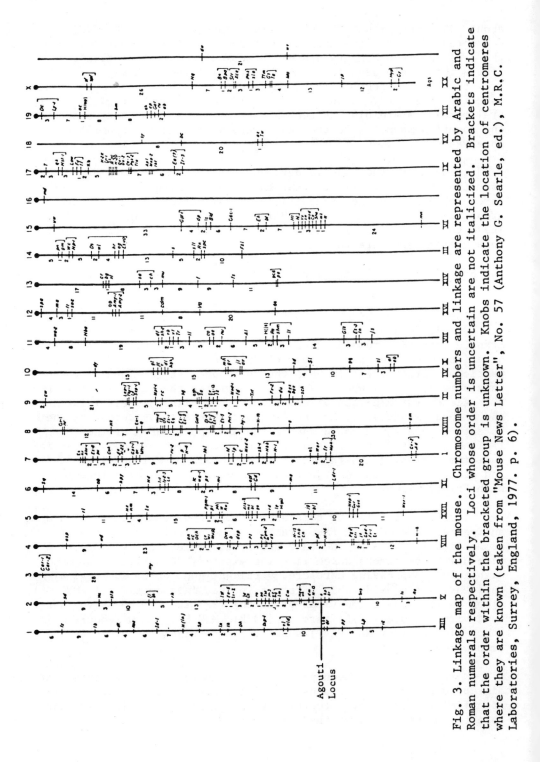

Fig. 3. Linkage map of the mouse. Chromosome numbers and linkage are represented by Arabic and Roman numerals respectively. Loci whose order is uncertain are not italicized. Brackets indicate that the order within the bracketed group is unknown. Knobs indicate the location of centromeres where they are known (taken from "Mouse News Letter", No. 57 (Anthony G. Searle, ed.), M.R.C. Laboratories, Surrey, England, 1977. p. 6).

Table 7

SPECIFICITY OF PROTECTION SEEMS TO CORRELATE
WITH ONCORNAVIRUS ASSOCIATED ANTIGENS

	Associated Virus Type
1. Complete Cross-Protection Seen Between AD755a and:	
S-180a	FMR
EAC	FMR
C57B1 (MSV HA) FLV	FMR
2. No Cross-Protection Seen Between AD755a and:	
6C3HED	Gross – AKR
EL-4	Gross – AKR
C57B1 (MSV HA) NP	None
3. Immunization Against AD755a was Possible with:	
Intact FLV Disrupted	
But Not with:	
Intact AKR Disrupted AKR	

Table 8

EFFECTIVENESS OF ANTI-TUMOR VS. ANTI-VIRAL ANTIBODIES
IN ABROGATION OF AD755a TUMOR GROWTH

Antiserum	Specificities	Prevention of Tumor Growth
Anti-AD755a	Anti-Tumor, Anti-Virus	+
Anti-AD755a Abs. with FLV	Anti-Tumor	+
Anti-AD755a Abs. with AD755a Cells	?	+
Anti-FLV, Anti-FLV gp71	Anti-Virus	–
Anti-FLV Producing Cells	Anti-Cell, Anti-Virus	–

Attempts to Achieve Protection Against AD755a Tumor Challenge with Anti-Viral Antisera

The concordance between protection and the presence of FMR viruses suggested that a viral component might represent the target antigen on the tumor surface. The most likely candidate for this was the major surface glycoprotein of the virus, not only because of its strategic location but also because the anti-AD755a serum possessed a high antibody titer exclusively against this virion component. Thus, it was reasonable to attempt protection with hyper-immune antisera to gp71, virus, and non-transformed cells producing virus. These antisera had anti-gp71 titers equal to or in some cases, much greater than those of anti-AD755a antisera. The results of these studies (Table 8) were disappointing, however, since none of these antisera were able to mediate protection. Moreover, absorption of the protective anti-AD755a antiserum with Friend virus under conditions where all of the anti-gp71 activity is removed, had no effect on its ability to reject AD755a tumor challenge.

Attempts to Identify a Non-Structural Viral-Induced Antigen Associated with AD755a Tumor Cells

The results presented in the previous section could be inter-preted to signify the presence of a non-structural virus-associated antigen which was responsible for induction of the transferable pro-tective antibody population, as well as serving as a target antigen. Such virus-induced non-structural proteins have been identified on MLV-induced YAC lymphoma (5,6,7) and on feline leukemia and sarcoma cells (8). A direct attempt to immune precipitate an analogous com-ponent from surface labeled AD755a cells with various antisera was carried out. As is shown in Figure 4, the major component precipi-tated from surface iodinated AD755a cells with both mouse anti-FLV (Fig. 4A) and mouse anti-AD755a (Fig. 4B) antisera is represented by gp71. In fact, except for a minor component of about 45,000 MW, no other distinct molecular species are evident in the anti-AD755a antiserum immune precipitates. That the major component represents gp71 is substantiated by its nearly quantitative removal subsequent to absorption of the antiserum with purified Friend virus (Fig. 4C). Although a few minor components remain after this absorption, the results indicate that most of the reactivity of the anti-AD755a serum against iodinated species on the tumor cell surface is directed toward gp71. Similar results were obtained when the cell surface glycoproteins were labeled with galactose oxidase (data not shown). Thus these results indicate that antigens other than gp71 cannot be identified using these procedures. However, a second antigen could be either inaccessible to external labeling or inactivated following disruption of the cells prior to immune precipitation. Alternatively, gp71 may indeed represent the only relevant antigen involved in pro-duction and binding of protective antibody, as discussed below.

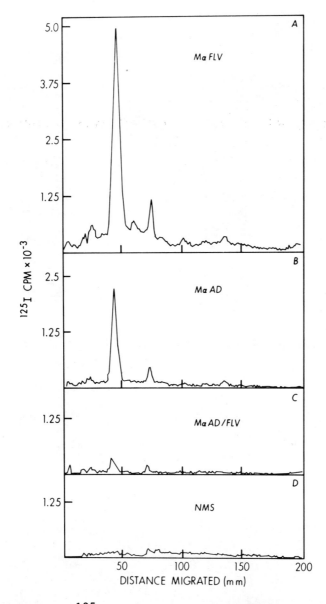

Fig. 4. Analyses of ^{125}I-labeled AD755a cells after immune precipitation with various mouse sera followed by electrophoresis on SDS polyacrylamide gels. (A) Mα FLV (B6 serum raised against purified Friend leukemia virus); (B) Mα AD (B6 anti-AD755a serum); (C) Mα AD/FLV (B6 anti-AD755a serum absorbed with FLV); and (D) NMS (normal mouse serum).

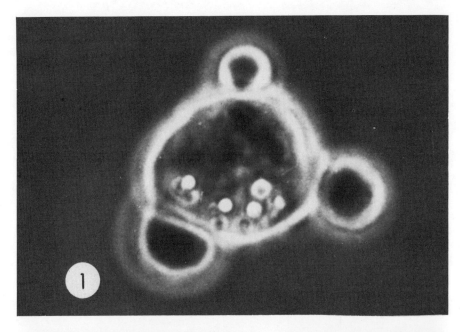

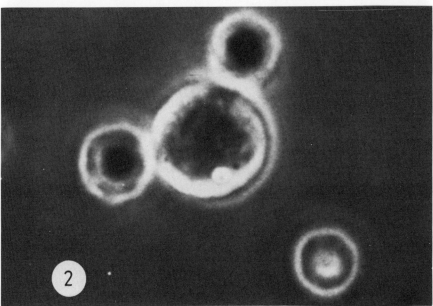

Fig. 5. Phase-contrast microscopic analysis of mouse peritoneal aspirates collected 2 hr. (1), 3 hr. (2) or 6 hr. (3) after ip inoculation of AD755a cells and B6 mouse anti-AD755a serum. <u>Note</u> that tumor cells (large granular cells) are bound to large mononuclear cells.

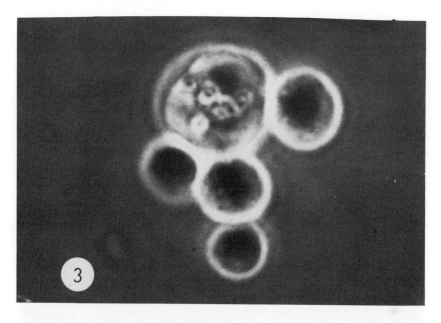

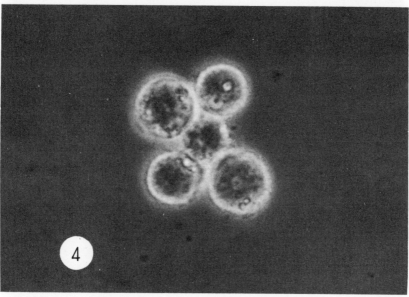

Similar analyses were carried out _in vitro_ by mixing AD755a cells, normal B6 mouse peritoneal exudate cells and B6 mouse anti-AD755a serum for 1 hr. _Note_ binding of tumor cells to a large mononuclear cell in a rosette formation, reverse of binding pattern seen _in vivo_ (see 1-3). This rosette reaction was not observed when normal B6 mouse serum was substituted for immune serum. X400 (reduced 20% for reproduction).

Protection Appears to Require a Cytophilic Antibody

    An observation which was made early in this study which bears
heavily on the mechanism of protection is that sequential absorption
of the hyperimmune anti-AD antiserum ten times with fresh AD755a
cells at its titer end point had no effect on the protective capacity
of the serum (see Table 8). Moreover, although antibodies absorbed
to the cell surface under conditions of great excess could yield
lysis in the presence of added complement; they were unable to provide protection when these antibody coated cells were inoculated as
tumor challenge. Thus, the protective function was not easily absorbed by the target cells.

    Along with the inability to directly absorb the protective
serum with the target cell, the potent protective capacity of small
volumes of the immune serum, as well as its apparent strain specificity, may be indicative of a cellular component in the passive
serum transfer process. Phase contrast microscopic analysis of
AD755a cells after interaction with the B6 immune serum and normal
B6 peritoneal exudate cells, both in vivo and in vitro, demonstrated
the induction of large mononuclear cell attachment to the tumor cells
(Fig. 5). This response was not observed when normal B6 mouse serum
was substituted and suggests that the B6 anti-AD755a serum may be
capable of activating macrophages or other mononuclear cells for
tumor cell destruction. It is of interest in this regard that antisera directed against FLV or FLV-producing cells which are not protective, also do not have the capacity to form rosettes in vivo. It
is thus possible that the protective factor is a cytophilic antibody
with affinity for a host effector cell, presumably a macrophage. Because of the previously described viral specificity of the tumor rejection process, we tentatively postulate that a viral component remains the principal candidate for the target antigen, but that its
function in this regard can only be demonstrated through a cooperative action between the antibody and the appropriate effector cell.
Studies are planned to identify this component and the corresponding
antibody population through in vitro and in vivo assays involving
effector cells.

CONCLUDING REMARKS

    In summary, AD755a can be used as an animal model system of
tumor rejection that involves lymphoid cell and serum factors.
This system can serve in the examination of the immune recognition
and immune response mechanisms participating in tumor rejection, as
well as in the study of mouse strain-specific interactions between
serum factors and lymphoid cells, which may possibly mediate the
observed transfer of tumor immunity.

The strain dependence of serum transfer protection was found to be controlled by a locus linked to agouti which itself is situated on linkage group V, chromosome 2. No function has been mapped in this region which could account for the phenomenon observed suggesting that the locus controlling protection by serum transfer is a new discovery. Extensive fine mapping using appropriate congenic and recombinant inbred strains is in progress to better establish its location.

Several parameters thus far noted in this system may reflect the function of this locus. These include (1) genes controlling various activities related to the virus associated with the AD755a tumors, particularly those which might affect the immune system of the recipient; or (2) immune response functions which regulate the cooperative effects between the protective antibody and the host effector cells, which might include factors such as Fc receptor specificity for the protective antibody. Based on recent studies by Greene et al. (9), an additional consideration might be a powerful effect of this serum on suppressor cells. These workers demonstrated a similarly potent anti-tumor effect using minute quantities of anti-suppressor cell antisera.

The question of antigenic specificity remains elusive. The data obtained thus far strongly suggest a viral related component as the antigen involved in both the generation of protective antibody and as a target for tumor rejection. The best candidate for the antigen at present is the gp71 surface glycoprotein of ADV. However, we would have to postulate that two forms of antibody to this antigen are produced during our immunization procedure. One is a classical antibody and can be measured in virus neutralization, cytotoxicity and radioimmunoassay analyses and can be efficiently absorbed with virus or target cells. The other is a cytophilic antibody with a weak affinity for the target cell in the absence of the effector cell. In the presence of lymphoid cells and target cells, however, this antibody induces rosette formation, linking the target and effector cells very efficiently. Antibodies with similar functions have also been described by Haskill and colleagues (10,11). Studies are now in progress to determine the nature of this antibody subclass and the mechanism by which it induces rosette formation.

Having noted the powerful protective function of antiserum prepared as described against AD755a tumor challenge, we have prepared similar antisera against other murine tumors. Such sera also demonstrate strong anti-tumor effects, particularly against virus associated sarcomas (see Table 8). Application of this principle to sarcomas in cats induced by the Snyder-Theilen strain of feline sarcoma virus caused a dramatic regression of lethal tumors in 8 of 9 cats at a relatively late stage of tumor growth, where the primary tumors were more than 7 cm in diameter and the animals were near death. Studies to determine whether cytophilic antibodies are involved in this form of tumor rejection are also in progress (de Noronha and Bolognesi, in preparation).

REFERENCES

1. Haagensen, Jr., D. E., Roloson, G., Collins, J. J., Wells, Jr., S. A., Bolognesi, D. P. and Hansen, H. J. (1978). J. Nat. Cancer Inst. 60:131-139.

2. Wolfe, H. G. and Coleman, D. L. (1966). In: "Biology of the Laboratory Mouse", 2nd Ed. (Earl L. Green, ed.), McGraw-Hill Book Company, New York, N. Y. pp. 405-425.

3. Brandes, D. and Groth, D. P. (1960). Cancer Res. 20:1205-1207.

4. Collins, J. J., Roloson, G., Haagensen, Jr., D. E., Fischinger, P. J., Wells, Jr., S. A., Holder, W. and Bolognesi, D. P. (1978). J. Nat. Cancer Inst. 60:141-152.

5. Siegert, W. E., Fenyo, E. M. and Klein, G. (1977). Int. J. Cancer 20:75-82.

6. Fenyo, E. M., Crundner, G. and Klein, E. (1974). J. Nat. Cancer Inst. 52:743-752.

7. Fenyo, E. M., Yefenof, E., Klein, E. and Klein, G. (1977). J. Exp. Med. 146:1521-1533.

8. Stephenson, J. R., Khan, A. S., Sliski, A. H. and Essex, M. (1977). Proc. Nat. Acad. Sci. USA 74:5608-5612.

9. Greene, M. I., Dorf, M. E., Pierres, M. and Benacerraf, B. (1977). Proc. Nat. Acad. Sci. USA 74:5118-5121.

10. Yamamura, Y. (1977). Int. J. Cancer 19:717-724.

11. Yamamura, Y., Virella, G. and Haskill, J. S. (1977). Int. J. Cancer 19:707-716.

12. This work is supported by NIH Grant No. CA19905; Contract No. NCI NO1 CP33308 of the Virus Cancer Program. D. P. Bolognesi is the recipient of an American Cancer Society Faculty Research Award, FRA-141.

THE ROLE OF EBV IN THE ETIOLOGY OF BURKITT'S LYMPHOMA (BL)

GEORGE KLEIN

Department of Tumor Biology

Karolinska Institutet

S 104 01 Stockholm 60, Sweden

Time-space clustering of highly malignant childhood lymphoma that appeared with a remarkably high frequency in the hot and humid regions of tropical Africa and had characteristic histological, cytological and clinical features have led Burkitt to propose that the disease was due to an insect transmitted virus (1). Subsequently, a tumor associated virus has been identified in a suspension culture derived from Burkitt lymphoma tissue, first by electron microscopy (2) and later by serological tests (3). Nucleic acid hybridization (4) and the detection of a virally determined nuclear antigen, EBNA (5), conclusively showed that 97% of the African Burkitt lymphomas from the high endemic regions carry multiple copies of the viral genome in a latent form (6). EBNA is reminiscent of the T-antigen of the small oncogenic DNA viruses. It is the only viral product regularly expressed in all virus-DNA positive cells in vitro and in vivo. Virus production has never been seen in the tumor tissue in vivo. Following in vitro explantation, the viral cycle is switched on in a minority of cells in some lines whereas others remain non producers (7). In some non-producer lines, it is possible to induce the viral cycle by the halogenated pyrimidines, BUDR and IUDR (8,9), and by exposure to certain tumor promotors such as phorbol esters (10).

The isolation of EBV from Burkitt lymphoma lines and its serological identification as a previously unknown herpesvirus that failed to cross react with any other member of the herpes group (11) has led to the rapid development of EBV-research. It has revealed some important facts about the biology of the virus and its interaction with its host, the B-lymphocyte. They will be summarized briefly since they are essential for a discussion of the etiological role of a virus in Burkitt's lymphoma.

Biology of EBV

The virus can infect human and some non-human primate B-lymphocytes in vitro but no other tissues so far tested. In vivo, the virus has only been found in one tissue that was not derived from B-lymphocytes, namely the epithelial cells of nasopharyngeal carcinoma (12).

EBV receptors have only been found on B-lymphocytes where they are intimately associated with the complement receptors (13, 14). All laboratory and natural isolates of EBV, with the exception of one laboratory strain (15) "transform" normal lymphocytes into permanently growing, EBV-DNA and EBNA positive lines (16).

Viral adsorption to B cells is followed by penetration and induction of the nuclear antigen, EBNA, as the earliest detectable event (17, 18), occurring after 24-48 hours, this is followed by polyclonal activation of immunoglobulin synthesis (19), and cellular DNA synthesis that appears to represent a true S-phase (18, 20). Subsequently, large cell clumps are formed and, in one or two weeks, an 100% EBNA positive cell line grows out. Established lines carry multiple viral genomes, as a rule, similarly to the Burkitt tumor in vivo (21, 22). In both types of cells, a few copies of the viral genome are covalently integrated with the host cell DNA, whereas the majority are present in the form of free plasmids with covalently closed circular DNA (23). The interrelationships of the integrated and the plasmid forms are not known.

In vitro EBV-transformed lymphoblastoid cell lines (LCL) are initially purely diploid (24). As long as they remain diploid, they fail to grow in nude mice and do not plate in agarose or only at a very low efficiency (25). After serial in vitro passage for several months or years, they tend to become aneuploid and acquire the ability to grow in agarose and cause tumors in nude mice. In contrast, Burkitt lymphoma biopsies and derived lines have not been found purely dipoloid in any case so far studied (24). Most of them carry the same characteristic chromosome aberration (see below). They are regularly tumorigenic in nude mice and grow in agarose. This implies that in vitro immortalization cannot be equated with in vivo tumorigenicity, although it may be a prerequisite for it. For malignant growth in vivo, additional changes appear to be required, at the cytogenetic level.

Phenotypic changes involved in EBV transformation have been most extensively studied by comparisons between EBV negative but EBV-convertible B-lymphoma lines and their in vitro converted EBNA-positive sublines. Changes detected include increased cellular resistance to saturation con-

ditions (26), decreased serum requirement (27), independence of a dia-
lysable serum factor (28), reduced lateral mobility (capping) of membrane
constituents (29), increased lectin agglutinability (30) and an increased
ability to activate the alternate complement pathway (31). These changes
are reminiscent of the events that are known to accompany the transformation of monolayer cultures by oncogenic DNA (polyoma, SV40) and
RNA (Rous) viruses. It is therefore likely that in vitro immortalization that
can be induced by different viruses and in very diverse target cells, is
accompanied by a characteristic set of phenotypic changes.

        EBV is oncogenic in certain New World monkeys, notably cotton
top marmosets (32) and owl monkeys (33,34,35). It is important to note
that no old World monkeys so far tested were susceptible to the oncogenic
effect of the virus. The reasons for this may be sought in the fact that all
large apes and old World monkeys tested carry EBV-related viruses that induce the formation of EBV-neutralizing cross reactive antibodies. New
World monkeys do not carry EBV-related viruses, although they have lymphotropic herpesviruses of their own (for review see 36). Three EBV-related Old World monkey viruses have been studied, an EBV-related chim-
panzee virus (37), a baboon virus, HVP (38) and an orangoutang (39).
Virus carrying B-cell lines have been isolated from seropositive normal
animals in all 3 systems. All 3 viruses show partial DNA homology and
partial antigenic cross reactivity with human EBV but virus-cell relation-
ships are remarkably similar with only some differences of detail (39,40,
41).

        While EBV fails to induce tumors in the Old World monkeys, The
susceptible New World monkey species respond with the development of
EBV-DNA and EBNA positive lymphomas (42). The success rate is not
100% and self-limiting lymphoproliferative lesions have been noted. While
the detailed mechanisms of the oncogenic process remain to be studied
further, the experiments already at hand clearly show the oncogenic potential of the virus.

EBV-related diseases

        Three diseases are clearly associated with EBV, infectious mononu-
cleosis (IM), Burkitt's lymphoma (BL) and nasopharyngeal carcinoma (NPC).

Infectious mononucleosis. It has been proven beyond doubt that the heterophile positive form of IM (and a proportion of the heterophile negatives)
is caused by EBV. The evidence is based on retrospective (43,44) and prospective (45) seroepidemiological data, together with the ready isolability
of infectious (transforming) EBV from the throat washings of IM patients
(46,47,48), the easy establishment of permanent EBV-carrying lines from
the peripheral blood of IM patients (49) and the demonstration of EBNA-

positive cells as a minority fraction of the circulating B-cells (50,51).
A fatal case of IM showed extensive infiltration of the lymphoid tissues
with EBNA-positive B-cells (52). The apparently "irrelevant" antibody formation of acute IM patients against a variety of unrelated antigens (including the heterophile reaction) may be due to the polyclonal B-cell activation that occurs during a primary EBV-infection.

During acute IM, EBV-specific killer T-cells appear in the peripheral circulation (53,54). They disappear in convalescence (55). They
kill EBV-carrying lines and EBV-positive Burkitt biopsies without any apparent HLA restriction but fail to kill EBV negative cell lines. It may be
surmised that the killer T cells play an important role in the rejection of
the EBV-transformed B-blasts. More or less malignant forms of IM, including chronic IM, have been described and may be related to a deficiency
of the normal rejection mechanism against EBV-transformed cells (56a,56b).

Burkitt's lymphoma. As already mentioned, 97% of the African Burkitt lymphomas examined were found to be EBV-DNA and EBNA positive (6). In
contrast, only 22% of the non-african (sporadic) BL cases were found to
carry the viral genome (57). This raises the important question whether
the virus carrying and the virus negative BL represents the same disease
entity. Since the histopathological diagnosis of BL is not based on sharply
defined criteria, it is concievable thet the virus positive and negative
forms represent two different diseases (58). The possibility that they may
represent the same disease is discussed in connection with the cytogenetic
evidence below. Whichever theory one favours, the fact that Burkitt's lymphoma was defined as a clinical and histopathological entity prior to the
discovery of EBV implies that the question is in reexamination, preferably
by unbiased histopathological and prospective clinical studies.

Burkitt's lymphoma is a uniclonal tumor, as conclusively shown by
the G6PD method (59) studies of immunoglobulin synthesis (60), and the
cytogenetic evidence discussed below. Fialkow et al. (59) have also approached the question whether recurring tumors represent regrowth of the
same original clone or, at least ocassionally, a new induction event. The
original clone recurred in all studied cases except one. In one case, a
tertiary tumor that arose in a patient exposed to heavy chemotherapy was
derived from a different clone, probably due to a second induction event.
BL-lines differ from EBV-transformed lymphoblastoid cell lines (LCL)
of non-neoplastic origin with regard to multiple phenotypic properties (61).
While different BL lines tend to be quite different among themselves, each
line is usually very uniform within itself. In contrast, LCL:s are rather heterogeneous within each line, but different LCL:s are very similar. These
differences may reflect the uniclonal vs. polyclonal nature of BL vs. LCL.

Cytogenetic features.

Approximately 90% of the in vivo BL tumors studied were found to contain the same 14q+ marker (24,62,63). The marker arises by the addition of an extra band at the end of the long arm of one No. 14. Zech et al. (24) showed that the extra material is consistently derived from the distal part of the long arm of No. 8. The remaining 10% BL that had no M14 had other chromosomal anomalies.

14q+ markers have been also found in EBV-negative Burkitt lymphomas (24). Also, 14q+ markers of similar or more or less similar appearance were found in non-Burkitt lymphomas of both lymphocytic and histiocytic types (24,64,66,67,68,69,70). These studies raised interesting questions concerning the origin of the extra material on No. 14 in these cases, and the cytogenetical relationship between different histopathological types of lymphomas.

Very recently, Mark et al. (71) studied the banding patterns in 6 histiocytic lymphomas. The authors reviewed their results together with data from 32 further non-Hodgkin and non-Burkitt lymphomas in the literature. They have drawn the following conclusions: i) No. 14 was most commonly affected, usually by structural deviations involving its long arm, preferentially band q32; this resulted in the formation of 14q+ markers, as a rule, found in 17 of the 45 cases: the extra material on No. 14 showed inconsistent derivation, in contrast to Burkitt lymphomas; ii) Nos. 3, 7, 8 and 11 were next in frequency of involvement; structural deviations predominated for Nos. 3 and 11, and some recurrent marker types were seen; Nos. 7 and 8 were mostly affected by numerical deviations, usually gains for No. 7 and losses for No. 8. iii) Structural deviations often affected Nos. 1, 6, 9 and 13 and recurrent marker types related to Nos. 6 and 13 were seen. iv) The centromeric and the light-staining regions were preferentially affected by the breakpoints.

While the significance of the chromosome 14 anomaly for Burkitt's and other lymphomas is not known, it is tempting to speculate that it may be related to the liberation of the normal human lymphocyte from superimposed growth control. In this respect, it is of interest that McCaw et al. (72) found a remarkable instability of chromosome 14 in ataxia teleangiectasia (AT), a condition that predisposes for leukemia, lymphomas and other neoplasias. Recently, Cohen et al. identified a 14q+ marker that closely resembled the BL associated marker, in mitogen stimulated peripheral lymphocytes of AT patients (73). The interpretation of the chromosome 14 anomaly in human lymphomas may be facilitated by considering some recent findings on murine lymphomas. The majority of T-cell derived mouse lymphomas of spontaneous (74), x-ray induced (75), viral (76), and chemical (DMBA) origin (77) had the same anomaly, chromosome 15-trisomy. T-cell

lymphomas with rearranged (translocated) karyotypes had a cryptic 15-tri-
somy (77). In contrast, murine non-T cell lymphomas had no 15-trisomy.

Etiology of BL.

Several questions can now be asked that may illuminate the etiology
of BL. Most of them are answerable by available evidence and/or by further studies.

a) Is EBV a passenger in BL that is picked up after the tumor has
been induced by other agents or is it present from the inception of the
tumor ?

EBV-negative but in vitro EBV-convertible B-cell lymphomas have
been found in EBV-seropositive (i.e. infected) patients (78,79). This shows
that an EBV infection does not readily "jump" onto lymphomas that arise
for other reasons. This is understandable since chronically EBV-infected
persons have high neutralizing antibody levels that can stop in vitro infection with great efficiency (80,81). It appears more likely that the EBV-
carrying monoclonal lymphomas arise oroginally from an EBV positive cell.
It is clear that the virus can remain latent indefinitely in B-lymphocytes.
In vitro, such lymphocytes are immortal and they probably have long life
span in vivo as well. Under certain conditions, e.g. prolonged growth stimulation, they may undergo secondary changes and occasionally give rise
to an autonomous clone.

b) What is the EBV-infection status of an African child prior to BL
development, in comparison with healthy controls from the same area ?

This question is now partially answerable by the recent prospective
seroepidemiological study of de The' and Geser (81). Anti-EBV (VCA) antibody titers of children who developed BL 7-21 months after the bleeding
were significantly higher than in controls from the same region. Invariably,
they showed signs of chronic EBV-infection with IgG anti VCA and anti-
EBNA antibodies but no IgM anti VCA. This is clearly different from the
serological picture seen in acute primary infection (in the course of IM)
where IgM anti VCA is the predominating antibody and anti-EBNA antibodies are absent, as a rule. It is therefore clear that Burkitt's lymphoma
clone arises in chronically EBV-infected children, in contrast to IM. It is
likely that the pre-BL child carries a higher virus load than controls. This
would fit with the role postulated for EBV-carrying preneoplastic cells in
the genesis of BL, as postulated under a) above.

c) What is the explanation for the peculiar geographical pathology
of high endemic BL ?

Burkitt (82) has suggested that an insect transmitted co-factor, probably chronic holoendemic malaria, precipitates the development of BL.

His reasoning is suggestive but not conclusive. It is quite concievable that chronic malaria or other insect vectored diseases act as "promotors", if the word is used in the same sense as in experimental carcinogenesis. Promoting agents would be expected to exert a chronic growth stimulation on the "dormant" or preneoplastic cells. In addition, they may delay or inhibit differentiation and also act as immunosuppressants. In the actual context, the heavy chronic proliferation of holoendemic malaria would urge the long-lived EBV-carrying, preneoplastic B-lymphocytes to proliferate. This would increase the chances for the generation of chromosomal aberrations. When the "right" cytogenetic change arises by chance, postulated as the ultimate cause of the malignant growth, autonomous neoplasia would arise.

In conclusion, the genesis of Burkitt's lymphoma is visualized as proceeding in three steps:

I. Primary EBV infection affects the young child, probably at a relatively high multiplicity. It immortalizes a certain number of B-lymphocytes in vivo.

II. This is followed by the impact of an environmental promoting agent, perhaps chronic holoendemic malaria, providing a chronic stimulus to the proliferation of the EBV-carrying preneoplastic cells.

III. Chromosomally abnormal variants appear in the stimulated tissue by chance. After certain types of changes, particularly the 8 to 14 translocation that leads to the 14q+ marker, the affected B lymphocyte would no longer obey the negative feedback controls that would otherwise restrict its proliferation in vivo.

Since III is regarded as the essential, ultimate change, it follows that I and II are only facultative. This may explain the existence of EBV-negative Burkitt lymphomas where initiation may have been due to other, viral or non-viral agents. It also explains the fact that the high endemic, time-space clustered cases are not the only form of the disease. Sporadic cases occur all around the world, presumably through the impact of other promotors. Finally, the chromosomal aberrations (III) are also subject to certain variations, as shown by the 10% BL that carry no 14q+ marker but have other anomalies. It is well known, however, that the same phenotypic change can be brought about by multiple genetic changes.

Nasophryngeal carcinoma will not be discussed here in detail, since it is obviously outside the subject matter of this treatise. It may be sufficient to state that the association between the viral genome and the low differentiated or anaplastic form of the disease is 100% so far (83) and occurs equally in high and low incidence ethnic groups. The viral genome and EBNA are localized in the epithelial (carcinoma) cell, although it is not clear how it gets there. Explanations of NPC etiology meet a similar dilemma as BL since it is necessary to reconcile a relatively rare disease with a ubiquitous virus. Unlike BL, genetic rather than environmental co-factors must be envisaged in NPC (84).

REFERENCES

(1) Burkitt, D. In: Treatment of Burkitt's Tumours. (J.H. Burchenal and D.P. Burkitt, eds.), UICC Monogr. pp. 94-101. Springer-Verlag, Berlin and New York (1967).

(2) Epstein, M.A., Achong, B.G., and Barr, Y.M., Lancet, 1, 702 (1964).

(3) Henle, G. and Henle, W., J. Bacteriol., 91, 1248 (1966).

(4) zur Hausen, H., Schulte-Holthausen, H., Klein, G., Henle, W., Henle, G., Clifford, P. and Santesson, L., Nature, 228, 1056 (1970).

(5) Reedman, B.M. and Klein, G., Int. J. Cancer, 11, 499 (1973).

(6) Klein, G., Cold Spring Harbor Symp. on Quant. Biol., 39, 783 (1975).

(7) Nadkarni, J.S., Nadkarni, J.J., Klein, G., Henle, W., Henle, G. and Clifford, P., Int. J. Cancer, 6, 10 (1970).

(8) Gerber, P., Proc. Nat. Acad. Sci. USA 69, 83 (1972).

(9) Klein, G. and Dombos, L., Int. J. Cancer, 11, 327 (1973).

(10) zur Hausen, H., O'Neill, F.J., Freese, U.K. and Hecker, E., Nature, 272, 373 (1978).

(11) Henle, G. and Henle, W., Cancer Res., 27, 2442 (1967).

(12) Andersson-Anvret, M., Forsby, N. and Klein, G., In: Progr. Exp. Tumor Res., 21, 100, ed. Karger, Basel (1978).

(13) Yefenof, E., Klein, G., Jondal, M. and Oldstone, M.B.A., Int. J. Cancer, 17, 693 (1976).

(14) Yefenof, E., and Klein, G., Int. J. Cancer, 20, 347 (1977).

(15) Menzes, J., Leibold, W. and Klein, G., Exp. Cell Res., 92, 478 (1975).

(16) Miller, G., Yale J. Biol. Med., 43, 358 (1971).

(17) Leibold, W., Flanagan, T.D., Menezes, J. and Klein, G., J. Nat. Cancer Inst., 54, 65 (1975).

(18) Einhorn, L. and Ernberg, I., Int. J. Cancer, 21, 157 (1978).

(19) Rosen, A., Gergely, P., Jondal, M., Klein, G. and Britton, S., Nature, 267, 52 (1977).

(20) Robinson, J. and Miller, G., J. Virol. 15, 1065 (1975).

(21) Nonoyama, M., and Pagano, J.S., Nature New Biol. 233, 103 (1973).

(22) zur Hausen, H., and Schulte-Holthausen, H., Nature, 227, 245 (1970).

(23) Adams, A., In: The Epstein-Barr Virus, A.M. Epstein and R. Achong eds., in press.

(24) Zech, L., Haglund, U., Nilsson, K. and Klein, G., Int. J. Cancer, 17, 47 (1976).

(25) Nilsson, K., Giovanella, B.C., Stehlin, J.S. and Klein, G., Int. J. Cancer, 19, 337 (1977).

(26) Steinitz, M. and Klein, G., Proc. Nat. Acad. Sci. USA 72,3518 (1975).

(27) Steinitz, M. and Klein, G., Europ. J. Cancer, 13, 1269 (1977).

(28) Steinitz, M. and Klein, G., Virol., 70, 570 (1976).

(29) Yefenof, E., and Klein, G., Exp. Cell Res., 99, 175 (1976).

(30) Yefenof, E., Klein, G., Ben-Bassat, H. and Lundin, L., Exp. Cell Res., 108, 185 (1977).

(31) McConnell, I., Klein, G., Lint, T.F. and Lachmann, P.J., Europ. J. Immunol., in press.

(32) Shope, T., Dechairo, D., and Miller, G., Proc. Nat. Acad. Sci. USA 70, 2487 (1973).

(33) Epstein, M.A., Hunt, R.D. and Rabin, H., Int. J. Cancer 12, 309 (1973).

(34) Epstein, M. A., Rabin, H., Ball, G., Rickinson, A.B., Jarvis, L. and Melendez, L.V., Int. J. Cancer 12, 319 (1973).

(35) Epstein, M.A., zur Hausen, H., Ball, G., and Rabin, H., Int. J. Cancer 15, 17 (1975).

(36) Deinhardt, F.W., Falk, L.A. and Wolfe, L.G., Adv. Cancer Res., 19, 167 (1974).

(37) Gerber, P., Kalter, S.S., Schidlovsky, G., Peterson, W.D. Jr. and

Daniel, M.D., Int. J. Cancer 20, 448 (1977).

(38) Falk, L., Henle, G., Henle, W., Deinhardt, F. and Schudel, A., Int. J. Cancer, in press.

(39) Rabin, H., Neubauer, R.H., Hopkins, R.F. and Nonoyama, M., Int. J. Cancer, in press.

(40) Ohno, S., Luka, J., Falk, L. Klein, G., Int. J. Cancer 20, 941 (1977).

(41) Klein, G., Falk, L. and Falk, K., Intervirol., in press.

(42) Frank, A., Andiman, W.A. and Miller, G., Adv. Cancer Res. 23, 171 (1976).

(43) Henle, G., Henle, W. and Diehl, V., Proc. Nat. Acad. Sci. 59, 94 (1968).

(44) Evans, A.S., Niederman, J.C. and McCollum, R.W., New Engl. J. Med. 279, 1121 (1968)

(45) Niederman, J.C., Evans, A.S., Subrahmanyam, L. and McCollum, R.W., New Engl. J. Med. 282, 361 (1970).

(46) Gerber, P., Nkrumah, F.K., Pritchett, R., and Kieff, E., Int. J. Cancer 17, 71 (1976).

(47) Golden, H.D., Chang, R.S., Prescott, W., Simpson, E., and Cooper, T.Y., J. Infect. Dis. 127, 471 (1973).

(48) Niederman, J.C., Miller, G., Pearson, H.A., Pagano, J.S. and Dowaliby, J.M., New Engl. J. Med. 294, 1355 (1976).

(49) Diehl, V., Henle, G., Henle, W., and Kohn, G., J. Virol. 2, 663 (1968).

(50) Klein, G., Svedmyr, E., Jondal, M. and Persson, P.O., Int. J. Cancer 17, 21 (1976).

(51) Hinuma, Y. and Katsuki, T., Int. J. Cancer 21, 426 (1978).

(52) Britton, S., Andersson-Anvret, M., Gergely, P., Henle, W., Jondal, M., Klein, G., Sandstedt, B. and Svedmyr, E., New Engl. J. Med. 298, 89 (1978).

(53) Svedmyr, E. and Jondal, M., Proc. Nat. Acad. Sci. 72, 1622 (1975).

(54) Bakacs, T., Svedmyr, E., Klein, E., and Rombo, L. and Klein, G., submitted for publ.

(55) Svedmyr, E., Jondal, M., Henle, W., Weiland, O., Rombo, L.

and Klein, G., submitted for publ.

(56) Purtilo, D.T., Cassel, C. and Yang, J.P.S., New Engl. J. Med.,
      291, 736 (1974).

      Purtilo, D.T., Cassel, C. and Yang, J.P.S., Cassel, C., Allegra,
      S. and Rosen, F.S., Clin. Immunol. Immunopathol. 9, 147 (1978).

(57) Ziegler, J.L., Andersson, M., Klein, G. and Henle, W., Int. J.
      Cancer 17, 701 (1976).

(58) zur Hausen, H., Biochim. Biophys. Acta 417, 25 (1975).

(59) Fialkow, P.J., Klein, G., Gartler, S.M. and Clifford, P., Lancet,
      1, 384 (1970).

(60) Fialkow, P.J., Klein, E., Klein, G., Clifford, P. and Singh, S.,
      J. Exp. Med. 138, 89 (1973).

(61) Nilsson, K. and Ponten, J., Int. J. Cancer 15, 321 (1975).

(62) Manolov, G. and Manolova, Y., Nature 237, 33 (1972).

(63) Jarvis, J.E., Ball, G., Rickinson, A.B. and Epstein, M.A., Int.
      J. Cancer 14, 716 (1974).

(64) Reeves, B.R., Humangenetik 20, 231 (1973).

(65) Prigogina, E.L. and Fleischman, E.W., Humangenetik 30, 109 (1975).

(66) Mark, J., Hereditas 81, 289 (1975).

(67) Fukuhara, S., Shirakawa, S. and Uchino, H., Nature 259, 210
      (1976).

(68) Fleischman, E.W. and Prigogina, E.A., Humangenetik 35, 269 (1977)

(69) Mark, J., Adv. Cancer Res. 74, 165 (1977).

(70) Yamada, K., Yoshioka, M. and Oami, H., J. Nat. Cancer Inst.,
      59, 1193 (1977).

(71) Mark, J., Ekedahl, C. and Dahlenfors, R., Hereditas, in press.

(72) McCaw, B.K., Hecht, F., Harnden, D. and Teplitz, R.L., Proc.
      Nat. Acad. Sci. 72, 2071 (1975).

(73) Cohen, M.M., personal communication.

(74) Dofoku, R., Biedler, J.L., Spengler, B.A. and Old, L.J., Proc.
      Nat. Acad. Sci. 72, 1515 (1975).

(75) Chang, T.D., Biedler, J.L., Stockert, E. and Old, L.J., Proc.
      Am. Assoc. Cancer Res., abstract 225 (1977).

(76) Wiener, F., Ohno, S., Spira, J., Haran-Ghera, N. and Klein, G.
      J. Nat. Cancer Inst., in press.

(77) Wiener, F., Spira, J., Ohno, S., Haran-Ghera, N. and Klein, G.,
      submitted for publ.

(78) Klein, G., Giovanella, B., Westman, A., Stehlin, J.S. and
      Mumford, D., Intervirol., 5, 319 (1975).

(79) Menezes, J., Leibold, W., Klein, G. and Clements, G., Biomed.
      22, 276 (1975).

(80) de Schryver, A., Klein, G., Hewetson, J. Rocchi, G., Henle, W.,
      Henle, G., Moss, D.J. and Pope, J.H., Int. J. Cancer 13, 353
      (1974).

(81) de Thé, T. and Geser, A., C.R. Acad. Sc. Paris 282, 1387 (1976).

(82) Burkitt, D., J. Nat. Cancer Inst., 42, 19 (1969).

(83) Andersson-Anvret, M., Forsby, N., Klein, G. and Henle, W.,
      Int. J. Cancer 20, 486 (1977).

(84) Ho, J.H.C., Adv. Cancer Res. 15, 57 (1972).

FELINE LEUKEMIA AND IMMUNOLOGICAL SURVEILLANCE

M. Essex,[1] C.K. Grant,[1] A.H. Sliski,[1] and
W.D. Hardy, Jr.[2]

[1]Department of Microbiology, Harvard University School
of Public Health, Boston, Massachusetts 02115
[2]Memorial Sloan Kettering Cancer Center, New York
New York 10025 USA

INTRODUCTION

According to the immunological surveillance hypothesis, newly
arising clones of tumor cells will be recognized as foreign and
subsequently eliminated (Burnet, 1970). When proposed, this concept
seemed simple and logical even though evidence for effective tumor
immunity was not available at the time. As homograft rejection was
immunologically mediated, however, the most rational phylogenetic
purpose for this phenomenon was the development of immunological
surveillance to control or prevent tumor cell growth.

Contrary to expectation, clear support for the immunosurveillance hypothesis was hard to find, especially when considered in
relation to spontaneous tumors. Numerous explanations were provided
for the absence of supporting evidence, and by the time a given case
of cancer was diagnosed it was clear that the individual being
studied had lost the battle and that the immune response had failed.
If immune resistance toward transformed cell clones was being exer-
cised under normal circumstances, this resistance must have been
functional when numbers of malignant cells were large enough to
exert an immunogenic effect (e.g., 10^4-10^6), but small enough to be
controlled by a successful response (e.g., not more than 10^7-10^9).
Until tumor cell surface antigen markers are available for seroepidemiologic studies, it will obviously be difficult to identify
those individuals who experience successful immunosurveillance
responses.

Surface changes on cells transformed with chemicals or irra--
diation are generally antigenically specific for each primary clone
of tumor cells (Klein, 1968). Conversely, virus-transformed cells
or virus-induced tumors express group specific cell surface antigens that cross react for all cells altered by a given virus, regardless of individual, strain, or specie characteristics. This
property obviously makes the virus--associated models more adaptable
for experimental studies in tumor immunology. Detracting from the
usefulness of these tumor models is the concern expressed by many
that the virus induced tumors are "laboratory artifacts," occurring
only with artificially selected viruses and/or in artificially
selected strains of mice.

In at least one outbred free-living mamalian species, the cat,
spontaneous lymphomas, leukemias, and fibrosarcomas are caused by
infectious agents under natural conditions (Hardy et al., 1973;
Jarrett et al., 1973; Essex 1975a). The etiologic agents that cause
these malignancies are RNA tumor viruses (see Essex 1975a for review).
If a virus-induced tumor model is to be representative of the situation in man where replicating oncogenic viruses are not found,
then virus-associated tumor antigens must be expressed independently
from virus replication and the antigens must be distinct from the
virus structural proteins.

In the feline model these criteria are met. The target for
tumor immunity is the feline oncornavirus associated cell membrane
antigen (FOCMA) which is expressed independently from the virus
structural proteins and from virus replication (Essex et al., this
volume). FOCMA is highly immonogenic under natural conditions, and
an effective response to FOCMA appears to protect animals from
development of tumors. Thus, a strong case exists for a natural
immunosurveillance mechanism in at least one outbred mammalian
specie (Essex et al., 1975e; Essex 1977).

NATURAL HISTORY OF THE DISEASES

Feline lymphoid malignancies occur primarily as thymic, multicentric, or alimentary lymphomas, or as acute lymphoblastic leukemia (for review see Essex, 1975b). The tumor target cell is
usually, though not always, a T (thymus-derived) cell (Hardy et al.,
1977). These diseases occur in both young and old cats, at a
relative frequency of at least 40 cases per 100,000 per year (Dorn
et al., 1967). In the majority of cases (70-75%) the feline leukemia virus (FeLV) is readily detectable in animals with tumors
(Essex et al., 1975b) replicating both from tumor cells and epithelial tissues (Jarret et al., 1977). Infectious FeLV is excreted
in high levels in saliva (Francis et al., 1977).

The majority of cats living under free-roaming or group conditions have serologic evidence of previous exposure to FeLV (Essex
et al., 1975a; Rogerson et al., 1975; Grant et al., 1978a). Most
cats exposed to FeLV under natural conditions only undergo transient
viremia and either eliminate the virus or suppress replication with
an efficient virus neutralizing antibody response (Francis and
Essex, 1978). In unusual cases, persistent viremia develops (Hardy
et al., 1973, 1976; Essex et al., 1975c,d), which may last at least
5 years before the cat succumbs to leukemia or other virus-related
diseases (Francis and Essex, 1978). The time period between initial
virus infection and subsequent disease development is usually prolonged many months or several years, and the major factors which
influence disease outcome are age of the animal at the time of
initial exposure, the dose and strain of FeLV involved, and probably
the genetic background of the animal. Resistance to both viremia
and disease development appear to be immunologically mediated.

Fibrosarcoma occurs less frequently than leukemia (Essex, 1975b).
Most cases of multicentric fibrosarcoma that occur in young cats
readily yield replication-defective transforming feline sarcoma
virus(es) (FeSV) that exist in conjunction with helper FeLV-type
viruses (Essex and Snyder, 1973; Hardy 1974). The incubation period
for this disease under natural conditions is unknown. When young
kittens are inoculated with FeSV they usually develop rapidly progressing tumors that subsequently metastasize and kill the animal
(Essex and Snyder, 1973; Snyder and Dungworth, 1973). When adult
animals are inoculated with the same doses of FeSV they ordinarily
develop either no visible tumors, or tumors that grow only transiently and subsequently regress (Essex et al., 1971b).

DISTINCTION BETWEEN ANTI-VIRAL AND ANTI-TUMOR RESPONSES

Unlike the situation with the murine oncornaviruses, all FeLV
antigens appear to be immunogenic for the feline host under optimal
conditions (Essex et al., 1977a,b; Stephenson et al., 1977a,b).
The gag gene virus core proteins, designated p15, p12, p30 and p10,
all elicit antibodies which can be detected by radioimmunoprecipitation or by fixed-cell immunofluorescence with FeLV producer target
cells (Stephenson et al., 1977a,b). The pol gene product, reverse
transcriptase, also elicits antibodies in cats that resisted persistent infections while residing in households that provide constant horizontal exposure to FeLV (Jacquemin et al., 1978). The
same cats readily produce high levels of antibodies to gp70, the
main envelope gene product, which occurs both on the surface of
FeLV particles and on membranes of FeLV-producer cells (Essex et al.,
1977a,b, 1978a,b; Stephenson et al., 1977a,b). Anti-gp70 antibody
activity neutralizes the virus, and appears to be responsible for
the termination and/or prevention of persistent viremia (Hardy et
al., 1976; Noronha et al., 1978).

Cats inoculated with FeSV elicit high titers of FOCMA antibody if they resist development of progressive fibrosarcomas (Essex et al., 1971a,b; Essex and Snyder 1973). See Table 1. A similar correlation was found between resistance to development of FeLV induced leukemia (Jarrett et al., 1973; Essex 1974), and cats with naturally occurring leukemia and lymphoma regularly lacked significant levels of FOCMA antibody (Essex et al., 1975b). See Table 1.

In the case of laboratory induced tumors, it was clear that the inadequate anti-FOCMA response preceded and/or predisposed the animal to the growing tumor burden rather than simply resulting from it, as it might occur due to a soaking up of antibody by the tumor cells (Schaller et al., 1975). To evaluate the same question in cats with naturally occurring lymphoid malignancies a long-term prospective serological study was conducted among cats known to be at high risk for leukemia development (Cotter et al., 1974; Essex et al., 1975c). In support of the immunosurveillance hypothesis, cats that subsequently developed malignancies also lacked protective levels of anti-FOCMA for varying intervals before the malignancies were clinically apparent (Essex et al., 1975e).

Healthy cats, under continuous exposure to FeLV in leukemia cluster households, often resist the development of persistent viremia and have serologic evidence for antibodies to all virion proteins. In such cases, the same animals usually have high antibody titers to FOCMA, the transformation and tumor specific antigen (Sliski et al., 1977, 1978; Stephenson et al., 1977b; Essex et al., this volume). In the same leukemia cluster households a minority population (e.g., 20-30%) of the healthy cats remain persistently viremic for at least several years, harboring high levels (10^4-10^6/ml) of infectious virus in both plasma and saliva (Essex et al., 1975c; Francis et al., 1977). Such cats never have significant levels of free antibody to any of the virus structural proteins described above (which may be at least partly due to a soaking up of any antibodies that are produced by circulating virus) but they do have significant antibody titers to FOCMA (Essex 1977, Essex et al., 1977b). Additionally, cats which resist the development of FeSV-induced progressing fibrosarcomas and develop high plasma levels of anti-FOCMA antibodies may still maintain a persisting viremia (Aldrich and Pedersen, 1974).

An effective immune response to FeLV gp70 presumably provides some degree of protection against tumor development by eliminating the oncogenic agent before significant numbers of tumor cells are transformed within the animal (Hardy et al., 1976; Noronha et al., 1978). The FeLV gp70 is also expressed on the membranes of FeLV producer cells (Ruscetti and Parks, 1977; Noronha et al., 1977; Essex et al., 1978a,b). Additionally, goat antibody to gp70 will lyse these cells in the presence of complement, and passive administration has been shown to cause regression of growing FeSV induced

TABLE 1. ANTIBODY TITERS TO FOCMA ACCORDING TO HEALTH STATUS
AND ENVIRONMENTAL EXPOSURE

Description	Number and Percent of Cats with FOCMA Antibody Titer of:			Total Tested	Geo-metric Mean
	<4	4–16	16		
FeSV inoculated regressors[a]	0	20(61)	13(39)	33	20.3
FeSV inoculated progressors	37(88)	5(12)	0	42	0.6
Spontaneous leukemia	37(82)	8(18)	0	45	0.8
Spontaneous lymphoma	42(95)	2(5)	0	44	0.3
Subsequently developed leukemia	8(100)	0	0	8	1.4
Healthy FeLV-exposed field controls	6(14)	28(65)	9(21)	43	11.0
Healthy unexposed laboratory cats	218(99)	3(1)	0	221	0

[a] Either tumors originally developed and subsequently regressed
(25 animals), or no palpable tumors were observed at inoculation
site (8 animals).

fibrosarcomas (Noronha et al., 1977). Anti-gp70 antisera are not
specific to tumor cells, however, and they lyse all virus producer
cells, whether normal or malignant. Nevertheless, an anti-gp70
response could provide an important first line of defense against
FeLV associated diseases and thereby provide the rational for
virus vaccination in this species. Wherever the anti-FeLV response
is ineffective, however, the anti-FOCMA response remains functional,
and this accounts for the population of FeLV carrier animals that
resist tumor development.

Using serum samples from viremic and non-viremic cats demonstrating tumor immunity, we compared anti-FOCMA titers for the
cultured cat lymphoma cells (which are positive for FOCMA, FeLV gp70,
and FeLV p30), to titers obtained on FeSV transformed mink nonproducer cells (FOCMA positive, but negative for FeLV gp70 and p30
antigens) (Sliski et al., 1977,1978). See Table 2. In the case
of viremic cats, the titers seen on FOCMA positive virus producer
cat lymphoma cells were similar to those found on FOCMA positive
virus negative FeSV-transformed mink nonproducer cells. The same
anti-FOCMA containing viremic sera showed no reactivity for control
FeLV producer FOCMA negative nontransformed cells. Conversely,
antisera from nonviremic animals sometimes contained slightly higher
antibody titers when assayed on FOCMA positive FeLV producer cells.

If anti-FOCMA and anti-gp70 responses are controlled by independent immune response genes, then an effective anti-FOCMA response
in the absence of an effective anti-gp70 response might be expected
in some cats. Equally, we might also expect that some animals would
have anti-gp70 virus neutralizing responses in the absence of anti-
FOCMA responses, especially if the anti-gp70 response was so effective that virus and virus infected normal cells were totally eliminated before any transformed FOCMA positive cells were produced.
If, however, a reasonable number (e.g., 10^3-10^5) of FOCMA positive
cells were generated before the anti-FeLV response took effect, then
in vivo immunoselection might eliminate the gp70 positive FeLV producer cells while allowing FOCMA positive gp70 negative non-producer
tumor cells to "sneak through" and develop into "virus negative"
tumors (Essex et al., this volume).

In the case of RNA sarcoma viruses of mammals and Friend spleen
focus forming leukemia virus, the transforming viruses are a minority
"replication defective" population, existing in the presence of an
excess of replication competent helper virus which is non-transforming for the same target cells (Stephenson et al., 1978). When
cells become infected with only the replication defective transformation competent virus, transformed nonproducer cell clones may
result. Whether or not leukemogenic populations of FeLV might contain a transformation competent (for lymphoid cells), replication
defective minority population of particles is of course unknown.
Quite aside from this possibility, however, various restriction

TABLE 2.   CORRELATION BETWEEN FOCMA ANTIBODY TITERS AS ASSAYED BY
INDIRECT MEMBRANE IMMUNOFLUORESENCE ON VARIOUS
TARGET CELL LINES

Virus Status	Cat Number	Norm[a] Uninf. Mink	Anti-FOCMA Titer on: Nontrans. FeLV Prod. Mink	Trans. Nonprod. Mink	Trans. FeLV Prod. Mink	Trans. FeLV Prod. Cat
Positive	1	<2	<2	16	8	8
	2	<2	<2	16	8	16
	3	<2	<2	32	16	32
	4	<2	<2	32	64	64
	5	<2	<2	16	16	32
	6	<2	<2	16	32	32
	7	<2	<2	16	8	16
	8	<2	<2	16	16	16
	9	<2	<2	32	32	32
	10	<2	<2	32	32	32
	11	<2	<2	32	32	32
	12	<2	<2	16	32	16
	13	<2	<2	64	64	64
	g.m.	<2	<2	23.2	23.2	25.9
Negative	1	<2	128	16	256	256
	2	<2	64	32	256	256
	3	<2	128	32	256	256
	4	<2	64	32	256	256
	5	<2	32	16	128	128
	6	<2	32	32	128	128
	7	<2	64	64	128	256
	8	<2	32	32	128	128
	9	<2	64	16	128	128
	10	<2	32	8	128	128
	11	<2	32	16	64	128
	12	<2	8	8	64	64
	13	<2	32	32	64	64
	14	<2	16	16	32	128
	15	<2	16	32	64	128
	16	<2	8	16	16	8
	17	<2	8	8	16	16
	g.m.	<2	32.2	20.4	92.4	108.7

[a] Abbreviations: norm = normal, uninf. = uninfected, nontrans. =
nontransformed, prod. = producer, trans. = transformed,
nonprod. = nonproducer, g.m. = geometric mean.

mechanisms have been described in murine oncornavirus systems, and
these block the replication of integrated DNA proviruses at both
the transcriptional and translational levels (Aaronson and Stephenson,
1976). Accordingly, it is possible that the anti-viral response
could provide an in vivo immunoselection mechanism for virus negative
tumors.

IMMUNE EFFECTOR MECHANISMS

Systems which allow the study of immune effector mechanisms
directed to well defined tumor specific antigens of spontaneous
tumors have generally not been available. Largely because of this,
most studies of tumor immunity have employed transplantable lines
of tumor cells, or virus-induced tumors where the anti-viral response could not be distinguished from the tumor specific response.
Studies with these models, when successful in identifying any particular immune effector mechanism, have generally implicated the T
cell response, as was predicted on the basis of work done with homograft rejection (Burnet, 1970). A positive correlation between
antibody to tumor cells and tumor resistance was rarely observed
(Essex and Lamon, 1976). Thus, our observation that elevated levels
of anti-FOCMA antibody were correlated with resistance to tumor
development were unexpected.

Because of the close correlation between anti-FOCMA antibody
and tumor resistance, antisera from resistant cats were analyzed
for antibody which was cytotoxic for FOCMA positive lymphoma cells
(Grant et al., 1977a,b, 1978a). A close correlation was observed
between titers of anti-FOCMA antibody, as determined by indirect
membrane immunofluorescence, and complement dependent antibody (CDA)
which specifically directed to the tumor target cell (Grant et al.,
1977a, 1978a). See Table 3. This correlation was significant when
comparing FOCMA antibody titers to CDA titers using either guinea
pig or cat serum as the complement source. The correlation was
closest when cat complement was employed, although lysis occurred
more slowly than might be predicted (Grant et al., 1977a). The
possibility that CDA antibody represents anti-FOCMA as opposed to
antibody to FeLV is greatly strengthened by the observation that
anti-FOCMA containing healthy viremic cats consistently have significant levels of CDA (Grant et al., 1977a, 1978a), since such cats
do not have detectable antibody to any of the FeLV structural proteins (Essex et al., 1977a,b; Stephenson et al., 1977a,b).

Anti-FOCMA tumor immunity is mediated primarily by antibody
plus complement, though we have not ruled out the possibility that
mechanisms such as antibody-dependent cell cytotoxicity
or a T-cell mediated mechanism of immunity might also be important.
However, since the tumor target cell expressing FOCMA is most often
a T lymphocyte, it seems logical that evolutionary pressure would be

TABLE 3.   CORRELATION BETWEEN ANTI-FOCMA AND COMPLEMENT-DEPENDENT
LYTIC ANTIBODIES IN CAT SERA

CDA[a] Titer	Viremia	<4	Anti-FOCMA Titer of:		
			4-8	16-32	>32
<5	+	21(8.1)[b]	1(0.4)	0	0
	−	89(34.4)	7(2.7)	0	0
5	+	1(0.4)	2(0.8)	0	0
	−	4(1.5)	12(4.6)	2(0.8)	0
25	+	1(0.4)	11(4.2)	5(1.9)	3(1.2)
	−	2(0.8)	18(6.9)	19(7.3)	2(0.8)
125	+	0	3(1.2)	5(1.9)	2(0.8)
		0	3(1.2)	23(8.9)	23(8.9)

[a] Complement dependent lytic antibody. Titers of both CDA and anti-FOCMA represent the reciprocal of the highest five-fold or two-fold dilution giving a positive result as determined on FeLV producer lymphoid cells.

[b] Number of cats and percentage of total. A total of 259 cats were tested.

exerted to develop immune effector mechanism(s) that were not T cell dependent.

Since complement alone appears to have an anti-viral (Welsh et al., 1976) and/or an anti-tumor effect (Kassel et al., 1973) in some species, the question might be raised about whether or not leukemic cats, which are generally deficient in both anti-FOCMA and CDA, have normal complement levels. However, cats with leukemia were found to have levels of lytic complement comparable to those found in virus-free healthy cats, suggesting that complement alone is not sufficient to prevent or reverse the leukemic disease process (Grant et al., 1978b). Healthy cats which maintain high anti-FOCMA and CDA titers in the presence of persistent viremia are occasionally deficient in complement, possibly due to the presence of antigen-antibody complexes. The possibility remains that transient complement depletions in preclinical disease stages may contribute to occasional failures in immune surveillance (Grant et al., 1978b).

SUMMARY

The immunosurveillance hypothesis predicts that transformed cells will be recognized as antigenically distinct, and eliminated before sufficient replication has occurred to create a clinically recognizable tumor. In at least one outbred mammalian specie, the cat, there is strong evidence to support this hypothesis. Although the lymphoproliferative neoplasms in this species are caused by horizontally transmitted oncornaviruses, the immune response directed to the tumor specific antigen, FOCMA, is readily distinguishable from the immune response to the virus structural proteins, including the virus neutralizing antibody response. A close correlation exists between anti-FOCMA activity and the presence of complement dependent antibodies in the same serum samples, suggesting that these antibody activities are overlapping or identical. The complement dependent antibodies, which lyse cultured lymphoma cells, function best in the presence of cat complement.

ACKNOWLEDGEMENTS

Work done in the laboratories of the authors was supported by National Cancer Institute grants CA-13885, CA-18216, CA-16599, CA-18488, and CA-08748, contract CB-64001 from the National Cancer Institute, grant DT-32 from the American Cancer Society, and grants from the Cancer Research Institute and the Massachusetts Branch of the American Cancer Society. C.K.G. is a Scholar of the Massachusetts Branch of the American Cancer Society and W.D.H. is a Scholar of the Leukemia Society of America.

REFERENCES

Aaronson, S.A., and Stephenson, J.R., 1976, Endogenous type-C viruses
of mammalian cells, Rev. on Cancer 458:323.

Aldrich, C.D., and Pederson, N.C., 1974, Persistent viremia after
regression of primary virus-induced feline fibrosarcomas, Am. J.
Vet. Res. 35:1383.

Burnet, F.M., 1970, The concept of immunological surveillance,
Prog. Exp. Tumor Res. 13:1.

Cotter, S.M., Essex, M., Hardy, W.D., Jr., 1974, Serological studies
of normal and leukemic cats in a multiple case leukemia cluster,
Cancer Res. 34:1061.

Dorn, C.R., Taylor, D.O.N., Schneider, R., Hibbard, H.H., and
Klauber, M.R., 1968, Survey of animal neoplasms in Alameda and
Contra Costa Counties, California. II. Cancer morbidity in dogs
and cats from Alameda County, J. Natl. Cancer Inst. 40:307.

Essex, M., 1974, The immune response to oncornavirus infections,
in: Viruses, Evolution and Cancer (E. Kurstak and K. Maramorosch,
eds.), pp. 513-548, Academic Press, New York.

Essex, M., 1975a, Horizontally and vertically transmitted oncornaviruses of cats, Advan. Cancer Res. 21:175.

Essex, M., 1975b, Tumors induced by oncornaviruses in cats,
Pathobiol. Ann. 5:169.

Essex, M., 1977, Immunity to leukemia, lymphoma and fibrosarcoma
in cats: A case for immunosurveillance, Contemp. Topics in
Immunobiol. 6:71.

Essex, M., and Snyder, S.P., 1973, Feline oncornavirus associated
cell membrane antigen. I. Serological studies with kittens exposed to cell-free materials from various feline fibrosarcomas,
J. Natl. Cancer Inst. 51:1007.

Essex, M., and Lamon, E.W., 1976, Host immune response to oncornavirus-induced tumors, in: Comparative Leukemia Research, 1975
(J. Clemmesen and D.S. Yohn, eds.) pp. 166-172, S. Karger, Basel.

Essex, M., Klein, G., Snyder, S.P., and Harrold, J.G., 1971a,
Antibody to feline oncornavirus-associated cell membrane antigen
in neonatal cats, Int. J. Cancer 8:384.

Essex, M., Klein, G., Snyder, S.P., and Harrold, J.G., 1971b, Feline
sarcoma virus (FSV) induced tumors: Correlations between humoral
antibody and tumor regression, Nature 233:195.

Essex, M., Cotter, S.M., Carpenter, J.L., Hardy, W.D., Jr., Hess, P., Jarrett, W., and Yohn, D.S., 1975a, Feline oncornavirus-associated cell membrane antigen. II. Antibody titers in healthy cats from pet household and laboratory colony environments, J. Natl. Cancer Inst. 54:631.

Essex, M., Hardy, W.D., Jr., Cotter, S.M., Jakowski, R.M., and Sliski, A., 1975b, Naturally occurring persistent feline oncornavirus infections in the absence of disease, Infect. Immun. 11:47.

Essex, M., Jakowski, R.M., Hardy, W.D., Jr., Cotter, S.M., Hess, P., and Sliski, A., 1975c, Feline oncornavirus-associated cell membrane antigen. III. Antibody titers in cats from leukemia cluster household, J. Natl. Cancer Inst. 54:637.

Essex, M., Cotter, S.M., Hardy, W.D., Jr., Hess, P., Jarrett, W., Jarrett, O., Mackey, L., Laird, H., Perryman, L., Olsen, P.G., and Yohn, D.S., 1975d, Feline oncornavirus associated cell membrane antigen. IV. Antibody titers in cats with naturally occurring leukemia, lymphoma, and other diseases, J. Natl. Cancer Inst. 55:463.

Essex, M., Sliski, A., Cotter, S.M., Jakowski, R.M., and Hardy, W.D., Jr., 1975e, Immunosurveillance of naturally occurring feline leukemia, Science 190:790.

Essex, M., Cotter, S.M., Sliski, A.H., Hardy, W.D., Jr., Stephenson, J.R., Aaronson, S.A., and Jarrett, O., 1977a, Horizontal transmission of feline leukemia virus under natural conditions in a feline leukemia cluster household, Int. J. Cancer 19:90.

Essex, M., Stephenson, J.R., Hardy, W.D., Jr., Cotter, S.M., and Aaronson, S.A., 1977b, Leukemia, lymphoma, and fibrosarcoma of cats as models for similar diseases of man, Cold Spring Harbor Proc. on Cell Proliferation 4:1197.

Essex, M., Hoover, E.A., and Hardy, W.D., Jr., 1978a, manuscript in preparation.

Essex, M., Sliski, A.H., Hardy, W.D., Jr., Cotter, S.M., and Noronha, F. de, 1978b, Feline oncornavirus associated cell membrane antigen: Specificity for transformation or tumor induction, in Comparative Leukemia Research, in press.

Essex, M., Sliski, A.H., and Hardy, W.D., Jr., FOCMA: A transformation specific RNA sarcoma virus encoded protein, this volume.

Francis, D.P., and Essex, M., 1978, Leukemia and lymphoma, infrequent manifestations of common viral infections?, submitted for publication.

Francis, D.P., Essex, M., and Hardy, W.D., Jr., 1977, Excretion of feline leukemia virus by naturally infected pet cats, Nature 269:252.

Grant, C.K., Worley, M.B., and DeBoer, D.J., 1977a, Detection of complement dependent lytic antibodies in sera from feline leukemia virus-infected cats by the chromium-51 release assay, J. Natl. Cancer Inst. 58:157.

Grant, C.K., DeBoer, D.J., Essex, M., Worley, M.B., and Higgins, J., 1977b, Antibodies from healthy cats exposed to feline leukemia virus lyse feline lymphoma cells slowly with cat complement, J. Immun. 119:401.

Grant, C.K., Essex, M., Pedersen, N.C., Hardy, W.D., Jr., Stephenson, J.R., Cotter, S.M., and Theilen, G.H., 1978a, Lysis of feline lymphoma cells by complement-dependent antibodies in feline leukemia virus contact cats. Correlation of lysis and antibodies to feline oncornavirus-associated cell membrane antigen, J. Natl. Cancer Inst. 60:161.

Grant, C.K., Ramaika, C., Madewell, B.R., Pickard, D.K., and Essex, M., 1978b, Lytic complement levels in cats with lymphoid malignancies and variations in activity associated with feline leukemia virus infection, submitted for publication.

Hardy, W.D., Jr., 1974, Immunology of oncornaviruses, Vet. Clinics of N. Amer. 4:133.

Hardy, W.D., Jr., Old, L.J., Hess, P.W., Essex, M., and Cotter, S.M., 1973, Horizontal transmission of feline leukemia virus in cats, Nature 244:266.

Hardy, W.D., Jr., Hess, P.W., MacEwen, E.G., McClelland, A.J., Zuckerman, E.E., Essex, M., and Cotter, S.M., 1976, The biology of feline leukemia virus in the natural environment, Cancer Res. 36:582.

Hardy, W.D., Jr., Zuckerman, E.E., MacEwen, E.G., Hayes, A.A., and Essex, M., 1977, A feline leukemia virus- and sarcoma virus-induced tumor-specific antigen, Nature 270:249.

Jacquemin, P., Saxinger, C., Gallo, R.C., Hardy, W.D., Jr., and Essex, M., 1978, An immune response in serum of cats to feline leukemia virus reverse transcriptase, submitted for publication.

Jarrett, W., Jarrett, O., Mackey, L., Laird, H.M., Hardy, W.D., Jr., and Essex, M., 1973, Horizontal transmission of leukemia virus and leukemia in the cat, J. Natl. Cancer Inst. 51:833.

Kassel, R.L., Old, L.J., Carswell, E.A., Fiore, N.C., and Hardy, W.D., Jr., 1973, Serum-mediated leukemia cell destruction in AKR mice. Role of complement in the phenomenon, J. Exp. Med. 138:925.

Klein, G., 1968, Tumor-specific transplantation antigens: G.H.A. Clowes memorial lecture, Cancer Res. 28:625.

Noronha, F. de, Baggs, P., Schäfer, W., and Bolognesi, D.P., 1977, Therapy with anti-viral antibodies of oncornavirus-induced sarcoma in cats, Nature 267:54.

Noronha, F. de, Schäfer, W., Essex, M., and Bolognesi, D.P., 1978, Influence of antisera to oncornavirus glycoprotein (gp71) on in vivo infections, Virology, in press.

Rogerson, P., Jarrett, W., and Mackey, L., 1975, Epidemiological studies on feline leukemia virus infection. I. A serological survey in urban cats, Int. J. Cancer 15:781.

Ruscetti, S.K., and Parks, W.P., 1977, Characterization of a feline leukemia viral cell membrane antigen reactive with feline sera, J. Immun. 119:2194.

Schaller, J.P., Essex, M., Yohn, D.S., and Olsen, R.G., 1975, Feline oncornavirus-associated cell membrane antigen. V. Humoral immune response to virus and cell membrane antigens in cats inoculated with Gardner-Arnstein feline sarcoma virus, J. Natl. Cancer Inst. 55:1373.

Sliski, A.H., Essex, M., Meyer, C., and Todaro, G., 1977, Feline oncornavirus-associated cell membrane antigen: Expression in transformed nonproducer mink cells, Science 196:1336.

Sliski, A.H., and Essex, M., 1978, Comparison of FOCMA expression on feline sarcoma virus vs. feline leukemia virus transformed cells, submitted for publication.

Snyder, S.P., 1971, Spontaneous feline fibrosarcomas: Transmissibility and ultrastructure of associated virus-like particles, J. Natl. Cancer Inst., 47:1079.

Snyder, S.P., and Dungsworth, D.L., 1973, Pathogenesis of feline viral fibrosarcomas. Dose and age effects, J. Natl. Cancer Inst. 51:781.

Stephenson, J.R., Essex, M., Hino, S., Aaronson, S.A., and Hardy, W.D., Jr., 1977a, Feline oncornavirus-associated cell-membrane antigen (FOCMA): Distinction between FOCMA and the major virion glycoprotein, Proc. Natl. Acad. Sci. 74:1219.

Stephenson, J.R., Khan, A.S., Sliski, A.H., and Essex, M., 1977b, Feline oncornavirus-associated cell membrane antigen (FOCMA), Identification of an immunologically cross-reactive feline sarcoma virus-cod ed protein, Proc. Natl. Acad. Soc. 74:5608.

Stephenson, J.R., Devare, S.G., and Reynolds, F.H., 1978, Translational products of Type C RNA tumor viruses, Advan. Cancer Res., in press.

Welsh, R.M., Jr., Jensen, F.C., Neil, R.C., and Oldstone, M.B.A., 1976, Inactivation and lysis of oncornavirus by human serum, Virology 74:432.

SECTION V

Molecular approaches to active intervention into oncogenesis by tumor viruses

Convenor

Dr. Prakash CHANDRA

Gustav-Embden-Zentrum der Biologischen
Chemie

Abt. für Molekularbiologie

Klinikum der Johann-Wolfgang-Goethe
Universität

Theodor-Stern-Kai 7

6000 Frankfurt am Main 70

W-Germany

THE ROLE OF THE PHARMACEUTICAL INDUSTRY IN THE DEVELOPMENT OF POTENTIAL ANTICANCER DRUGS

Mario Ghione

Montedison Pharmaceutical Division

Milan, Via B. Crespi 27

The study of a new drug is a cumbersome and time-consuming task involving the investigation of a galaxy of biomedically oriented problems in the dim light of sometimes inadequate and perplexing socioeconomic information. These difficulties are particularly evident in the search for new anticancer agents, owing to our basic ignorance of cancer etiology and pathogenesis, as well as the high prevalence and strong emotional impact of the disease.

In countries where the problems of infectious and parasitic diseases and of unbalanced diet have been successfully solved, or at least contained within reasonable limits, malignant tumors have gained the front rank among leading causes of morbidity and mortality, competing only with cardiovascular diseases. The story of modern cancer chemotherapy begins immediately after World War II, and is characterized by a joint effort carried out by academic institutions, government agencies, scientific foundations, and pharmaceutical industry research groups. The latter have played an important role in developing this sector. In the United States the trend was pioneered by Lederle Laboratories, which established a major screening program, and by Burroughs Wellcome. In the United Kingdom a relevant drug development program was started by Imperial Chemical Industries (Zubrod et al., 1977). With improvement in the economy after the war, the European and Japanese pharmaceutical companies invested heavily in the search for new therapeutic agents and pursued an aggressive research program connected with the development of potential antitumor compounds. No attempt will be made to name them all, but as examples we can mention Hoffman La Roche (5-fluorouracil), Bayer (Trenimon), Kyowa (Mitomycin C), Rhône Poulenc (Rubidazone), Chinoin (Dibromo-mannitol), and Farmitalia (Adriamycin). Many pharmaceutical companies participated in this effort by submitting material to the

445

screening programs spearheaded in the USA by Rhoad at the Sloan-
Kettering Institute and to this day actively carried out by the
National Cancer Institute in the USA, the European Organization for
Research and Treatment of Cancer, the Mario Negri Institute of
Milan, etc.

The role of the pharmaceutical industry in implementing cancer
therapy research is highly varied and can only be outlined briefly.
The long journey toward clinical application starts obviously with
the discovery of a new biologically active chemical entity or a new
and previously unsuspected biologic activity of an old structure.
New chemical entities may be obtained by synthesis or isolated from
microorganisms, plants, or animal metabolites.

In providing new compounds the pharmaceutical and chemical
industries play an overwhelming role in comparison with other
sources. This is illustrated by an analysis according to origin of
new single entities submitted for screening during 1975 to the U.S.
National Cancer Institute (Wood, 1977). Of the 21,295 crystalline
materials evaluated, industry provided 73.0%. The absolute number
of active compounds among them is surpassed only by the number of
active substances found among the new chemicals synthesized under
contract, the latter consisting chiefly of analogues of already
known active principles.

A closer analysis of these data shows the overall yield of the
anticancer screening. Approximately one out of every thousand
screened crystalline compounds was selected as a candidate for
preclinical toxicologic evaluation and clinical trials in 1975 by
the Developmental Therapeutics Program of the U.S. National Cancer
Institute. The ratio is higher for fermentation and animal products
(1.8% and 2.6%, respectively) and lower for plant and synthetic
products (0.6 and 0.06%, respectively). For a very few products
(slightly less than one in five thousand) an Investigational New Drug
(IND) application for clinical trials could be filed with the Food
and Drug Administration during the above-mentioned time period.

In spite of the many thousands of compounds screened every
year, the field is only marginally explored. Only 11-12% of the
approximately 36,000 unique ring systems described in the literature
reviewed by Chemical Abstracts have been tested. A substantially
lower aliquot (0.2%) has been submitted to a statistically adequate
sampling by examining at least 200 compounds belonging to each class.

The scanty crop harvested from the blind screening and random
selection pointed the way to a different approach. An attempt toward
a rational development was carried out by many pharmaceutical
research groups through what was defined as an enlightened empiric
philosophy consisting chiefly in synthesizing and testing analogues
and derivatives of active compounds. The task appears to be particu-

larly appropriate to the skills and means of pharmaceutical industry researchers. Moreover, an endeavor in this direction seems to be warranted by the success of the same methodological approach in many other fields of pharmacological research. The development of the sulfonamides and the production of semisynthetic penicillins are just two among the many examples offered by the history of the closely related realm of antibacterial chemotherapy.

The extensive search for new analogues is, therefore, one of the peculiar aspects of the role played by the pharmaceutical industry in exposing the capabilities of potential anticancer agents. In this kind of research not only the cytocidal and toxic activities of a new compound but even its pharmacokinetic properties are taken into consideration. The aim is to discover particular characteristics which may permit its use by new ways of administration in new schedules of treatment, or which may allow it to reach parts of the body inaccessible to the parent compound or to avoid dangerous accumulations.

In the study of cytotoxic compounds great care is devoted to an exploration of their immuno-interfering properties.

The research relevant to the characterization of new analogues and the tedious but essential ancillary work supporting every step of the main line of research will either be carried out by the pharmaceutical industry researchers directly or closely followed up by them when the task is allotted to extramural groups. Experience has demonstrated that even apparently minor or supposedly trival modifications of the chemical structure of an active compound can induce new and unexpected biological properties and, in some cases, even drastic alterations in clinical activity. A good example is the work that has been done on the anthracyclines. These glucosidic antibiotics possessing a dihydroxyanthraquinone tetracyclic aglycone are produced by many strains of Streptomyces. Their chemistry has been reviewed by Brockmann (1963) and more recently by Arcamone (1977). Daunorubicin (DNR), a compound belonging to this class (comtemporaneously and independently discovered by Farmitalia and Rhône Poulenc research groups), was the first anthracycline derivative thoroughly studied by the pharmaceutical industry from the point of view of its potential anticancer activity (Di Marco et al., 1963). The good clinical efficacy displayed by DNR in the treatment of leukemias encouraged many research groups to look for analogues. Adriamycin (ADM), a compound closely related to DNR, was identified by the Farmitalia group and developed in close connection with the U.S. National Cancer Institute, the Istituto Nazionale per lo Studio e la Cura dei Tumori of Milan, and other academic and research institutes throughout the world (Ghione, 1975). The experimental research gave evidence that in spite of the apparently minor modification of the chemical structure, ADM is endowed with biological properties which are quite different from DNR (Di Marco, 1975). The clinical trials supported the preclinical data and substantiated the outstanding potency of ADM in the treatment of solid tumors (Carter, 1975).

In this sphere the main effort of the Farmitalia research group has been directed toward the synthesis and investigation of ADM derivatives. Through a rationally planned approach a multifaceted chemical manipulation has been carried out in the aglycone and/or in the sugar moiety of the antibiotic molecule (Arcamone et al., 1977).

A few of the numerous compounds obtained to date have displayed interesting properties (Casazza, 1975). The most promising substances have been submitted to preclinical tests in laboratory animals. One of these (4'-epiadriamycin) has already satisfactorily gone through the preclinical test system. Other compounds are presently progressing along a standard protocol designed to gather information on the pharmacodynamic, pharmacokinetic, and toxic properties of this class of anticancer drugs.

The proper design and execution of such preclinical tests constitute a very important facet of the role played by the pharmaceutical industry in the development of potential antitumor compounds. The number of animals required, the intricacy of the test array, as well as the protracted period of time required for the completion of long-term treatment studies call for the availability of suitably organized facilities that can be found only on the premises of ad hoc planned laboratories.

Particular stress should be placed on the fact that the execution of these tests, even if it involves a great but unavoidable amount of repetitive work, demands all the skill and ingenuity of experienced researchers to observe and interpret correctly the sometimes subtle and elusive signs of an unexpected biologic activity displayed by a new product. These observations assume a particular relevance for the prediction of the clinical tolerance of the new drug in man. The pharmaceutical industry researcher has to make a careful evaluation of this body of information in order to be able to forewarn the physician of the development of critical organ system toxic effects.

A stage of research and development which clearly forms part of the role of the pharmaceutical industry is the preparation of a clinically acceptable pharmaceutical form of the new drug. In some cases the task can be relatively simple, while in others it may require all the dexterity and versatility of the expert in pharmaceutical technique. The production of sterile i.v. injectable forms of water-insoluble or of highly unstable compounds can demand extensive research and a sound basic knowledge of highly complex phenomena. In every instance for all types of pharmaceutical preparations the pharmaceutical industry researcher is expected to provide an analytical system suitable for the estimation of the purity and assay of the drug as well as of the excipients and solvents. Suitable analytical procedures must also be developed for the determination of the drug in feces, urine, blood, and tissues, as a basis for pharmacokinetic studies.

The establishment of an analytical protocol is an essential prerequisite for the execution of stability tests, for the setting up of a quality control system, and for a study of the compatibility of the new drug with other compounds. The latter is of paramount importance in the research of cancer chemotherapy, where the administration of a multiple drug combination is much more the rule than the exception.

One of the tasks of the pharmaceutical industry researcher is to establish the necessary connections with clinicians for the design of a protocol and the organization of clinical trials. These trials will allow determination of the clinical tolerance of the new drug (phase I), its therapeutic activity (phase II), and the presence or absence of a clear advantage over existing and clinically tried and proven drugs (phase III). To accomplish this task, the sequential approach outlined by the above-mentioned phase system has been developed in close connection with the medical researchers of the pharmaceutical industry.

Much more troublesome are the problems associated with the international extension of the clinical trials with anticancer drugs. In designing multicentric trials or in comparing their results, not only the difficult to define epidemiological, environmental, ethical, and nutritional differences but also the even more intricate cultural peculiarities of the countries or regions involved in the trial have to be taken into consideration. All these aspects are of concern to the medical researchers working in the pharmaceutical industry owing to the fact that any phase III study is likely to be not only a multicentric and multinational study, but a transcultural study as well (Joyce, 1976). This remark assumes a particular weight when the trials are carried out with drugs which, like many antitumor compounds, may produce significant side effects that can evoke strong emotional reactions, whose emergence is modulated through the peculiar culture indigenous to the target population.

The problem of clinical tolerance of a new drug therefore has to be examined in a very broad context. A reappraisal of the multicentric trials carried out with Adriamycin and/or combined chemotherapy on a worldwide basis furnishes some good examples of special features emerging from transcultural trials. Many patients in countries of the Far East and Southeast Asia strongly object to, or even decline, the countinuation of therapy in spite of improvement of their morbid conditions only because of the appearance of a drug-induced alopecia. Alopecia, a spontaneously regressing side effect which occurs quite frequently with the administration of a number of

antitumor drugs (Adriamycin, Vincristine, Cyclophosphamide + Meto-
trexate + 5-fluorouracil, etc.), can cause such misery and unbearable
anguish to female and male patients of this cultural area that
therapy has to be interrupted. The same symptom has very seldom been
considered as a serious hindrance by patients in Western countries,
perhaps because they are more familiar with the problems of baldness
and anyway willing to avail themselves, if necessary, of wigs or
headdresses. In other instances an exactly opposite psychological
phenomenon has been observed, that is, the fall of hair represents
for the patient a sign of "potency" of the therapy. This belief has
been so ingrained that those few patients who escaped alopecia com-
plained to the physician, wanting to know why they were supposedly
deprived of a treatment as active as that administered to other
patients.

These examples stress the need for a detailed exploration of
cross-cultural trials. Similar considerations are relevant for
every kind of drug though research on highly active compounds like
the antitumor agents tends to magnify phenomena which in other cases
may go unnoticed but nevertheless can play a basic role in determining
the fate of the drug. Generally, multinational pharmaceutical
industry research groups are best qualified to take care of this
important aspect of the problem, as well as other problems connected
with international liaison in clinical testing of anticancer drugs
(Carter, 1976).

Another task of pharmaceutical industry researchers is to collect
all the information generated during preclinical and clinical trials.
This evidence has to be submitted to the regulatory agencies of the
various countries to get approval for marketing of the drug. To cope
with the sometimes tiring bureaucratic burden imposed by certain
national regulations (Lasagna, 1976) requires not only a bit of spirit
of self-sacrifice but a complex organization.

Definitely more exciting for the researchers is the determinant
role the pharmaceutical industry can play in the long-term monitoring
of delayed drug-induced side effects. This phase IV monitoring is
carried out after the introduction of the drug on the market. It can
be aimed either at ascertaining the emergence of unexpected occur-
rences or at checking the real incidence of an already known and
undesired outcome of the drug therapy. Research-oriented pharmaceutical companies use various approaches to cope with these problems
(Ghione, 1971). Usually a regular system of early warning follow-up
and feedback is framed by company agents scattered throughout the
country and acting in liaison with a centralized medico-toxicological
advisory service. A well designed product-oriented and cross-
sectional (in time) drug monitoring experiment organized by a pharmaceutical industry has been described by Ferrari (1976). Bearing
directly upon the theme of this lecture is the international
multicentric monitoring system organized by the Medical Direction of

the pharmaceutical company Farmitalia (Praga et al., 1978). The aim of this retrospective analysis (designed in cooperation with the National Cancer Institute) is to collect information from European oncological centers on the risk factors connected with Adriamycin-associated cardiomyopathy. In spite of the fairly low incidence of this problem, the Farmitalia research group has devoted great effort to it by studying the pathogenetic factors and looking for antidotes (Fioretti et al., 1976; Bertazzoli and Ghione, 1977).

Another consideration arises if the whole picture is examined from another point of view. Malignant tumors are one of man's oldest, most persistent, most costly, and most frequent diseases. According to statistics, one out of every four U.S. citizens will develop cancer (Zubrod et al., 1977). But even though tumors are in the front rank among the leading causes of morbidity and mortality, the number of compounds specifically prepared and studied as potential antitumor agents by the most active pharmaceutical industries around the world is disappointingly small. The five most important fields of research in the pharmaceutical industry in 13 countries (Europe, Japan, and USA), deduced by Struller (1976) from a patent survey (1970–74), involve neurotropic, analgesic, cardiovascular, and antimicrobial drugs and drugs active against metabolic disorders. These five most important fields represent 64–89% of the total pharmaceutical industry research (see the incisive discussion of this point by Gross, 1976). However, a survey we recently carried out on a fairly large sample of the scientific literature has demonstrated that the number of compounds reported to have been somehow examined from the point of view of potential antitumor activity has changed considerably in the last three years. In the sample examined the number of such compounds out of the total number of compounds cited as having been examined for all types of biologic activity was 10/1079 for 1975, 49/1763 for 1976, and 90/1203 for 1977. The percentage values go from 0.926 (1975) to 2.78 (1976) and rise to 7.48 (1977). A substantial share of these compounds originated in pharmaceutical industry research laboratories. The trend is increasing, and this is a rewarding sign for those who for years have struggled in this direction.

REFERENCES

Arcamone, F. M., New antitumor anthracyclines, Lloydia 40, 45, 1977.

Arcamone, F. M., Di Marco, A., and Casazza, A. M., Chemistry and pharmacology of new antitumor anthracyclines, VIII Intern. Symposium of the Princess Takamatsu Cancer Res. Fund, Advances in Cancer Chemotherapy, Tokyo, November 15–17, 1977.

Bertazzoli, C., and Ghione, M., Adriamycin associated cardiotoxicity: research on prevention with coenzyme Q, Pharmacol. Res. Comm. 9, 235, 1977.

Brockmann, H., Anthracyclinone und Anthracycline, Fortschr. Chem. Org. Naturst. 21, 127, 1963.

Carter, S. K., Adriamycin--a review, J. Natl. Cancer Inst. 55, 1265, 1975

Carter, S. K., International liaison in clinical testing of new anticancer drugs, in: Rationality of Drug Development, P. E. Lucchelli, N. Bergamini, and V. Bachini, Eds., Excerpta Medica, Amsterdam - Oxford, and American Elsevier, New York, 1976, p. 35.

Casazza, A. M., Attività biologica dei farmaci antitumorali antraciclinici, Simp. Internaz. La ricerca scientifica nell'industria farmaceutica in Italia--Risultati e ruolo internazionale, Rome, October 2-4, 1975.

Di Marco, A., Gaetani, M., Dorigotti, L., Soldati, M., and Bellini, O., Studi sperimentali sull'attività antineoplastica del nuovo antibiotico daunomicina, Tumori 49, 203, 1963.

Di Marco, A., Adriamycin (NSC-123127): mode and mechanism of action, Cancer Chemoth. Rep. Part 3, 6, 91, 1975.

Ferrari, V., An experiment of drug monitoring by a pharmaceutical industry, in: Rationality of Drug Development, P. E. Lucchelli, N. Bergamini, and V. Bachini, Eds., Excerpta Medica, Amsterdam - Oxford, and American Elsevier, New York, 1976, p. 59.

Fioretti, A., Ghione, M., Pozzoli, E., and Lambertenghi-Deliliers, G., Autoantibodies and spleen-cell-mediated cytotoxicity in Adriamycin-induced myocardiopathy in rabbits, Cancer Res. 36, 1462, 1976.

Ghione, M., Il "monitoring" su larga scala per la si curezza dei farmaci, Boll. Chim. Farmaceut. 110, 573, 1971.

Ghione, M., Development of Adryamicin (NSC-123127), Cancer Chemoth. Rep. Part 3, 6, 83, 1975.

Gross, F., The present dilemma of drug research, Clin. Pharmacol. Therap. 19, 1, 1976.

Joyce, C. R. B., International cooperative clinical trials and other behavioural sciences, in: Rationality of Drug Development, P. E. Lucchelli, N. Bergamini, and V. Bachini, Eds., Excerpta Medica, Amsterdam - Oxford, and American Elsevier, New York, 1976, p. 17.

Lasagna, L., International cooperation in drug testing in a changing world, in: Rationality of Drug Development, P. E. Lucchelli, N. Bergamini, and V. Bachini, Eds., Excerpta Medica, Amsterdam - Oxford, and American Elsevier, New York, 1976, p. 3.

Praga C., Lenaz, G., and Soldati, M., Miocardiotossicità da farmaci antiblastici--Revisione critica, Sillabus del IV° corso di aggiornamento in oncologia AIOM, Genoa, January 18-21, 1978, p. 917.

Struller, T., Problems of medical practice and of medical-pharmaceutical research, in: Progress in Drug Research, Vol. 20, E. Jucker, Ed., Birkhäuser Verlag, Basel-Stuttgart, 1976, pp. 491-519.

Wood, H. B. Jr., Selection of agents for the tumor screening of potential new antineoplastic drugs, National Cancer Institute Monograph 45, 15, 1977.

Zubrod, C. G., Schepartz, S. A., and Carter, S. K., Historical background of the National Cancer Institute's drug development thrust, National Cancer Institute Monograph 45, 7, 1977.

CHEMICAL CARCINOGENESIS IN NON-HUMAN PRIMATES AND

ATTEMPTS AT PREVENTION

S. M. Sieber and R. H. Adamson

Lab. of Chemical Pharmacology, National Cancer Inst.

NIH, Building 37, Room 5A13, Bethesda, Md. 20014

INTRODUCTION

Studies in non-human primates of the potential carcinogenicity of various chemicals and other substances have been underway in our laboratory for approximately 16 years. A wide variety of substances have been, or are being, evaluated. These substances can be categorized as follows (Table 1): model rodent carcinogens (3-methylcholanthrene, dibenz(a,h)anthracene, 3,4,9,10-dibenzpyrene, N-2-fluorenylacetamide, N,N-2,7-fluorenylenebisacetamide, N,N'-dimethyl-p-phenylazo-analine, N,N'-dimethyl-p-($\underline{m}$-tolylazo)-analine, ethyl carbamate); food additives and environmental contaminants (cyclamate, saccharin, aflatoxin B_1, methylazoxymethanol-acetate, sterigmatocystin, DDT, arsenic, cigarette smoke condensate, low density polyethylene plastic); therapeutic agents (procarbazine, azathioprine, Adriamycin, 1-phenylalanine mustard); and nitroso-compounds (1-methylnitrosourea, N-nitrosodiethylamine, N-nitroso-dipropylamine, 1-nitrosopiperidine, and N-methyl-N'-nitro-N-nitro-soguanidine).

The objectives of this program are: to obtain comparative data on the response of non-human primates to substances known to be carcinogenic in rodents and to materials suspected of being carcinogens in man, to evaluate the long-term effects of clinically useful antineoplastic and immunosuppressive agents, to develop model tumor systems in primates for evaluating the potential usefulness of new antitumor agents active against rodent tumors before these agents are administered to cancer patients, to make available normal and tumor bearing primates for pharmacological, biochemical, immunological and therapeutic studies, to develop

biological markers and other diagnostic tests for detecting preneoplastic changes as well as overt neoplasia, and to explore the
possibility of preventing and/or reversing the process of carcinogenesis - i.e., "chemoprevention" instead of chemotherapy.

Table 1: Substances Tested for Carcinogenic
Activity in Non-Human Primates

Model Rodent Carcinogens

    3-methylcholanthrene
    dibenz(a,h)anthracene
    3,4,9,10-dibenzpyrene
    N-2-fluorenylacetamide
    N,N-2,7-fluorenylenebisacetamide
    N,N'-dimethyl-p-phenylazo-analine
    N,N'-dimethyl-p-(m-tolylazo)-analine
    ethyl carbamate

Food Additives and Environmental Contaminants

    cyclamate
    saccharin
    aflatoxin B_1
    methylazoxymethanol-acetate
    sterigmatocystin
    DDT
    arsenic
    cigarette smoke condensate
    low density polyethylene plastic

Therapeutic Agents

    procarbazine
    azathioprine
    Adriamycin
    1-phenylalanine mustard

Nitroso- Compounds

    1-methylnitrosourea
    N-nitrosodiethylamine
    N-nitrosodipropylamine
    1-nitrosopiperidine
    N-methyl-N'-nitro-N-nitrosoguanidine

In this paper, we summarize some of the data obtained thus far on chemical carcinogenesis in non-human primates. Earlier reports from this laboratory describing results from ongoing studies of chemical carcinogenesis in non-human primates, the relationship of serum alpha-fetoprotein levels to the growth of hepatocellular carcinomas, and the therapy of chemically-induced tumors in monkeys, have been published (1-11).

MATERIALS AND METHODS

Animals

The present colony consists of approximately 600 animals; 80 of these monkeys are adult breeders which supply the newborn animals for experimental studies. The monkeys represent four species: approximately 48% are Macaca mulatta (rhesus), 42% are Macaca fascicularis (cynomolgus), 8% are Cercopithecus aethiops (African green), and 2% are the prosimian Galago crassicaudatus (bushbabies). The majority of the animals are housed in an isolated facility which contains only animals committed to this study, and, with the exception of the monkeys in the breeding colony, most animals are housed in individual cages. Details of maintenance and management procedures, and the method used to rear neonates have been described elsewhere (1,5). Newborns produced by the breeding colony are taken within 12 hours of birth to the nursery which is staffed on a 24 hour basis. In most cases, the administration of test compounds is initiated within 24 hours of birth, although adult monkeys have been utilized in some experiments. Dosing continues until a tumor is diagnosed or until a predetermined exposure period has been completed. A minimum of 30 animals is usually allotted to each treatment group, since in a sample of this size it is possible to detect a tumor incidence of 10% within 95% confidence limits.

A number of clinical, biochemical and hematological parameters are monitored weekly or monthly, not only to evaluate the general health status of each animal, but also for the early detection of tumors. Surgical procedures are performed under phencyclidine hydrochloride, Ketamine or sodium pentobarbital anesthesia. All animals which die or are sacrificed are carefully necropsied and their tissues subjected to histopathologic examination.

Administration of test compounds

The compounds are administered subcutaneously (sc), intravenously (iv), intraperitoneally (ip) or orally (po). For po

administration to newborn monkeys, the compound is added to the
Similac formula at the time of feeding; when the monkeys are 6
months old, carcinogens given po are incorporated into a vitamin
mixture which is given to monkeys as a vitamin sandwich on a half
slice of bread. The dose level chosen is dependent on the chemical under evaluation. The therapeutic agents under test are
administered at doses likely to be encountered in a clinical
situation; other substances, such as environmental contaminants
and food additives, are usually given at levels 10-40 times
higher than the estimated human exposure level. The remainder of
the chemicals tested are administered at maximally tolerated doses
which, on the basis of weight gain, blood chemistry and hematology
findings, and clinical observations, appear to be devoid of acute
toxicity.

RESULTS AND DISCUSSION

Since the inception of this program, studies on the carcinogenic effects of 26 substances have been initiated; treatment with
7 of these has been associated with an increased incidence of
tumors, and 19 of the substances either have failed to induce
tumors or have not been under test for a sufficient length of
time. The compounds which have not demonstrated carcinogenic
activity after evaluation periods of 5 years or longer include 3-
methylcholanthrene, dibenz(a,h)anthracene, 3,4,9,10-dibenzpyrene,
N-2-fluorenylacetamide, N,N-2,7-fluorenylenebisacetamide, ethyl
carbamate, N,N'-dimethyl-p-phenylazoanaline, N,N'-dimethyl-p-(m-
tolylazo)-analine, cyclamate, saccharin and dichlorodiphenyl-
trichloroethane. The compounds which have not induced tumors
after evaluation periods of less than 5 years include N-methyl-N'-
nitro-N-nitrosoguanidine, low density polyethylene plastic, cigarette smoke condensate, arsenic, sterigmatocystin, azathioprine,
Adriamycin and 1-phenylalanine mustard.

During the past 16 years, 2 spontaneous tumors have developed
in 211 non-treated breeders and vehicle-treated controls, yielding
a tumor incidence of less than 1%. The tumors were diagnosed as a
reticulum cell sarcoma and a carcinoma of the gallbladder. The 7
chemicals found to be carcinogenic in non-human primates produced
tumors in 14-100% of treated animals (Table 2). The carcinogens
include N-nitrosodiethylamine (DENA), 1-nitrosopiperidine (PIP),
N-nitrosodipropylamine (DPNA), aflatoxin B_1 (AFB_1), methylazoxymethanol-acetate (MAM-acetate), procarbazine, and 1-methylnitro-
sourea (MNU).

Aflatoxin and cycasin are both known to be contaminants of
human foodstuffs. Table 3 summarizes our results with regard to
the carcinogenicity of AFB_1 in non-human primates. Nine of 45

Table 2. Summary of Compounds Inducing Tumors in Monkeys*

Compounds	Route of Administration	Total Treated	No. Alive	No. Dead (%) With Tumor	No. Dead (%) Without Tumor
Controls†	--	211	145	2 (0.9)	64
N-nitrosodiethylamine	ip	122	2	98 (80)	22
N-nitrosodipropylamine	ip	6	0	6 (100)	0
1-nitrosopiperidine	po	12	0	11 (92)	1
Aflatoxin B_1	po & ip	45	17	9 (20)	19
MAM-acetate	po & ip	26	11	7 (27)	8
MNU	po	43	25	6 (14)	12
Procarbazine	sc, po & ip	50	13	11 (22)	26

*In rhesus, cynomolgus and African green monkeys surviving longer than 6 months following treatment.

†Includes both non-treated breeders and vehicle treated controls.

Table 3. Tumors Induced in Monkeys Treated with Aflatoxin B_1 (AFB_1)*

Monkey Number	Species	Sex	Age at first dose	Route	Total dose (mg)	Latent period (mo)†	Histological diagnosis
692I	Rh	♀	at birth	ip & po	99.19	48	hepatic cell carcinoma
680H	Rh	♂	3 days	ip & po	119.44	51	hemangioendothelial sarcoma, liver
488F	Cyno	♂	13 mo.	ip	130.80	50	olfactory neuroepithelioma
590G	Afr Gr	♂	at birth	ip & po	291.83	107	hemangioendothelial sarcoma, pancreas
582G	Cyno	♂	9 days	ip & po	411.52	115	osteosarcoma, tibia
500F	Rh	♀	9.5 mo.	ip & po	463.55	118	adenocarcinoma, intrahepatic bile duct with wide metastases
454F	Rh	♀	8 days	po	842.36	74	hepatic cell carcinoma
479F	Rh	♂	at birth	po	1252.28	130	adenocarcinoma, gall bladder with invasion of liver and lung metastases
374E	Rh	♀	at birth	po	1354.24	134	adenocarcinoma, bile duct

*AFB_1 was administered weekly by ip (0.125-0.250 mg/kg) or po (0.2-0.8 mg/kg) routes.
†Latent period is the time in months from the first dose of AFB_1 until the clinical diagnosis of tumor.

monkeys (20%) treated with AFB_1 for longer than 2 years have
developed tumors. Two of the tumors were primary liver carcinomas
and 3 were adenocarcinomas of the bile duct or gall bladder; in
addition, single cases of hemangioendothelial sarcoma of the
liver, hemangioendothelial sarcoma of the pancreas, olfactory
neuroepithelioma, and osteosarcoma of the tibia were diagnosed.
The latent period for tumor induction ranged from 48 months to 134
months, averaging 92 months; the average total dose given to
monkeys developing tumors was 551.7 mg (range 99-1,354 mg).

MAM-acetate, the aglycone of the active carcinogen in the
cycad nut (cycasin), is also a carcinogen in non-human primates,
as shown in Table 4. A total of 26 rhesus, cynomolgus and African
green monkeys were given this substance by weekly ip injections
(10 mg/kg) or were given compound orally (3 mg/kg, 5 days every
week). To date, 7 animals (27%) have developed primary liver cancer; in 2 of these monkeys, bilateral renal carcinomas, squamous
cell carcinoma of the esophagus, and liver hemangiosarcomas were
also found. Six of the 7 monkeys developing tumors were given the
compound by the ip route; for these 6 monkeys the average latent
period for tumor induction was 81 months (range 50-100 months),
and the average total dose received was 6.1 gm (range 3.58-9.66
gm).

Among the series of chemicals classified as therapeutic agents, only procarbazine has as yet induced malignant neoplasms in
monkeys (Table 5). Fifty monkeys have survived for longer than 6
months after receiving procarbazine by sc, ip and/or po routes at
doses of 5-50 mg/kg, and 37 of these monkeys have been necropsied.
Eleven out of the 50 animals (22%) have had malignant neoplasms.
Six of the 11 cases (54.5%) were classified as acute leukemia, all
but one of the myelogenous type; the other acute leukemia was
undifferentiated. The 5 solid tumors were a poorly differentiated
lymphocytic lymphoma, 2 hemangiosarcomas and 2 osteosarcomas. The
tumors were diagnosed after treatment for periods ranging from 16
to 108.5 months, and averaging 75 months. Total doses of procarbazine received by these monkeys averaged 36 gm, and ranged from
2.69 to 101.65 gm. No specificity with regard to sex was noted
for tumor development. The neoplasms were approximately evenly
divided between rhesus and cynomolgus monkeys, with none appearing
in African green monkeys. Other adverse effects of long-term
procarbazine treatment included vomiting, myelosuppression and
testicular atrophy with complete aplasia of the germinal epith-
lium.

The nitroso- compounds as a class appear to be potent carcinogens in non-human primates. Forty-three monkeys have received
oral doses (10-20 mg/kg) of MNU, and 18 monkeys have been necropsied to date. Squamous cell carcinomas of the mouth, pharynx, and

Table 4. Liver Carcinomas Induced with MAM-acetate[*]

Monkey Number	Species	Sex	Total Dose (gm)	Latent period(mo)[†]	Histological diagnosis
671H	Rh	♂	3.58	50	Primary liver carcinoma
664H	Afr Gr	♂	3.88	63	Adenocarcinoma, liver
670H	Cyno	♀	5.06	83	Hepatoma & liver hemangiosarcoma with lymph node metastases; bilateral renal carcinoma; squamous cell carcinoma, esophagus
672H	Rh	♀	6.27	93	Hepatic cell carcinoma
665H	Rh	♀	8.38	100	Hepatic cell carcinoma; bilateral renal carcinoma; adenocarcinoma, small intestine; squamous cell carcinoma, esophagus
669H	Rh	♂	9.66	89	Hepatic cell carcinoma
309D	Cyno	♂	48.53	95	Hepatic cell carcinoma

[*]Monkeys received the initial dose of MAM-acetate at birth; all received MAM-acetate by weekly intraperitoneal injections (10 mg/kg) except for #309D, which was given compound orally (3 mg/kg) on a vitamin sandwich 5 times every week.

[†]Latent period is the time in months from the first dose of MAM-acetate until the clinical diagnosis of tumor.

Table 5. Tumors Induced in Monkeys by Procarbazine[*]

Monkey Number	Species	Sex	Total Dose (gm)	Latent period (mo) [†]	Histological Diagnosis
267D	Rh	♀	2.64	16	acute myelogenous leukemia
733I	Cyno	♂	7.29	57	acute undifferentiated leukemia
726I	Cyno	♂	16.24	68	acute myelogenous leukemia
734I	Rh	♂	17.17	71	hemangioendothelial sarcoma, kidney
731I	Rh	♀	24.22	68	osteosarcoma, humerus, with lung metastases
314E	Cyno	♀	32.88	97	hemangiosarcoma, spleen, liver, intestine, kidney, & ovaries
313E	Rh	♀	37.26	68	acute myelogenous leukemia
567G	Rh	♀	49.99	77	acute myelogenous leukemia
315E	Cyno	♂	50.19	98	lymphocytic lymphoma
333E	Cyno	♀	57.04	103	osteosarcoma, jaw
13T	Rh	♂	101.65	109	acute myelogenous leukemia

[*] Monkeys were treated with procarbazine by sc, ip or oral routes at 5-50 mg/kg; all monkeys received the initial dose of procarbazine within 48 hours of birth except for #13T, which received the first dose at the age of 5 months.

[†] Latent period is the time in months from the first dose of procarbazine until the clinical diagnosis of tumor.

Table 6. Tumors in Monkeys Receiving 1-Methylnitrosourea
          (MNU) by the Oral Route*

Monkey Number	Species	Sex	Total dose (gm)	Latent period (mo)[†]	Histological diagnosis
617H	Cyno	♂	53.21	63	SCA[††], pharynx & esophagus with invasion of mediastinal lymph nodes; squamous metaplasia, trachea
622H	Rh	♀	65.73	57	SCA, soft palate, tongue & esophagus with invasion into stomach
539G	Rh	♀	108.15	72	SCA, mouth; SCA in situ, pharynx; squamous papillomas, tongue, pharynx & esophagus; dyskeratosis, esophageal mucosa
540G	Rh	♂	129.28	83	SCA, mouth & esophagus; squamous papilloma & hyperkeratosis, buccal mucosa
538G	Rh	♂	133.81	72	SCA, mouth, pharynx & esophagus; multiple squamous papillomas, pharynx & esophagus
539G	Afr Gr	♂	137.20	124	SCA, mouth, pharynx & esophagus

*MNU (10-20 mg/kg) was incorporated into a vitamin sandwich and given daily 5 times every week; dosing was initiated within 1 week of birth.

†Latent period is the time in months from the first dose of MNU until the clinical diagnosis of tumor.

††SCA = squamous cell carcinoma.

esophagus have been diagnosed in 6 of the monkeys (Table 6), yielding an overall tumor incidence of 14%. All but one of the monkeys that have received total doses of MNU exceeding 50 gm have developed carcinoma, whereas no malignant tumors have developed in monkeys receiving cumulative doses less than 50 gm. The average latent period for tumor development was 78 months, and ranged between 63 and 124 months.

The severity of the esophageal lesions seen in this group of monkeys appeared roughly proportional to both the total dose of MNU ingested and the time interval over which MNU was given (Table 7). No esophageal lesions were noted at necropsy in 2 monkeys that received an average total MNU dose of 15.3 gm for an average of 26 months. Esophagitis, atrophy of the esophageal mucosa, and esophageal candidiasis were found in 3 monkeys necropsied after receiving an average total MNU dose of 14.1 gm over a period of 59 months. In 4 monkeys dosed for an average of 52 months and receiving average cumulative MNU doses of 58.7 gm, various more severe lesions were noted at necropsy, including dysplasia, dys-keratosis, hyperkeratosis and ulceration of the esophageal mucosa. And finally, 6 monkeys treated for an average of 78 months with average cumulative MNU doses of 104.6 gm developed squamous cell carcinoma of the esophagus.

Table 7. Esophageal Lesions Found At Necropsy in Monkeys Given 1-Methylnitrosourea (MNU)*

No. of Monkeys	Av. Total Dose (gm)	Months Dosed	Esophageal Pathology
2	15.3	26	none
3	14.1	59	atrophy, esophagitis, candidiasis
4	58.7	52	hyper- or dys-keratosis, ulceration
6	104.6	78	squamous cell carcinoma

*MNU (10-20 mg/kg) was given orally 5 days/week

A number of similarities between the esophageal tumors developing in our monkeys and human esophageal carcinoma were apparent. The order of appearance of the esophageal lesions in our monkeys, as well as the clinical manifestation of the tumors, resembled those seen in man, and included difficulty in swallowing, frequent vomiting and subsequent weight loss, and sialorrhea. The common complications of esophageal carcinoma in man (regurgitation, aspiration, sepsis and hemorrhage) were also noted in these monkeys. In addition, histological examination revealed a morphology similar to that seen in human esophageal carcinoma, despite the highly variable nature of such tumors in both monkeys and man. In view of these similarities between human esophageal carcinoma and those noted in the present study, we feel that MNU-induced esophageal carcinoma may prove to be a valuable model for the study of the human tumor.

The remainder of the carcinogenic nitroso- compounds are hepatocarcinogens, at least in Old World monkeys. Twelve monkeys have received po doses of PIP (400 mg/kg), and 11 (92%) have developed hepatic cell carcinomas (Table 8). In addition, 11 monkeys have been treated with PIP (40 mg/kg) by the ip route, and 4 (36%) have developed hepatocellular carcinomas. The average cumulative dose of PIP given orally was 1706.1 gm, and when given ip it was 60.95 gm; the average latent period for tumor induction ranged between 22 and 101 months, depending on the route of administration and the sex and the species of the monkey. However, the number of animals in each group was too small to draw any conclusions with regard to differences between species or sex in tumor susceptibility.

N-nitrosodipropylamine (DPNA) induced primary liver cancer in rhesus and cynomolgus monkeys when given bimonthly at ip doses of 40 mg/kg (Table 9). All monkeys treated with this chemical developed hepatic cell carcinoma after receiving average cumulative doses of 7.0 gm; the average latent period for tumor development was 28.5 months, ranging between 22 and 33 months.

N-nitrosodiethylamine (DENA) is also a carcinogen in non-human primates, inducing tumors when given either by the ip or po routes (Table 10). Twenty-eight out of 41 monkeys (68%) receiving po doses of DENA (40 mg/kg, 5 times every week) developed hepatocellular carcinoma. DENA given by bimonthly ip injection (40 mg/kg) induced hepatocellular carcinoma in 96 out of a total of 120 monkeys (80%). When administered po, DENA induced tumors earlier and at a lower cumulative dose in cynomolgus monkeys as compared to African greens, with the group of rhesus monkeys intermediate between the two species. This apparent species difference was not observed, however, when DENA was given by the ip route.

Table 11 shows that DENA is also carcinogenic in the prosimian, Galago crassicaudatus (bushbaby). It is interesting to note that the tumors induced in this species are primarily mucoepidermoid carcinoma of the nasal cavity rather than the hepatocellular carcinoma found in Old World monkeys. Ten out of 12

Table 8. Hepatic Cell Carcinoma Induced By Oral or Intraperitoneal Doses of 1-nitrosopiperidine (PIP)*

Species	Sex	Number of Animals	Cumulative Dose (gm)	Latent Period (mo)[†]
Oral Administration				
Rh	♀	1	177.0	36.0
	♂	5	1968.6	89.0
Cyno	♀	3	1535.4	101.0
	♂	2	2070.7	85.5
Intraperitoneal Administration				
Rh	♂	2	50.4	90.0
Cyno	♀	2	71.5	22.3

*For oral administration, PIP (400 mg/kg) was incorporated into a vitamin sandwich and given 5 days every week; for intraperitoneal administration, the dose was 40 mg/kg given once every week.

†The latent period is the time in months from the initial dose of PIP until the clinical diagnosis of a tumor.

Table 9. Hepatic Cell Carcinoma Induced by
Intraperitoneal Injections of N-
nitrosodipropylamine (DPNA)*

Species	Monkey Number	Sex	Total dose(gm)	Latent Period(mo)[†]
Rh	816J	♀	6.06	26
	815J	♂	6.56	27
	817J	♂	6.59	22
	811J	♀	7.25	31
Cyno	812J	♀	7.60	33
	814J	♀	7.96	32

*DPNA was given bimonthly at a dose of 40 mg/kg.

†Latent period is the time in months from initiation of treatment
until clinical diagnosis of tumor.

Table 10. Hepatocellular Carcinoma Induced by N-nitrosodiethylamine (DENA)*

Species	No. of Animals	Av. Latent Period (mo)	Av. Total Dose (gm)
Oral Administration			
Cyno	14	25.8	18.0
Rh	11	40.0	26.4
Afr Gr	3	105.0	55.1
Intraperitoneal Administration			
Cyno	36	16.9	1.54
Rh	49	16.9	1.93
Afr Gr	11	16.3	1.40

*40 mg/kg; oral doses 5 days/week; ip doses bimonthly.

Table 11.   Nasal Cavity Muco-epidermoid Carcinomas Induced in
            Bushbabies (Galago crassicaudatus) by IP Injections
            of N-nitrosodiethylamine (DENA)*

Monkey Number	Sex	Age at first dose (mo)	Total dose (gm)	Latent period (mo) [†]	Characteristics of tumor
838K	♂	1	0.295	13	Invasion of cranial bones & meninges; lung metastases
935M	♀	1	0.498	22	Well differentiated
939M	♂	3	0.525	19	Well differentiated, with invasion of bone & soft tissue of skull
907L	♂	1	0.614	12	Poorly differentiated, with metastases to brain
933M	♀	1	0.636	22	Invasion of brain
934M	♂	1	0.730	27	Well differentiated; also liver carcinoma with lung metastases
940M	♂	3	0.769	16	Well differentiated
936M	♂	1	0.786	22	Anaplastic adenoca., with invasion of bone & soft tissue of skull; metastases to cervical lymph nodes
904L	♂	1.5	1.130	22	Well differentiated
937M	♂	5	1.485	25	Invasion of bones & cartilage; also anaplastic carcinoma, liver with metastases to peri-gastric & -pancreatic lymph nodes

*DENA was given bimonthly at doses of 10-30 mg/kg: [†]Latent period is
the time in months from initiation of treatment until clinical diagnosis of tumor.

bushbabies (83%) given bimonthly ip doses of DENA (10-30 mg/kg)
developed tumors of the nasal cavity; in 2 of these animals,
carcinoma of the liver was also present, and in both cases metastases to the lungs or to intestinal lymph nodes were noted. The
first clinical symptom of the nasal cavity tumors was sneezing,
followed by audible nasal respiratory sounds, lacrimation and a
serous nasal discharge. Nodular development then became apparent
on the nose just anterior to the medial canthus. The tumors
continued to grow, often into the brain through the cribriform
plate or into the postorbital sinus.

The average total dose of DENA inducing tumors in the bushbabies (0.747 gm) is considerably lower than that required to
induce tumors in Old World monkeys, and reflects the lower body
weight of bushbabies. The average latent period for tumor induction in this species (20 months) is comparable to that in Old
World monkeys. There is no obvious reason for the marked difference noted between Old World monkeys and the bushbabies with
regard to the site of DENA-induced tumors. It is possible that it
is related to differences in the metabolism and/or distribution of
DENA, and this possibility is currently being investigated in our
laboratory.

We have also been evaluating the utility of determining serum
levels of the oncofetal protein, alpha-fetoprotein (AFP), as a
marker for hepatocellular carcinoma in tumor-bearing monkeys.
Results to date indicate that it has potential usefulness both in
diagnosis of tumors and in monitoring the success of surgery or
chemotherapy used to treat such tumors. Serum AFP levels are
determined by a double-antibody radioimmunoassay; the sensitivity
of the assay (lower level of detection is 5 ng/ml) has enabled us
to determine serum AFP levels in normal monkeys as well as in
monkeys being treated with carcinogens. The median value of
normal rhesus monkeys is 15.5 ng/ml (range 12.5-22 ng/ml), and in
cynomolgus is 13.0 (range 9.0-16.5 ng/ml).

The serum AFP levels of the majority of the monkeys in our
colony are determined every 6-12 months; however, in the groups of
monkeys at high risk of developing tumor, e.g., those receiving
DENA, AFP levels are monitored at monthly or bimonthly intervals.
In these monkeys, a rising serum AFP level precedes the clinical
and histologic diagnosis of hepatocellular carcinoma by several
months. Furthermore, we have found that all monkeys showing
elevated AFP levels (> 2,000 ng/ml) are destined to develop liver
carcinoma.

In addition to being a marker for the early detection of
tumors, AFP is also useful for following the course of therapy in
tumor-bearing monkeys. Figure 1 shows the AFP levels in a monkey

developing hepatocellular carcinoma after treatment with aflatoxin B_1. Approximately 46 months after initiation of aflatoxin B_1 treatment, AFP levels began to rise, and remained elevated until surgery, when the larger of 2 tumor nodules was removed at laparotomy. The AFP levels fell after tumor resection, although they never attained a normal level. At 60 days after surgery, serum AFP levels began a definitive rise in the absence of clinical signs of tumor recurrence. A second laparotomy was performed, and 2 small tumor nodules were resected. Serum AFP levels again fell after surgery, but the animal became progressively weaker and was sacrificed 20 days after surgery. At autopsy residual tumor was found in the liver, and it had invaded the wall of the stomach. Such studies suggest that serum AFP levels are a valid reflection of tumor growth and tumor activity.

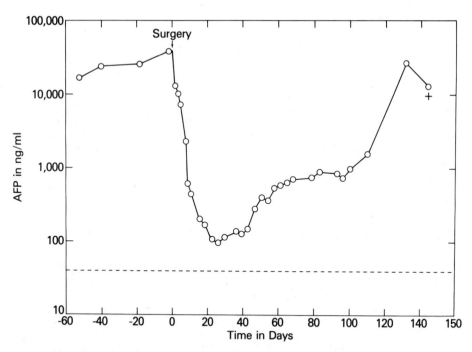

Figure 1. Serum AFP levels (ng/ml) as determined by radioimmunoassay prior to resection of aflatoxin B_1-induced hepatocellular carcinoma and during tumor regrowth. The zero on the abscissa represents the day tumor was resected.

DENA is highly predictable as a hepatocarcinogen in Old World monkeys, and accordingly we have accumulated a relatively large amount of information on its carcinogenic effects in these animals. We are therefore currently using this chemical as a model carcinogen to investigate two questions of importance to chemical carcinogenesis.

The first question pertains to whether there is a specific total dose of carcinogen which, within the lifespan of the test animal, reproduceably induces tumor. Asked another way, the question is, can the latent period for tumor induction be lengthened by reducing the dose of carcinogen to which the animal is chronically exposed? In order to evaluate this question, groups of monkeys are being given bimonthly ip injections of DENA at doses of 1, 5, 10, 20 and 40 mg/kg, and are observed for the appearance of tumor. In the 4 groups of monkeys in which tumors have developed, we have found that the latent period increases as the mg/kg dose decreases (Table 12). The study is as yet incomplete and in some groups the proportion of tumor-bearing animals is small, so that it is not yet possible to report a precise value for the carcinogenic dose of DENA. However, it appears that this value will lie between 1.2 and 2.2 gm.

Table 12. Hepatocellular Carcinomas Induced in Monkeys by Bimonthly IP Doses of N-Nitrosodiethylamine (DENA)

DENA Dose (mg/kg)	No. with Tumors/ No. Treated	Av. Total Dose (gm)[†]	Av. Latent Period (mo)[†]	Months on Study
1[*]	0/10	--	--	68
5	2/10	2.24	55	56
10	5/10	1.67	35	53
20	3/14	1.18	22	96
40	96/122	1.72	17	96

[*] Monkeys in this group have received an average total DENA dose of 0.373 gm for an average of 52 months; [†]for tumor-bearing animals.

The second question revolves about the issue of whether chemically-induced cancer can be prevented or reversed by other chemicals, either administered simultaneously with the carcinogen, or following carcinogen exposure. It is now recognized that the reactive forms of most chemical carcinogens are strong electrophiles (12). Although the carcinogenic alkylating agents, being electrophilic reactants, are already in their final reactive forms, most other chemical carcinogens require in vivo activation to this state. Thus it is frequently the case that the parent unreactive carcinogen or precarcinogen must be converted through a series of metabolic reactions into its ultimate carcinogenic species, e.g., a reactive electrophile capable of attacking tissue nucleophiles (12,13). Taking into consideration these concepts, there are a number of approaches to the prevention or reversal of chemical carcinogenesis that are possible, at least in theory, and these have been aptly reviewed recently (14,15).

In brief, these approaches involve: (A) altering the metabolism of the carcinogen by effecting changes in the hepatic mixed function oxidase systems; such an approach could either enhance detoxification of the carcinogen or suppress its activation to the ultimate carcinogenic species (16); (B) blocking the formation of the carcinogen; thus Mirvish et al. (17), found that sodium ascorbate blocks the induction of adenomas in mice given dietary amines or ureas plus $NaNO_2$ (combinations which form nitrosamines); (C) inhibiting the promotion and/or progression of tumors already formed, as is thought to be the action of retinoids against some forms of epithelial malignancies (18); and (D) "scavenging" the reactive electrophilic species of carcinogens once formed, using non-critical nucleophiles such as sulfhydryl reagents, to react with these electrophiles (12). It is the potential utility of the latter approach that we have chosen to evaluate in DENA-treated monkeys.

Two groups of monkeys are receiving bimonthly ip doses of DENA at 10 mg/kg or 5 mg/kg. In both groups, the DENA dose is given 10 minutes after an ip injection of a "protective cocktail" (Table 13). For the monkeys receiving DENA at 10 mg/kg, the "protective cocktail" consists of l-cysteine (20 mg/kg), cysteamine (20 mg/kg) and reduced glutathione (150 mg/kg). The "protective cocktail" given the monkeys receiving DENA at 5 mg/kg is composed of N-acetylcysteine (50 mg/kg). These substances were chosen as nucleophilic chemoprotectants for two reasons. First, they do not reduce the antitumor effects of various clinically useful alkylating agents and therefore could be used to protect against the carcinogenicity of these drugs without interfering with their therapeutic effects (19). Secondly, both N-acetyl-cysteine and cysteamine have been shown to prevent the covalent binding of acetaminophen to tissue, and for this reason have been

used in humans to reverse the hepatotoxic effects of acute acetaminophen poisoning (20). By analogy, it is hoped that these
sulfhydryl reagents will prevent the covalent binding of the
activated form of DENA to critical macromolecules of liver tissue,
an event which is thought to be a prerequisite for hepatocarcin-
ogenesis by a variety of chemicals including DENA. To date, none
of the monkeys have received the minimum cumulative dose of DENA
(1.2 gm) required for tumor development. The monkeys on this
study longest are those receiving DENA at 10 mg/kg. In this
group, the average cumulative DENA dose to date is 0.759 gm, and
the highest total dose given a monkey is 0.950 gm.

Table 13. Summary of Monkeys Receiving "Protective Cocktails"
to Prevent DENA-Induced Tumors

No. of Animals	DENA Dose (mg/kg)	Av. mg DENA Given to Date	Components of "Protective Cocktail"[*]
9	10	759	ℓ-cysteine(20 mg/kg), cysteamine (20 mg/kg) & GSH (150 mg/kg)
8	5	56	N-acetylcysteine (50 mg/kg)

[*]"Protective cocktails" are given ip 10 min before each bimonthly
dose of DENA

CONCLUSIONS

Carcinogenesis studies in non-human primates are expensive,
time consuming and require relatively large amounts of test chemical; thus, monkeys will probably never replace rodents as the
primary species for screening large numbers of chemicals for
carcinogenic activity. However, the use of non-human primates in
carcinogenesis studies has several advantages over rodent species.
One of these advantages is the comparatively low incidence of
spontaneous neoplasms in monkeys. In our colony, the tumor incidence in untreated breeders and vehicle-treated controls during
the past 16 years has been less than 1%. In contrast, results of
rodent carcinogenesis testing are frequently obscured by the high
incidence of tumors observed in control animals; in one rodent
colony, this incidence was 26% for control mice and 46% for control rats (21).

In addition, monkeys are phylogenetically closer to man than
are rodents, thus obviating some of the difficulties in extrapola-

ting rodent carcinogenesis data to the human. Certain metabolic pathways in non-human primates resemble those of humans more closely than do those of rodents. Smith and Caldwell (22) summarized the adequacy of the rhesus monkey, the rat, and other non-primate mammalian species as metabolic models for man; the comparisons were made on the basis of pathways of metabolism rather than kinetic or excretion differences. For the 23 compounds evaluated, the best metabolic model for man was provided by the rhesus monkey on 17 occasions. In contrast, other non-primate species (dog, guinea pig and rabbit) provided good metabolic models for only 5 compounds, and the rat for only 4 chemicals. Such considerations are of particular importance in chemical carcinogenesis, where metabolic activation of a precarcinogen to its ultimate reactive species is frequently a prerequisite for the manifestation of its carcinogenic effects.

The relatively longer life span of monkeys makes it possible to administer test compounds at doses equivalent to estimated human exposure levels; furthermore, it provides a more reasonable estimate of the latent period for tumor development following exposure to potential carcinogens than is possible with rodents. For example, the average latent period for the procarbazine-induced acute leukemia noted in our monkeys was approximately 5 1/2 years. This interval corresponds well with the latent period of a known human leukemogen, X-irradiation, which has been estimated to be approximately 4-8 years (23). In contrast, mice treated with po or ip doses of procarbazine develop leukemia within an average of only 20 weeks after initiation of treatment (24).

The site of tumor development in primates exposed to carcinogens also appears to parallel the human situation more closely than is the case with rodents, as exemplified by the studies with MNU. Nitrosamines may be synthesized in the upper GI tract of man (25), and MNU is final product of a reaction between nitrites in human saliva and methylguanidine, a constituent of several human foods (26). Therefore MNU or related nitroso compounds have been implicated as etiologic factors in human GI tract cancer (11,27). In fact, MNU induced squamous cell carcinomas of the oropharynx and/or esophagus in non-human primates, whereas rats treated orally with MNU developed kidney, skin and jaw tumors as well as tumors of the gastrointestinal tract (28). This similarity between non-human primates and man with regard to site of chemically-induced tumors also suggests that monkeys might represent a valuable model tumor system for the study of the corresponding human tumor. For example, many parallels were noted between the esophageal squamous cell carcinomas observed in the MNU-treated monkeys and human esophageal carcinoma; these parallels included the clinical manifestations of the tumor and its complications, radiographic appearance, and morphology.

In addition, results from studies with the hepatocarcinogens aflatoxin B_1, MAM-acetate, and the nitrosamines have made it possible to develop the alpha-fetoprotein assay as a tool for the early diagnosis of primary liver tumors and for monitoring the regrowth of hepatomas after surgical removal of the tumor or after chemotherapy. It is likely that other diagnostic tests, including additional onco-fetal antigens, will be developed in non-human primates and will prove useful for the detection of preneoplastic lesions in man.

And finally, the wealth of data already accumulated regarding DENA-induced hepatocellular carcinomas in Old World monkeys has enabled us to initiate studies on chemoprevention, utilizing exogenous nucleophiles such as N-acetylcysteine and cysteamine. It is to be hoped that information derived from such studies will ultimately be applicable to the prevention of cancer in human populations exposed to known chemical carcinogens.

REFERENCES

(1)   KELLY MG, O'GARA RW, ADAMSON RH, et al: Induction of hepatic cell carcinomas in monkeys with N-nitrosodiethylamine. J Natl Cancer Inst 36:323-351, 1966

(2)   O'GARA RW, ADAMSON RH, KELLY MG, et al: Neoplasms of the hematopoietic system in non-human primates: report of one spontaneous tumor and two leukemias induced by procarbazine. J Natl Cancer Inst 46:1121-1130, 1971

(3)   ADAMSON RH: Carcinogenicity studies with procarbazine. In Proceeding of the Chemotherapy Conference on Procarbazine (Matulane: NSC-77213): Development and Application March 13, 1970. US Dept of Hlth Educ and Welfare, PHS, Bethesda, Md., 1971, pp 29-33

(4)   O'GARA RW, ADAMSON RH: Spontaneous and induced neoplasms in non-human primates. In Pathology of Simian Primates (Fiennes RN T-W, ed.). Basel, New York, S. Karger, 1972, pp 190-238

(5)   ADAMSON RH: Long-term administration of carcinogenic agents to primates. In Medical Primatology 1972 - Proc 3rd Conference on Experimental Medicine and Surgery in Primates part III (Goldsmith EI, Moor-Jankowski J, eds.). Basel, Switzerland, S. Karger, 1972, pp 216-225

(6)   , CORREA P, DALGARD DW: Occurrence of a primary liver carcinoma in a rhesus monkey fed aflatoxin B_1. J Natl Cancer Inst 50:549-553, 1973

(7)   , SMITH CF, DALGARD DW: Induction of neoplasms in non-human primates by chemical carcinogens - correlation of serum alpha-fetoprotein and appearance of liver tumors. In Embryonic and Fetal Antigens in Cancer, Vol 2, February 14-16, 1972 (Anderson N-G, Coggin JH Jr, Cole E, Holleman JW, eds.). Oak Ridge, Tennessee, Oak Ridge National Laboratory, 1973, pp 331-337

(8)   DALGARD DW, MCINTOSH CL, MCINTIRE KR, et al: Hepatic carcinogenesis and serum alpha-fetoprotein in non-human primates. In Alpha-Feto-Protein (Masseyeff R, ed.). Paris, France, Proc Internatl Conf Inst Natl de la Sante et de la Recherche Medicale, 1974, pp 211-216

(9)   MCINTIRE KR, ADAMSON RH, WALDMAN TA, et al: Metabolism of alpha-fetoprotein in non-human primates. In Alpha-Feto-Protein (Masseyeff R, ed.). Paris, France, Proc Internatl Conf Inst Natl de la Sante et de la Recherche Medicale, 1974, pp 301-312

(10) ADAMSON RH, CORREA P, SIEBER SM, et al: Carcinogenicity of aflatoxin B_1 in rhesus monkeys: two additional cases of primary liver cancer. J Natl Cancer Inst 57:67-78, 1976.

(11)   , KROLIKOWSKI FJ, CORREA P, et al: Carcinogenicity of 1-methyl-1-nitrosourea in non-human primates. J Natl Cancer Inst 59:415-422, 1977.

(12) MILLER JA: Carcinogenesis by chemicals: An Overview. Cancer Res 30:559-576, 1970

(13)   , MILLER EC: Chemical carcinogenesis: Mechanisms and approaches to its control. J Natl Cancer Inst 47:5-14, 1971

(14) WATTENBERG LW: Inhibition of chemical carcinogenesis. J Natl Cancer Inst 60:11-18, 1978

(15) MILLER EC, MILLER JC: Approaches to the mechanisms and control of chemical carcinogenesis. In Environment and Cancer (The University of Texas M.D. Anderson Hospital and Tumor Institute at Houston), 24th Annual Symposium on Fundamental Cancer Research, Williams and Wilkins Co., Baltimore, 1972, pp 5-39

(16)   MAGEE PN: Activation and inactivation of chemical carcin-
       ogens and mutagens in the mammal. In Essays in Biochemistry,
       Vol. 10, (Campbell, PN and Dickens, F, eds.), London, Aca-
       demic Press, 1974, pp 105-136

(17)   MIRVISH SS, CARDESA A, WALLCAVE L, et al: Induction of
       mouse lung adenomas by amines or urea plus nitrite and by
       N-nitroso compounds: Effects of ascorbate, gallic acid,
       thiocyanate, and caffeine. J Natl Cancer Inst 55:633-636,
       1975

(18)   SPORN MB, DUNLOP NM, NEWTON DL, et al: Prevention of chem-
       ical carcinogenesis by vitamin A and its synthetic analogs
       (retinoids). Fed Proc 35:1332-1338, 1976

(19)   ADAMSON RH: Unpublished observations

(20)   PRESCOTT LF, NEWTON RW, SWAINSON CP, et al: Successful
       treatment of severe paracetamol overdosage with cysteamine.
       Lancet 1: 588-592, 1974

(21)   WEISBURGER JH, GRISWOLD DP, PREJEAN JD, et al: The carcino-
       genic properties of some of the principle drugs used in
       clinical cancer chemotherapy. Recent Results in Cancer Res
       52:1-17, 1975

(22)   SMITH RL, CALDWELL J: Drug metabolism in non-human pri-
       mates. In Drug Metabolism - From Microbe to Man (Parke
       DV, Smith RL, eds.). London, Taylor and Francis, Ltd.,
       1977, pp 331-356

(23)   UPTON AC: Radiation. In Cancer Medicine (Holland JF, Frei
       E, eds.). Philadelphia, Lea & Febiger, 1973, pp 90-101

(24)   KELLY MG, O'GARA RW, YANCEY ST, et al: Comparative carcin-
       ogenicity of N-isopropyl-α-(2-methylhydrazino)-p-toluamide.
       HCl (procarbazine hydrochloride), its degradation products,
       other hydrazines, and isonicotinic acid hydrazide. J Natl
       Cancer Inst 42:337-344, 1969

(25)   CORREA P, HAENSZEL W, CUELLO C, et al: A model for gastric
       cancer epidemiology. Lancet 2:58-60, 1975

(26)   ENDO H, TAKAHASHI K: Methylguanidine, a naturally occur-
       ring compound showing mutagenicity after nitrosation in
       gastric juice. Nature 245:325-326, 1973

(27)   MAGEE PN: Nitrosamines: ubiquitous carcinogens? New Sci
       59:432-434, 1973

(28)   LEAVER DD, SWANN PF, MAGEE PN: The induction of tumors in
       the rat by a single oral dose of N-nitrosomethylurea. Brit
       J Cancer 23:177-187, 1969

NUCLEOTIDES, NUCLEOSIDE PHOSPHATE DIESTERS AND PHOSPHONATES

AS ANTIVIRAL AND ANTINEOPLASTIC AGENTS - AN OVERVIEW

Jaroslaw T. Kusmierek & David Shugar

Institute of Biochemistry & Biophysics

Academy of Sciences, 02-532 Warsaw (Poland)

A wide variety of nucleoside analogues are now known which exhibit significant antiviral or/and antineoplastic activity (Hermann, 1977; Cohen, 1977; Prusoff & Ward, 1976; Bloch, 1975; Shugar, 1974). The basic concept behind the development of such analogues, as well as other agents, is that they may specifically interfere with some stage(s) of the nucleic acid metabolism of the virus (or tumour cell) without undue toxicity towards the host (or normal) cell. In view of the known marked differences amongst various viruses, as well as their mode of replication (e.g. Dales, 1973), it is not at all surprising that the activity of a given analogue may be specific for a certain virus or class of viruses. Furthermore, it is now reasonably well established that the active agent is usually a product of intracellular metabolism, e.g. the antiviral activity of 5-iodo-2'-deoxyuridine is associated with its conversion to the 5'-triphosphate by intracellular kinases, followed by its incorporation into DNA (Prusoff & Goz, 1975). One of the newer, and most interesting, of such analogues is 5'-amino--2',5'-dideoxy-5-iodouridine, which is apparently selectively taken up by herpes simplex virus type 1 (HSV-1) infected cells, initially phosphorylated by HSV-1 thymidine kinase, and subsequently by the host cell kinases (Chen et al., 1975). By contrast 5'-amino-5'-deoxy-araC is active against vaccinia virus, but not HSV-1 (Prusoff & Ward, 1976).

The extensive efforts devoted to the synthesis of a multitude of nucleoside analogues, involving modifications of the heterocyclic base or the sugar moiety, are understandable in view of the relative ease with which nucleosides are transported across cell membranes. But this approach frequently suffers from some limitations, as illustrated by the intracellular deamination of araC to

481

the inert araU, or of araA to araHx which, in some instances, is
less active as an antimetabolite. These limitations may be
circumvented occasionally by the synthesis of more sophisticated
analogues, such as the cytidine deaminase resistant 2,2'-anhydro-
-araC or 2,2'-anhydro-5-fluoro-araC (which are really depot forms
of araC and 5-fluoro-araC, respectively) (Fox et al., 1972) or the
deaminase resistant carbocyclic araA (Vince and Daluge, 1977).
The use, in such instances, of deaminase inhibitors (Cohen, 1977;
Henderson, 1978), although widely contemplated, is subject to the
serious reservation that these may interfere with the normal
metabolic processes of the cell.

NUCLEOTIDES AS ANTIMETABOLIC AGENTS

The generally accepted view that cellular membranes are fully
impermeable to nucleotides was at least rendered dubious by the
demonstration by Ortiz et al. (1972) that 5'-araAMP is more lethal
to mouse fibroblasts than the parent nucleoside, and that this
lethal effect is accompanied by transport of the <u>intact</u> nucleotide
across the cell membrane, albeit much less effectively than the
nucleoside, followed by further phosphorylation and incorporation
of the nucleotide into cellular DNA (Plunkett et al., 1974). This
phenomenon is not necessarily a general one since araC, under
these conditions, is more effective than the 5'-, 2'- or 3'-
araCMP, or the 2',5'-cyclic phosphate of araC (Ortiz et al., 1972).
On the other hand 2',3'-dideoxyadenosine-5'-phosphate, the
triphosphate of which is an obvious chain terminator, is lethal
to L cells under conditions where the nucleoside itself exhibits
minimal toxicity, and in accordance with the observation that the
latter is not significantly phosphorylated by crude extracts of
the cells (Plunkett & Cohen, 1975; Cohen, 1977).

The foregoing should not be confused with the well-known
results of LePage et al. (1972) on the use of 5'-nucleotides in
man, which was in fact dictated by the premise that nucleotides
would not enter intact cells. The use of nucleotides (of araA and
ara-6-mercaptopurine) in this instance was based on the observation that phosphomonoesterase levels in human kidney were much
lower than in the mouse and other small mammals. Administration
of the foregoing nucleotides to patients therefore led, in
accordance with expectations, to sustained blood plasma levels of
the nucleosides, as well as better dosage formulations because of
the higher solubility of nucleotides.

A number of reported, but generally overlooked, examples of
transport of organic phosphates across cell membranes have been
cited by Cohen (1975). A recent striking example is a mutant yeast
strain which actually requires thymidine-5'-phosphate for growth,
and has been shown to be deficient in thymidylate synthetase

(Bisson & Thorner, 1977).

Interest has also developed in the use of nucleotides as antiviral agents by the observation that the corresponding nucleoside analogues must usually be converted to the nucleotides before exhibiting biological activity. The higher solubility of nucleotides is an additional distinct advantage. Furthermore nucleotides may by-pass metabolic pathways responsible for resistance to nucleosides, such as high cellular nucleoside deaminase activity, or low levels of nucleoside kinase. A number of nucleotide analogues have consequently been tested for <u>in vitro</u> antiviral activity (see Revankar et al., 1976 for references). In no instance, however, was activity significantly superior to that of the parent nucleoside, and usually it was considerably lower. In the case of HSV-1 experimental keratitis, the activity of araAMP was comparable to that of araA itself, but the higher solubility of the former suggests that it may have a significant advantage over the nucleoside (Kaufman & Varnell, 1976).

In none of the foregoing, however, were attempts made to establish whether the observed activity was due to transport of the nucleotide across the cell membrane; and it is conceivable that, in those instances where the level of antiviral activity was comparable to that of the nucleoside, this may have been due to dephosphorylation by membrane-localized phosphomonoesterases or 5'-nucleotidase, followed by transport of the nucleoside into the cell. In fact, earlier findings with ^{32}P-labelled nucleotides (see

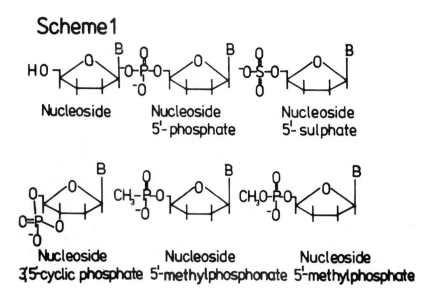

Scheme 1

Nucleoside   Nucleoside 5'-phosphate   Nucleoside 5'-sulphate

Nucleoside 3'5'-cyclic phosphate   Nucleoside 5'-methylphosphonate   Nucleoside 5'-methylphosphate

Plunkett et al., 1974) suggested that such is usually the case.

ALKYL ESTERS OF NUCLEOTIDES

If it is, in fact, the diionized phosphate group of a nucleotide which hinders its transport across the cell membrane at physiological pH, it should theoretically be feasible to at least partially overcome this by blocking one of the phosphate hydroxyls to yield an alkyl ester. Such a nucleoside-5'-alkylphosphate could conceivably be hydrolyzed to the nucleotide by membrane-localized phosphodiesterase I, and subsequently to the nucleoside by 5'-nucleotidase, during transport. Or it could be transported intact across the membrane, its subsequent fate being determined by the intracellular enzyme machinery. Although it has long been known that nucleoside-5'-methylphosphates are substrates for phosphodiesterase I (Szer & Shugar, 1961), and thymidine-5'-(p-nitrophenyl)phosphate has been employed for years as a presumed specific substrate for this enzyme (Razzell, 1963), more recent developments call for some revision of these concepts (see below). Furthermore, insofar as we are aware, no attempts appear yet to have been made to examine directly the fate of a nucleoside-5'-alkylester at a cellular membrane. An analogue of a monoionized nucleotide and potential antimetabolite, 5-fluoro-2'-deoxyuridine-5'-sulfate, was synthetized some time ago and reported to penetrate cell membranes (Wigler & Lozzio, 1972).

In a series of in vitro tests against HSV-1, HSV-2 and vaccinia viruses on KB and RK-13 cells, Revankar et al. (1975) found araA, araAMP and araHxMP to exhibit comparable levels of activity against all three viruses, as did also the methyl ester of araAMP. By contrast, the methyl ester of araHxMP was totally inactive against HSV-2 and only 50% as active against HSV-1 and vaccinia. The relevance of the results to the possible mode of action of the esters was not considered. It is somewhat odd that the methyl ester of araAMP was no more effective than araAMP itself, and even more so that the activity of ara-Hx-5'-methyl phosphate was so low compared to the parent araHxMP.

In a series of earlier studies on in vitro cytotoxicity vs L1578Y and KB cells the Upjohn group (Wechter, 1967; Smith et al., 1967) compared araCMP and its methyl and phenyl esters with the parent araC. AraCMP (whether the 5'-, 3'- or 2'- phosphate) exhibited activity comparable to that of araC. The methyl and phenyl esters of 5'-araCMP also were quite active as cytotoxic agents, the phenyl ester being superior to the methyl. This is in accord with the higher susceptibility of the phenyl ester to phosphodiesterase I (Richards et al., 1967; Zeleznick, 1969). Since deoxycytidine was able to reverse the above effects, and the compounds were inactive against kinase-deficient cells, the conclusion was drawn that these were enzymatically degraded before entering the cell to release araC, which then acted subsequently as such.

Inhibition of incorporation of ^{14}C-formate into DNA thymine of Ehrlich ascites cells was used as a test system by Mukherjee & Heidelberger (1962) to compare the cytotoxic activities of various 5-fluorouracil nucleosides and nucleotides. The 5'-phosphate of 5-fluorodeoxyuridine was 10-fold less effective than the nucleoside, but simple alkyl esters of the nucleotide were even less active. These findings do not appear readily interpretable; at best they point to the difficulty of drawing generalizations for different cell systems.

The comparative effects of araC, araA, and their 5'-nucleotides and methyl esters on the growth of a human hemopoietic cell line (SK-L7) have been examined by Dr. Z. Darzynkiewicz of Sloan-Kettering. At 10^{-6} M and slightly higher concentrations of the araC analogues, the cells were found to slowly traverse through the S phase of the cell cycle and were blocked in G_2 + M. At 10^{-5} M, and slightly higher concentrations, the cells were blocked in early S phase. AraC was found to be markedly more effective than its nucleotide or methyl ester. By contrast, the perturbing effects of araA and its nucleotide and methyl ester (at concentrations in the range 3×10^{-5} to 3×10^{-4} M) were manifested by a block in late S or G_2 + M, with the nucleotide and methyl ester being more effective than the nucleoside. The comparative effects of araA and araAMP, in this instance, are therefore qualitatively similar to those reported by Ortiz et al. (1972) in the case of mouse L cells.

Cytotoxicity of araC, 5'-araCMP, and the methyl, ethyl and glycol esters of the latter, has also been examined with L5178Y cells by Dr. J. Koziorowska of the Pharmaceutical Institute in Warsaw. The nucleotide and its methyl ester exhibited cytotoxic effects comparable to those of araC at concentrations of 10^{-7} M, whereas the ethyl and glycol esters were only slightly less effective, notwithstanding our observation that these are more slowly hydrolyzed by PDase I than the corresponding methyl ester. Controls treated with equivalent concentrations of the methyl esters of 5'-CMP and 5'-AMP exhibited no adeverse effects on cell growth.

In studies still in progress on the antiviral activities of araA, araC and their nucleotides and methyl esters, by Dr. E. De Clercq, the order of activity against vaccinia virus on PRK cells was nucleoside > nucleotide > methyl ester. By contrast, activities against the same virus on HSF cells were similar for the nucleoside, nucleotide and methyl ester of both series of compounds.

Scheme 2

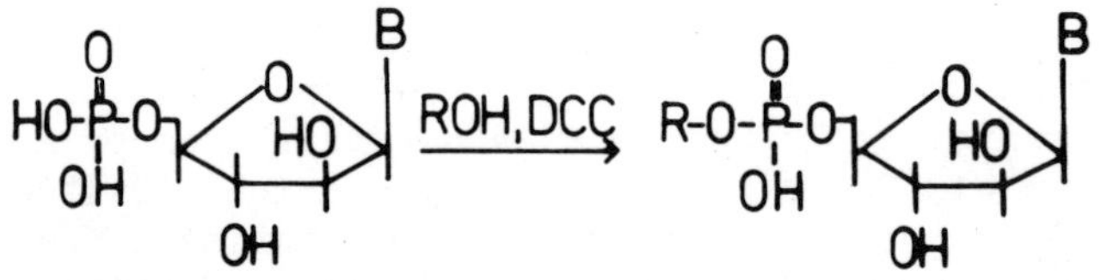

B= cytosine, adenine
R=CH$_3$-, C$_2$H$_5$- , HO-CH$_2$ CH$_2$-

Further studies with alkyl esters of nucleotides might profitably be extended to the use of such groups as phenyl, p-nitrophenyl, etc., characterized by higher leaving tendencies. For example the p-nitrophenyl ester of 5'-TMP is cleaved at a much higher rate by PDase I than simple alkyl esters. Such trials are now under way in our laboratories.

Synthesis of Alkyl Esters of 5'-Nucleotides

These are readily prepared in good yield (Scheme 2) according to the procedure of Khorana (1959), by reaction of the 5'-nucleotide with the corresponding alcohol (e.g. with methanol for 20 hrs at 37°C; with ethanol for 2 hrs at 80°C; with glycol for 1 hr at 100°C) in the presence of an excess of dicyclohexyl-carbodiimide (DCC). The ester is isolated by chromatography on a column of Dowex 1x2 (HCO$_3$⁻) by elution with a linear gradient of 0.0 - 0.5 M triethylammonium carbonate. The isolated ester is converted to the free acid by passage over Dowex (H⁺), and then precipitated from concentrated aqueous solution by addition of acetone. In routine preparations we have obtained overall yields ranging from 70-90% for esters of 5'-araCMP and 5'-araAMP.

NUCLEOSIDE-3',5'-CYCLIC PHOSPHATES

Like ribonucleoside-2',3'-cyclic phosphates, these compounds are diesters of phosphoric acid and, at physiological pH, carry a single negative charge, and so should more readily penetrate the cell membrane. This has been shown to apply also to a variety of cAMP analogues (LePage & Hersh, 1972). Furthermore they are hydrolyzed by specific phosphodiesterases, in mammalian cells, to the corresponding nucleoside-5'-phosphates. Although cyclic PDases active against pyrimidine-3',5'-cyclic phosphates have been described, these are probably present at low levels, so that pyrimidine analogues are usually relatively resistant, a fact frequently ignored, but of some significance.

The 3',5'-cyclic phosphates of araA, and the ribosides of 6-mercaptopurine and 6-methylmercaptopurine, were all inhibitory in several tumour lines resistant to the parent nucleosides or heterocyclic bases because of lack of essential enzymes (such as hypoxanthine-guanine phosphoribosyl pyrophosphate transferase, necessary for conversion of 6-methylmercaptopurine to the 5'-nucleotide; or adenosine kinase necessary for conversion of nucleosides to the 5'-phosphates) (LePage and Hersh, 1972). The araA analogue was rapidly converted to 5'-araAMP by L1210 cell homogenates, which also rapidly deaminated araA, but not araAMP or its cyclic phosphate. It would consequently appear that the active inhibitors are the 5'-phosphates.

Consistent with the foregoing are the results of Hughes & Kimball (1972), who showed that araA-3',5'-cyclic phosphate inhibited DNA (but not RNA) synthesis in L1210 cells, and was readily hydrolyzed by cell homogenates. However, some direct effect of the cyclic phosphate itself was not excluded. The same analogue inhibits growth of mice fibroblasts, but with activity not exceeding that of araAMP, and under conditions where cAMP is without effect (Plunkett & Cohen, 1975); the inactivity of the 2',5'-cyclic phosphate of araA can probably be ascribed to the absence of known enzymes active against this linkage.

It had earlier been shown that the 3',5'-cyclic phosphate of 5-fluorodeoxyuridine was inactive against mouse fibroblasts, whereas the parent nucleoside and nucleotide were potent inhibitors (Ortiz et al., 1972). This is probably related to the relative resistance of pyrimidine 3',5'-cyclic phosphates to mammalian cyclic PDases, referred to above.

By contrast, Long et al. (1972) reported that araC-3',5'-cyclic phosphate was as active as araC in inhibiting the growth of several DNA viruses, exhibited appreciable toxicity against leukemia L1210 in vivo, and was markedly effective in treatment of HSV-1 keratitis in the eyes of rabbits. Using a partially purified rabbit kidney cAMP phosphodiesterase, they demonstrated appreciable hydrolysis rates for a number of pyrimidine 3',5'-cyclic phosphates, e.g. araC-3',5'-P was cleaved at 5% the rate of cAMP. These findings merit further examination. The same authors refer to antiviral activity of some analogues of cAMP resistant to enzymatic cleavage, suggesting, as did Hughes and Kimball (1972), the possibility of some direct effect by the cyclic phosphates. It would clearly have been desirable for Long et al. (1972) to examine cyclic PDase activities of the homogenates of cells employed in

their investigation, since both the nature and level of cyclic
PDase activities may vary with cell type.

Independently Kreis & Wechter (1972) examined the activities
of araC-3',5'-P against P815/S cells (sensitive to araC) and
P815/R cells (resistant to araC and lacking araC/dC kinase
activity). The compound was about half as effective as araC
against the sensitive strain, and somewhat more effective than
araC against the resistant strain. However, the concentrations
required for measureable inhibition against the resistant strain
were about 100-fold higher. It was assumed that activity was due
to passage of araC-3',5'-P through the cell membrane, followed by
hydrolysis to araCMP. If this were the case, one might have
expected the cyclic phosphate to be much more effective than araC
in the resistant cells than actually observed. It clearly would
have been extremely useful in this case to have compared the rates
of hydrolysis of araC-3',5'-P by homogenates of sensitive and
resistant cells. In in vivo experiments with mice bearing P815 R
or S neoplasms, the cyclic phosphate was as ineffective against
P815/R as araC, and appreciably less effective than araC against
P815/S. The poor results obtained with the cyclic phosphate were
ascribed to its hydrolysis by phosphodiesterase in the serum, but
no measurements on this were reported.

The synthesis, and in vitro antiviral activity, of a series
of purine nucleoside 3',5'-cyclic phosphates, has been described
by Robins' group (Revankar et al., 1976). Several of these were
also tested by intracerebral administration in mice with HSV-1
induced encephalitis, but the highest therapeutic index attained
was about 4, as compared to 30 for araA in the same system. The
utility of such results, even though partially negative, would be
considerably enhanced if accompanied by concomitant biochemical
studies of mechanisms.

Of some interest also is the 3',5'-cyclic phosphate of
ribavirin, which exhibits potent in vitro activity against a
variety of RNA and DNA viruses. The cyclic phosphate is readily
cleaved by kidney or brain cyclic PDase, but its activity is lower
than that of ribavirin itself. Somewhat surprisingly, its spectrum
of activity is also reduced relative to that of ribavirin (Simon
et al., 1973), a phenomenon worthy of further study.

PHOSPHONATES

Phosphonates have for some years been employed as analogues
of naturally occurring phosphates because of their possible use
for perturbation or regulation of metabolic processes, and their
potential use for studies of reaction mechanisms, while naturally
occurring phosphonates have been isolated from numerous organisms.

The chemistry of phosphonates, and their biological aspects and implications, have recently been extensively reviewed by Engel (1977). The presumption that some organisms could hydrolyze the carbon-phosphorus bond was initially strengthened by the isolation of E. coli mutants capable of using simple phosphonic acids as a source of phosphorus, and has been reinforced by further developments (see Engel, 1977). The synthetic 4-nitrophenyl and 2-naphthyl monoesters of phenylphosphonic acid are excellent substrates for phosphodiesterase I (Kelly et al., 1975; Kelly and Butler, 1977), although the specificity is not as narrow as originally proposed (see below). Extension of these studies showed that some synthetic phosphonothioates are likewise good phosphodiesterase substrates (Dudman and Benkovic, 1977). A variety of phosphonates have now been shown to be suitable phosphate analogues in the reactions catalyzed by yeast glyceraldehyde-3-phosphate dehydrogenase and calf spleen nucleoside phosphorylase (Gardner and Byers, 1977). Finally, phosphonoacetate has proven effective against a number of viruses in animal studies; its mechanism of action in the case of herpes simplex virus is through blocking of HSV DNA synthesis by a specific effect on the HSV-induced DNA polymerase. Phosphonoformate is as effective as phosphonoacetate (see Boezi, 1978, for review).

Nucleoside-5'-Methylphosphonates

There are two well-documented examples of the use of such analogues as antimetabolites. Wigler and Lozzio (1972) demonstrated that 5-bromo-2'-deoxyuridine-5'-methylphosphonate was cytotoxic to Chinese hamster (V-79) cells at concentration as low as 10 uM. Reversal of cytotoxicity by thymidine was observed only when added to the medium at the same time as the phosphonate. Evidence for penetration of the analogue, and its incorporation into cellular DNA, was based on the observation that cells with sublethal damage were sensitive to near UV light. Such behaviour, however, is consistent only with the incorporation of 5-bromouracil residues into DNA. Interaction of the analogue with the cells was shown by its disappearance from the growth medium and the absence of degradation products such as 5-bromouracil and 5-bromodeoxyuridine. But this does not constitute evidence for intracellular phosphorylation of the analogue to the triphosphate (see below) and its incorporation as such into cellular DNA. It is unfortunate that the authors did not compare the cytotoxicity of the analogue with that of 5-bromodeoxyuridine and 5-bromodeoxyuridine-5'-phosphate.

In a more recent study, Gormley et al. (1977) examined the cytotoxicity of the 5'-methylphosphonate of araC (araCMeP) against leukemia P388 cells. An almost 100-fold greater concentration of the analogue, relative to araC, was required for comparable cell inhibition. Both araCMeP and araCMP were equally effective competitive inhibitors of dCMP kinase from leukemic L1210 cells,

but only the latter was a substrate for this enzyme. This was
taken to indicate that araCMeP could not as such enter the
triphosphate pool and that a 1% conversion to araC might account
for its observed toxicity; but an equally plausible interpretation
is the inhibition of dCMP kinase. Our own observations on the slow
hydrolysis of araCMeP by 5'-nucleotidase (see below) could account
for the 1% hydrolysis. Here again it would have been useful to
have employed araCMP (in addition to araC) as a control, in view
of the known lethality of araAMP against L cells (Plunkett et al.,
1974).

Dr. J. Koziorowska has tested the cytotoxicity of araCMeP
against L1578Y cells, using araC as a control. Under conditions
where araC exhibited observable cytotoxicity at a level of 10^{-8} M,
araCMeP was without effect at a level of 10^{-6} M.

In retrospect, it appears to us that it would be logical to
also examine the potential antimetabolic properties of 5'-deoxy-
nucleoside-5'-phosphonates and their monoalkyl esters. Such phosphonates, but not their esters, have been synthezied and extensively employed, particularly as the polyphosphates, in studies on
the mechanisms of protein biosynthesis (Kurland, 1972), reactions
of NAD utilizing enzymes (Hampton et al., 1972), etc.

Synthesis of 5'-Methylphosphonates of Cytidine and AraC

This procedure, based on the conversion of cytidine-5'-methyl-
phosphonate to araC-5'-methylphosphonate, via a 2,2'-anhydro
derivative (Scheme 3), is simpler than that described by Gormley

Scheme 3

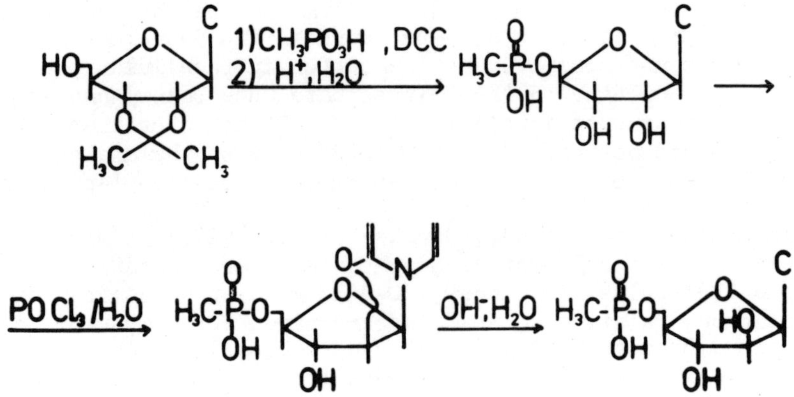

et al. (1977) for araC-5'-methylphosphonate, and simultaneously
makes available cytidine-5'-methylphosphonate, as well as its
2,2'-anhydro derivative, which could conceivably serve as a depot
form of araC-5'-methylphosphonate.

Cytidine-5'-methylphosphosphonate is prepared by reaction of
2',3'-O-isopropylidenecytidine with methylphosphonic acid in the
presence of DCC in dimethylformide (DMF) solution at 37°C for
40 hrs. Following removal of solvent, isopropylidene blocking
group is removed by heating in 20% aqueous acetic acid for 1.5 hrs
at 100°C. The product is isolated by chromatography on a Dowex 1x2
(HCO_3^-) column by elution with a linear gradient of 0.0 - 0.5 M
triethylammonium carbonate, is then converted to the free acid by
passage over Dowex (H^+), and precipitated from concentrated
aqueous solution by addition of acetone. Yield is about 70%.

O^2,2'-cyclocytidine-5'-methylphosphonate is prepared as
described for the corresponding O^2,2'-cyclocytidine-5'-phosphate
(Kanai et al., 1971). Cytidine-5'-methylphosphonate in ethyl
acetate, in the presence of partially hydrolyzed $POCl_3$, is heated
for 1 hr at 60°C. Following addition of water, the mixture is
chromatographed on a Dowex 50W (H^+) column by elution with a
linear gradient of 0.0 - 0.1 M HCl. The appropriate fractions are
pooled, brought to dryness, taken up in the minimal volume of
methanol, and the desired product precipitated by addition of
acetone. Yield, 40%.

AraC-5'-methylphosphonate is obtained quantitatively from
O^2,2'-cyclocytidine-5'-methylphosphonate by hydrolysis of the
latter in 1 N NaOH for 1 hr at 37°C. The product is passed over
Dowex (H^+) to obtain the free acid, and precipitated from concentrated aqueous solution with acetone.

DINUCLEOSIDE MONOPHOSPHATES

A dinucleoside monophosphate may be considered as a nucleoside ester of a nucleotide, so that the phosphate of the latter
bears a single negative charge at physiological pH. Analogues of
the dinucleoside monophosphates shown in Scheme 4, in which one or
both of the nucleoside components are known antimetabolites, were
synthesized and examined for antimetabolic activity during the
1960's. Some of the reported findings are undoubtedly of more than
historic interest, and are briefly summarized here. It should be
noted that all three types of dinucleoside monophosphates shown
in Scheme 4 may be regarded as "nucleoside esters" of nucleoside-
5'-monophosphates and are therefore potentially good substrates
for phosphodiesterase I.

The following dinucleoside monophosphates, containing

Scheme 4

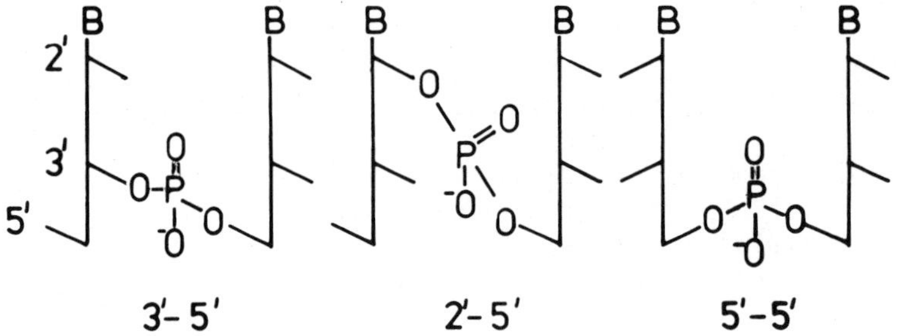

Dinucleoside monophosphates

5-fluorodeoxyuridine (FUdR) and 6-mercaptopurine riboside (MPR) were synthetized and examined for growth inhibition of HEp-2/S cells (sensitive to 6-mercaptopurine) and HEp-2/MP cells (resistant to 6-mercaptopurine): FUdR5'-5'MPR, FUdR3'-5'MPR, MPR5'-5'MPR (Montgomery et al., 1963). All three proved to be effective inhibitors of both types of cells, whereas MPR and MP inhibited only the HEp-2/S cells. Inhibition of HEp-2/MP cells by the dinucleoside monophosphates containing FUdR may be interpreted as due to liberation of FUdR prior to and/or following transfer through the cell membrane. The activity of MPR5'-5'MPR against resistant cells, which were not affected by exogenous MP, MPR and MPR-5'-phosphate, is explicable on the assumption that the dinucleoside monophosphate penetrated the cell intact, and was intracellularly hydrolyzed to MPR-5'-phosphate and MPR, the former of which would be the active antimetabolite in such cells. It should be noted that the lack of any effect of MPR-5'-phosphates on the resistant cell line indicates that the intact nucleotide does not adequately penetrate the cell membrane, in contrast to the results of Ortiz et al. (1972) with 5'-araAMP and mouse fibroblasts.

Several dinucleoside monophosphates containing 5-fluorouridine and 5-fluorodeoxyuridine residues were tested by Mukherjee & Heidelberger (1962) and Parsons & Heidelberger (1966) as inhibitors of ^{14}C-formate incorporation into DNA thymine of Ehrlich ascites cells, relative to a number of 5-fluorouracil nucleoside analogues. The most potent inhibitors were 5-fluorodeoxyuridine and 5-fluorodeoxycytidine, with 5-fluorodeoxyuridine-5'-phosphate about 10-fold less active. None of the dinucleoside monophosphates was more active than the latter. By contrast, chemically synthesized oligonucleotides containing 5-fluorodeoxyuridine residues were somewhat more effective than 5-fluorodeoxyuridine-5'-phosphate, but was apparently not considered sufficiently promising to pursue further. Similar dinucleoside monophosphates were examined as growth inhibitors in a bacterial system, Streptococcus faecalis (Bloch et al., 1966); the overall data, based in part on cross--resistance and uptake measurements, suggested that observed inhibition was due to nucleoside degradation products of the dinucleoside monophosphates, formed probably at the cell surface.

The Upjogn group synthesized a large group of of dinucleoside monophosphates containing araC residues, and with 2'-5', 3'-5' and 5'-5' diester linkages (Wechter, 1967) and tested these as inhibitors of cell growth (Smith et al., 1967) or of in vitro virus multiplication (Renis et al., 1967). A number of the dinucleoside monophosphates exhibited appreciable antimetabolic activity, but in no instance did this exceed that of the parent araC itself. In the majority of cases the activity of a given dinucleoside monophosphate correlated with its susceptibility to PDase I (Richards et al., 1967; Zeleznick, 1969). Furthermore the cytotoxic effects of the compounds could be reversed by deoxycytidine, while the compounds were inactive against kinase-deficient cells. The overall results are consequently consistent with the view that the mechanism of action involves hydrolysis of the dinucleoside monophosphates to araC outside the cells, and any subsequent effect is due to entry of araC as such. The difference between these findings, and those of Montgomery et al. (1963) referred to above, are rather puzzling. However, the cell systems employed, L1578Y and KB, were different.

ENZYMOLOGICAL ASPECTS

Attempts at applications of nucleoside alkylphosphates or phosphonates as potential antimetabolic agents necessarily requires some prior knowledge of the susceptibilities of these compounds to various enzymes, such as phosphatases, nucleases, phosphodiesterases, etc. likely to be encountered in normal, tumour and virus--infected cells. For this reason we have begun a qualitative survey of some readily accessible purified and crude enzyme systems against these classes of analogues. We briefly summarize some preliminary findings, together with several previously reported literature results which have hitherto received little attention.

Following a series of syntheses of nucleotides with modified phosphate substituents, Holy & Hong (1972) reported that the 5'-methylphosphonates of adenosine and uridine were degraded by snake venom 5'-nucleotidase to the nucleosides and methylphosphonic acid, but at rates considerably lower than for the parent nucleotides. We have found that snake venom purified 5'-nucleotidase is active against the 5'-nethylphosphonates of cytidine and araC, the rates of hydrolysis being 100-fold lower than for 5'-CMP; the products of hydrolysis were directly identified as the nucleosides and methylphosphonate. No hydrolysis was observed with a crude extract of normal human erythrocytes, known to contain a pyrimidine specific 5'-nucleotidase (Torrance et al., 1977).

Further trials with cytidine-5'-methylphosphonate showed slight susceptibility to wheat germ extracts, to commercial wheat germ acid phosphatase, and to purified potato acid phosphatase, but complete resistance to a highly purified acid phosphatase (Ostrowski and Barnard, 1973) from human prostate.

Highly purified nucleotide pyrophosphatase from potatoes (Kole et al., 1976), an enzyme with a broad range of specificity, also purified from cultured tobacco cells (Shinshi et al., 1976), exhibits feeble activity against cytidine-5'-methylphosphonate. There are reports on the isolation from mammalian sources of analogous pyrophosphatase activities (e.g. Nuss and Furuichi, 1977; Lavers, 1977) considered to be involved in the decapping of the 5'-terminal $m^7G(5')$pppN- of viral and mammalian mRNA; and a study has recently appeared on the distribution of such activity in various organs and body fluids (Haugen and Skrede, 1977). Like the plant enzyme, its mammalian counterpart appears to exhibit PDase I activity, but its range of specificity has not been as extensively studied.

Relevant to the foregoing are the results of Hickey et al. (1976) on a purified preparation of wheat germ phosphatase, which hydrolyzed nitrophenyl esters of alkyl and aryl phosphonates at rates comparable to those for phosphomonoesters. The procedure for isolation of the enzyme, and a description of its properties, has not yet appeared. We have found that potato acid phosphatase exhibits only low activity against p-nitrophenyl phenylphosphonate, relative to p-nitrophenylphosphate. It is rather surprising that acid phosphatases from two plant sources exhibit such marked differences in specificity, and this is being further investigated. Of possible significance in this regard is our observation that p-nitrophenyl phenylphosphonate and p-nitrophenylphosphate are hydrolyzed at equal rates by potato nucleotide pyrophosphatase. It should be recalled that p-nitrophenyl phenylphosphonate was initially proposed by Kelly et al. (1975) as a specific substrate for 5'-nucleotide phosphodiesterase (PDase I). We have found the 5'-methylphosphonates of cytidine and araC to be resistant to PDase I.

The 5'-methylphosphonate of araC was not a substrate for leukemia L1210 dCMP kinase, but was a competitive inhibitor of this enzyme, with a K_i value identical to that for araCMP (Gormley et al., 1977). However 6'-deoxyhomoadenosine-6'-phosphonates (compounds isosteric with 5'-AMP) have been shown to exhibit both substrate and inhibitor properties towards rabbit and pig AMP kinases (Hampton et al., 1973), and it is somewhat surprising that such analogues have not received more attention as potential anti-metabolites.

As regards the alkyl esters of nucleotides, the methyl, ethyl and glycol esters of 5'-araCMP are substrates for PDase I, but are hydrolyzed at 5 to 10-fold lower rates than the methyl ester of 5'-CMP. The relative rates of hydrolysis decrease in the order methyl > ethyl > glycol. The susceptibility to PDase I of alkyl esters of 5'-araCMP, as well as of dinucleoside monophosphates containing this residue, had been earlier reported by Richards et al. (1967) and Zeleznik (1969).

Somewhat unexpected, on the other hand, was our observation that alkyl esters of 5'-CMP and 5'-araCMP were, like the 5'-methyl-phosphonates of cytidine and araC (see above), susceptible to snake venom 5'-nucleotidase. The rates of hydrolysis of these esters are about 100-fold lower than for the nucleotides, the esters of 5'-araCMP being hydrolyzed more slowly than the methyl ester of 5'-CMP. This reaction is not an artifact resulting from potential contamination of the 5'-nucleotidase by PDase I (a possibility that cannot be ignored, since both enzymes are present in the crude snake venom) since, in the case of the methyl ester of 5'-CMP, it was established that the products of hydrolysis are cytidine and methylphosphate. Hence 5'-nucleotidase (at least that from snake venom) is capable of cleaving from 5'-nucleotides not only a phosphate group, but also an alkylphosphate and an alkyl-phosphonate.

CONCLUDING REMARKS

Considerable attention and effort have been, and continue to be, devoted to the synthesis of more sophisticated analogues of nucleosides in the search for more effective antimetabolic agents. These involve extensive modifications of the heterocyclic base moieties or/and the sugar rings. If we bear in mind the fact that most of these are active as antiviral or antineoplastic agents only following their intracellular conversion to a nucleotide form, it is indeed surprising that so little attention has been consciously devoted to the design of nucleotides with modified phosphate groups. Possibly this has been due, as underlined by Cohen (1977), to the widely accepted dogma of the impermeability of cellular membranes to natural nucleotides.

The foregoing, rather brief, presentation underlines our view that the potential antimetabolic properties, not only of nucleot-ides, but also of their alkyl esters and phosphonates, merit further exploitation, particularly if accompanied by investigat-ions of their metabolic fate at cellular membranes, their substrate and inhibitor properties with cellular enzyme systems and, in general, their metabolism in the specific cellular system in which their potential antimetabolic properties are being surveyed. The organic chemist is frequently concerned mainly as to whether a new analogue is more effective. But at the present stage of development of the field, it is frequently just as useful to establish why a given designed analogue does not fulfil the functions anticipated for it.

ACKNOWLEDGMENTS

We are indebted to Prof. W. Ostrowski for a gift of human prostatic phosphatase, to Dr. Magdalena Zan-Kowalczewska for potato nucleotide pyrophosphatase, to Dr. Jadwiga Koziorowska for cytotoxicity tests, and to Dr. Halina Sierakowska for some enzymatic tests. The original research reported here was supported by the Polish National Cancer Research Program (PR/6-1701).

REFERENCES

Bisson, L. & Thorner, J. (1977), J. Bacteriol., 132, 44-50.
Bloch, A. (Ed.) (1975), "Chemistry, Biology and Clinical Uses of Nucleoside Analogues", Ann. N. Y. Acad. Sci., Vol. 255.
Bloch, A., Fleysher, M.H., Thedford, R., Mane, R.J. & Hall, R.M. (1966), J. Med. Chem., 9, 886-887.
Boezi, J.A. (1978), Pharmacol. and Therapeutics, A, in press.
Chen, M.S., Ward, D.C. & Prusoff, W.H. (1976), J. Biol. Chem., 251, 4833-4838.
Cohen, S.S. (1975), Biochem. Pharmacol., 24, 1929-1932.
Cohen, S.S. (1977), Cancer, 40, 509-518.
Dales, S. (1973), Bacteriol. Rev., 37, 103-135.
Dudman, N.P. & Benkovic, S.J. (1977), J. Am. Chem. Soc., 99, 6113-6115.
Engel, R. (1977), Chem. Rev., 77, 349-367.
Fox, J.J., Falco, E.A., Wempen, I., Pomeroy, D., Dowling, M.D. & Burchenal, J.H. (1972), Cancer Res., 32, 2269-2272.
Gardner, J.H. & Byers, L.D. (1977), J. Biol. Chem., 252, 5925-5927.
Gormley, P.E., Benvenuto, J. & Cysyk, R.L. (1977), Biochem. Pharmacol., 26, 1291-1294.
Hampton, A., Sasaki, T. & Paul, B. (1972), J. Am. Chem. Soc., 95, 4404-4414.
Haugen, H.F. & Skrede, S. (1977), Clin. Chem., 23, 1531-1537.
Henderson, J.F. (1978), Pharmacol. and Therapeutics, A, in press.
Hermann, E.C. (Ed.) (1977), "Third Conference on Antiviral Substances", Ann. N. Y. Acad. Sci., Vol. 284.
Hickey, M.E., Waymack, P.P. & Van Etten, R.L. (1976), Arch. Biochem. Biophys., 172, 439-448.
Holy, A. & Hong, N.D. (1972), Coll. Czech. Chem. Commun., 37,

2066-2076.

Hughes, R.G. & Kimball, A.P. (1972), Cancer Res., 32, 1791-1792.

Kanai, T., Ichino, M., Hoshi, A. & Kuretani, K. (1971), Tetrahed. Lett., 1965-1968.

Kaufman, H.E. & Varnell, E.D. (1976), Antimicrob. Agents Chemother., 10, 885-888.

Kelly, S.J. & Butler, L.G. (1977), Biochemistry, 16, 1102-1104.

Kelly, S.J., Dardinger, D.E. & Butler, L.G. (1975), Biochemistry, 14, 4983-4988.

Khorana, H.G. (1959), J. Am. Chem. Soc., 81, 4657-4660.

Kole, R., Sierakowska, H. & Shugar, D. (1976), Biochim. Biophys. Acta, 438, 540-550.

Kreis, W. & Wechter, W.J. (1972), Res. Commun. Pathol. Pharmacol., 4, 631-640.

Kurland, C.G. (1972), Ann. Rev. Biochem., 41, 377-393.

Lavers, G.C. (1977), Mol. Biol. Rep., 3, 413-420.

LePage, G.A. & Hersh, E.M. (1972), Biochem. Biophys. Res. Commun., 46, 1918-1922.

LePage, G.A., Lin, Y.T., Orth, E. & Gottlieb, J.A. (1972), Cancer Res., 32, 2441-2444.

Long, R.A., Szekers, G.L., Khwaja, T.A., Sidwell, R.W., Simon, L.N. & Robins, R.K. (1972), J. Med. Chem., 15, 1215-1218.

Montgomery, J.A., Dixon, G.J., Dulmage, E.A., Thomas, H.J., Brockman, W. & Skipper, H.E. (1963), Nature, 199, 769-772.

Mukherjee, K.L. & Heidelberger, C. (1962), Cancer Res., 22, 815-822.

Nuss, D.L. & Furuichi, Y. (1977), J. Biol. Chem., 252, 2815-2823.

Ortiz, P.J., Manduka, M.J. & Cohen, S.S. (1972), Cancer Res., 32, 1512-1517.

Ostrowski, W. & Barnard, E.A. (1973), Biochemistry, 12, 3893-3898.

Parsons, D.G. & Heidelberger, C. (1966), J. Med. Chem., 9, 159.

Plunkett, W. & Cohen, S.S. (1975), Cancer Res., 35, 1547-1554.

Plunkett, W., Lapi, L., Ortiz, P.J. & Cohen, S.S. (1974), Proc. Natl. Acad. Sci., 71, 73-77.

Prusoff, W.H. & Goz, B. (1975), in "Antineoplastic and Immuno-suppressive Agents" (Eds. A.C. Sartorelli & D.G. Johns), Vol. 2, p. 272, Springer, Berlin.

Prusoff, W.H. & Ward, D.C. (1976), Biochem. Pharmacol., 25, 1233-1239.

Razzel, W.E. (1963), in "Methods in Enzymology" (Eds. S.P. Colowick & N.D. Kaplan), Vol. 6, p. 236, Academic Press, N.Y.

Renis, H.E., Hollowell, C.A. & Underwood, G.E. (1967), J. Med. Chem., 10, 777-782.

Revankar, G.R., Huffman, J.H., Allen, L.B., Sidwell, R.W., Robins, R.K. & Tolman, R.L. (1975), J. Med. Chem., 18, 721-726.

Revankar, G.R., Huffman, J.H., Sidwell, R.W., Tolman, R.L., Robins, R.K. & Allen, L.B. (1976), J. Med. Chem., 19, 1026-1028.

Richards, G.M., Tutas, D.J., Wechter, W.J. & Laskowski Sr., M. (1967), Biochemistry, 6, 2908-2914.

Shugar, D. (1974), FEBS Lett., <u>40</u>, S48-S62.
Simon, L.N., Shuman, D.A. & Robins, R.K. (1973), in "Advances in
     Cyclic Nucleotide Research" (Eds. P. Greengard & G.A.
     Robison), Vol. 3, p. 332, Raven Press, New York.
Sinshi, H., Miwa, M., Kato, K., Noguchi, M., Matsushima, T.
     & Sugimura, T. (1976), Biochemistry, <u>15</u>, 2185-2190.
Smith, C.G., Buskirk, H.M. & Lummis, W.L. (1967), J. Med. Chem.,
     <u>10</u>, 774-776.
Szer, W. & Shugar, D. (1961), Biokhimija, <u>26</u>, 840-845.
Torrance, J.D., Whittaker, D. & Beutler, E. (1977), Proc. Natl.
     Acad. Sci., <u>74</u>, 3701-3704.
Vince, R. & Daluge, S. (1977), J. Med. Chem., <u>20</u>, 612-613.
Wechter, W.J. (1967), J. Med. Chem., <u>10</u>, 762-773.
Wigler, P.W. & Lozzio, C.B. (1972), J. Med. Chem., <u>15</u>, 1020-1024.
Zeleznick, L.D. (1969), Biochem. Pharmacol., <u>18</u>, 855-862.

A NEW TEST MODEL FOR THE IDENTIFICATION OF ENVIRONMENTAL CARCINOGENS

N. Nashed and P. Chandra

Gustav-Embden-Zentrum der Biologischen Chemie

der Univ. Frankfurt, 6 Frankfurt/M., W. Germany

According to one estimate there may be at least 25,000 environmental chemicals awaiting carcinogenicity testing, the number increasing by about one thousand every year. To tackle this job, we have at present a whole battery of carcinogenicity test systems. The question would therefore be justified if one asked "What is the sense of developing a new test?" The answer lies in the fact that, inspite of their multiplicity, the available test systems do not as yet offer an optimal solution to the complex problem of evaluating human risk. The model we are now studying is an in vivo-in vitro system meant to combine the advantages of an in vivo application with the short duration of an in vitro cell culture.

Before going into the details of our model, it might be useful to give a brief review of the pros and cons of the present major test systems. At one end of the scale we have the extremely costly standard animal test with its requirement for hundreds of animals maintained for 2-3 years. Although this might be the most relevant system in terms of human risk, it is becoming a formidable barrier against a speedy testing of present and future environmental agents. At the other extreme we have a series of short-term and inexpensive tests which, while being suitable for a primary screening, they have a limited relevance to carcinogenicity in man. What is now needed is an adequate assay between these two extremes which would, at a bearable cost in time and money, serve to confirm the primary screening test results. The in vivo-in vitro transplacental system proposed by DiPaolo et al. (1973) could be considered as a serious attempt to satisfy this requirement. The model we are

presenting is another variation of this system in which the
transplacental approach is avoided.

We could now take a closer look at the available test
systems starting with the simplest microbial screening tests.
Here, we shall concentrate our discussion on the Ames test.
Judging by the results of the 300 agents tested so far, the
Ames **test** should be considered one of the most promising screening tests developed so far. Inspite of this, the Ames test
results can have no significant relevance to the evaluation
of the carcinogenicity risk in man before they are comfirmed
in an animal system.   There are several reasons for this:

(i) Malignant transformation cannot be explained away
as a simple reversion in a gene locus of a naked
DNA molecule in a repair-deficient bacterium.
The risk is too high that, among the 25,000 unknowns, many agents exist which induce cancer by
other mechanisms e.g. regulation mutations, virus
activation or suppression of the immune system,to
name a few.   These would not be detected by the
Ames test.   Among the false negatives recently
reported for the Ames test are: butter yellow
(Hay, 1977) and hexamethylphosphoramide (Ashby et
al., 1977), both being strong carcinogens.

(ii) The mutation frequency observed in the Ames test,
usually somewhere around 10^{-5}, is several orders
of magnitude lower than the 1-5% frequency commonly
observed in transformation tests (Cleaver, 1976).
This major discrepancy is further aggravated by
the poor correlation reported by Ashby and Styles
(1978) between the mutagenic potency observed in
the Ames test and the carcinogenic potency of the
same agents observed in animals.

(iii) An in vitro system can only represent a rough appro-
ximation of the situation in vivo.   The immersion
of cells in the test solution has little in common
with an in vivo application involving such complex
processes as absorption, distribution, conjugation
with various serum proteins, activation and/or detoxification in the living cells of the liver and
other tissues; all this taking place under the influence of homeostatic, immune and repair processes.

This criticism should, however, in no way diminish the value
of the Ames test as a proven and very useful primary screening system.

Next, we could look at another useful in vitro system, this time using mammalian cells. In the transformation test, mammalian cell lines or embryonal cells are treated in culture and then observed for signs of abnormal growth. As a mammalian system, this test has a certain advantage over bacterial systems. However, if established cell lines are used, we know that these are not to be regarded as normal cells; they often show aberrant chromosome numbers as well as metabolic deviations. Where fresh fetal cells are used, the results might not necessarily be applicable to cells of the adult in view of their poorly developed activating and repair systems. Due to inadequate activation, no transformation could be observed after the treatment of Syrian hamster embryo cells with the carcinogens urethan and dimethylnitrosamine (DMN) (DiPaolo et al., 1972).

In an attempt to compensate for this deficiency in fetal cells, Styles (1977) proposed the addition of the S-9 rat liver fraction to the treatment solution. Using a baby hamster kidney cell line, Styles was able to show an improved accuracy in the prediction of the carcinogenicity of tested agents.

In an effort to improve the relevance of in vitro test systems, the host-mediated assay was developed by Legator (see Legator and Malling, 1973). In its classical form the host-mediated assay involves the injection of Salmonella cells in a mouse, treatment of the mouse in vivo with the test agent and finally withdrawal of a sample of the injected bacteria and testing it for reversion. Among the drawbacks later noticed in this system are the following:

(i) The test has to be usually conducted under lethal or even supralethal conditions; the injected 10^9 Salmonella cells being by themselves lethal to the mouse. If we now consider the added toxicity of the near-lethal dose of the test agent which has to be used to ensure reaching the bacterial cells, it becomes clear that the main objective of this assay in achieving a normal metabolism of the test agent could never be achieved under such conditions.

(ii) A selection in the recovered bacterial sample can hardly be avoided; the majority of the injected bacteria is either phagocytized or taken up by the different membranes, and is thus not available for sampling.

(iii) Using the host-mediated assay it was possible to detect fewer than one half of the carcinogens tested (Poirier, 1976).

An interesting modification of the host-mediated assay was developed by DiPaolo et al. (1973).   Rather than using intrahost bacteria, fetal cells of a treated pregnant animal are homogenized, cultured and tested for transformation and colony growth in soft agar.   This transplacental system has several points in its favour.   It allowed an adequate in vivo activation of such agents as DMN, urethan and vinyl chloride aerosol, thus permitting the observation of transformed fetal cells in culture (DiPaolo and Casto, 1977). This approach proved also useful in the study of organotropic transplacental carcinogenesis in the case of the brain carcinogen ethyl nitroso urea (Laerum and Rajewsky, 1975). The main drawback of this system, however, lies in the placental barrier.   This endocrine organ exerts an unknown   influence on both the dose and types of metabolites reaching the fetus. Furthermore, fetal cells might not represent an optimal model for cells of the adult as mentioned earlier.

In a more recent modification where nonpregnant rats were used, kidney cells took the role of the fetal cells in the DiPaolo model, (Hard et al., 1971).   Male 6 week old rats were treated with a single dose of 60 mg/kg of DMN while being maintained on a protein-free diet to ensure the induction of kidney cancer in all survivors (Swan and McLean, 1968).   Seven days later, kidney tissue was treated with 0.1% trypsin for 1 hour to obtain a cell suspension. The cells were then cultured and observed for transformation.   Clusters of piled-up cells were observed in the treated and to some extent in the control cultures.   It is possible that the cell clustering observed both in the treated and control cultures was due to the long trypsin treatment.   Proteolytic enzymes were reported by Sefton and Rubin (1970) to induce, even at low doses, a cell growth free from density inhibition. It is obvious therefore that if non-dividing cells such as those of the adult kidney are to be stimulated, other more suitable mitogens have to be found which do not influence the transformation results.

In our search for more suitable mitogenic agents, we discovered that low doses of aluminium hydroxide plus lithium carmine permitted freshly collected rat peritoneal macrophages to form clones or aggregates within 4 days on a solid medium (Fig.1a and 1b).   This compares well with the aggregates formed by established cell lines on a comparable solid medium without mitogen which were described by Steuer et al.(1977a). Our solid medium is composed of TC 199, 10% bovine calf serum, 0.8% agar plus 100 mg/l of $Al(OH)_3$ and 5mg/l lithium carmine. Aluminium hydroxide was previously shown to stimulate cell division of rat peritoneal cells in vivo (Nashed, 1975a).

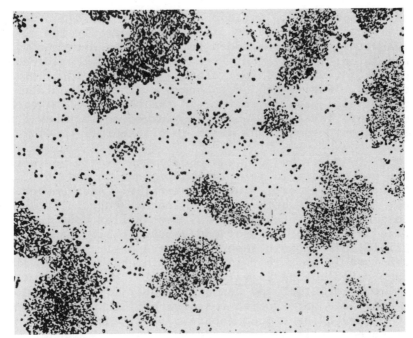

Fig.1a: Rat peritoneal macrophage clones after 4 days of
        growth on the mitogenic solid medium.

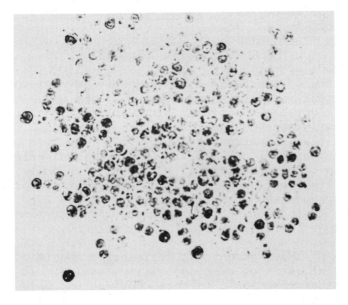

Fig.1b.: One macrophage clone at a higher magnification

We failed, however, to achieve a similar stimulation in vitro
using Al(OH)$_3$ alone. In an experiment where lithium carmine,
a known vital stain, was added to facilitate microscopy, we
noticed to our suprise that this addition of the stain now permitted the formation of cell clones from the freshly collected
macrophages. Peritoneal macrophages collected from adult rats
do not normally grow in culture in the absence of mitogenic
stimulation. The cell clones we observed so far showed no
signs of spontaneous transformation or abnormal growth.

Now, to describe our test model, the general plan provides
for the use of mice to test inhalation agents and rats to test
substances applied orally or parenterally. Adult nonpregnant
animals are used in both cases. Mice are especially suited for
inhalation experiments in view of the smaller dose to be prepared in the form of aerosol and because their lungs are less
suscptible to pneumonia than rats. The Snell mouse might offer
an advantage in this test in view of the high sensitivity of
its lung cells to the in vitro transforming action of cigarette
smoke (Leuchtenberger and Leuchtenberger, 1974). Rats on the
other hand, are more suited for oral application by stomach
tube and they offer a good source of peritoneal cells which can
be collected repeatedly from the same animal (Nashed, 1975b).
However, other laboratory animals can also be used in both
tests. After an in vivo application, mouse lung cells or rat
peritoneal cells, both being predominantly composed of macrophages, are collected, cultured in vitro and watched for signs
of abnormal growth.

THE CHOICE OF MACROPHAGES

The macrophages used in this test have several advantages:
they are present in nearly every tissue in the body; they can
be easily collected without need for such injurious procedures
as trypsinization or homogenization. They are known to undergo malignant transformation both in vivo in the form of mono-
cytic leukemia as well as in vitro in the form of colonies
growing in soft agar (Metcalf et al., 1969). Finally, a macrophage epithelioid culture should be a better indicator for carcinogenesis in man than the fibroblasts commonly used, since
85% of human cancers arise from epithelial rather than fibroblastic tissues (Cairns, 1975).

In view of these advantages macrophages should offer a
suitable target cell for carcinogenicity testing. In describing a test model comparable to ours, Borland and Hard (1974)
proposed the use of kidney cells as the target in vitro system.
Their choice was based on experiments with DMN using a protocol
which guaranteed the induction of kidney cancer in each surviving animal. However, since no such guarantee for kidney

organotropy can be expected of the unknown agents to be tested,
it would probably be more advisable to use a more universal
type of cell like the macrophage rather than those of a specific organ like the kidney.

THE TRANSFORMATION TEST

Among the criteria for cell transformation which could be
considered in our test model is the maintenance of a high rate
of viable cells during the first 4 days of growth on the solid
medium. This criterion was reported by Steuer et al., (1977)
to be well correlated with tumor formation in transplanted
syngeneic animals.

COLONY FORMATION ON SOFT AGAR

This has been shown to be a reliable indicator of cell
transformation induced by chemicals (DiPaolo et al., 1969) as
well as by virus (MacPherson and Montagnier, 1964; Shin et al.,
1975). This criterion was reported to apply both to fibroblasts as well as to epithelial cells (Steuer and Ting, 1977).
In our model the cells are seeded in a 0.35% agar layer on top
of the solid medium and observed for colony formation.

THE MOUSE INHALATION TEST

In this test (Fig. 2) inhalation is applied daily for 30
days after which the mouse is killed and its lungs removed
asceptically. The lung tissue is teased gently with two fine
forceps in the 199 medium. The cells, which usually contain
a majority of macrophages, are centrifuged, washed, counted
and seeded on the solid and in the soft agar media. Signs of
abnormal growth and the rate of viable cells are examined on
the solid medium whereas the soft agar is watched for colony
growth. A further confirmatory test can be performed by the
transplantation of the cells in syngeneic young animals and
palpating for subcutaneous tumors.

THE RAT PERITONEAL TEST

As in the mouse test, the agent to be tested is applied
daily for 30 days (Fig. 3). The peritoneal cells are collected twice, the first before the start of treatment to serve as
a control and then a month later, 6 hours after the last application. Peritoneal cell collection is performed in the living
animal using lavage by a special glass pipette (Fig. 4). The
operation is very simple and lasts only about 1 min. per rat.
The trick is to use a large volume of a warm physiological
solution (we now use 35 ml. of TC 199) which is injected intraperitoneally and is immediately withdrawn by mild suction

carrying with it about 20 million macrophages per rat (Nashed, 1975b). By taking simple precautions e.g. shaving the skin and cleaning it with alcohol before inserting the needle and using a sterile pipette, it is possible to obtain peritoneal cells completely free of infection. This cell collection procedure has been performed in a great number of rats with no visible harmful effects.

Daily inhalation dose

for 30 days

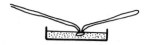

Solid Medium	Soft agar
Test : 1. Abnormal growth 2. % viable cells during 4 days	3. Colony growth

Transplantation in syngeneic mice

Fig. 2:   The mouse inhalation test

Control cell collection

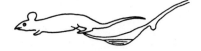

Treatment

(p. o. or parenteral)

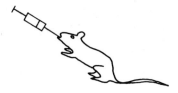

Post – treatment cell collection

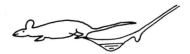

Washed peritoneal cells

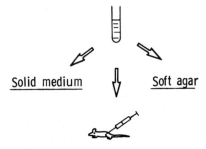

Solid medium   Soft agar

Transplantation in syngeneic rats

Fig.3: The rat peritoneal test

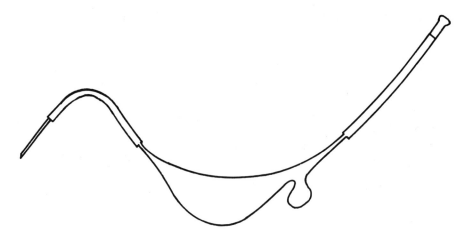

Fig. 4:   The rat peritoneal pipette

THE EXPERIMENTAL PLAN

The animals are devided into 3 treatment groups (high, medium and low) plus a positive and negative control groups. In
the case of the rat test the negative control group can be om-
mited since each animcl serves as its own control. Each group
comprises 3♂ and 3♀ adult animals. The total number of animals
required would thus be 24 in the rat test and 30 in the mouse
test.

Cell collection is done 6 hours after the last dose. The relatively long treatment period of 30 days serves an important
purpose. It covers the cancer initiation phase usually considered to last about one month (see Falk, 1971). During this
phase, which corresponds to the mutation fixation period in
mutagenesis (Auerbach, 1966), the induced lesion has not yet
acquired its stable irreversible status; it could thus be strongly influenced by factors in the cellular environment e.g.
temperature or the presence of antimutagens or anticarcinogens
in the medium such as SH-groups or vitamins. There are several
examples in the literature (see Nashed, 1976) showing a partial or total inhibition of carcinogenesis when anticarcinogens were applied to the treated animal during the labile cancer
initiation phase. Since SH-groups and vitamins are present in
different levels in each culture medium, a too early exposure
of the cells to the in vitro culture conditions could probably
explain some of the reproducibility problems encountered in
transformation experiments.

ADVANTAGES OF THE PROPOSED MODEL

The proposed model has several attractive features:

(i) It is an animal system using adult rather than fetal cells.

(ii) Cells are cultured after and not during the labile cancer initiation phase.

(iii) Inhalation agents, including air pollutants and aerosol drugs, are tested in the target organ, the lung.

(iv) Each rat serves as its own control thus giving more weight to the observed treatment effect while minimizing the number of required animals.

REFERENCES

Ashby, J., J. A. Styles D. Anderson. 1977. Br. J. Cancer 36:564.

Ashby, J. and J. A. Styles. 1978. Nature 271:452.

Auerbach, C. 1966. Proc. Roy. Phys. Soc. 29.

Borland, R. and G. C. Hard. 1974. Europ. J. Cancer 10:177.

Cairns, J. 1975. Nature 255:197.

Cleaver, J. E. 1976. In: Screening Tests in Chemical Carcinogenesis. Montesano, Bartsch and Tomatis (Eds.). IARC Publ. No.12 p. 18, Lyon, France.

DiPaolo, J. A., R. L. Nelson and P. J. Donovan. 1969. Science 165:917.

DiPaolo, J. A., R. L. Nelson and P. J. Donovan. 1972. Nature 233:278.

DiPaolo, J. A., R. L. Nelson, P.J. Donovan and C. H. Evans. 1973. Arch. Pathol. 95:380.

DiPaolo, J. A. and B. C. Casto. 1977. In: Recent Advances in Cancer Research v.1. R.C. Gallo (Ed.) pp. 17-47 CRC Press, Ohio, USA.

Falk, H. L. 1971. Progr. Exp. Tumor Res. 14:105.

Hard, G. C., R. Borland and W. H. Butler. Experientia 27:1208.

Hay, A. 1977. Nature 269:468.

Laerum, O. D. and R. F. Rajewsky. 1975. J. Natl. Cancer Inst. 55:1177.

Legator, M. S. and H. V. Malling. 1973. In: Chemical Mutagenesis v.2. A. Hollaender (Ed.), Plenum Press, New York.

Leuchtenberger, C. and R. Leuchtenberger. 1974. Oncology 29:122.

MacPherson, I. and L. Montagnier. 1964. Virology 23:291.

Metcalf, D., M. A. S. Moore and N. L. Warner. 1969. J. Natl. Cancer Inst. 43:983.

Nashed, N. 1975a. Mutation Res. 30:407.

Nashed, N. 1975b. Lab. Animal Sci. 25:225.

Nashed, N. 1976. Environm. Health Perspect. 14:193.

Poirier, L. A. 1976. In: Screening Tests in Chemical Carcinogenesis. Montesano, Bartsch and Tomatis (Eds.) IARC Publ. No. 12 p. 18, Lyon, France.

Sefton, B. and H. Rubin. 1970. Nature 227:843.

Shin, S. V. H. Freedman, R. Risser and R. Pollack. Proc. Natl. Acad. Sci. USA. 72:4435.

Steuer, A. F., J. S. Rhim, P. M. Hentosh and R. C. Ting. 1977 J. Natl. Cancer Inst. 58:917.

Steuer, A. F. and R. C. Ting. 1977. In: Recent Advances in Cancer Res. v.1. pp. 67-77. R.C. Gallo (Ed.), CRC Press, Ohio, USA.

Swann, P. F. and A. E. M. McLean. 1968. Biochem J.107: 14P.

Styles, J. A. 1977. Br. J. Cancer 36:558.

SYNTHESIS AND ANTIHERPETIC PROPERTIES OF SOME 5-ALKYL SUBSTITUTED PYRIMIDINE NUCLEOSIDES

Tadeusz Kulikowski, Zbigniew Zawadzki and David Shugar

Institute of Biochemistry and Biophysics Polish Academy

of Sciences, 02-532 Warsaw (Poland)

Considerable interest has centred around the use of 5-alkyl-pyrimidine deoxynucleosides as antiherpes agents following the demonstration that 5-ethyluracil (an obvious thymine analogue) may be incorporated into bacterial DNA (1), 5-ethyldeoxyuridine into phage DNA (2), and that the latter is a reasonably good _in vitro_ and _in vivo_ inhibitor of HSV and vaccinia viruses (3-6). It has been demonstrated that 5-EtdUrd also undergoes incorporation into human lymphocytes (7) and mouse melanoma B59 cells (8), does not produce chromosomal aberrations (7), is non-mutagenic (4) and does not display immunosuppressive activity (9). Its cytotoxicity, at the levels required for virus inhibition, is also very low; it is inhibitory to HSV transformed HeLaTK$^-$ (10), and mouse B$_5$59 melanoma, cells (8), and (unlike 5-halogenopyrimidine-2'-deoxy-nucleosides) apparently does not act as an inducer of oncogenic viruses (11).

A number of additional 5-alkyl thymidine analogues have now been investigated with a view to obtaining one with increased antiviral activity, viz. 5-allyl (10), 5-propyl (10,12), 5-vinyl (10), 5-ethynyl (13), etc. The interest in these is further enhenced by the fact that 5-halogenopyrimidine-2'-deoxynucleosides have hitherto been effective therapeutically only against herpetic keratoconjunctivitis.

Concurrently with the foregoing, it was found that the 5-methyl derivative of araU, i.e. araT, originally isolated from marine sponges (14), exhibited selective _in vitro_ activity against HSV 1 and 2 (15) at levels non-toxic to the host chinese hamster cells, and under conditions where the parent araU is inactive. It was proposed that, as in the case of 5-substituted pyrimidine

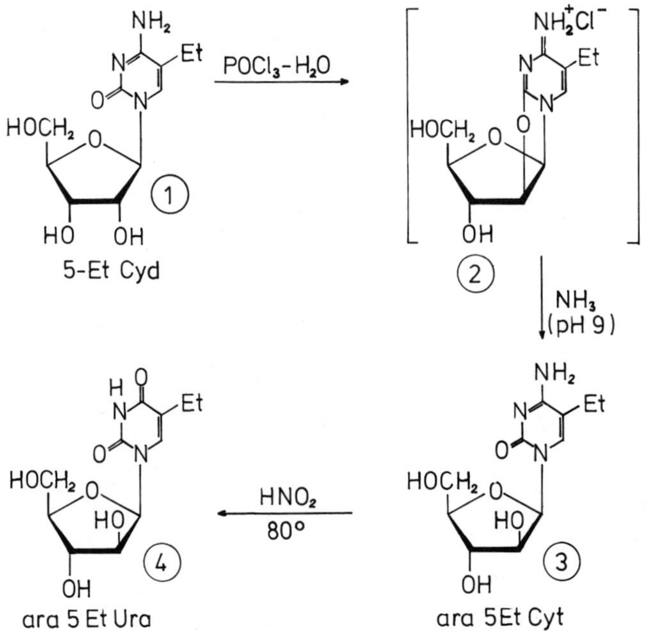

Scheme 1. Synthesis of 1-β-D-arabino-5-ethylcytosine (5EtaraC) and 1-β-D-arabinofuranosyl-5-ethyluracil (5EtaraU) via "inversion".

deoxynucleosides (16), araT is a substrate for HSV-1 and HSV-2
induced deoxythymidine kinases. It was subsequently demonstrated
that 5-methyl-araC, earlier claimed to be inactive as an antiviral
agent (17), is, in fact, an antiherpes agent in cell systems
endowed with a high level of cytidine deaminase, such as HEp-2
cells of human laryngeal epidermoid carcinoma. In such systems,
5-MearaC would act as a depot form of 5-MearaU (araT), which would
then undergo phosphorylation by kinases to the 5'-phosphates (18).

In view of the foregoing, it appeared logical to synthesize
additional 5-alkyl derivatives of araC with increased (or decreased) susceptibilities to cytidine deaminase, as well as corresponding analogues of araT with substrate properties towards viral
induced dT kinase(s).

CHEMISTRY

Two such analogues would be 1-β-D-arabinofuranosyl-5-ethyl-
uracil (5-ethylaraC, 5-EtaraC), and its deamination product,
5-ethylaraU (5-EtaraU). We have prepared both of these by different
routes.

Reaction of partially hydrolyzed $POCl_3$ with the previously
synthesized (19) 5-ethylcytidine (1) gave 2,2'-anhydro-5-ethyl-
cytidine (2), which is a depot form of 5-EtaraC. Hydrolysis of 2
with ammonia gave the desired 5-EtaraC (3) in 53% yield (Scheme 1).
Nitrous acid deamination of this product led to 5-EtaraU (4) in
92% yield.

Larger scale syntheses of the foregoing were based on several
variants of the Hilbert-Johnson condensation reaction. The first
of these involved the non-catalyzed reaction of 2,3,5-tri-O-
benzoyl-α-D-arabinofuranosyl bromide (5) with a large excess of
2,4-diethoxy-5-ethylpyrimidine (6) at room temperature to give
1-(2,3,5-tri-O-benzoyl)-β-D-arabinofuranosyl)-4-ethoxy-5-ethyl-
2(1H)pyrimidone (7) in 40% yield (Scheme 2). The absence of the
α-anomer was verified by chromatography and CD spectroscopy,
testifying to the SN_2 character of the reaction. Ammonolysis of 7
gave 1-(2,3,5-tri-O-benzoyl-β-D-arabinofuranosyl)-5-ethylcytosine
(8) in 65% yield. This intermediate readily underwent catalytic
hydrogenation to the required 5-EtaraC in 80% yield.

The foregoing procedure suffers from the disadvantage that it
requires a large excess of the pyrimidine derivative 6, the synthesis of which involves several steps starting from thiourea or
barbituric acid (19).

An alternative route is based on the condensation of
di-O-TMS-5-ethyluracil (10) with equimolar proportions of 2,3,5-

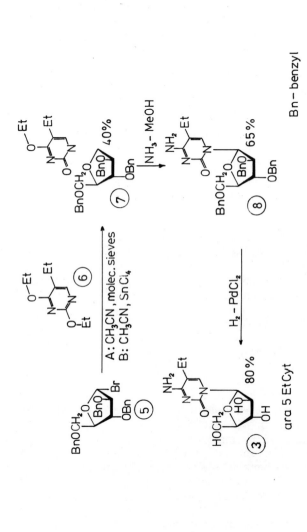

Scheme 2. Synthesis of 1-β-D-arabinofuranosyl-5-ethylcytosine via Hilbert—Johnson reaction.

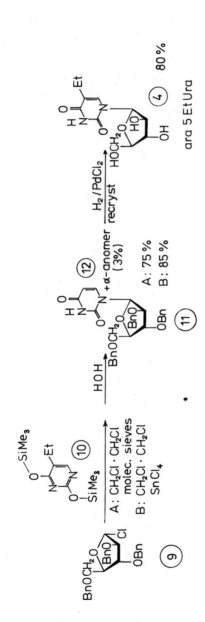

Scheme 3. Synthesis of 1-β-D-arabinofuranosyl-5-ethyluracil via catalysed Hilbert–Johnson reaction.

tri-O-benzoyl-α-D-arabinofuranosyl chloride (9) in the presence of
molecular sieves or SnCl$_4$ (Scheme 3). Both of these variants gave
good yields (70% and 85%, respectively) of the β-anomer of
1-(2,3,5-tri-O-benzoyl-D-arabinofuranosyl)-5-ethyluracil (11), but
containing 3-4% of the corresponding α-anomer (12). Desilylation
and catalytic hydrogenolysis of the products yielded a mixture of
the α and β anomers of 5-EtaraU in 80% yield. With a view to
obtaining a higher yield of the α-anomer (which is occasionally
desirable in view of demonstrated instances of biological activity
of the α-anomers of several nucleosides) the silylated pyrimidine
derivative 10 was condensed with the bromide of the benzoylated
sugar, 10, as shown in Scheme 4. This gave a mixture of the α and
β anomers of the benzoylated 5-EtaraU in which the former
predominated.

Since isolation of the individual anomers is technically
difficult (20,21), this was carried out on the basis of a previous
observation (22). The mixture of anomeric O'-benzoylated nucleosides was thiated with P$_2$S$_5$ in dioxane. The resulting O'-benzoylated
4-thio anomeric derivatives exhibit more marked differences in R$_f$
values on tlc chromatography with silica gel than the 4-keto
derivatives, so that they can be quantitatively resolved.

Table 1. Spectrophotometrically determined apparent pKa values
of 5-ethylpyrimidine nucleosides.

Compound	pKa value at 20°C (±0.05)
Cytidine	4.17
1-β-D-arabinosylcytosine (araC)	4.19
1-β-D-arabinosyl-5-methylcytosine (5MearaC)	4.28
1-β-D-arabinofuranosyl-5-ethylcytosine (β-5EtaraC)	4.39
1-α-D-arabinofuranosyl-5-ethylcytosine (α-5EtaraC)	4.40
1-β-D-arabinosyluracil (araU)	9.3
1-β-D-arabinosylthymine (araT)	9.80
1-β-D-arabinosyl-5-ethyluracil (5EtaraU)	9.9
5-Ethyl-2'-deoxyuridine (5EtdUrd)	9.9
5-Ethyl-2'-deoxycytidine (5EtdCyd)	4.5

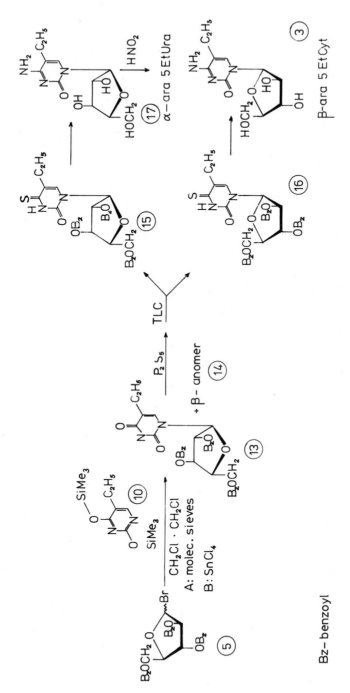

Scheme 4. Synthesis of α – and β –anomers of 1– –D–arabinofuranosyl–5–ethylcytosine and uracil via catalysed Hilbert–Johnson reaction.

Subsequent treatment of each of the fractions with methanolic
ammonia gave the α (17) and β (3) 5-EtaraC, and deamination of
these led to the   and   anomers of 5-EtaraU. As anticipated, the
CD spectra of these nucleosides (Fig. 1 and 2) and pKa values
(Table 1) were virtually similar with those for the corresponding
5-methyl derivatives, i.e. 5-MearaC (23,24) and araT (23,25).

It is worth noting that, since completion of the foregoing
syntheses, Bergstrom (26) has described a fairly general procedure
for the 5-alkylation of pyrimidine ribo and deoxyribonucleosides.
It is our feeling that application of this procedure to ribonucle-
osides, followed by inversion of the configuration at $C(2')$, may
in future be the most effective route to 5-alkylpyrimidine
arabinosides, including the 5-ethyl derivatives.

BIOLOGICAL ASPECTS

Preliminary results on the antiviral activity of 5-EtaraC
and 5-EtaraU indicated that 5-EtaraU exhibits marked activity
against HSV-1 (strain KOS) virus in both primary rabbit kidney
(PRK) and human skin fibroblast (HSF) cell systems, but is totally
inactive against vaccinia virus. Further trials are under way by
Dr. E. De Clercq.

The activity of 5-EtaraU is comparable to that of 5-ethyl-
deoxyuridine (6) and, relative to other analogues, is in the order
araT > 5-EtdUrd > 5-EtaraU > araU. However, it should be noted
that 5-EtdUrd was equally effective against HSV-1 and vaccinia
(6), whereas 5-EtaraC was considerably less effective than araC
and only slightly more active than 5-EtdCyd, which had been
previously investigated (22). This is readily explicable if the
mechanism of action of 5-EtaraC is similar to that proposed for
5-MearaC (18), viz. that 5-EtaraC is deaminated by the host cell
deaminase to 5-EtaraU which, in turn, is phosphorylated by the HSV
induced kinase to the 5'-phosphate. It was earlier shown (26) that
introduction of a 5-alkyl substituent to a cytosine nucleoside led
to a decrease in the rate of deamination by S. typhimurium cytidine
deaminase in the order Cyd(dCyd) > 5-MeCyd(5-MedCyd) > 5-EtCyd(5-
MedCyd). In more recent trials, using crude deaminase preparations
from S. typhimurium and   B.subtilis, the same order of rates
of hydrolysis was found for the corresponding araC nucleosides,
5-EtaraC being hydrolyzed at a rate three-fold lower than that for
5-MearaC. Hence 5-EtaraC would behave, in cellular systems with
moderate or high levels of deaminase activity, as a depot form of
5-EtaraU.

Preliminary measurements by Dr. E. Krajewska have shown that
the rates of deamination of 5-MearaC and 5-EtaraC, relative to
araC, by extract of human kidney cells are appreciably lower, and

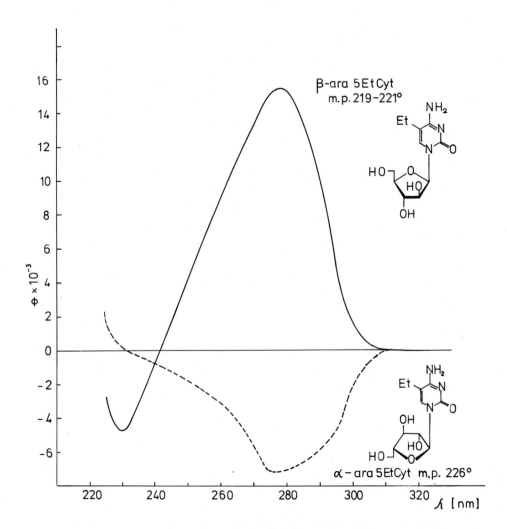

Figure 1. The circular dichroism spectra of 1-β-D-arabino-furanosyl-5-ethylcytosine (——) and its α-anomer (- - -).

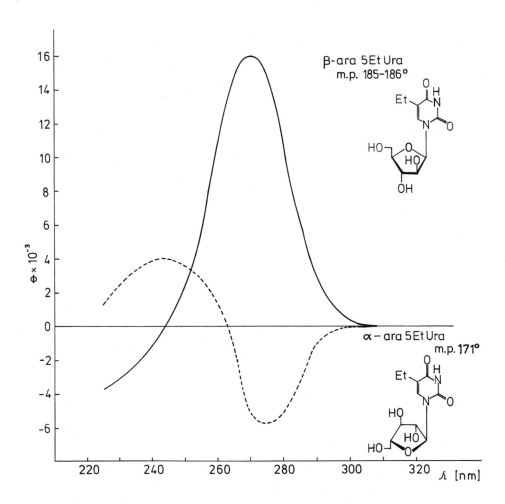

Figure 2. The circular dichroism spectra of 1-β-D-arabino-
furanosyl-5-ethyluracil (———) and its α-anomer (- - -).

even less with human leukocyte extracts. Consequently the effectiveness of a given analogue will be related to the level of
deaminase in the host cells, and will decrease with increasing
length of the 5-alkyl side chain. In the uracil nucleoside series,
an increase in the length of the chain would lead to an increase
in antiherpes specificity, araU analogues being more selective
than the corresponding deoxynucleosides.

REFERENCES

(1) Piechowska, M. and Shugar, D. (1965) Biochem. Biophys. Res.
Commun., 20, 768.

(2) Pietrzykowska, I. and Shugar, D. (1967) Acta Biochim. Polon.,
14, 169-181.

(3) Gauri, K.K. and Malorny, G. (1967) Naunyn Schmiedeberg Arch.
Pharmacol. Exp. Pathol., 257, 21-22.

(4) Świerkowski, M. and Shugar, D. (1969) J. Med. Chem., 12,
533-534.

(5) Martenet, A.-C. (1975) Ophtalmic Res., 7, 170-180.

(6) De Clercq, E. and Shugar, D. (1975) Biochem. Pharmacol., 24,
1073-1078.

(7) Świerkowska, K.M., Jasińska, T.K. and Steffen, J.A. (1973)
Biochem. Pharmacol., 22, 85-93.

(8) Silagi, S., Balint, R.F. and Gauri, K.K. (1977) Cancer Res.,
37, 3367-3373.

(9) Gauri, K.K., Malorny, G. and Schiff, W. (1969) Chemotherapy
14, 129-132.

(10) Cheng, Y.C., Domin, B.A., Sharma, R.A. and Bobek, M. (1976)
Antimicrob. Agents Chemother., 10, 119-122.

(11) Shugar, D. (1974) FEBS Lett., 40, S48-62.

(12) De Clercq, E., Descamps, J. and Shugar, D. (1978) Antimicrob.
Agents Chemother., in press.

(13) Barr, P.J., Jones, A.S. and Walker, R.T. (1976) Nucleic Acid.
Res., 3, 2845-2850.

(14) Bergman, W. and Feeny, R.J. (1950) J. Amer. Chem. Soc., 72,
2809-2810.

(15) Gentry, G.A. and Aswell, J.P. (1975) Virology 65, 294-296.

(16) De Clercq, E., Descamps, J., Torrence, P.F., Krajewska, E.
and Shugar, D. (1977) Proceedings of the Tenth International
Congress of Chemotherapy, Zurich, Switzerland, Sept. 18-23,
No. 450.

(17) Renis, H.E., Underwood, G.E. and Hunter, J.H. (1967)
Antimicrob. Agents Chemother. 675-679.

(18) Aswell, J.P. and Gentry, G.A. (1977) Ann. N.Y. Acad. Sci.
342-350.

(19) Kulikowski, T. and Shugar, D. (1971) Acta Biochim. Polon.,
17, 209-236.

(20) Kulikowski, T. and Shugar, D. (1973) J. Chromat., 79, 353-356.

(21) Kulikowski, T. and Shugar, D. (1974) Acta Biochim. Polon., 21,
169-186.

(22) Kulikowski, T. and Shugar, D. (1974) J. Med. Chem., <u>17</u>, 269-273.

(23) Rabczenko, A., Ph.D. Theses Institute of Biochemistry and Biophysics, Polish Academy of Sciences, Warsaw 1972.

(24) Fox, J.J., Van Praag,D., Wempen, I., Doerr, I.L., Cheong, L., Knoll, J.E., Eidinoff, M.L., Bendich, A. and Brown, G.B. (1959) J. Amer. Chem. Soc., <u>81</u>, 178.

(25) Fox, J.J. and Shugar, D. (1952) Biochim. Biophys. Acta <u>9</u>, 369-384.

(26) Bergstrom, D.E. and Ruth, J.L. (1976) J. Amer. Chem. Soc., <u>98</u>, 1587-1589.

(27) Krajewska, E. and Shugar, D. (1975) Acta Biochim. Polon., <u>22</u>, 185-194.

MOLECULAR MECHANISMS FOR CONTROL OF RNA TUMOR VIRUSES

Prakash Chandra, Uwe Ebener and Dietmar Gericke

Gustav-Embden-Zentrum der Biologischen Chemie
Abteilung für Molekularbiologie
Klinikum der J.W. Goethe-Universität
6 Frankfurt/Main 70, W. Germany

A great many factors, such as ionizing radiation, environmental carcinogens, hormones, genetic factors, etc. are known to be involved in the etiology of cancer.Viruses are well documented as causative agents of tumors in animals. One needs only to review the role of viruses in the malignant neoplasia of rodents, cats, fowls, frogs, bovines and non-human primates. The viral "footprints" in several human malignant cells and tissues (see sections II and III) lead us the idea that tumor viruses may be involved in human cancer as well. Available data support the concept that the major element among many in cancer may be a virus or viral-related genetic material; and that all other factors may play a secondary role. This concept is favored by evidence that cancer cells usually have a new genetic input that allows them to make new and unique virus-specific antigens. These antigens have been detected in transformed cells and on their surfaces. In contrast, carcinogenic chemicals and radiations do not provide such genetic input. These agents rearrange the output by modification of nucleic acid bases (e.g. translocation, inversion etc.), or by causing chain breaks in the genomic DNA of the host (chromosomal imbalance). If it be true that viral infection (directly or indirectly initiated endogenously by chemical and physical agents) is necessary to cause cancer, then the search for a "target" in preventing viral infection or negating the viral effect, would ultimately lead to the development of potential anticancer drugs. This paper will describe our efforts in developing some useful compounds against RNA tumor viruses.

S T R A T E G Y

The present state of our knowledge on the replicative cycle of oncornaviruses, and the molecular events involved in cell transformation by such viruses, suggests several points of attack in blocking the oncornavirus-induced cell transformation or the expression of integrated viral information (oncogene) in the genome of the host cell (Fig. 1)

CONTROL   OF   RNA   TUMOR   VIRUSES

A. FORMATION OF THE DNA PROVIRUS

    a. Inactivating, or modifying HMW RNA

    b. Inhibiting the Viral DNA Polymerase

B. INTEGRATION OF THE PROVIRUS
    INTO HOST CELL DNA

    e. g. Modifying the proviral DNA

C. EXPRESSION OF THE PROVIRUS

    a. Selective modification of the integrated
    Provirus

    b. RNA - Processing
    e. g. polyadenylation

    c. Translation of mRNA in a specific manner

FIG. 1

    The life cycle of the oncornaviruses involves the following sequential events: 1) Adsorption and penetration of the virus into the host cell; 2) Release of viral components followed by the synthesis of proviral DNA; 3) Integration of the proviral DNA segment into the host genome; 4) Transcription and processing of viral-related RNA ; 5) Translation of viral proteins; 6) Assembly of proteins and RNA ;

7) The envelopment and release (budding) of the virus particles.

Adsorption is mainly dependent on the recognition of the host cell surface receptors by the viral envelope proteins. Our present knowledge about the factors which govern the relationship between the viral envelope proteins and the cell surface receptors is still in its infancy; hence a molecular strategy to block this process is difficult. However, this process is amenable to specific immuno-logical control.

The next step in the life cycle, formation of proviral DNA, is unique to this class of viruses and is therefore most amenable to chemical control(Fig. 1, A). One of the major concerns of our labora-tory is the development of chemical inhibitors which block the synthe-sis of proviral DNA (Chandra et al., 1977). These studies will be described in detail in the next section.

After the initial synthesis of proviral DNA, this DNA is covalent-ly circularized, and processed further for its integration into the genomic DNA of the host cell (Fig. 1, B). It has been reported(Varmus et al., 1974; Guntaka et al., 1975) that this step can be chemically blocked by ethidium bromide, an intercalative drug. In the absence of integration, transformation of cells and the production of virus are blocked (Varmus et al., 1974; Guntaka et al., 1975).

The next step, the synthesis of viral RNA by transcription of proviral DNA (Fig. 1, C), offers another attractive site for mole-cular manipulation. Of the three possibilities mentioned in Fig 1 (C), the RNA-processing step seems to be most attractive. Gillespie and Gallo (1975 and 1977) have suggested that the viral RNA does not under-go the same processing observed in cellular RNA (messenger) prior to its appearance in the cytoplasm. Within the nucleus, mRNA receives a polyadenylic acid (poly A) tail; approx. 2oo adenylic acid residues are attached to its $3'-$ OH end. During the process of transport to the cytoplasm, about 50 AMP residues are lost from this terminal tract. While the polyadenylated mRNA exists in the cytoplasm of the cell, AMP residues are gradually lost, so that the poly A stretches at any given time are of heterogeneous length. In contrast, the poly A stretches in the cytoplasmic viral RNA are 200 or more residues in length. These authors suggest that either the poly A sequences of viral RNA are not "tailored" during the transport process from nucleus to the cytoplasm, or the polyadenylation of viral RNA takes place in the cytoplasmic fraction. Experimentally, Wu et al. (1972) could show that $3'$-deoxyadenosine (cordycepin) is able to block the induction of virus production by 5-iodo-2'-deoxyuridine (IDU); other adenine con-taining nucleosides did not block this induction. This however, is no proof that cordycepin is acting only at the polyadenylation step; as an analog of adenosine it may also interfere in the transcriptional event of the integrated viral DNA.

CHEMICAL CONTROL OF DNA SYNTHESIS IN RNA TUMOR VIRUSES

Compounds that inhibit DNA synthesis in RNA tumor viruses may
be divided, according to their mode of action, into several classes.
The important ones are listed in Table 1.

TABLE 1

INHIBITORS OF VIRAL REVERSE TRANSCRIPTASES

Mode of Action	Compounds

Enzyme-binding compounds	Ansa macrolides
	  Rifamycins
	  Streptovaricins
	  Ca-Elenolate
	  Alkaloids

Substrate analogs	Ara-CTP 5-Mercapto-desoxy-uridine triphosphate

Template-primer analogs	Oligothymidylate derivatives
	Polyribonucleotides
	Modified Polynucleotides
	  ϵ-Poly(A), 70-S RNA
	Vinyl analogs
	Partially thiolated
	  polycytidylate

Template-binding compounds	Actinomycin D Chromomycin Olivomycin Daunomycin, adriamycin, and derivatives Cinerubin Distamycin-A and analogs Ethidium bromide Proflavine Tilorone and congeners Fagaronine (alkaloid)
Divalent cation-binding agents	O-Phenanthroline Thiosemicarbazones
Miscellaneous	Pyran copolymers Streptonigrin and analogs 2-Oxopropanol Silicotungstate 5-Tungsto-2-animoniate

For references see Chandra et al. (1977)

Although it has been only recently recognized that the reverse transcription offers a unique target for drug design, the number of compounds reported to inhibit this process has exceeded expectations, as one sees from Table 1. It is indeed very encouraging that this approach has been endowed with so much experimentation in a number of laboratories; however, the critical analysis of the "*en block*" progress leaves a big gap.

The *in vitro* assay systems employed for reverse transcriptase determination reveal a variety of substrates, template-primers, and interacting compounds that can modulate the catalytic rate of DNA synthesis (reviewed by Temin and Baltimore, 1972; Gillespie, Saxinger and Gallo, 1975). Some examples of this type of modulation are: the detergent effect on the activity of rifamycins (Thompson et al.,1972), the influence of divalent cations (Mg^{++} or Mn^{++}) on the rate of DNA synthesis with different substrates, and the role of chelates or cation binders in buffering agents (Waters and Yang, 1971), and the interaction of thiols with some potential inhibitors (or the direct influence thereof) on measured DNA synthesis (Levinson et al.,1973). Thus, slight variations in assay conditions may lead to wrong interpretations with respect to the specificity of a particular inhibitor in the viral DNA polymerase system.

The second problem is the interpretation of enzymatic data with respect to the antiviral activity of these inhibitors. This is particularly the case with compounds that exert their inhibitory action by complexing with one or the other of the synthetic templates. This may be due to lack of specificity of such inhibitors for the viral enzyme. Drugs either exhibiting cytotoxic activities to the extent of causing a delayed death or intervening in the replicative cycle of the host cell may give erroneous information about the specific antiviral activity of the compound. Thus, the antiviral studies *in vitro* should be carried out under conditions (and at inhibitor concentrations) that have no or little effect on the replicative cycle of the cell. The molecular manipulations of the parent compounds have proved to be very useful in several instances in developing inhibitors of viral DNA polymerases that exhibit a low cytotoxicity and at the same time gain a high antiviral potential. This is evidenced by our studies with distamycin derivatives and tilorone congeners (reviewed by Chandra et al., 1977).

Further efforts to develop compounds that inhibit viral DNA polymerases by interacting with templates may lead to the discovery of useful compounds exhibiting a higher therapeutic index, i.e., a low cytotoxicity and a high antiviral activity. This approach, however, will not lead to the development of a specific inhibitor of the viral enzyme unless one finds a compound that specifically binds to the 70-S RNA. Though 70-S RNA is a novel feature of oncornaviruses, from the chemical and physical standpoint it does not offer any uniqueness

to distinguish it from the cellular nucleic acids. Thus, the stra-
tegical approach to develop an inhibitor of this type is, at the
present state of our knowledge, unthinkable.

The second molecular approach, which has proved to be more useful and relatively specific in developing such inhibitors, is to design compounds that bind to the viral enzyme. One of these compounds
is the polycytidylic acid containing 5-mercapto-substituted cytidy-
late units (Fig. 2). The mode of action of this compound as an inhibitor of the viral DNA polymerase, and its biological implications
will here be described.

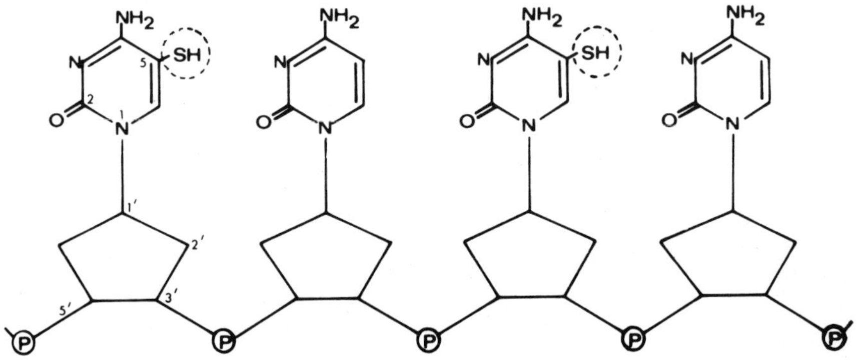

FIG. 2   SCHEMATIC PRESENTATION OF MPC STRUCTURE

INHIBITION OF ONCORNAVIRAL DNA POLYMERASE BY MPC

MODE OF ACTION :The inhibition of DNA polymerases from RNA tumor
viruses by 5-mercapto-polycytidylic acid (MPC) was described earlier
(Chandra & Bardos, 1972; Chandra, Ebener & Götz, 1975; Chandra, 1974
and Chandra, 1977). Partially thiolated polycytidylic acid preparations, MPC I-III (containing 1.7 %, 3.5 % and 8.6 % 5-mercaptocyti-
dylate units, respectively) inhibited the DNA polymerase of Friend
leukemia virus (FLV) in the endogenous reaction as well as in the
presence of poly rA. (dT)$_{14}$, or poly rC.(dG)$_{12-18}$; the inhibitory
activities were directly related to the percent of thiolation.

The mode of inhibition of viral DNA synthesis by MPC was investigated by product analysis of the DNA polymerase reaction in the
absence or in the presence of MPC, as described elsewhere(Chandra,
Ebener & Götz, 1975). The reaction mixtures were dissolved with

Na-dodecyl sulfate (1 %, wt/wt, final concentration), loaded on a hydroxylapatit column (1g, Bio-Rad Lab., Munich), eluted with a Na-phosphate gradient (0.05-0.4 M), collected into about 40 tubes (total vol. approx. 100 ml), and the TCA-insoluble radioactivity collected on GF/C filters (Whatman) and counted in a liquid scintillation counter.

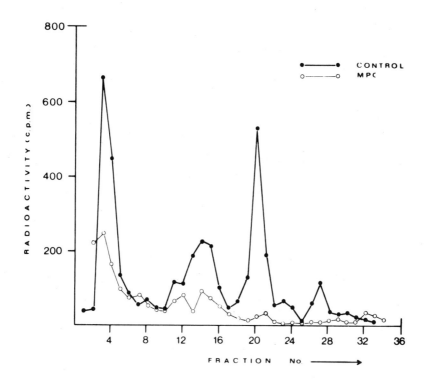

FIG. 3   ANALYSIS OF THE DNA SPECIES SYNTHESIZED BY FLV-DNA POLYMERASE BY ELUTION FROM HYDROXYLAPATIT COLUMN.
Each column was filled with 1g of hydroxylapatit and carefully washed with 0.05 M Na-phosphate (approx. 50 ml). The columns were loaded with the reaction products, as described in text. The columns were washed with 0.05 M Na-phosphate buffer, pH 6.8, until equilibrium reached. Macromolecular species were eluted from the column by a linear gradient of Na-phosphate (0.05-0.4 M). The first species to be eluted from the column contained ss-DNA, the second contained hy-DNA and finally, the ds-DNA, eluted in the last species.The concentration of MPC in the reaction mixture was 20 mcg/ reaction mix.

Analysis of the endogenous products of the detergent disrupted virions exhibits 3 DNA specis: single stranded DNA (ss-DNA), RNA-DNA hybrids (hy-DNA) and the double stranded DNA (ds-DNA). As follows from Fig. 3, in the presence of MPC (open circles) there is an over-all inhibition of ^{3}H-dTMP incorporation, indicating that the forma-

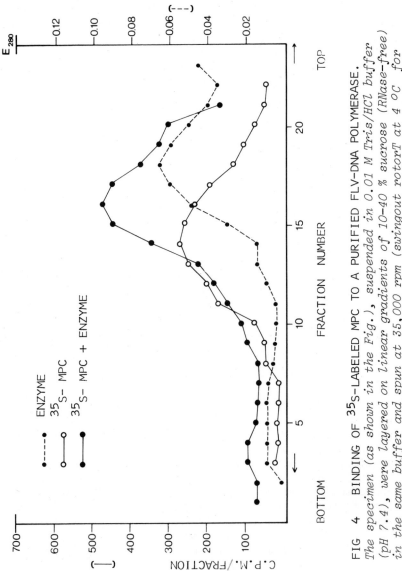

FIG 4   BINDING OF ^{35}S-LABELED MPC TO A PURIFIED FLV-DNA POLYMERASE.
The specimen (as shown in the Fig.), suspended in 0.01 M Tris/HCl buffer (pH 7.4), were layered on linear gradients of 10-40 % sucrose (RNase-free) in the same buffer and spun at 35,000 rpm (swingout rotorT at 4 °C for 20 h. The gradients were dripped from below, fractions collected and after dilution, were analyzed for their radioactivity or absorption at 280 nm. The radioactivity was measured using Brays scintillation fluid. The sp.activity of 35S-MPC was 141 c.p.m./ µg MPC; and the specimen contained 20 ug of MPC. The MPC preparation contained 10.1 % of thiolated Cytosine residues.

tion of all the 3 species is blocked. This is to be expected since
the inhibitor binds to the enzyme. This has been confirmed by ultracentrifugation studies in which the binding of ^{35}S-labeled MPC to a
purified FLV enzyme fraction was investigated (Fig. 4).

In view of the fact that all of the oncornaviral DNA polymerases
examined so far do require a primer-template-like double-stranded
secondary structure for the initiation of DNA synthesis, it is no
surprise that single stranded synthetic polynucleotides(unprimed
templates) can act as inhibitors of the polymerization reaction. This,
presumably, is due to hydrogen bonding of the base sequences between
the added polymer and the functional tmplate. Thus, the specificity
of inhibition by such polymers is not limited to the viral enzyme
system only. On the other hand, minor modifications in the chemical
structure of synthetic polynucleotides might be useful to develop
inhibitors that interact directly with the enzyme but fail to be transcribed, i.e. they function as "dead template" for the enzyme. The data
from our laboratory have shown (Chandra, Ebener & Götz, 1975) that the
partially thiolated polymer of cytidylic acid is functioning as a"dead-
template" in the DNA polymerase system of FLV. The results of these
studies can be summarized as follows: 1) The incorporation of ^{3}H-dGMP
into DNA by the viral enzyme is stimulated to about 9-fold(compared
to the endogenous value) in the presence of poly rC.(dG)$_{12-18}$. However,
under similar conditions a hybrid of MPC.(dG)$_{12-18}$ failed to stimulate
the incorporation of ^{3}H-dGMP into DNA; 2) In the presence of this
hybrid, MPC.(dG)$_{12-18}$, the increasing concentrations of poly rC.(dG)$_{12}$
in the reaction mixture have no effect on the activity of the enzyme;
however, at higher enzyme concentrations the stimulatory effect of
poly rC.(dG)$_{12-18}$ gradually reappears. These data indicate that the
viral enzyme has a higher binding affinity towards MPC than to its
optimal template poly rC. The presence of zinc in reverse transcriptase
makes it attractive to suggest that the mercapto group may undergo an
interaction with zinc to form a stable complex.

SELECTIVITY OF MPC ACTION:In order to determine the selectivity
of MPC action, further studies were conducted using DNA polymerases
from different sources.As follows from Table 2, the viral DNA polymerases are most sensitive towards inhibition by MPC, whereas MPC is
completely unable to inhibit the bacterial DNA polymerase. Enzymes from
human lymphocytes are more sensitive twoards MPC inhibition than the
DNA polymerase I of regenerating rat liver. In spite of the fact that
the experiments were carried out in different laboratories, a comparative evaluation shows that the viral enzymes are at least twice as
sensitive as DNA polymerase from any other source.

Similar results were obtained with enzymes from human spleen
of a patient with myelofibrosis (see Chandra et al., in this volume).
The effect of MPC (SH = 15 %) on the activity of cellular enzymes
(α-, β- , γ- DNA polymerases) and on the reverse transcriptase acti-

T A B L E 2

EVALUATION OF THE INHIBITORY RESPONSE OF PARTIALLY THIOLATED (SH = 13%) POLYCYTIDYLIC ACID ON DNA POLYMERASE FROM VARIOUS SOURCES

Source of DNA Polymerase	Type of DNA Polymerase	Template Used	Compound Required to Inhibit 50% of the Reaction ($\mu g/ml$)
Human lymphocytes* (1788)	I	Poly(dA) · (dT)$_{12-18}$	30
	II	Poly(dA) · (dT)$_{12-18}$	38
Regenerating rat liver	I	CT-DNA	>100 (38% inhibition at 78 $\mu g/ml$)
E. coli K$_{12}$	I	Poly(dA-dT)	No inhibition >100
RMuLV*	Reverse transcriptase	Poly(rA) · (dT)$_{12-18}$	20
FLV	Reverse transcriptase	Poly(rA) · (dT)$_{12-18}$	19.2

*These studies were done by Dr. R. Graham Smith at the Laboratory of Tumor Cell Biology of the National Cancer Institute, Bethesda, Md.

vity was investigated (Chandra, Steel and Ebener, manuscript in preparation). At a concentration of 1 µg/reaction mixture, none of the
cellular enzymes was inhibited. In contrast, the reverse transcriptase activity was inhibited to approx. 20 %.At a concentration of 16
µg, the reverse transcriptase activity was inhibited to 80 %, whereas
the cellular enzymes lost only 25-40 % of their activity.

BIOLOGICAL EFFECTS OF MPC

To measure the effect of MPC (SH = 8.6 %) on the production of
splenomegaly by FLV, we first incubated the cell-free extracts of
spleen from mice (Groppel strain) with 100 ug/ml of MPC at 37 °C for
1 hr. In the control group, where no compound was used, the cell-free
spleen suspension was preincubated with Tris buffer(0.01 M,pH 7.4),
the solvent for MPC. The aliquots of this suspension were injected
(0. 2 ml, LD90) into each group, consisting of 10 animals. The spleen
weights were analyzed on the 8th or the 12th day after infection.

As follows from Fig. 5 there is a 60 % reduction of spleen
weights (arithmatic mean of five individual values) in the MPC-

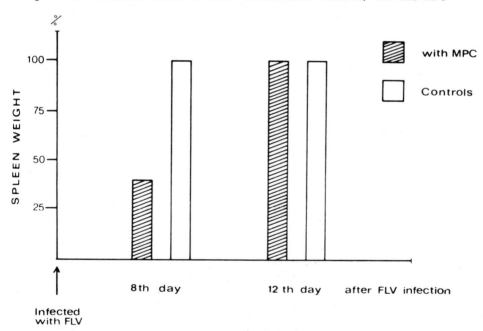

FIG. 5   INHIBITION OF FLV-LEUKEMOGENESIS BY IN VITRO   TREATMENT
OF THE VIRUS WITH MPC. *The studies were carried out on male and
female albino mice (Groppel strain) weighing 20-30 g. FLV suspensions were prepared by filtering the homogenates from infected
spleens through Seitz K-filters (Seitz Company, Bad Kreuznach,
Germany). This suspension was diluted with Hanks solution to give
a LD90 in 0.2 ml. Each column represents an arithmatic mean of five
individual values.*

treated group, measured on the 8th day after FLV-infection. However, no differences in spleen weights in the treated and the control group were observed on the 12th day. This is probably due to fact that at this MPC concentration the whole of virus is not inactivated, so that the residual active virus particles lead to potentiation of leukemogenesis.

To ensure that the splenomegaly is an actual indicator of leukemogenesis, and that the effects obtained on the 8th day were due to MPC inhibition of the viral activity, cell-free spleen extracts from FLV-infected mice, treated in-vitro/vivo with MPC, were injected into normal mice, and their leukemogenic potential was indexed by various parameters (see Table 3). The animals were divided into 4 groups of 5 each (donors): 1) Group 1 was injected with a viral suspension (citrate plasma from FLV-infected animals, dose LD_{90}) preincubated with tris/HCl buffer, pH 7.6 for 30 min. at 37 $^{\circ}C$; 2) Group 2 was injected with the viral suspension, as in 1, but preincubated with MPC (200 ug per 0.2 ml of suspension) at 37$^{\circ}C$ for 30 min. These animals received, in addition, on day 5 and day 9 (post infection), 50 ug of MPC, injected intraperitoneally; 3) Group 3 was treated similar to group 1, except that the viral suspensions were preincubated for 2 hr.; 4) Group 4 was treated in a similar manner as group 2, except that viral suspensions were preincubated for 2 hr. at 37 $^{\circ}C$. On the 10th day, animals were sacrificed and spleen extracts were prepared, as cited elsewhere (Chandra et al., 1975). The spleen extract from each mouse was then analyzed individually, with respect to their leukemogenic potentiality. Each "donor" spleen specimen was reinjected to a different mouse (20 in total), and the leukemogenesis was followed, as shown in Table 3.

All the animals in groups i and 3 developed splenomegaly and died between 40-60 days; whereas, in the MPC treated groups, of the 10 animals only 3 showed signs of splenomegaly. In group 2, 2 animals had splenomegaly but in spite of that, all animals survived till the 123rd day, at which time our experiment was terminated. Similarly, in the last group 4 animals survived till the 123rd day; one died on the 97th day. The spleen weights, shown in the last column, also exhibit large differences between the MPC-treated group, and the control group.In another study we have analyzed the effect of MPC on normal mice of the same strain. We failed to observe any effect of MPC on the spleen weights of non-infected mice. These studies were followed up to analyze the in-vivo effect of MPC on leucocytes of mice infected with the active Friend virus. Within 12 hr. after the MPC injection a dramatic fall in the leucocyte count of animals infected with FLV was observed; MPC failed to reduce the leucocyte number in mice not infected with the virus. This indicates that MPC acts primarily on the leukemic cells without damaging the normal leucocytes. Similar behavior of MPC has been observed by us in patients with ALL and AML demonstrating leucocytosis (see Kornhuber and Chandra, in this volume).

T A B L E 3

ASSAY FOR LEUKEMOGENIC POTENTIAL OF SPLEEN EXTRACTS FROM FLV-INFECTED MICE AFTER THEIR IN-VITRO/VIVO TREATMENT WITH MPC.

TREATMENT OF DONOR MICE	LEUKEMOGENESIS IN RECEPIENT MICE AFTER INFECTION WITH SPLEEN EXTRACT[1]		
	NO. OF POSITIVE / TOTAL NO. OF MICE	MEAN SURVIVAL TIME (DAYS)	MEAN SPLEEN WEIGHT(g)
Virus Suspension[2] (0.2 ml) + Tris buffer (37°C,30 min)	5/5	47	2. 41
Virus Suspension + 200 µg of MPC (37 °C, 30 min.) + 50 µg MPC,i.p.(day 5 & 9)	2/5	123[3]	1. 05 (1.78, 2.10, 0.52,0.41,0.44)
Virus Suspension + Tris buffer (37 °C, 2hr)	5/5	52.2	1. 80
Virus Suspension + 200 µg of MPC (37 °C, 2 hr) + 50 µg MPC,i.p.(day 5 & 9)	1/5	110 4 (123)[3] 1 (97)	0. 38 (0.74,0.29,0.34, 0.22, 0.31)

(1) Cell-free spleen extracts were prepared(described under Fig.5) from spleens of individual donors on the 10th day after being challenged with the virus, or other treatments as shown.

(2) Citrate plasma from FLV-infected mice was used as the source of visus (LD90).

(3) The experiment was terminated on day 123 and all animals were sacrificed on this day.Therefore, the term "mean survival period" does not apply to these animals.

536

Our experimental studies have lead us to postulate the following working hypothesis: The selective cytolysis of leukemic cells by MPC indicates that this compound binds to some "novel" component present in these cells, which may be the viral-related reverse transcriptase. The reason for this selectivity may be the concentration range, which does not effect the normal cellular polymerases, as indicated by our enzymatic data. Once the compound is bound to this "target" the cytotoxicity could then be a secondary event, probably by release of lysosomal enzymes. This is supported by two facts: 1) The lysosomal membranes of tumor cells are less stable than those of normal liver cells (Taniguchi et al., 1976), and 2) after treatment with antitumor agents the lysosomal enzyme activities in tumor cells are higher than in normal cells (Haddow, 1947). Taniguchi et al. (1976) have shown that lysosome labilizers, plasmin and lipoprotein-lipase, are capable of enhancing the cytocidal effect of mitomycin-C on tumor cells. The advantage of our compound is that unlike other lysosome labilizers which can not distinguish between the normal and the tumor cells, this compound could act more specifically on cells which bear its specific receptor, the reverse transcriptase.

ACKNOWLEDGEMENTS

This work was supported by grants from Stiftung Volkswagenwerk (grant No. 14 0305), Kind-Philipp-Stiftung and Riese Stiftung.

REFERENCES

1. CHANDRA,P. & T.J. BARDOS (1972): Res.Commun.Chem.Path.Pharmacol. 4, 615.
2. CHANDRA,P. (1974):in, Topics in Current Chemistry(Medicinal Chem.) 52, 99. Springer-Verlag,Berlin-Heidelberg-New York.
3. CHANDRA,P., U. EBENER & A. Götz (1975): FEBS-Letters 53, 10.
4. CHANDRA, P., L.K. STEEL, U. EBENER, M. WOLTERSDORF, H. LAUBE & G. WILL (1976):Progr. in Molecular & Subcell. Biology 4, 167.
5. CHANDRA,P., B. KORNHUBER, D. GERICKE, A. GÖTZ & U. EBENER (1975): Z. Krebsforschung Klin. Onkol. 83, 239.
6. CHANDRA,P., L.K.STEEL, U. EBENER, M. WOLTERSDORF, H. LAUBE, B. KORNHUBER, B. MILDNER & A. GÖTZ(1977):Pharm.Ther.A 1 ,231.
7. GILLESPIE, D., W.C. SAXINGER & R.C. GALLO (1975): Progr. Nucl. Acid Res. & Mol. Biol. 15, 1
8. GILLESPIE, D. & R.C. GALLO(1975): Science 188, 802.
9. GILLESPIE, D. & R.C. GALLO(1977): Ann. N.Y.Acad.Sci. 284,576.
10. GUNTAKA,R.V., B.W.J. MAHY, J.M. BISHOP & H.E. VARMUS (1975): Nature(Lond.) 235, 507.
11. LEVINSON,W., A. FARAS, B. WOODSON, J. JACKSON & J.M. BISHOP(1973): Proc.Natl.Acad.Sci.,U.S.A. 70, 164.

12. TEMIN,H.M. & D. BALTIMORE (1972): Adv.Virus Res. 17, 129.
13. THOMPSON, F.M., L.J. LIBERTINI, U.R. JOSS & M. CALVIN (1972):
       Science 178, 505.
14. VARMUS, H.E., R.V. GUNTAKA, W.J.W. FAN, S. HEASLEY & J.M. BISHOP
       (1974): Proc.Natl.Acad.Sci.,U.S.A. 70, 3874.
15. WATERS, L.C. & W.K. YANG (1971): Fed. Proc. 30(II), 1163 A.
16. Wu, A.M., R.C. TING, M. PARAN & R.C. GALLO (1972):Proc.Natl.Acad.
       Sci., U.S.A. 69, 3820.

Additional References

17. HADDOW, A. (1947): Growth 11, 339.
18. TANIGUCHI, T., H.Nitani, A. SUZUKI, N. SAIJO, I. KAWASE &
       K. Kimura (1976): in, Chemotherapy (Edt. K. Hellmann & T.A.Connors)
       Vol. 8 , 175.

INHIBITION OF ONCORNAVIRUS ACTIVITIES BY POLYNUCLEOTIDE ANALOGUES

Erik de Clercq

Department of Human Biology, Division of Microbiology
Rega Institute, University of Leuven
B-3000 Leuven, Belgium

Polynucleotides are endowed with a variety of biologic activities. For double-stranded RNAs the most characteristic biologic functions are interferon induction and inhibition of protein synthesis (1). For single-stranded RNAs the most prominent features are an inhibitory effect on complement activity (2) and inhibition of the reverse transcriptase (RNA-directed DNA polymerase) activity associated with oncornaviruses. The latter properties will be reviewed here.

Tuominen and Kenney (3) were first to report that single-stranded homopolyribonucleotides such as (U)n could inhibit the DNA polymerase of RNA tumor viruses. These observations were later confirmed and extended to various other synthetic polyribonucleotides and analogues thereof. The polynucleotide inhibitors of oncornavirus DNA polymerase could be divided into four classes : (A)n analogues (Fig. 1), (I)n analogues (Fig. 2), (U)n analogues (Fig. 3) and (C)n analogues (Fig. 4).

The full designations of these polynucleotides and the leading references pertaining to their anti-reverse transcriptase activity are as follows :

- (A)n, polyadenylic acid (3-9)
- (aza^{2}A)n, poly(2-azaadenylic acid) (10)
- (i-pro^{2}A)n, poly(2-isopropyladenylic acid (11)
- (ms^{2}A)n, poly(2-methylthioadenylic acid (12)
- (es^{2}A)n, poly(2-ethylthioadenylic acid) (12)
- (c^{3}A)n, poly(3-deazaadenylic acid) (13)
- (c^{7}A)n, poly(7-deazaadenylic acid) (13,14)

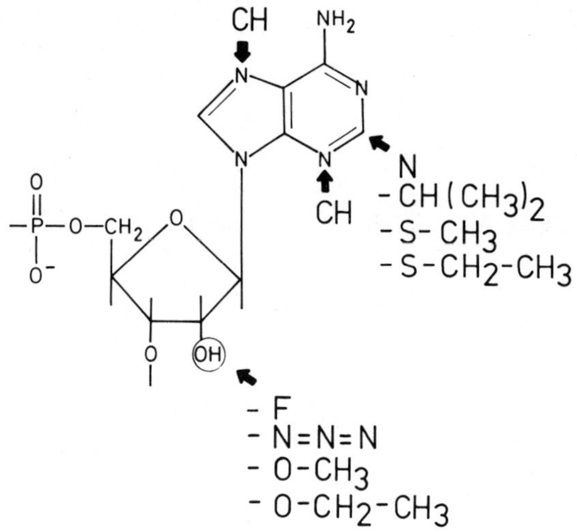

FIGURE 1

(A)$_n$ analogues with anti-reverse transcriptase
         activity

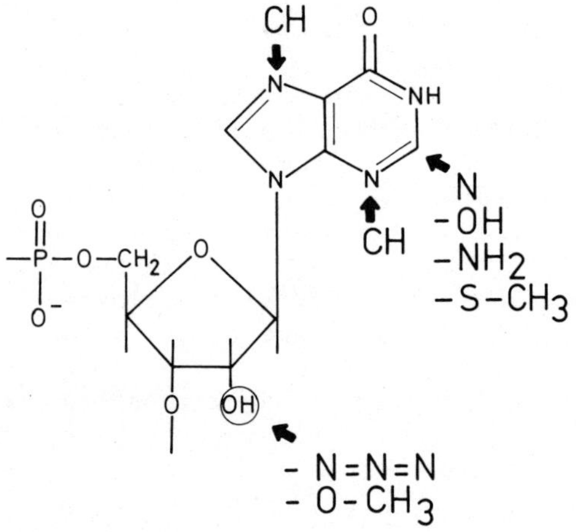

FIGURE 2

(I)$_n$ analogues with anti-reverse transcriptase
         activity

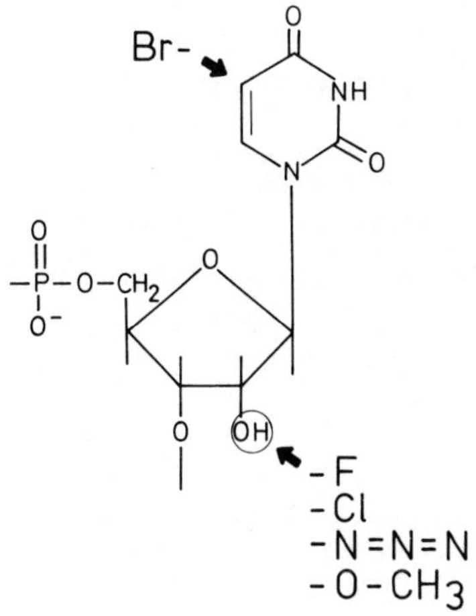

FIGURE 3

(U)$_n$ analogues with anti-reverse transcriptase activity

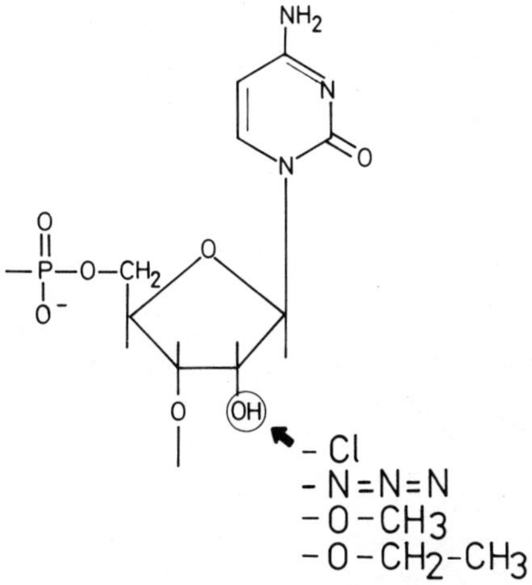

FIGURE 4

(C)$_n$ analogues with anti-reverse transcriptase activity

- (dAfl)n, (poly(2'-fluoro-2'-deoxyadenylic acid (12)
- (dAz)n, poly(2'-azido-2'-deoxyadenylic acid) (12)
- (Am)n, poly(2'-O-methyladenylic acid (4-8,15)
- (Ae)n, poly(2'-O-ethyladenylic acid) (6-8)
- (I)n, polyinosinic acid (6,8,16,17)
- $(aza^2I)n$, poly(2-azainosinic acid) (10)
- (X)n, polyxanthylic acid (18)
- (G)n, polyguanylic acid (3,18)
- $(ms^2I)n$, poly(2-methylthioinosinic acid) (19)
- $(c^3I)n$, poly(3-deazainosinic acid) (13)
- $(c^7I)n$, poly(7-deazainosinic acid) (13,14)
- (dIz)n, poly(2'-azido-2'-deoxyinosinic acid) (12)
- (Im)n, poly(2'-O-methylinosinic acid) (8,16)
- (U)n, polyuridylic acid (3,9,20-24)
- $(br^5U)n$, poly(5-bromouridylic acid) (11,22)
- (dUfl)n, poly(2'-fluoro-2'-deoxyuridylic acid) (22)
- (dUcl)n, poly(2'-chloro-2'-deoxyuridylic acid) (22)
- (dUz)n, poly(2'-azido-2'-deoxyuridylic acid) (24)
- (Um)n, poly(2'-O-methyluridylic acid) (8,16)
- (C)n, polycytidylic acid (3,24)
- (dCcl)n, poly(2'-chloro-2'-deoxycytidylic acid) (22)
- (dCz)n, poly(2'-azido-2'-deoxycytidylic acid) (24)
- (Cm)n, poly(2'-O-methylcytidylic acid) (8)
- (Ce)n, poly(2'-O-ethylcytidylic acid) (25)

Many of these polynucleotide analogues proved to be effective inhibitors of the in vitro DNA polymerase activity of Moloney murine leukemia virus (MuLV (Moloney) (Table 1)). Note that for the experiments reported in Table 1 no exogenous template-primer was added to the reaction mixtures, so that only endogenous viral RNA-directed DNA synthesis was measured. While inactive by itself, (A)n became markedly inhibitory upon introduction of an ethylthio group at C-2 or an azido group at C-2'. Similarly, substitution of 2'-azido for 2'-hydroxyl markedly enhanced the anti-reverse transcriptase activities of (I)n, (U)n and (C)n (Table 1). The inhibitory activity of the 2'-azido polymers specifically resided in the homopolymer structure, since no inhibition was observed when the 2'-azido polymer (e.g. (dUz)n) had been annealed with a complementary polymer (e.g. (A)n) before addition to the DNA polymerase assay mixture.

For a few selected compounds, (I)n, (A)n, (dIz)n and (dAz)n, the time-response relationship of MuLV DNA polymerase inhibition is presented in Figure 5. The inhibitory effects of (dIz)n and (dAz)n on DNA synthesis gradually increased with the time of incubation. Similar time-response curves have been obtained previously for other polynucleotide analogues, viz. $(ms^2I)n$ (19), $(c^7A)n$, $(c^7I)n$ (13), $(aza^2A)n$ and $(aza^2I)n$ (10).

TABLE 1. Effect of Various Polynucleotide Analogues on DNA
Polymerase Activity of MuLV (Moloney), in the Absence
of (A)n.oligo(dT) as Template-Primer

Polynucleotide	Extent of inhibition noted at a polynucleotide concen- of 70 µg/ml ($\sim$0.2 µmol/ml)	References
(A)n	0 %	10,13,14
(aza^{2}A)n	35 %	10
(es^{2}A)n	90 – 95 %	12
(c^{3}A)n	20 %	13
(c^{7}A)n	50 %	13,14
(dAz)n	60 %	12
(I)n	15 – 25 %	10,13,14,19
(aza^{2}I)n	55 %	10
(ms^{2}I)n	70 %	19
(c^{3}I)n	5 %	13
(c^{7}I)n	20 – 35 %	13,14
(dIz)n	40 – 50 %	12
(U)n	25 %	24
(dUz)n	70 %	24
(C)n	5 %	24
(dCz)n	55 %	24

The assay mixtures contained (in a total volume of 280 µl)
200 µl of a solution which was 40mM Tris-HCl (pH 7.8), 50mM
NaCl, 1.6mM dithiothreitol, 4mM MnCl$_2$, 0.64mM each in dATP,
dCTP and dGTP, 0.035mM ^{3}H-dTTP (specific activity: 11-50
Ci/mmol, depending on the batch) and 0.0125 % (v/v) Triton
X-100, 20 µl of polynucleotide stock solution (1 mg/ml),
20 µl of Carbopol (carboxypolymethylene) stock solution
(4 mg/ml) and 20 µl MuLV (Moloney) virus stock (Electro-
Nucleonics Laboratories, catalog no. 1021). The data
reported here refer to assay mixtures which were incubated
at 37° for 60 minutes.

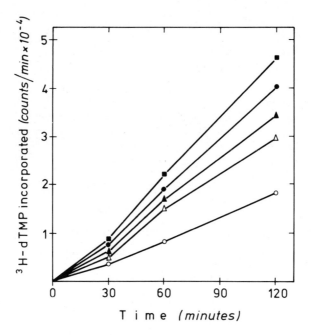

Effect of $(A)_n$ (●), $(dAz)_n$ (○), $(I)_n$ (▲) and $(dIz)_n$ (△)
on DNA polymerase activity of MuLV (Moloney). Control: ■
No template-primer added. DNA synthesis measured
at different times of incubation (as indicated on the
abscissa). Final concentration of the polymers:
70 µg/ml.

FIGURE 5

In several other studies in which polynucleotides were evaluated for their inhibitory effects on oncornaviral DNA polymerases, a template-primer such as (A)n.oligo(dT) was generally added
to the assay mixture (6,16,18,20,22). This addition renders the
DNA synthesis much more sensitive to inhibition. As shown in
Table 2, various polynucleotides including (I)n and (U)n, brought
about a dramatic reduction in (A)n.oligo(dT)-directed DNA synthesis, even when added at a concentration as low as 1 µg/ml. For
compounds such as (dAz)n and (dUz)n, the extent of inhibition
approached 99 % (at a polynucleotide concentration of 10-100 µg/
ml) (Table 2). In an endogenous RNA-directed DNA polymerase reaction, (dAz)n and (dUz)n did not effect an inhibition greater than
60-70 % (at a polynucleotide concentration of 70 µg/ml, Table 1).

Figure 6 clearly demonstrates the differences in inhibition
of DNA synthesis obtained with (dAz)n in the presence and absence
of (A)n.oligo(dT) as template-primer. The same behavior was noted
for (I)n, (X)n, (U)n, (dUz)n and (br[5]U)n, as they all inhibited
the (A)n.oligo(dT)-directed DNA synthesis to a considerably

TABLE 2. Effect of Various Polynucleotide Analogues
on (A)n.oligo(dT)-Directed DNA Polymerase
Activity of MuLV (Moloney)

Polynucleotide	^{3}H-dTMP incorporated (%)		
	Polynucleotide concentration:		
	1 µg/ml	10 µg/ml	100 µg/ml
(A)n	220	283	340
(dAz)n	91	1.8	1.5
(i-pro^{2}A)n	19	5.5	4.4
(I)n	57	14	5.7
(X)n	43	14	7.9
(ms^{2}I)n	97	81	9.5
(U)n	84	46	2.8
(dUz)n	6.3	1.4	1.3
(br^{5}U)n	105	18	1.0

The assay mixtures contained (in a total volume of
100 µl) 25mM Tris-HCl (pH 8.3), 100mM NaCl, 5mM
dithiothreitol, 0.5mM Mn(OOC-CH$_3$)$_2$, 7.5 µM (A)n, 2 µM
oligo(dT), 0.04 % (v/v) Triton X-100, 5.0 µCi ^{3}H-dTTP,
varying amounts of polynucleotide (as indicated) and
0.5 µl MuLV (Moloney) virus stock, containing 1.8 x
10^{11} virus particles (1.7 mg/protein) per ml (Elec-
tro-Nucleonics Laboratories, catalog no. 1024, lot
no. 5004-26-56). The assay mixtures were incubated
at 37° for 60 minutes.

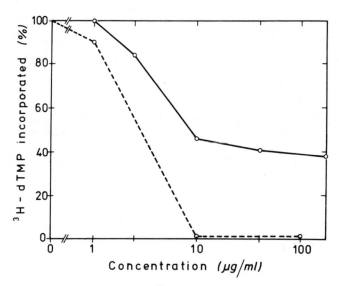

Effect of (dAz)n on DNA polymerase activity of MuLV (Moloney),
in the absence (——) or presence (----) of (A)n· oligo (dT) as
template - primer. DNA synthesis measured at different concentrations of (dAz)n (as indicated on the abscissa). Incubation
time of assay mixtures : 60 minutes.

FIGURE 6

greater extent than the endogenous RNA-directed DNA synthesis. One
may wonder, however, whether the potent inhibitory effects that
polynucleotides such as (I)n, (X)n, (U)n, (dUz)n and (br⁵U)n
exert on the (A)n.oligo(dT)-directed DNA synthesis (as reported
herein and previously (6,16,18,20,22)), are not due to a direct
interaction of the polynucleotide with the (A)n template rather
than with the DNA polymerase itself. All these polynucleotides
are indeed known to form rather stable double- and/or triple-
stranded complexes with (A)n. The latter reasoning does, of
course, not apply for (dAz)n and the other (A)n analogues.

    One might expect that the (A)n analogues would compete with
the (exogenously) added (A)n for the template binding site of the
DNA polymerase. Accordingly, the kinetics of inhibition of the
(A)n.oligo(dT)-directed MuLV DNA polymerase by (Am)n and (Ae)n
appeared entirely consistent with a simple competitive inhibition
(as judged from Lineweaver-Burk (1/v versus 1/(A)n.oligo(dT))
plots (6)). For (I)n, (Im)n and (X)n the kinetics of inhibition
were neither simply competitive nor noncompetitive; it appeared
to be a mixed type of inhibition (6,16,18). Obviously, these
kinetics may have been influenced by a direct interaction (complex formation) between template ((A)n) and inhibitors ((I)n,
(Im)n, (X)n).

TABLE 3. Structural Requirements for Synthetic
Polynucleotides to Act as Reverse
Transcriptase Inhibitors

---

1. Sufficiently high molecular size

2. Single-strandedness (as opposed to double- or
    triple-strandedness)

3. Intact or, preferably, modified purine or
    pyrimidine moieties

4. Intact or, preferably, substituted 2'-hydroxyl
    groups

5. Purine polyribonucleotides more potent than
    pyrimidine polyribonucleotides

The inhibition of the RNA-directed DNA polymerase of RNA
tumor viruses by synthetic polynucleotides depends on some structural requirements, as summarized in Table 3. The molecular size
requirement was assessed with (U)n as inhibitor. Erickson et al.
(21) found that the inhibitory effect of (U)n on the viral DNA
polymerase dropped sharply at chain lengths below approximately
200 nucleotide residues per (U)n molecule. Unlike interferon
induction, which critically depends on the double-stranded character of the polyribonucleotide, inhibition of the reverse transcriptase require a single-stranded polynucleotide (14,19,24). The
anti-reverse transcriptase activity of the polynucleotide is not
impaired or rather increased upon modifications of the purine ring
(e.g. substituion of CH for N-7 in (I)n or introduction of a
2-methylthio or 2-ethylthio substituent in either (I)n or (A)n
(Table 1)) or modifications of the pyrimidine ring (e.g. substitution of a bromo group at C-5 of (U)n (Table 2)). Other modifications which have been shown to enhance the inhibitory effects of
polynucleotides on oncornavirus DNA polymerases are the introduction of a 1,N^6-ethenobridge in (A)n (26) and the introduction of
5-mercapto groups in (C)n (27,28). An intact 2'-hydroxyl group is
not a requisite for the anti-reverse transcriptase activity of
polyribonucleotides. In fact, replacement of the 2'-OH group by a
fluorine or chlorine (as in (dUfl)n, (dUcl)n and (dCcl)n (22)),
or an azido (as in (dUz)n, (dCz)n, (dAz)n and (dIz)n (12,24)), or
a methoxy or ethoxy group (as in (Am)n and (Ae)n (4,6)) greatly
increased the inhibitory activity of the polymers. In contrast,
2'-O-methylation of (I)n and (U)n decreased the inhibitory potency
of these polynucleotides (16). The reasons for this discrepancy
are not clear. They may be related to the use of (A)n.oligo(dT)
as template-primer in the DNA polymerase reactions. Finally, Arya

et al. (18) postulated that purine polyribonucleotides may be more
potent inhibitors of viral DNA polymerase (and viral replication)
than pyrimidine polyribonucleotides. This contention certainly
holds for a limited set of polynucleotides including (G)n, (X)n,
(I)n, (C)n and (U)n, but cannot as yet be generalized to other
polynucleotide analogues.

Are polynucleotides selective in their anti-reverse transcriptase activity or do they inhibit viral and cellular DNA polymerases to the same extent ? (U)n was originally reported to
specifically inhibit the DNA polymerase of Rauscher leukemia virus,
without affecting the DNA polymerases from mouse embryos or
Escherichia coli (3). However, the prospect that (U)n may discri-
minate between viral DNA polymerases and cellular DNA polymerases
did not appear justified, since Abrell et al. (20) found that (U)n
inhibited some cellular DNA polymerases as much as the viral enzymes. (Am)n and (Ae)n have also been reported to inhibit MuLV DNA
polymerase with no effect on E.coli or mouse spleen DNA polymerase
(6). However, the effect of these (A)n analogues on DNA polymerases from several other sources will need to be investigated
before a definitive conclusion regarding specificity of inhibition
can be reached. The same situation applies to (I)n, (X)n and (G)n
which have also been shown to inhibit MuLV DNA polymerase to a
considerably greater extent than cellular DNA polymerase (17,18).
The latter specificity may at least partially be influenced by a
direct interaction of the inhibitor with the template, as different template-primers $\left[(A)n.oligo(dT)\ and\ d(A-T)n.d(A-T)n\right]$ were
employed to monitor the viral and cellular DNA polymerase reactions.

If (Am)n, (Ae)n, (I)n, (X)n, (G)n and their congeners are
selective inhibitors of viral RNA-directed DNA polymerase, one
may expect these polynucleotides to inhibit the replication of
RNA tumor viruses in cell cultures at concentrations which are
not toxic for the host cells. These expectations have been fulfilled for quite a variety of polynucleotide analogues (Table 4).
Some polymers such as (Am)n and (Ae)n were also effective in mice,
in inhibiting the replication of Friend leukemia virus (7) and/or
Moloney sarcoma virus (15). In several instances, the polynucleotides exhibited a reasonably good correlation between their
effects on virus replication in vivo and their effects on virion-
associated RNA-directed DNA polymerase in vitro : e.g. for (A)n
and its analogues (Am)n and (Ae)n, the order of inhibitory potency
was (Ae)n > (Am)n > (A)n, both in vitro (6) and in vivo (7). These
observations are consistent with the hypothesis that the inhibition of virus replication by polynucleotides may be mediated by an
inhibitory effect on viral RNA-directed DNA synthesis. This hypothesis is further supported by the observation that the polynucleotides are most effective when added prior to or just after

TABLE 4. Polynucleotide Analogues which have been
shown to Inhibit (murine) Leukemia and/or
Sarcoma Virus Replication in Cell
Cultures and/or Mice

Polynucleotide	Active in cell cultures	Active in mice	References
(A)n	+	+	4,5,7-9,23
(Am)n	+	+	4,5,7,8,15
(Ae)n	+	+	7,8
(I)n	+	?	8,17,19
(X)n	+	?	18
(G)n	+	?	18
$(ms^2 I)n$	+	−	19
(Im)n	+	?	8
(U)n	+	?	8,9,23
(dUz)n	+	?	24
(Um)n	+	+	8,15
(dCz)n	+	?	24
(Cm)n	+	?	8

virus infection (5,23), which suggests that an early stage in
virus infection is affected. The polynucleotides do not suppress
the formation of oncornavirus particles in persistently infected
cells (24). Nor do they suppress the activation of endogenous
oncornaviruses by 5-iodo-2'-deoxyuridine (5,29). Thus, the target
for the inhibition of RNA tumor virus replication by polynucleotides may well be the synthesis of proviral DNA.

There are, however, inconsistencies in the in vitro and in
vivo behavior of some polynucleotides : while showing little, if
any, activity on viral DNA polymerase activity in vitro (3,6,10,
13,14), (A)n markedly inhibits virus replication in vivo (7,8,23).
An equally potent in vivo activity is observed for (Cm)n (8),
although (Cm)n is notoriously inactive as an in vitro reverse
transcriptase inhibitor (16). In fact, (Cm)n acts as an ideal

template for the RNA-directed DNA polymerase of RNA tumor viruses
(30). Hence, additional factors should be considered in correlating the in vitro potency of polynucleotides as reverse transcriptase inhibitors with their in vivo effects on virus replication.
These additional factors may be related to the fate of the polynucleotide within cells or biological fluids (as determined by
the resistance of the polynucleotide to enzymatic degradation),
or, alternatively, the virion-associated RNA-directed DNA polymerase may not be the only target for the in vivo inhibition of
oncornavirus replication by polynucleotides.

Acknowledgments. The original investigations reported herein
were supported by grants from the F.G.W.O. (Fonds voor Geneeskun-
dig Wetenschappelijk Onderzoek, krediet nr. 3.0048.75) and the
Geconcerteerde Onderzoeksacties, Conventie nr. 76/81-IV. The
editorial help of Janine Putzeys is gratefully acknowledged.

REFERENCES

1. Carter, W.A. and De Clercq, E. (1974) Science, 186, 1172-
    1178.
2. De Clercq, E., Torrence, P.F., Hobbs, J., Janik, B.,
    De Somer, P. and Witkop, B. (1975) Biochem. Biophys. Res.
    Commun., 67, 255-263.
3. Tuominen, F.W. and Kenney, F.T. (1971) Proc. Nat. Acad. Sci.
    USA, 68, 2198-2202.
4. Tennant, R.W., Kenney, F.T. and Tuominen, F.W. (1972) Nature,
    238, 51-53.
5. Tennant, R.W., Farrelly, J.G., Ihle, J.N., Pal, B.C., Kenney,
    F.T. and Brown, A. (1973) J. Virol., 12, 1216-1225.
6. Arya, S.K., Carter, W.A., Alderfer, J.L. and Ts'o, P.O.P.
    (1974) Biochem. Biophys. Res. Commun., 59, 608-615.
7. Arya, S.K., Carter, W.A., Alderfer, J.L. and Ts'o, P.O.P.
    (1975) Molec. Pharmacol., 11, 501-505.
8. Arya, S.K., Carter, W.A., Alderfer, J.L. and Ts'o, P.O.P.
    (1976) Molec. Pharmacol., 12, 234-241.
9. Arya, S.K. and Chawda, R. (1977) Molec. Pharmacol., 13, 374-
    377.
10. De Clercq, E., Huang, G.-F., Torrence, P.F., Fukui, T.,
    Kakiuchi, N. and Ikehara, M. (1977) Nucleic Acids Res., 4,
    3643-3653.
11. De Clercq, E., Hattori, M. and Pfleiderer, W. (1978)
    Unpublished observations.
12. De Clercq, E., Fukui, T., Kakiuchi, N. and Ikehara, M. (1978)
    Unpublished observations.
13. De Clercq, E., Torrence, P.F., Fukui, T. and Ikehara, M.
    (1976) Nucleic Acids Res., 3, 1591-1601.

14. De Clercq, E., Billiau, A., Torrence, P.F., Waters, J.A. and Witkop, B. (1975) Biochem. Pharmacol., 24, 2233-2238.
15. Tennant, R.W., Hanna Jr., M.G. and Farrelly, J.G. (1974) Proc. Nat. Acad. Sci. USA, 71, 3167-3171.
16. Arya, S.K., Carter, W.A., Alderfer, J.L. and Ts'o, P.O.P. (1975) Molec. Pharmacol., 11, 421-426.
17. Arya, S.K. (1977) Molec. Pharmacol., 13, 585-597.
18. Arya, S.K., Helser, T.L., Carter, W.A. and Ts'o, P.O.P. (1976) Molec. Pharmacol., 12, 844-853.
19. De Clercq, E., Billiau, A., Hattori, M. and Ikehara, M. (1975) Nucleic Acids Res., 2, 2305-2314.
20. Abrell, J.W., Smith, R.G., Robert, M.S. and Gallo, R.C. (1972) Science, 177, 1111-1114.
21. Erickson, R.J., Janik, B. and Sommer, R.G. (1973) Biochem. Biophys. Res. Commun., 52, 1475-1482.
22. Erickson, R.J. and Grosch, J.C. (1974) Biochemistry, 13, 1987-1993.
23. Pitha, P.M., Teich, N.M., Lowy, D.R. and Pitha, J. (1973) Proc. Nat. Acad. Sci. USA, 70, 1204-1208.
24. De Clercq, E., Billiau, A., Hobbs, J., Torrence, P.F. and Witkop, B. (1975) Proc. Nat. Acad. Sci. USA, 72, 284-288.
25. Mikke, R., Kielanowska, M., Shugar, D. and Zmudzka, B. (1976) Nucleic Acids Res., 3, 1603-1611.
26. Chirikjian, J.G. and Papas, T.S. (1974) Biochem. Biophys. Res. Commun., 59, 489-495.
27. Chandra, P. and Bardos, T.J. (1972) Res. Commun. Chem. Pathol. Pharmacol., 4, 615-622.
28. Srivastava, B.I.S. (1973) Biochim. Biophys. Acta, 335, 77-84.
29. Pitha, P.M., Pitha, J. and Rowe, W.P. (1975) Virology, 63, 568-572.
30. Gerard, G.F. (1975) Biochem. Biophys. Res. Commun., 63, 706-711.

DIFFERENTIAL AND SELECTIVE CONTROL OF DNA SYNTHESIS OF NONINFECTED AND HERPES SIMPLEX VIRUS INFECTED CELLS BY ARABINOFURANOSYLADENINE

Werner E. G. Müller and Rudolf K. Zahn

Institut für Physiologische Chemie, Abteilung "Angewandte Molekularbiologie" , Universität
Duisbergweg, 6500 Mainz, WEST GERMANY

ABSTRACT

9-D-Arabinofuranosyladenine occurs in the α (αaraAdo) as well as in the ß (ßaraAdo) anomeric form. These two compounds act differentially on host cell- and Herpes simplex virus (HSV) DNA synthesis.

αAraAdo strongly inhibits cell proliferation of noninfected L5178y cells. At cytostatic concentrations αaraAdo selectively blocks the incorporation rate of thymidine into DNA but not the incorporation rates of precursors into RNA or protein. In the intact cell system αaraAMP is incorporated into DNA to a low extent. αAraAdo is intracellularly phosphorylated to αaraATP. Enzymatic studies revealed that αaraATP has no effect on the HSV DNA polymerase system but a high inhibitory potency in the host cell DNA polymeraseα system.

ßAraAdo reduces HSV DNA synthesis at low concentrations with a high selectivity compared to the cellular DNA synthesis. On molecular basis, the specific anti-HSV effect of ßaraAdo seems to be explainable on the level of the DNA polymerase. The HSV enzyme is 120-fold more sensitively inhibited by ßaraATP than the polymerase α . Higher concentrations of ßaraAdo are needed to inhibit cell proliferation; this reduction of cell proliferation is a consequence of a competitive inhibition of DNA polymeraseα by ßaraATP. In intact cell system ßaraAMP is incorporated not only into cellular DNA but also into HSV-DNA. In the case of cellular DNA the drug is incorporated in internucleotide linkage while the incorporated compound is present in HSV DNA in terminal positions.

The results obtained demonstrate αaraAdo to be an absolute specific inhibitor of cellular DNA synthesis and in consequence a potent inhibitory cytostatic compound; it has no influence on HSV growth. In contrast, ßaraAdo is a relatively specific virostatic compound; the differential inhibition is due to a differential sensitivity of host cell- and HSV DNA synthesizing system towards ßaraATP.

INTRODUCTION

It seems to be well established that Epstein-Barr virus in man (1, 2), Marek's disease herpesvirus in chicken (3), herpesvirus saimiri and ateles in monkeys (4, 5), and some Herpes simplex virus (HSV) defective mutants (6) interact oncogenetically with various animal or human target cells. Even though some new information about the molecular biology of tumor viruses has appeared, the enzymic process of cellular transformation is hardly understood. One critical difference between transformed and untransformed cells lies in the fact that untransformed cells go into a resting G_1-state under suboptimal conditions while transformed cells continue to grow. The time point in the cell cycle at which cells rest is somewhere during G_1 but not at the border G_1-S phase. For that reason it appears that the initial event of transformation is not a process involving the control of cellular DNA synthesis (7). It remains still an open question what controls the expression of viral DNA and triggers transformation. Therefore, at the present stage, experimental studies about a therapy and control of herpesvirus-caused transformation must be restricted to a prevention of a transmission of the virus. One approach to block horizontal spread is an inhibition of virus growth. This aim could be achieved e. g. by compounds which inactivate key enzymes for virus growth. However, these compounds must be at least relatively selective in such a way that they affect the function of viral molecules more sensitively than the analogous host molecules. This task can be accomplished with some hope if compounds are available which inhibit the HSV-induced enzymes, e. g. the deoxypyrimidine kinase and the DNA polymerase.

In the last four years two antimetabolites were found which exert an anti-herpesvirus activity of some selectivity: Arabinofuranosylthymine (araThd) (8, 9) and arabinofuranosyladenine (araAdo) (10, 11). The mode of action of these compounds is known to some extent. It was suggested that the selective inhibitory effect of araThd is due to the fact that the mammalian host cell deoxythymidine kinase does not have the capacity to phosphorylate araThd to araTMP (12), while the HSV-induced deoxypyrimidine kinase (which is essential for virus replication under certain conditions; Ref. 13) uses araThd as substrate. However, in later studies (14, 15) it could be clearly shown, using L5178y mouse lymphoma cells, that araThd acts cytostatically by a selective block of DNA synthesis. This blocking of cellular DNA synthesis is due to a competitive inhibition of cellular DNA polymeraseα by the intracellularly formed araTTP with respect to the analogous substrate (dTTP) and to a non-competitive inhibition if non-analogous substrate (dATP) is used. Thus the anti-herpesvirus specificity of araThd is most likely cell type- and/or cell function dependent.

The mode of action of the anti-herpesvirus compound araAdo is described in the following in more detail.

COMPOUNDS

The group of arabinosyl nucleosides is distinguished from the ribosyl- and deoxyribosyl nucleosides by the sugar moiety arabinose which is altered in the 2' position. As shown in Fig. 1 the arabinose molecule resembles ribose by the identical formula but arabinose is distinguished from ribose by its trans-glycol configuration. Compared to deoxyribose the arabinose molecule has the identical cis configuration at the 2' and 3' position but a different formula due to the presence of the hydroxyl group at carbon 2'.

9-ß-D-arabinofuranosyladenine (ßaraAdo) was found in an antibiotic concentrate from Streptomyces antibioticus; this compound is formed by enzymic epimerization of the 2'-hydroxyl group of adenosine (16). 13 years ago, ßaraAdo was already chemically synthesized by Goodman's group (17).

Only ß-D-sugar nucleosides have been found naturally. Therefore it was of interest to clarify whether arabinosylnucleosides in a different isomeric form, exert biological activity. Among the derivatives synthesized (18), 9-α-D-arabinofuranosyladenine (α araAdo) (Fig. 1) gained some interest in the aspect of a selective control of DNA synthesis of noninfected and Herpes simplex-infected cells. α AraAdo was chemically synthesized.

TARGET ENZYMES

Cellular Enzymes

Both ßaraAdo and αaraAdo are metabolically activated via araAMP (adenosine kinase) and araADP (adenylate kinase) to araATP (nucleoside-diphosphate kinase). Besides these three enzymes mentioned, which could be influenced by the ara-nucleosides or ara-nucleotides, the DNA - as well

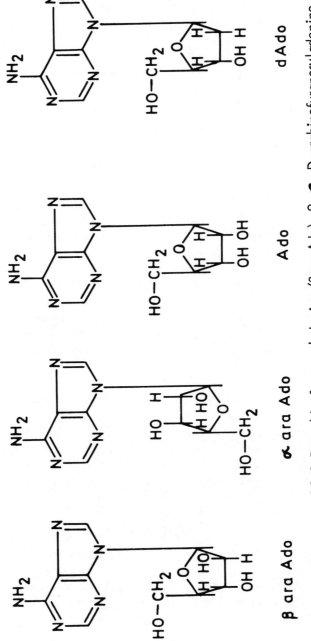

Fig. 1 :   Structures of 9-ß-D-arabinofuranosyl adenine (ß araAdo), 9-α-D-arabinofuranosyl adenine
(α araAdo), adenosine (Ado) and deoxyadenosine (dAdo).

as the RNA polymerases are the possible target enzymes for an inhibition.

DNA polymerases. Uninfected eukaryotic cells contain three major distinct DNA-dependent DNA polymerases. The DNA polymeraseα was found to be the DNA replication enzyme (19), the DNA polymerase ß is probably the DNA repair enzyme (19) and the DNA polymerase γ is mito-chondria associated (20).

RNA polymerases. Eukaryotic cells contain three species of DNA-dependent RNA polymerases, termed I, II and III. Polymerase I is involved in rRNA synthesis (21), enzyme II is thought to synthesize cellular pre-mRNA (21) and RNA polymerase III is responsible for the synthesis of pre-tRNA (22).

Viral Enzymes

Among the proteins induced in HSV-infected cells the following proteins could be established as metabolically active; a DNA exonuclease (23), a deoxypyrimidine kinase (24) and a DNA-dependent DNA polymerase (25, 26, 27). The RNA polymerases as well as the poly (adenosine diphosphate ribose) polymerase (28, 29) are obviously not virus-induced proteins. Among these enzymes the DNA polymerase seems to be the promising target enzyme for a possible influence of araATP because the function of this enzyme is a prerequisite for the onset and the continuation of HSV DNA synthesis (13, 29). Fig. 2 shows a close correlation between the pattern of HSV-DNA synthesis and of the appearance of the HSV-induced DNA polymerase in infected BHK cells.

9-ß-D-ARABINOFURANOSYLADENINE

Cytostatic Activity

Studies with intact cell systems. The compound ßaraAdo has a considerable influence on cell proliferation; the 50 % inhibition concentration (ED50) was found in the case of L5178 y cells at 2.9 μM (30). ßAraAdo acts cytostatically in a limited concentration range; e. g. after exposure of cells for 24 hrs. to 3 times the ED50 of the drug, viability drops to 44 %. After incubation of the cells with the compound the average volume increases by 40 % (30). This observed increase of the cellular volume ("unbalanced growth") is the first clue that the drug inhibits primarily DNA synthesis. Incorporation studies with uninfected L 5178y cells revealed (30) that up to at least twice the ED50 concentration ßaraAdo inhibits the rate of DNA

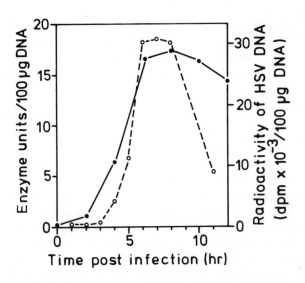

Fig. 2 :
Induction of HSV DNA polymerase (●—●) and the appearance of HSV
DNA (o——o) in infected BHK cells in dependence on the time post infection. HSV (type 1) strain Lennette was used (28, 29). The details of the enzyme assay (^{3}H-dCMP incorporation) and the procedure of isolation of
HSV DNA are essentially as described earlier (28, 29). The enzyme activity is refered to 100 µg DNA of the infected cells (ordinate, left). The
values, indicating the amount of ^{3}H-dThd incorporated into HSV DNA at
the end of the pulse (1 hr), are given on the right ordinate, they are refered to 100 µg DNA in one centrifugation tube which was analyzed in a
CsCl gradient centrifugation tube.

synthesis selectively, whereas RNA synthesis and protein synthesis are not influenced significantly. In order to rule out the possibility that mRNA synthesis is blocked by the drug, the amount of polysomes in cells treated with the compound was compared with the amount present in control cells; no reduction in drug-treated cells was found (30).

The compound exerts a synchronizing effect in the L5178y cell system (31). After treatment of the cells with two ßaraAdo blocks a 62 % synchronization was achieved. The drug affects the cells during the transition from G_1 to S phase.

Highly synchronized L5178y cells were used for the studies. DNA synthesis in these cells, as measured by thymidine incorporation, could be halted almost completely by ßaraAdo (31). The level of thymidine incorporation was used to determine the extent of cellular DNA synthesis only qualitatively; with this method alone it is not possible to determine the synthesis quantitatively, because of the unknown intracellular thymidine pool. Alterations of dATP and ara-ATP pool sizes and fluctuations of DNA and RNA polymerase activities, both of which are involved in cellular DNA synthesis, were studied in the absence and presence of ßaraAdo. Thus, these experiments were performed to answer the question of whether cellular RNA and/or protein synthesis occurs as a possible consequence of ßaraAdo incubation. Such an event could deplete enzymes and substrates necessary for the DNA-synthesizing system. Our previous data, mentioned above, showed that both uridine incorporation into RNA and synthesis of mRNA are not influenced in ßaraAdo-treated cells. Now, despite a nearly complete inhibition of cellular DNA synthesis by the compound, the alterations of the pool sizes and enzyme activities preceding cellular DNA synthesis occured to the same extent as in the untreated controls. As shown in Fig. 3, a multifold increase of DNA polymeraseα activity (during progression of the cells from G_1 to S phase) was not altered after incubation with ßaraAdo. During G_1 phase, the absolute level of DNA polymeraseα activity in L5178y cells (82 units/10^8 cells) was somewhat lower than that (112 units/10^8 cells) in mouse L-cells (Earle's L-cells, clone 929) (19). However, the induction rate of DNA polymeraseα in L5178y cells at the beginning of the S phase was as high as in mouse L-cells (32). The alteration of DNA polymerase ß activity seems to be influenced during ara-A incubation. In untreated controls, the enzyme level did not change during transition of the cells from G_1 to S phase; however, during incubation of L5178y cells with ßaraAdo, the absolute amount of DNA polymerase ß increased by 105 %. Future experiments are necessary to study whether this increase is a reflection of the DNA repair synthesis, induced by the observed (30) incorporation of ara-AMP moieties into cellular DNA during DNA synthesis in vivo.

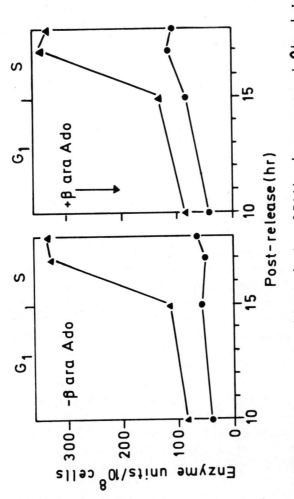

Fig. 3 : Alterations in dependence on ßaraAdo incubation of DNA polymerase *α* and *β* levels in synchronized L 5178 y cells. Lower abscissa, time after release of the 2nd thymidine block, upper abscissa, cell cycle phase. At different times after release, cells were taken and extracted, and the 2 polymerases were separated by a sucrose gradient. The activities of the *α* and *β* enzyme obtained were plotted. At the time indicated by the arrow, ßaraAdo was added in a concentration of 25 μg/ml. ● , ß enzyme, ▲ , *α* enzyme. The values represent the means of 4 parallel determinations of 1 gradient, the standard deviation does not exceed 8 %.

It is well known that ßaraAdo is readily converted into its corresponding 5'-mono-, di-, or triphosphates (33, 31). The araATP formed intracellularly in L5178y cells is incorporated into DNA but not into RNA (30). At
non-cytostatic concentrations (0.4 µM of ßaraAdo) 8430 moles of dAMP are
incorporated per 1 mole of ßaraAMP. Enzymatic digestion of ßaraAdo-label-
led DNA clearly indicated that ßaraAMP is incorporated via internucleotide
linkage.

An incubation of L5178y cells with dAdo at concentrations up to 40µM
had no influence on cell growth. However, exogenous administered dAdo
increases the intracellular pool size of dATP; see Fig. 4. Coincubation of
the cells with dAdo (30 µM) and ßaraAdo (39 µM) had no influence on the
pool size of ßaraATP. Parallel with the pool size determination of dATP and
ßaraATP in cells incubated with dAdo, the cell proliferation was determined.
In all experiments, ßaraAdo was used at a concentration of 39 µM. This
ßaraAdo concentration caused a 76 % reduction in cell proliferation, which
is equal to a reduction of the doublings (34) from 1.10 to 0.35. The ßaraAdo-
caused inhibition of cell proliferation could be negated to some extent by
coincubation with dAdo (Fig. 4). At a dAdo concentration of 32 µM, an increase in cell proliferation from 0.35 to 0.82 doublings occured. The similarity in direction of slope of the curve representing the changes of the pool
size of dATP to that showing the increase of the cell proliferation seems to
indicate strongly that the ßaraAdo caused inhibitory influence on cell proliferation is reduced at higher intracellular dATP concentrations.

Studies with isolated enzyme systems. The mentioned data led us to
assume that the primary site of action of the compound must be on the level
of DNA- and RNA synthesizing enzyme systems. A prerequisite to proof
this assumption is the availability of the triphosphate derivative of ßaraAdo.
Systematic studies about the influence of ßaraATP on the isolated nucleic
acid synthesizing enzyme system have been performed by the group of Cohen
(35) and by us (30, 36, 37). In detailed studies it could be shown that the
eukaryotic DNA-dependent RNA polymerases I, II and III as well as the
poly(A) polymerase (Mg^{2+}-dependent enzyme) are not affected at all by
ßaraATP; see Table 1. However, ßaraATP inhibits the activity of eukaryotic DNA polymerases (Table 1). All the DNA polymerases tested are inhibited by ßaraATP in a purely competitive way with respect to dATP. As a
measure for the relative affinities of the enzyme for inhibitor and substrate
in competitive inhibition, the ratio $K_i : K_m$ can be adopted (38); the lower
this ratio the higher is the potency of the inhibitor to reduce the enzyme
activity. The highest affinity of ßaraATP is observed with the DNA polymerase ß; the ratio amounts to 0.39 (Table 1). A 3-fold lower affinity is observed for DNA polymerase α .

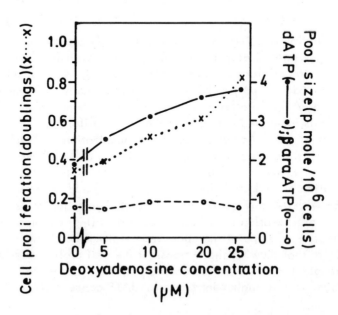

Fig. 4 :   Negation of the ßaraAdo-caused inhibition of cell proliferation
of unsynchronized L 5178 y cells by coincubation with deoxyadenosine. The experiments were performed for 24 hr with logarith-
mically growing cultures of a cell concentration of 2×10^5/ml.
Abscissa, final deoxyadenosine concentration in the cultures.
All cultures were incubated in the presence of ßaraAdo at 10.5
μg/ml (39 μM). At the different deoxyadenosine concentrations
indicated, the pool sizes for both dATP (•) and ara-ATP (○)
and the degree of cell proliferation, expressed in doublings(×),
were determined.

Table 1 : Influence of βaraATP and αaraATP on different polymerases.

Enzyme	Form of the enzyme	Source of the enzyme	Michaelis constant (μM) dATP	Michaelis constant (μM) ATP	Inhibitor constant (μM) βaraATP	Inhibitor constant (μM) αaraATP	$K_i : K_m$ βaraATP	$K_i : K_m$ αaraATP
DNA-dependent DNA polymerase	α	rabbit kidney cells	6.4±1.3		7.4 ±1.2	3.1±0.7	1.16	0.48
	β	rabbit kidney cells	14.3±2.1		5.6 ±1.3	no inhibition	0.39	–
		HSV	13.9±2.2		0.14+0.02	no inhibition	0.01	–
DNA-dependent RNA polymerase	I	rabbit kidney cells		17.4±2.9	no inhibition		–	–
	II	rabbit kidney cells		26.4±3.1	no inhibition		–	–
	III	rabbit kidney cells		31.9±3.0	no inhibition		–	–
Poly(A) polymerase		quail oviduct		41.2±6.3	no inhibition		–	–

By a calculation using the Michaelis constant for dATP and the inhibitor constant for ßaraATP of DNA polymerase α , as well as the intracellular dATP and ßaraATP pool sizes, it can be concluded that the ßaraAdo-caused reduction of cell proliferation is a consequence of a competitive inhibition of DNA polymeraseα by ßaraATP (31).

Antiviral Activity

Studies with intact cell systems. The anti-herpesvirus activity of ßaraAdo is known for some time (see: Ref. 10, 11). ßAraAdo inhibits growth of both HSV-type 1 (Lennette) and HSV-type 2 (D-316) (39); see Table 2. However, till recently the biochemical reason for this antiviral activity of the compound was not known. It was the work of Shannon (40) which indicated that the anti-herpesvirus activity of ßaraAdo is due to its action on the processes causing initiation of viral DNA synthesis. The suggestion that ßaraAdo is a relatively herpesvirus-specific agent came from the observations of Shipman et al. (41) demonstrating that this drug causes a rapid inhibition of DNA synthesis, while cellular DNA synthesis is inhibited only after a lag phase. A further indication that ßaraAdo causes an inhibition of HSV-DNA synthesis came from the observation that by coincubation of the drug with equimolar concentration of dAdo, the inhibitory effect of ßaraAdo can be abolished completely, while a coincubation with Ado was without this reducing inhibitory effect (39).

During HSV-DNA synthesis ßaraAdo is incorporated into HSV-DNA (37). It was found that during the period of HSV-DNA synthesis 1 mole of ßaraAMP is incorporated per about 4000 moles of dAdo if HSV-infected cells are incubated in the presence of 0.2 μM ßaraAdo.

In a recent study (42) we could show that ßaraAdo acts as a chain terminator for newly synthesized HSV-DNA strands. This is in contrast to the effect of the incorporated ßaraAMP into cellular DNA, where it is incorporated in internucleotide linkages (30). HSV-DNA from HSV-infected cells was separated by isopycnic centrifugation in neutral CsCl gradient into two peaks which are distinguished by their percental content of native DNA. The light HSV-DNA consisted of 62 % native DNA, while the heavy HSV-DNA contained only 12 %. From the enzymatic digestion studies with micrococcal nuclease and spleen phosphodiesterase, it could be shown that the araAMP moieties incorporated into newly synthesized DNA strands are localized at terminal 3'-hydroxyl positions. Further assembly of the observed low molecular weight DNA, with a maximal molecular weight of 2.6×10^6, to high molecular weight "intact" strands (molecular weight, 35×10^6) is not observed even after removal of the araAdo (Fig. 5). Thus it is most

Table 2: Influence of ßaraAdo and ⲁaraAdo on the synthesis of infective Herpes virus. Rabbit kidney cells were infected with either HSV-type 1 (Len) or D-316 (type 2) in a concentration of 1×10^5 PFU. 24 hrs. after infection the newly synthesized infective particles were determined. N. d.: not determined.

Treatment	PFU / 0.2 ml	
	Type 1	Type 2
Virus control	2.0×10^5	4.7×10^4
ⲁ araAdo: 370 µM	3.0×10^5	4.0×10^4
110 µM	2.2×10^5	6.0×10^4
37 µM	1.0×10^5	5.0×10^4
11 µM	3.5×10^5	4.0×10^4
ßaraAdo: 370 µM	4.0×10^2	2.0×10^2
110 µM	9.0×10^2	6.0×10^2
37 µM	1.5×10^4	1.3×10^2
11 µM	8.0×10^4	2.0×10^4
Ado: 370 µM	3.0×10^5	n. d.
dAdo: 370 µM	1.7×10^5	n. d.

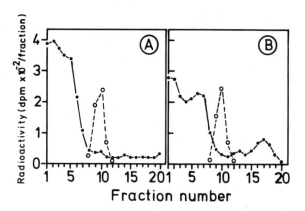

Fig. 5 : Analysis of the location of ßaraAMP moieties incorporated into
HSV-DNA. The HSV (type 1, Lennette)-infected cells were incubated 7 hrs. p. i. with 1.9 μM ^{3}H-ßaraAdo, and incubated
as follows : Experiment 1, incubation for 1 hr. followed by harvesting and Experiment 2, incubation for 1 hr., then washing
the cells free of unincorporated ßaraAdo and a subsequent incubation for an additional 5 hrs. The cells were harvested, DNA
was extracted, and HSV-DNA was separated from cellular DNA
by CsCl gradients. Viral DNA from CsCl gradients was analyzed
on alkaline sucrose gradients. Alkaline sucrose sedimentation
from Experiment 1 (A), and from Experiment 2 (B). Direction of
sedimentation is from left to right. As marker DNA, ^{14}C -
labeled T 7 phage DNA (o--o) was used, ^{3}H-ßaraAdo-labeled
HSV-DNA (•—•).

likely that in intact HSV-infected cells, ßaraATP blocks the synthesis of HSV-DNA rather than the synthesis of the ribonucleotide initiator. This conclusion is also supported by the finding, that the ßaraAMP moieties, incorporated into HSV-DNA, do not become acid soluble in alkali.

Studies with isolated enzyme systems. The first experimental evidence that ßaraATP is a strong inhibitor for HSV-DNA polymerase was published 1977 (37). It was clearly documented that HSV-induced DNA-dependent DNA polymerase was 39-fold more sensitive to ßaraATP than was cellular DNA polymerase ß and 116-fold more sensitive to DNA polymeraseα (Table 1). This observation was confirmed later by others (43). The type of inhibition of HSV-DNA polymerase by ßaraATP was of a competitive one with respect to dATP. The affinity of this HSV-induced enzyme for ßaraATP was only slightly influenced by the use of different template/initiators in the enzyme assays (37).

9-α-D-ARABINOFURANOSYLADENINE

Cytostatic Activity

Studies with intact cell systems. Only very recently the influence of α araAdo on the proliferation of non-infected cells was studied (14); the model cell system used was the mouse lymphoma line L5178y. This nucleoside, in the unusual α-glycosidically linked form, has been found to be an effective inhibitor of cell proliferation. The ED_{50} concentration was found to be 11.9 μM. Complete cytostasis is observed up to 2.3 times the ED_{50} concentration. After exposure of the cells to 4 times the ED_{50} of αaraAdo viability of the cells drops to 85 % after an incubation period of 24 hrs. Alike ßaraAdo also αaraAdo causes "unbalanced growth" of the cells.

The compound inhibits selectively DNA synthesis, as shown by incorporation experiments with the precursors dThd, Urd and Trp; RNA - as well as protein synthesis are not affected (Fig. 6).

Intracellularly araAdo is rapidly phosphorylated via αaraAMP and αaraADP to αaraATP (Table 3). In exponentially growing cells 63 % of the α araAdo uptaken is present as αaraATP after an incubation time of 30 min; 7 % was found to be αaraAdo, 14 % αaraAMP and 9 % αaraADP.

In a series of experiments it was checked, whether αaraAdo affects the phosphorylation of the naturally occuring nucleosides Ado and dAdo (Table 3). Even in the presence of a 10-fold excess of exogenous αaraAdo, Ado as well as dAdo are phosphorylated in the cells to the same amount as

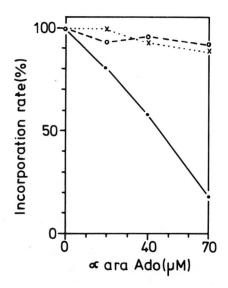

Fig. 6 : Effect of α araAdo on the synthesis of macromolecules in exponentially growing L 5178 y cells. Incorporation of dThd into
DNA (●——●), of Urd into RNA (o— —o) and of Trp into
protein (x····x).

Table 3: Phosphorylation of radiolabeled α araAdo, Ado and dAdo in L 5178 y cells in the absence as well as in the presence of additional unlabeled nucleosides.

Labeled compound (µM)	Additional compound (µM)	Distribution in the methanol-soluble fraction (10^6 cells)				
		Total (pmoles)	Nucleoside	Mono-phosphate	Diphosphate	Triphosphate
α araAdo: 0.5	-	0.9	0.06	0.13	0.08	0.57
	Ado: 5	1.1	0.20	0.18	0.07	0.61
	dAdo: 5	0.9	0.11	0.10	0.07	0.59
Ado: 0.5	-	6.9	1.7	0.1	0.3	4.7
	αaraAdo: 5	6.3	1.2	0.2	0.4	4.3
dAdo: 0.5	-	1.3	0.49	0.03	0.04	0.69
	αaraAdo: 5	1.5	0.61	0.07	0.02	0.74

in the control cultures.

In exponentially growing L5178y cells radiolabeled ɑaraAdo is incorporated into DNA. It was found that after incubation of the cells with
ɑaraAdo at non-cytostatic concentrations and subsequently performed isolation and purification of cellular DNA, 1 mole of ɑaraAMP is incorporated
per 14,000 moles of dAMP moieties.

The ɑaraAdo-caused inhibition of cell proliferation could be negated
by coincubation with the natural nucleoside dAdo; under the conditions
used (14) the cell doublings increase from 0.76 in the absence of dAdo to
1.63 in the presence of the natural nucleoside; in the controls (culture
without ɑaraAdo) the value for the cell doublings was found to be 1.79. The
inhibitory potency of the compound can not be abolished by coincubation
with Ado.

Studies with isolated enzyme systems. From the mentioned in vivo experiments it is obvious that the main site of action of ɑaraAdo is on the
level of DNA synthesis. Therefore the effect of ɑaraATP on the activity of
the isolated cellular DNA polymerases was tested (28, 18); see Table 1. It
was found that the DNA polymerase ß is insensitive towards ɑaraATP. However, the DNA polymerase ɑ is strongly inhibited by ɑaraATP; this compound inhibits the enzyme in a purely competitive way with respect to
dATP. The affinity of ɑaraATP towards DNA polymerase ɑ is 2.4-fold higher
compared with that determined in the inhibition assays with ßaraATP (Table
1). The three cellular DNA-dependent RNA polymerases are not affected by
ɑaraATP.

Antiviral Activity

Studies with intact cell systems. The compound ɑaraAdo does not exert any effect on growth of HSV both type 1 (Lennette) and type 2 (D-316)
even at the very high concentration of 370 µM (Table 2); Ref. 39. In contrast to the effect of ɑaraAdo on the incorporation rate of dThd into cellular
DNA, the compound shows no effect on the incorporation rate of the precursor into HSV-DNA; Fig. 7. The amount of acid-soluble radioactivity is
not influenced if the cultures are incubated with ßaraAdo or with ɑaraAdo.

During HSV-DNA synthesis ɑaraAdo is not incorporated both into
HSV-DNA and into RNA.

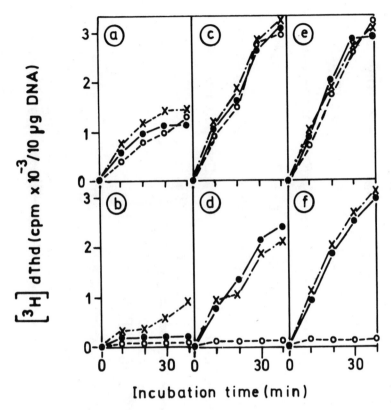

Fig. 7 :   Influence of αaraAdo and ßaraAdo on uptake as well as on incorporation of dThd in noninfected (a, b) and HSV-infected
cells type 1 Lennette (c, d) and type 2 D-316 (e, f). 5 hrs.
after infection no drug (x - · - x), ßaraAdo (o - - o) or αaraAdo
(●——●) at concentrations of 100 uM were added. 7 hrs. after
infection dThd was added and incubation was proceeded for
0 - 40 min. Acid-soluble (a, c, e) as well as acid-insoluble
radioactivity (b, d, f) was determined.

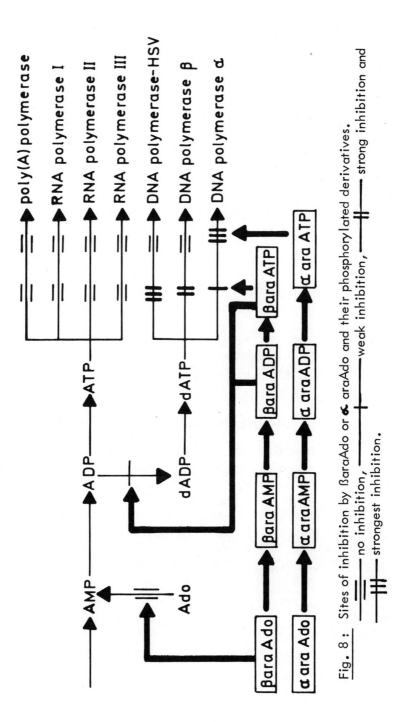

Fig. 8 : Sites of inhibition by βaraAdo or α araAdo and their phosphorylated derivatives. — no inhibition, — weak inhibition, — strong inhibition and — strongest inhibition.

Studies with isolated enzyme systems. Only in analogy we studied the influence of αaraATP on HSV-DNA polymerase (Table 1). We found that the activity of this enzyme is not affected at all by this triphosphate (28, 18).

CONCLUSION

ßAraAdo is one of the most promising anti-HSV drugs available. On enzymic level (Fig. 8) some remarkably strong differences exist between its influence on host cell metabolism and on herpes virus growth (differential inhibition of DNA-dependent DNA polymerase systems and difference in the kind of linkage of the ßaraAMP molecules, which have been incorporated into the DNA). Therefore it is not surprising that in intact cells which are infected by this virus, the drug inhibits the two biological systems selectively, depending on the dose used.

This observed selectivity of the drug, as documented on the biochemical level, should make it possible to draw advantage for human use especially in the case of herpes virus infection. This promising outlook is supported by one paper (44) demonstrating that upon successful treatment of HSV-infected mice with the compound a rechallenge of the test animal showed high resistance against the homologous virus.

α AraAdo is absolutely inefficient in preventing HSV growth; the compound exerts only a cytostatic influence. This in vivo finding is supported, in an excellent way, by the studies performed in isolated enzyme systems. There it could be demonstrated that αaraATP was inactive in the HSV polymerase system, while this triphosphate exerts a strong inhibitory influence on cellular DNA polymeraseα .

REFERENCES

1. Pagano, J. S. : Cold Spr. Harb. Symp. quant. Biol. 34: 797 (1975).

2. Klein, G. : Cold Spr. Harb. Symp. quant. Biol. 34 : 783 (1975).

3. Churchill, A. E. : J. Natl. Cancer Inst. 41: 939 (1968).

4. Falk, L. A., Stephen, M. N., Deinhardt, F., Wolfe, L. G.,
    Cooper, R. W. and Hernandez-Camacho, J. : Int. J. Cancer 14 :
    473 (1974).

5. Melendez, L. V., Hunt, R. D., King, N. W., Barahona, H. H.,
    Daniel, M. D., Fraser, C., E. O. and Garcia, F. G. : Nature
    New Biol. 234 : 182 (1972).

6. Rapp, F. and Li, J. L. H. : Cold Spr. Harb. Symp. quant. Biol.
    34 : 747 (1975).

7. Baltimore, D. : Cold Spr. Harb. Symp. quant. Biol. 34 : 747
    (1975).

8. Gentry, G. A. and Ashwell, J. F. : Virology 65: 294 (1975).

9. Miller, R. L., Iltis, J. P. and Rapp, F. : J. Virol. 23 : 679
    (1977).

10. Sidwell, R. W., Dixon, G. J., Schabel, F. M. and Kaump, D.H.:
    Antimicr. Agents and Chemotherapy 1968 : 148 (1968).

11. Müller, W. E. G., Zahn, R. K., Bittlingmaier, K. and Falke,D. :
    Ann. N. Y. Acad. Sci. 284 : 34 (1977).

12. Kit, S., Torres, R. A. and Dubbs, D. R. : Cancer Res. 26 :
    1859 (1966) .

13. Subak-Sharpe, J. H., Brown, S. M., Ritchie, D. A., Timbury,
    M. C., Macnab, J. C. M., Marsden, H. S. and Hay, J. :
    Cold Spr. Harb. Symp. quant. Biol. 34 : 717 (1975).

14. Müller, W. E. G., Zahn, R. K., Maidhof, A., Beyer, R. and
    Arendes, J. : Biochem. Pharmacol., in press.

15. Müller, W. E. G., Zahn, R. K. and Arendes, J. : submitted.

16. Anderson, M. M. and Suhadolnik, R. J. : In: IUB-Ninth Interna-
    tional Congress of Biochemistry; p. 3r10. Aktiebolaget Egnellska
    Boktryckeriet, Stockholm (1973).

17. Lee, W. W., Benitez, A., Goodman, L. and Baker, B. R. :
    J. Amer. Chem. Soc. 82 : 2648 (1960).

18. Müller, W. E. G.: Japan. J. Antib. 30 Suppl.: in press (1977).

19. Bollum, F. J. : Progr. Nucleic Acid. Res. Molec. Biol. 15 : 105 (1975).

20. Bolden, A., Noy, G. P. and Weissbach, A. : J. Biol. Chem. 252 : 3351 (1977).

21. Chambon, R. : In: The Enzymes (P. D. Boyer, ed.) Vol. 10; pp. 261 - 331. Academic Press, New York (1974).

22. Weil, P. A. and Blatti, S. P.: Biochem. 14 : 1636 (1975).

23. Morrison, J. M. and Keir, H. M. : J. Gen. Virol. 2 : 337 (1968).

24. Hay, J. P., Perera, A. J., Morrison, J. M., Gentry, G. A. and Subak-Sharpe, J. H. : Ciba Foundation Symp. (Strategy of the viral genome) pp. 355 - 376 (1971).

25. Keir, H. M., Hay, J., Morrison, J. M. and Subak-Sharpe, J. H. : Nature 210 : 369 (1966).

26. Weissbach, A., Hong, S. C. L., Aucker, J. and Miller, R. : J. Biol. Chem. 248 : 6270 (1973).

27. Müller, W. E. G., Falke, D. and Zahn, R. K. : Arch. ges. Virusforsch. 42 : 278 (1973).

28. Müller, W. E. G., Zahn, R. K. and Falke, D. : Virology, 84 : in press (1978).

29. Müller, W. E. G., Falke, D., Zahn, R. K. and Arendes, J. : submitted.

30. Müller, W. E. G., Rohde, H. J., Beyer, R., Maidhof, A., Lachmann, M., Taschner, H. and Zahn, R. K. : Cancer Res. 35 : 2160 (1975).

31. Müller, W. E. G., Maidhof, A., Zahn, R. K. and Shannon, W. M. : Cancer Res. 37 : 2282 (1977).

32.   Chang, L. M. S., Brown, M. and Bollum, F. J.: J. Mol. Biol.
      74 : 1 (1973).

33.   Brink, J. J. and Le Page, G. A. : Cancer Res. 24 : 312 (1964).

34.   Müller, W. E. G., Rohde, H. J., Steffen, R., Maidhof, A.,
      Lachmann, M., Zahn, R. K. and Umezawa, H. : Cancer Res. 35 :
      3673 (1975).

35.   Furth, J. J. and Cohen, S. S. : Cancer Res. 28 : 2061 (1968).

36.   Müller, W. E. G. : Experientia 32 : 1572 (1976).

37.   Müller, W. E. G., Zahn, R. K., Bittlingmaier,   K. and Falke,
      D. : Ann. N. Y. Acad. Sci. 284 : 34 (1977).

38.   Webb, J. L. : In: Enzyme and Metabolic Inhibitors, Vol. 1; pp.
      104 - 105. Academic Press, New York (1963).

39.   Falke, D., Ronge, K., Arendes, J. and Müller, W. E. G. :
      submitted.

40.   Shannon, W. M. : In: Adenine Arabinoside: An Antiviral Agent
      (D. Pavan-Langston, R. A. Buchanan and C. A. Alford, eds.)
      pp. 1 - 43. Raven Press, New York (1975).

41.   Shipman, C. and Drach, J. C. : Abstr. Ann. Mtg., Amer. Soc.
      Microbiol. 97 (1974).

42.   Müller, W. E. G., Zahn, R. K., Beyer, R. and Falke, D. :
      Virology 76 : 787 (1977).

43.   Reinke, C. M., Drach, J. C., Shipman, C. and Weissbach, A. :
      Third Int. Symp. on Oncogenesis and Herpesviruses; p. 122.
      Cambridge, July 25 - 29, 1977.

44.   Miller, F. A., Sloan, B. J. and Silberman, C. A. : Antimicr.
      Agents and Chemother. 1969 : 192 (1970).

A REPORT ON THE CLINICAL APPLICATION OF A PARTIALLY THIOLATED POLY-CYTIDYLIC ACID IN THE TREATMENT OF CHILDHOOD LEUKEMIA[(x)]

BERNHARD KORNHUBER[+] AND PRAKASH CHANDRA[++]

Zentrum der Kinderheilkunde[+](Abt. Päd. Onkologie) and Zentrum der Biologischen Chemie[++] (Abt. Molekularbio - logie), University Medical School, Theodor-Stern-Kai 7, 6 Frankfurt 70, W. Germany

SINCE the introduction of chemotherapeutic "cocktails", poly-chemotherapy has become the choice of therapyto treat malignant di-seases. In recent years this type of therapy has shown a great deal of success in the treatment of childhood acute lymphocytic leukemia (ALL)

Before the introduction of the folic acid antagonists by Farber in 1948 (Farber et al., 1948), there was no effective treatment for children with leukemia other than supportive therapy with blood trans-fusions and the few antibiotics that were available at that time. Early deaths were inevitable, although a few children had short re-missions as a result of blood transfusions.Since 1948 there has been a steady improvement in the length and quality of survival of chil-dren with acute leukemia. Fig. 1 illustrates the evolution of anti-leukemic therapy and the improvement in patient survival that each new advance has brought with it. The introduction of monotherapy with the folic acid antagonist, methotrexate, given orally every day (curve 1, Fig. 1), showed a median remission period of approx. 3 months. The same compound given at higher doses twice a week intra-muscularly (Fig. 1, curve 2) increased the median remission period to about 1 year. A real advance in the chemotherapy of leukemia was the introduction of a polychemotherapy protocol by Pinkel (1971), now known as Memphis-study VII.Treatment according to this regime

(x) Dedicated to Professor Helmut Martin on his 60th birthday.

ADVANCES   IN   ALL   CHEMOTHERAPY

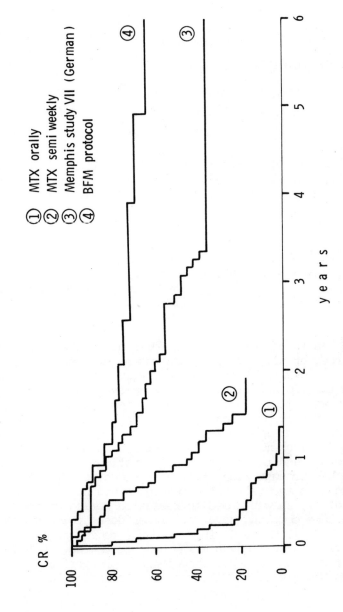

① MTX orally
② MTX semi weekly
③ Memphis study VII (German)
④ BFM protocol

Fig. 1 MEDIAN REMISSION IN CHILDREN WITH ACUTE LYMPHOCYTIC LEUKEMIA UNDER
DIFFERENT CHEMOTHERAPEUTIC TREATMENTS.
CR = Complete Remission; MTX = Methotrexate.

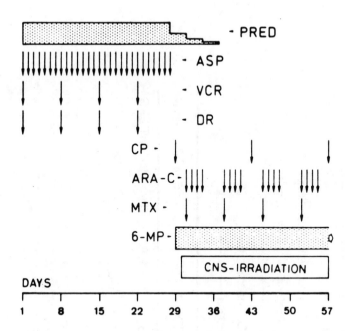

FIG. 2 INTENSIVE MULTIPLE DRUG CHEMOTHERAPY AND CNS-IRRADI-
ATION IN CHILDREN WITH ACUTE LYMPHOCYTIC LEUKEMIA, ADAPTED
FROM RIEHM ET AL.(1974): A COOPERATIVE STUDY IN BERLIN, FRANK-
FURT AND MÜNSTER (BFM).

led to long-term remissions in about 30 % cases(results from a
German study of Pinkel´s protocol). This protocol was modified and
intensified by Riehm (1974) as shown in Fig. 2; and jointly adopted
by the clinicians at Berlin, Frankfurt and Münster (BFM Protocol).
The treatment according to this protocol led to long-term remissions
in more than 60 % cases of childhood ALL.

The intensification of polychemotherapy, although increasing
the effectivity of ALL-treatment, at the same time led to an increasing number of side effects; particularly, the susceptibility
to infection. Such infections have in some cases led to death, even
during the remission period. The most common side effects known to
occur during the polychemotherapy are shown in Fig. 3.

The fact that ALL is potentially curable, and that all effective
therapies currently employed involve toxic side effects; has been
the rationale behind the development of specific treatment regimes,
under which, normals cells are not rendered to the toxic effects of

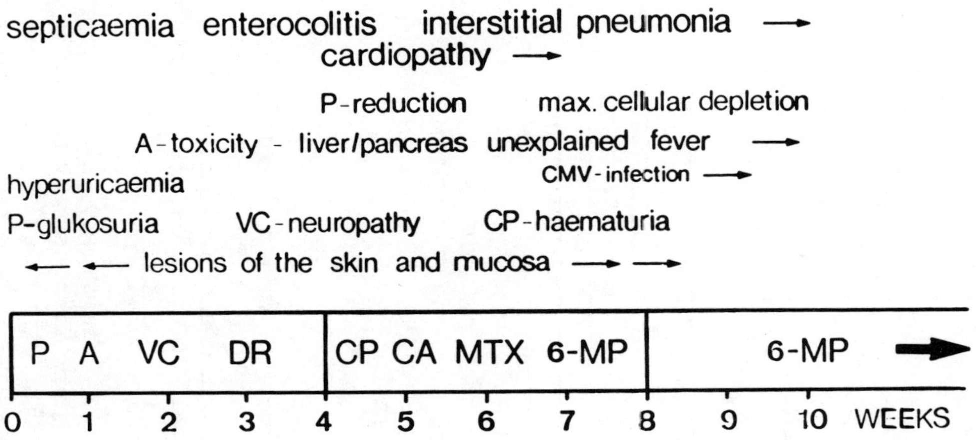

FIG. 3   MAJOR SIDE EFFECTS IN THE MULTIPLE DRUG TREATMENT OF ACUTE LYMPHOCYTIC LEUKEMIA.

The major side effects being the production of peripheral neuro-pathy by vincristine (VC); haematuria by cyclophosphamide (CP); glycosuria by prednisolone (P); cardiac toxicity by daunorubicin (DR); pancreatic damage by asparaginase (A); myelotoxicity by 6-mercapto purine (MP) and cytosine arabinoside (CA); and other toxic effects due to drug-drug interactions.

the drugs. In recent years, two major approaches have been adopted
to increase the specificity of leukemia treatment: a) the active
immune therapy with irradiated cells and BCG vaccination (reviewed
by Mathe, 1976), and b) the use of polynucleotide combinations with
interferon inducing potential (Krakoff et al., 1970; Mathe et al.,
1971 a, 1971 b).

Reproducibility of the beneficial effects of immune therapy in
the treatment of leukemia is a very controversal issue, if one surveys the literature carefully (Medical Res. Council Rep., 1971; Heyn
et al., 1973 and 1975; review by Mastrangelo et al., 1976).A similar
situation exists on the use of polynucleotide combinations, such as
poly (I : C), an effective inducer of interferon. This polynucleotide
combination was introduced to cancer therapy in the early 70's by
Krakoff (1970). Subsequently, poly (I : C) was used by Mathe and his
associated (1971 a, 1971 b), and simultaneously by our clinic in
Frankfurt. In 1972, Chandra and Bardos (1972) reported the inhibition
of oncornaviral reverse transcriptase by a structural analogue of polycytidylic acid (poly C), in which a part of cytosine residues were replaced by 5-mercapto cytosine bases, a partially thiolated polycytidylic acid (MPC). In subsequent studies, Chandra et al were able to
show that ^{35}S-labelled MPC binds tightly to the viral reverse transcriptase, and thereby inhibits the synthesis of all the three species
of DNA (ss-DNA, hy-DNA and ds-DNA) catalyzed by this enzyme under the
endogenous conditions (Chandra, Ebener & Götz, 1975). This compound
is endowed with many interesting biological properties, such as a)
its ability to induce interferon in combination with polyinosinic
acid (O'Malley et al., 1975), b) its ability to stimulate antibody
synthesis by spleen cells of mice (see Chandra et al., in this volume),
c) its ability to inhibit the oncogenic activity of FLV in mice (
Chandra et al., 1975), and the d) relative resistance of MPC, compared
to that of poly C, against the nucleolytic activity of human serum
(U. Ebener and P. Chandra, unpublished observations).The observations
of Chandra et al. (see in this volume) served the basis to substitute
poly C by MPC for further clinical trials. Thus, we used the combination of poly I:MPC to treat the terminal cases of ALL and AML
(Chandra et al., 1975). Subsequentyl, we were attracted by the idea
of using MPC alone in our terminal trials.Thus, the developmental
stages in the polynucleotide therapy were from poly (I:C) to poly-
I:MPC, and finally MPC alone.

E X P E R I M E N T A L

Poly C (Miles Chemicals GmbH, Frankfurt, Germany) was thiolated
by a procedure based on the conversion of pyrimidine nucleotides to
their 5-mercapto derivates (Bardos and Kalman, 1966; Szabo et al.,
1970); details are described elsewhere (Chandra et al., 1977). The

MPC preparation used in the clinical trials contained 15 % of thiolated cytosine bases. The lyophilized product (MPC) was dissolved
in 0.1 M Tris/HCl buffer, pH 7.6, and diluted further with 0.9 % NaCl
before use (final concentration 0.5 mg - 1.0 mg / ml). This solution
was sterilized by passing it through a membrane filter (Millipore
GmbH, Neu Isenburg, Germany). It was kept at 4 °C and used immediately,
or in the next five days; solutions older than 5 days were repreci-
pitated, redissolved and resterilized.

No.	Init.	Age	Sex	Diag.	Stage	Results
1	D. M.	8	♀	ALL	3rd rel.	PR , WBC ↓
2	T. I.	6 6/12	♀	ALL	2nd rel.	?
3	B. M.	6 7/12	♂	ALL	2nd rel.	?
4	M. M.	8 4/12	♂	ALL	2nd rel.	CR
5	J. O.	3 6/12	♂	ALL	2nd rel.	?
6	N. A.	10	♀	ALL	2nd rel.	CR
7	B. C.	5 8/12	♀	ALL	3rd rel.	CR
8	N. N.	7 11/12	♂	ALL	3rd rel.	?
9	M. A	12	♂	ALL	1st rel.	?
10	M. I.	8 6/12	♂	ALL	1st rel.	?
11	K. C.	11 3/12	♀	ALL	4th rel.	?
12	K. K.	10 9/12	♀	ALL	5th rel.	PR
13	L. J.	7	♂	ALL	3rd rel.	WBC ↓
14	F. D.	2 3/12	♂	ALL	init. ph.	WBC ↓
15	S. B.	7 11/12	♀	ALL	init. ph.	WBC ↓
16	H. B.	12 5/12	♀	ALL	init. ph.	WBC ↓
17	S. N.	4	♀	AML	init. ph.	WBC ↓
18	W. H.	5 6/12	♂	AML	init. ph.	WBC ↓

Ffm , II / 78

FIG. 4   CLINICAL DATAS OF PATIENTS WITH ALL AND AML SUBMITTED
         MPC TRAILS.

Prednisone

Vincristin

Daunorubicin

L - Asparaginase

Ara - C

6 - Mercaptopurine

Methotrexate (HD)

(Cyclophosphamide)

(Actinomycin D)

FIG. 5   DRUGS PREVIOUSLY USED FOR TREATMENT OF PATIENTS
WITH TERMINAL DISEASE

Clinical data of patients submitted to MPC trials are shown in
Fig. 4. To date, we have used MPC on 18 cases of acute leukemia, of
which 16 were ALL and the remaining two AML cases. Of the 18 cases
treated with MPC, 13 were in the terminal phase of the disease.
These were resistent to all previous chemotherapeutic regimes. Fig.
5 lists the drugs which had been used on these patients. The drugs
mentioned in parentheses were not used on all children.

In our clinical studies, MPC (1mg /ml, sterile) was given
intravenously at a dose of 0.5 - 1.0 mg /kg body weight. The injections were given once a week.

R E S U L T S

Of the 13 terminal cases, complete remission was achieved in
3, and a partial remission achieved in 2 other cases. In the terminal
cases, it is not possible to give an empirical evaluation of MPC-
effectivity, since these children either lived for a short time only,
or no remission could be achieved. The extent to which MPC affected
the survival period in these cases can not be evaluated, since the
patients were in a very heterogeneous state (1 to 5 relapses).

Fever, occasionally accompanied by shivering, was frequently

observed under MPC treatment in the first hour after injection. However, these symptoms never lasted more than the first hour, and no
other side effects could be observed.

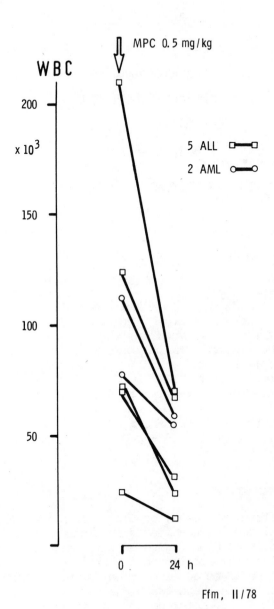

FIG. 6 MPC TRIALS IN THE INITIAL TREATMENT OF FRESH LEUKEMIC
CASES (DETAILS ARE GIVEN IN THE TEXT).

On the basis of our experience with MPC on terminal cases, we were motivated to give MPC a clinical trial in the beginning of leukemia. A monotherapy with MPC, as devised for terminal cases is, however, not possible. We therefore decided to introduce MPC (0.5 mg /kg body weight) therapy in the beginning of treatment of cases which at the time of diagnosis had leukocytosis. This initial treatment, a single injection of MPC, was then followed up by the usual Berlin-Frankfurt-Münster (BFM) protocol. As shown in Fig. 6, 24 h. after MPC injection, there was a dramatic reduction of leukemic cells in all the cases. Five of these seven children had ALL, and two AML.

We have shown that MPC is a very effective polynucleotide in the treatment of acute leukemias in children. It acts selectively on leukemic cells, probably by recognition of reverse transcriptase as target (Chandra et al., in this volume). The status of this drug in the chemotherapy of fresh leukemic cases, is not known, since monotherapy with MPC in such cases has not been done. The fact that under the present polychemotherapeutic protocols one can frequently achieve long-term remissions, hinders one ethically to use MPC as a montherapeuticum in fresh cases. However, its use in the initial phase of the acute disease, and its use as a monotherapeutic agent in terminal cases are very encouraging. On the basis of our to-date experience with MPC we could summarize by saying: a) MPC is useful to initiate the therapy in freshly diagnosed acute leukemic cases, b) It has shown promise as an effective treatment of leukemic cases in the terminal phase, and c) It could be used in the remission maintenance therapy. This aspect is yet to be investigated. This, as a matter of fact, is the rationale for its therapeutical application, since it is a potent inhibitor of reverse transcriptase.

A C K N O W L E D G E M E N T

This work was financially supported by the Stiftung Volkswagenwerk (grant No. 14 0305).

R E F E R E N C E S

1. BARDOS,T.J. & T.I. KALMAN (1966): J.Pharm.Sci. 55, 606.
2. CHANDRA,P. & T.J. BARDOS (1972):Res.Commun.Chem.Pathol.Pharmacol.
   4, 615.
3. CHANDRA,P., U. EBENER & A. GÖTZ (1975):FEBS-Letters 53, 10.
4. CHANDRA, P., B. KORNHUBER, D. GERICKE, A. GÖTZ & U. EBENER(1975):
   Z. Krebsforschung 83, 239.
5. CHANDRA,P. et al. (1977): in, Modulation of host immune resistance in the prevention or treatment of induced Neoplasia,Edt. M.A.-Chirigos,Fograty Intl. Center Proceedings 28 , 169.

6. FARBER,S., L.K. DIAMOND, R.D. MERCER, R.F. SYLVESTER & J.A.-
   WOLFF (1948): New Engl. J. Med. 238, 787.
7. HEYN, R., W. BORGES, P. JOO, M. KARON, R. SHORE, N. BRESLOW &
   D. HAMMOND (1973): Proc.Amer. Ass. Cancer Res. 14, 45.
8. HEYN, R., P. JOO, M. KARON, M. NESBIT, N. SHORE, N. BRESLOW,
   J. WEINER, A. RIED & D. HAMMOND (1975): Blood 46, 431.
9. KRAKOFF, I.H., C.W. YOUNG & M.R. HILLEMAN (1970): Proc.Amer.
                  Assoc.Cancer Res. 11, 45.
10. MASTRANGELO,M.J., D. BERD & R.E. BELLET (1976): Ann. N.Y. Acad.
                  Sci., 277, 94.
11. MATHE, G. (1976): Cancer Active Immunotherapy, Springer-Verlag
                  Berlin-Heidelberg-New York
12. MATHE, G., J.L. AMIEL, L. SCHWARZENBERG, M. SCHNEIDER, M. HAYAT,
    F DE VASSAL, C. JASMIN, C. ROSENFELD, M. SAKOUHI and J. CHOAY
    (1971 a): in, Biological Effects of Polynucleotides,Edts:R.F.-
    Beers and W. Braun,Springer-Verlag , pp. 225.
13. MATHE, G., M. HAYAT, M. SAKOUHI & J. CHOAY (1971 b): C.R. Acad.
                  Sci. (Paris) 272, 170.
14. MEDICAL RESEARCH COUNCIL (1971): Brit. Med. J. 4 , 189.
15. O'MALLEY, J.A., Y.K. HO, P. CHAKRABARTI, L. DIBERARDINO, P.-
    CHANDRA, D.A.O.ORINDA,D.M.BYRD,T.J.BARDOS & W.A.CARTER (1975):
                  Molec. Pharmacol. 11, 61.
16. PINKEL, D. (1971): J.Amer. Med. Assoc. 216, 648.
17. RIEHM,H., H. GADNER, K. JESSENBERGER & G. TARIVERDIAN (1974):
                  Proc.Am.Assoc. Cancer Res. 15, 58.
18. SZABO, L., T.I.KALMAN & T.J.BARDOS (1970):J.Org.Chem. 35,1434.

DEOXYNUCLEOTIDE-POLYMERIZING ENZYMES IN MAMMALIAN CELLS:

IMMUNOFLUORESCENCE

F. J. Bollum

Department of Biochemistry, Uniformed Services

University of the Health Sciences, Bethesda, MD 20014

INTRODUCTION

In the past ten years much new information about DNA replication, and the DNA polymerases thought to be involved in this process has become available. We now know that there are several deoxynucleotide-polymerizing enzymes present normally in cells and that under certain abnormal circumstances viral DNA polymerases may be found. The net result is a spectrum of DNA polymerases capriciously assigned to a spectrum of DNA replication processes. Faced with an increasing complexity in an already complex array we can do no better. There are several approaches that have been taken toward solving this problem, some that have not been taken, and some that cannot be taken, in complex cells.

Standard biochemical purification of proteins has been a most useful approach through most of the history of DNA polymerase research. Genetic analysis through mutation is not generally available in eukaryotic systems and may not be available for many years. With certain notable exceptions in viral polymerases, enzyme inhibition studies have not been especially helpful. I would like to discuss the application of immunological techniques to this problem and present some new results on the cytochemistry of deoxynucleotide-polymerizing enzymes. Immunological methods have wide applicability in research on deoxynucleotide-polymerizng enzymes and, used judiciously, should provide us with the best source of new information.

DNA POLYMERASE PROTEINS

The spectrum of known DNA polymerases in eukaryotic cells is presented in Table I.   The data presented is abbreviated in order to direct attention to a limited set of facts about these proteins. The first important fact is that DNA polymerases represent an exceedingly small fraction of the protein in a cell.   This means that if we are to take the standard biochemical approach toward purification of these proteins, rather large quantities of starting material must be obtained.   This places severe limitations on the systems amenable to standard purification procedures. In the set of DNA polymerases listed in Table I, DNA polymerase -β, TdT and certain reverse transcriptases are the only ones that are routinely studied as pure proteins.

A second type of information useful for the present discussion concerns the number of each kind of DNA polymerase molecule in a cell. Generally speaking one can estimate that there are between 10^3 and 10^6 copies of each kind of deoxynucleotide-polymerizing enzyme present in each cell.   The number of molecules present per cell should allow the use of cytochemical procedures, such as indirect immunofluorescence.   Immunological procedures can also be applied to increasingly sophisticated analyses of extracts of cells, but that is not the subject of the current discussion.

TABLE I.	CALF THYMUS DNA POLYMERASES		
	α	β	TdT
M_w	132 K	45 K	32 K
	(Single peptide)	(Single peptide)	(24 K + 8 K)
pH	7.2	8.6	7
pI	<7	>9	7.5
NEM	Sensitive	Resistant	Sensitive
Mg/kg	1	0.1	10
Molecules/cell	2×10^4	5×10^3	10^5

IMMUNOFLUORESCENCE OF DNA POLYMERASE-α

Immunological reagents for detection of DNA polymerase-α remain some what unsatisfactory, but some useful information can be obtained with these materials.   It is rather easy to develop neutralizing activity against non-homologous DNA polymerase-α in rabbits.   Since pure preparations of enzyme are not readily available the antibody produced in not immediately useful for cytochemical work. It is possible to use the polyvalent antiserum as an aid toward more specific reagents.

High titer rabbit antibody (1) against partially purified DNA polymerase-α (about 1% pure) is used to produce an immunoprecip-itate from more highly purified DNA polymerase-α (say 15% pure). The 132K polymerase is a good precipitin, leaving some contami-nating protein in the supernatant solution, and the precipitate is a good immunogen. The antibodies produced in the second rabbit by injection of an immunoprecipitate are called "second generation" antibodies. The second generation antibodies are produced with high titer and much greater species specificity than the first preoperation (2).

The second generation antibodies are then tested two ways for specificity. First they can be shown by immunoelectrophoresis of crude extracts and purified enzyme to contain only a single speci-ficity. Secondly, analysis of immune precipitates by SDS-poly-acrylamide gel electrophoresis shows only the 132K polymerase band, in addition to the heavy and light chain IgG bands. Further analysis of specificity can be done by adsorption, but the second generation anti DNA polymerase-α described is suitable for cellular immunofluorescence.

Early studies on DNA polymerase (now known to be α) by cellular fractionation (3, 4) demonstrated a cytoplasmic local-ization for a major fraction of the activity (>90%). These findings have been confirmed recently in many laboratories. Cytoplasmic location for a major DNA polymerase requires mech-anistic explanations and Littlefield (5) originally demonstrated the possibility of intracellular migration of enzyme. Actually some migration is a foregone conclusion since the enzyme must move from the ribosomes after synthesis.

The original findings on intracellular distribution were generally attributed to biochemical bungling and several types of experiment have been designed to prove the dogma that DNA poly-merase is in the nucleus, as it should be. Recent experiments with cytochalasin B (6) and non-aqueous solvents (7) are clearly designed to stamp out this biological heresy about cytoplasmic DNA polymerase, but the logic of these experiments is not quite so clear.

The results obtained by direct cytochemistry of DNA poly-merase-α are shown in Figure 1. The cells used are primary bovine fibroblasts (4 separate lines have been tested) fixed with methanol. The cytoplasmic localization of the major immunoreactive material is quite apparent. With imagination one can see some nuclear fluorescence in some rapidly dividing lines, but the predominant localization is cytoplasmic. Similar results have been observed in a chick embryo system by Chapeville and Brun (8).

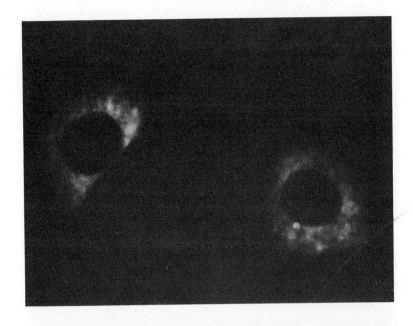

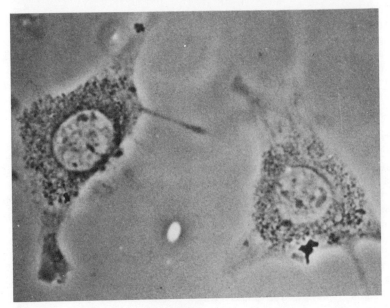

Figure 1.   Immunofluorescence of DNA polymerase-α in Primary
             bovine fibroblasts.

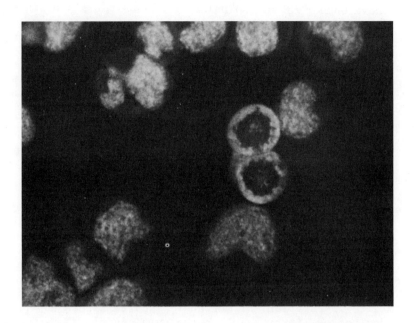

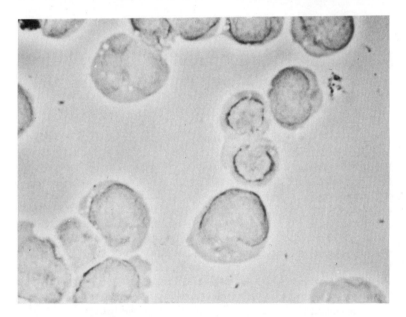

Figure 2.   Immunofluorescence of Terminal Transferease in
            continuous Human lymphoblastoid line 8402.

IMMUNOFLUORESCENCE OF TERMINAL DEOXYNUCLEOTIDLY TRANSFERASE (TdT)

The development of immunological reagents for a protein such as TdT is relatively straight forward. The enzyme has been purified to homogeneity from calf thymus gland (9), and having a pure antigen one should be able to develop a monovalent antiserum. After a certain amount of experimental immunization it was indeed found possible to develop such an antiserum (10).   The antiserum was produced in rabbits using TdT cross-linked with 0.1% gluta-raldehyde. This anti-TdT showed a rather broad cross-reactivity in neutralizing enzyme activity from such diverse species as humans, rodents and birds almost as well as from the homologous species. It should therefore be generally useful for studies on the localization of terminal deoxynucleotidyl transferase in various populations of cells.

The immunoglobulin fraction of the TdT antiserum was prepared and converted to homogeneous anti-TdT by adsorption and elution from a controlled pore glass column containing covalently coupled homogeneous TdT (11). The homogeneous, monovalent antibody obtained is then used as the primary reagent for immunofluorescence studies on cells, with a secondary reagent consisting of FITC-goat-F(ab')$_2$-anti-rabbit IgG. The use of these immunospecific reagents with preparations of methanol-fixed cells has now provided a great deal of new information on the cytology of TdT.

The photomicrograph in Figure 2 shows the presence of TdT in nuclei of a human lymphoblastoid line (8402) in interphase cells and liberation into the cytoplasm during mitosis. Other continuous cell lines (e.g. CEM-CCRF) are not so homogeneous and may show only 5% positive cells, consistent with the low level of enzyme present.

The next photomicrograph (Figure 3) shows the TdT fluores-cence in cryostat sections of thymus gland. As expected the fluorescence is limited to the cortical region of the thymus (11, 12) and no TdT positive cells appear to be located in the medulla. Cytospin preparations demonstrate a mixture of cytoplasmic and nuclear fluorescence. When rat embryo thymus is examined for TdT fluorescence an interesting difference in distribution appeared. The large immature thymocytes in the subcapsular region of the thymus have TdT immunofluorescence only in the nucleus (Figure 4). The more mature cortical thymocytes appear to have a mixture of cytoplasmic and nuclear fluorescence. It is therefore suggested that TdT shows a change in intracellular localization during maturation of the thymocyte. Ulitimately it must disappear from the thymocyte since no TdT is found in the medulla or in thoracic duct lymphocytes.

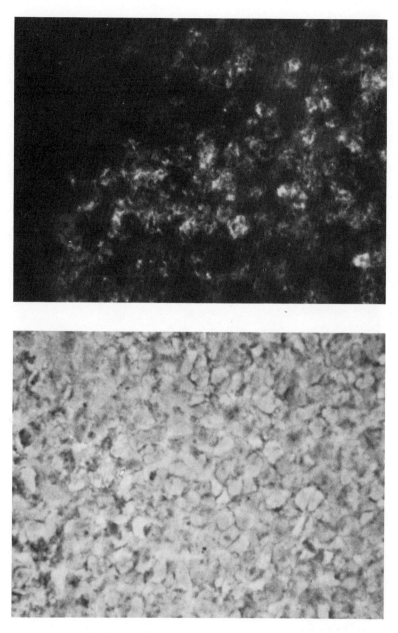

Figure 3.   Immunofluorescence of Terminal Transferase in a
cryostat section of mature rat thymus.

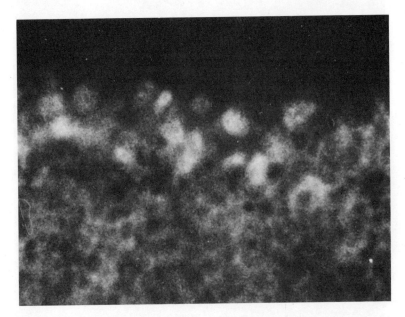

Figure 4.   Immunofluorescence of Terminal Transferase in a
cryostat section of rat embryo thymus.

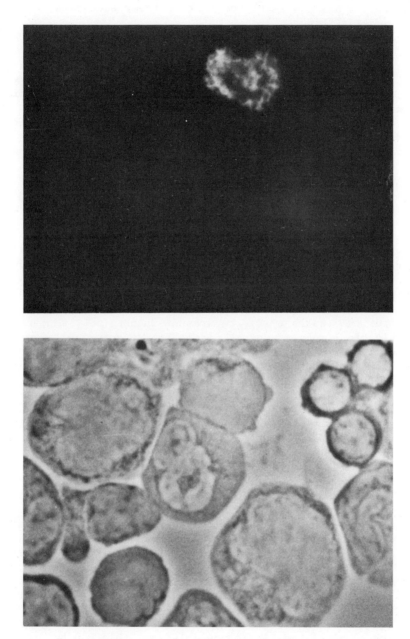

Figure 5.   Immunofluorescence of Terminal Transferase in a
cytospin preparation of rat bone marrow.

Bone marrow specimens show a low percentage of TdT positive cells, on the order of 1 to 2 percent depending upon species and age (13). In all cases the bone marrow fluorescence is exclusively nuclear (Figure 5).

The presence of TdT positive cells in a restricted set of tissues; thymus and bone marrow, and the change in the intracellular localization of TdT in thymus has interesting biological implications. I will not dwell on that matter further in this presentation. The results are presented to demonstrate the utility of the immunological method in surveying tissue distribution and the cellular localization of proteins of this kind. There are immediate applications for this kind of information.

Analysis for TdT activity has been demonstrated to be a useful marker for the diagnosis of lymphoblastic leukemias (14-19). Application of the immunofluorescence procedure to methanol-fixed peripheral blood and bone marrow specimens from leukemic patients opens up a new dimension in the diagnosis of leukemia. Generally speaking TdT is present in lymphoblastic cells, or perhaps a precursor of these cells. Thus large numbers of TdT positive cells are present in acute lymphoblastic leukemia (ALL) (Figure 6), in chronic myelogenous leukemia (CML) in blast crisis (Figure 7), and in certain lymphoblastic lymphomas (LBL, Figure 8). Normal numbers of TdT$^+$ cells (<1%) are present in AML, CGL, CML, non-lymphoblastic lymphomas and ALL patients in remission (Figure 9). The use of TdT immunofluorescence with standard blood and bone marrow specimens, as well as tissue sections, spinal fluid, and other effusions, provides a menas of assessing the presence of malignant lymphoblastic cells. The results are strikingly specific and can be performed on ordinary clinical specimens in a rather short time. All that is required is the highly specific monovalent antibody.

DISCUSSION

The results presented on TdT and DNA polymerase-α demonstrate a beginning in the use of immunological reagents for cytochemical studies on deoxynucleotide-polymerizing enzymes. These results are presented with full knowledge that use of this methodology is not a new suggestion. The reason for presenting these rather simple preliminary results is twofold. First of all it is clear that some of the results are new. Secondly, it is obvious to me that this is the only additional approach currently available for use in eukaryotic systems. The new information that can be obtained is essentially structural. Since eukaryotic replication units are rather large, it is possible that this can be a new window for examining the structure of replicating systems. The sensitivity of the immunological procedures is sufficient for this level of investigation, particularly the immuno-electron

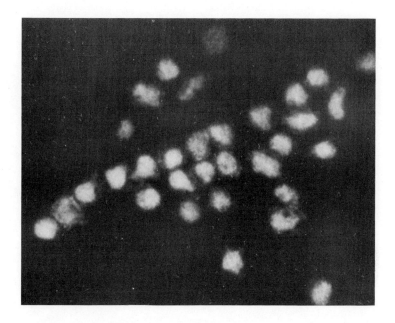

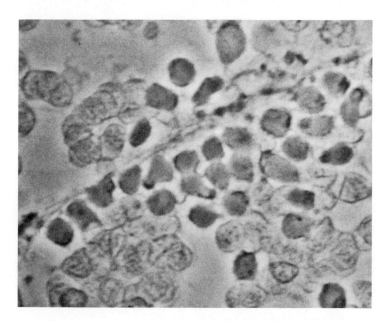

Figure 6.   Immunofluorescence of Terminal Transferase in a dried
bone marrow film from ALL patient.

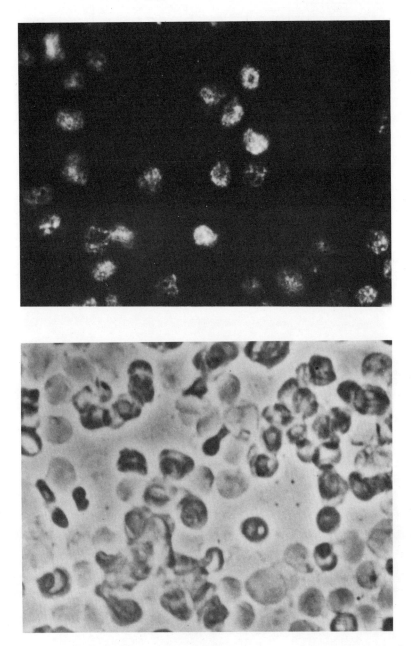

Figure 7.   Immunofluorescence of Terminal Transferase in a dried
bone marrow film from CML (blast crisis) patient.

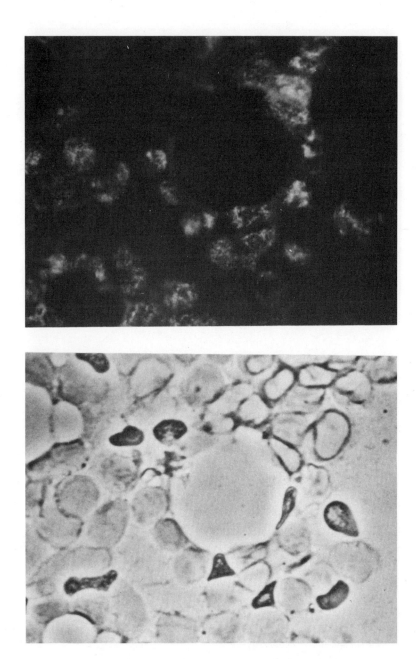

Figure 8.   Immunofluorescence of Terminal Transferase in a dried
bone marrow film from lymphoblastic lymphoma patient.

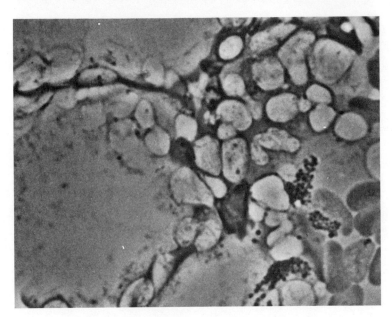

Figure 9.   Immunofluorescence of Terminal Transferase in a dried
bone marrow film from ALL patient in remission.

microscope procedures described by Sternberger (20).   Resolution in the electron microscope can proceed to the level of detecting single large molecules by appropriate amplification procedures.

It is important to note that the validity of the extremely sensitive immunological techniques is absolutely dependent upon the specificity of the immune reagents.   The specificity of the immune reagents depends upon the integrity of the preparations used for inciting the antibody and the investigators interpretation of his results.   I think in the future we will see wide application of immunological methods in elaborating the structures associated with deoxynucleotide polymerizing enzymes in eukaryotic systems.

REFERENCES

1. L. M. S. Chang and F. J. Bollum, Science 175:1116 (1972).
2. L. M. S. Chang and F. J. Bollum, unpublished results (1975).
3. F. J. Bollum and V. R. Potter, J. Biol. Chem. 233:478 (1958).
4. F. J. Bollum and V. R. Potter, Cancer Research 19:561 (1959).
5. J. W. Littlefield, A. P. McGovern, K. B. Margeson, Proc. Natl. Acad. Sci. U.S.A. 49:102 (1963).
6. G. Herrick, B. B. Spear and G. Veomett, Proc. Natl. Acad. Sci. U.S.A. 73:1136 (1976).
7. D. N. Foster and T. Gurney, J. Biol. Chem. 251:7893 (1976).
8. F. Chapeville and G. Brun, in "The organization and Expression of the Eukaryotic Genome" (E. M. Bradbury and K. Javakerian, Eds.), Academic Press, N.Y. (1977), p 261
9. L. M. S. Chang and F. J. Bollum, J. Biol. Chem. 246:909 (1971).
10. F. J. Bollum, Proc. Natl. Acad. Sci. U.S.A. 72:4119 (1975).
11. K. E. Gregoire, I. Goldschneider, R. W. Barton, and F. J. Bollum, Proc. Natl. Acad. Sci. U.S.A. 74:3993 (1977).
12. I. Goldschneider, K. E. Gregoire, R. W. Barton, and F. J. Bollum, Proc. Natl. Acad. Sci. U.S.A. 74:734 (1977).
13. K. E. Gregoire, I. Goldschneider, R. W. Barton, and F. J. Bollum, Federation Proceedings 36:1301 (1977).
14. R. McCaffery, D. F. Smoler, and D. Baltimore, Proc. Natl. Acad. Sci. U.S.A. 70:521 (1973).
15. M. S. Coleman, J. J. Hutton, P. DeSimone and F. J. Bollum, Proc. Natl. Sci. U.S.A. 71:4404 (1974).
16. M. S. Coleman, M. F. Greenwood, J. J. Hutton, F. J. Bollum B. Lampkin, and P. Holland, Cancer Research 36:210 (1976).
17. M. F. Greenwood, M. S. Coleman, J. J. Hutton, B. Lampkin, C. Krill, F. J. Bollum, and P. Holland, J. Clin. Invest. 59:899 (1977).
18. P. S. Sarin, P. N. Anderson, and R. C. Gallo, Blood 47:11 (1976).
19. J. A. Donlon, E. S. Jaffe and R. C. Braylon, New England J. Med. 297:461 (1977).
20. L. A. Sternberger, "Immuncytochemistry", Prentice-Hall Inc., Inglewood Cliffs, N.J. (1974).

EFFECT OF PHOSPHONOACETATE ON CELLULAR AND VIRAL DNA POLYMERASES

H. S. Allaudeen and J. R. Bertino

Departments of Pharmacology and Medicine

Yale University School of Medicine, New Haven, CT 06510

INTRODUCTION

Sodium phosphonoacetic acid (PAA) is an effective inhibitor of replication of herpes simplex virus in vitro (Overby et al., 1974; Yajima et al., 1976) and in vivo (Shipkowitz et al., 1973). The antiherpes virus effect of this compound was originally noticed by Abbott Laboratories during a random screening of compounds for antiviral activity. Subsequently, it has been shown that PAA inhibits reversibly the multiplication of a number of other herpes viruses tested including human cytomegalovirus, chicken Marek's disease virus, equine herpes virus, and a non-herpes, vaccinia virus.

The potent antiviral activity of this compound has stimulated considerable interest and led to studies on its mode of inhibition. The antiviral effect of PAA was found to be due to its ability to inhibit viral DNA synthesis (Mao et al., 1975). Herpes viruses, upon productive infection of cells, induce synthesis of virus specific DNA polymerase (Weissbach, et al., 1973). Genetic studies show that the structure of the herpes virus induced DNA polymerase is coded for by the viral genome and that the polymerase is essential in the viral DNA synthesis (Jofre et al., 1977). PAA was shown to be an effective inhibitor of activity of the herpes virus induced DNA polymerase (Mao et al., 1975; Mao and Robishaw, 1975; Leinbach et al., 1976). Studies to determine the mechanism of PAA inhibition showed that the compound brings about the inhibition presumably by interacting with the enzyme. The inhibition was non-competitive with deoxynucleoside triphosphate substrates and uncompetitive with DNA template (Mao and Robishaw, 1975; Leinbach et al.,

603

1976). Mao et al (1975) and Mao and Robishaw (1975) claimed that
PAA inhibited specifically the herpes virus induced DNA polymerase
activity. To evaluate the specificity of PAA, we examined its
effect on the activities of cellular DNA polymerases. We found
that the compound also inhibited the activities of the DNA polymerases purified from mammalian cells and RNA tumor viruses, and in
particular, DNA polymerase α is just as sensitive as the herpes
virus induced DNA polymerase. During the course of our study, Bolden et al (1975) reported that the DNA polymerase α of HeLa cells
was similar to the herpes and vaccinia virus induced DNA polymerases
in its sensitivity to PAA.

We studied the effect of PAA on the activities of the DNA polymerases α, β, and γ purified from a mouse lymphoid leukemia cell
line L1210, DNA polymerases α and β from leukocytes of a patient
with acute myelogenous leukemia (AML), and terminal deoxyribonucleo-
tidyl transferase (TdT) purified from leukocytes of a patient with
chronic myelogenous leukemia (CML) (blast crisis). Reverse transcriptase was purified from a type C virus of woolly monkey, Simian
sarcoma virus (SSV) and another type C virus released by L1210 cells
(Allaudeen and Bertino, 1977). These enzymes were purified using
procedures described earlier (Allaudeen and Bertino, 1977; Allaudeen
and Bertino, submitted for publication). Essentially, the cells
were extracted in the presence of salt and nonionic detergent, nucleic acids were removed by passing through a DEAE cellulose column,
and the DNA polymerases were separated on a phosphocellulose column
chromatography using a linear KCl gradient. The individual DNA polymerases used in this study were free from contamination of other
polymerase species. The purified DNA polymerases α, β, and γ
resemble the corresponding enzymes from other eukaryotic systems in
their general properties (Bollum, 1975; Weissbach, 1977). The reverse transcriptase of L1210 virus resembles the reverse transcriptase of R-MuLV in its biophysical, biochemical, and immunological
properties. Herpes simplex virus induced DNA polymerase, used as a
control, was prepared from HeLa cells after infecting with herpes
simplex virus type 1 (Weissbach et al., 1973).

Enzyme assays: DNA polymerase α activity was assayed in a
50 μl standard reaction mixture which contained 50 mM Tris.HCl,
pH 7.5, 2 mM dithiothreitol (DTT), 8 mM $MgCl_2$, 100 μM each of dATP,
dCTP, and dGTP, and 40 μM [^{3}H] dTTP (450 cpm/pmole), 10 μg of activated salmon sperm DNA, and enzyme. Incubation was at 37^0C for one
hour. Acid insoluble radioactivity was collected on a Gelman nitrocellulose filter, washed several times with 5% TCA containing
2 mM sodium pyrophosphate and measured in a liquid scintillation
counter. DNA polymerase β activity was assayed under similar conditions except pH 8.5 buffer and 40 mM KCl were used. The reaction
mixture for the HSV-DNA polymerase assay contained 50 mM Tris.HCl,
pH 8.0, 4 mM $MgCl_2$, and 150 mM potassium sulfate. Other ingredients
are the same. The reaction mixture for the assay of reverse

transcriptase activity contained the following ingredients in a total volume of 50 µl: 50 mM Tris.HCl buffer, pH 8.0, 1 mM $MnCl_2$, 80 mM KCl, 2 mM DTT, 20 µM [^{3}H] dGTP (900 cpm/pmole), 0.5 µg of $(dG)_{\sim15}\cdot(C^m)_n$ and enzyme. TdT activity was assayed in a 50 µl reaction mixture which contained 50 mM Tris.HCl, pH 8.0, 2 mM DTT, 0.6 mM $MnCl_2$, 2 µg of $(dA)_{\sim15}$, 200 µM of [^{3}H] dGTP (300 cpm/pmole) and enzyme.

RESULTS

Effect of PAA on the Activities of DNA Polymerases

The inhibition of DNA polymerases of L1210 cells by PAA is shown in Figure 1. Of the cellular enzymes, the DNA polymerase α was most sensitive to PAA inhibition, and DNA polymerases β and γ were least sensitive. Herpes simplex virus induced DNA polymerase (HSV-DP), used as a control, was slightly more sensitive than DNA polymerase α. For example, the DNA polymerases β and γ required 7-10 times more PAA than that required by the DNA polymerase α for a 50% inhibition of their activities. We obtained similar results with DNA polymerases α and β purified from human leukemic leukocytes (Figure 2). PAA was inhibitory to not only DNA dependent DNA polymerase activity but also RNA-dependent DNA polymerase as well as TdT activities were affected (Figure 3). However, PAA inhibited the activities of these enzymes only weakly. For example, PAA concentration required for a 50% inhibition of the activities of reverse transcriptases from SSV and L1210 virus was between $7\text{-}8 \times 10^{-5}$M whereas TdT required 2×10^{-4}M for a similar inhibition. The activities of DNA polymerase α and HSV-induced DNA polymerase were inhibited 50% by approximately 2.5×10^{-5}M of PAA.

Time Course of PAA Inhibition

To determine whether PAA could inhibit DNA synthesis even after the reaction was initiated, it was added to the ongoing reaction system at different time intervals and the activity was monitored. As shown in Figure 4, the compound caused an instantaneous inhibition whether it was added at the time of initiation or after the initiation of the reaction.

Effect of Substrate Concentration on PAA Inhibition

To characterize further the nature of the inhibition, we determined PAA inhibition with increasing substrate concentration. Tritiated dTTP was used as the rate limiting substrate, the other three triphosphates were in excess. When the data were plotted by

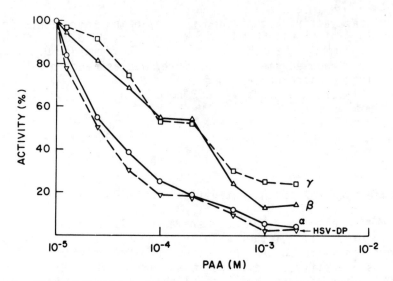

Figure 1: PAA inhibition of DNA polymerases of L1210 cells. Percentage of the remaining activity with increasing concentrations of PAA is shown. DNA polymerases α, β, and γ, and HSV-DNA polymerase contained 42, 33, 7, and 4 pmoles respectively, of the corresponding dNMP incorporated at 37° at 60 minutes under optimum assay conditions. Activated DNA was used as the template; other conditions of the assay are described in the text.

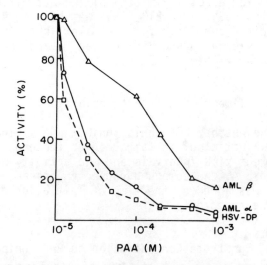

Figure 2: PAA inhibition of DNA polymerases of AML leukocytes. DNA polymerases α, β, and HSV-DNA polymerase contained 52, 46, and 4 pmoles respectively, of the enzyme activity in each experiment. Other conditions are described in Figure 1.

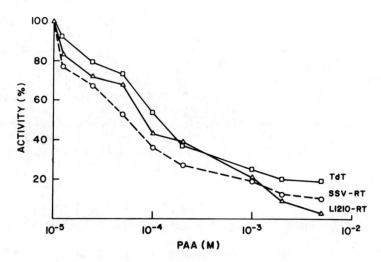

Figure 3: PAA inhibition of reverse transcriptases of SSV and L1210 virus and TdT of CML leukocytes. One hundred percent enzyme activity of SSV-reverse transcriptase, L1210 virus reverse transcriptase, and TdT represent 17, 21, and 9 pmoles of the enzyme activity, respectively. Other conditions are described in Figure 1.

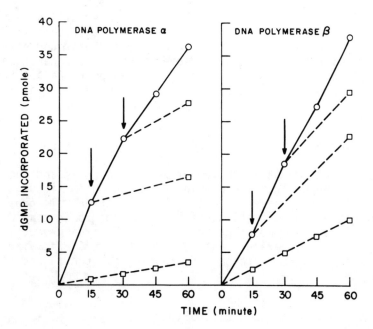

Figure 4: Time course of PAA inhibition. PAA at a final concentration of 5 x 10^{-4} M was added at the time interval as shown after the initiation of the enzyme reaction. Tritiated dGTP (450 cpm/pmole) was used in this experiment; all the other conditions are described in the text.

the method of Lineweaver and Burk (1934), straight lines could be drawn intersecting on the abscissa (Figure 5). These results indicate that the inhibition was noncompetitive with dTTP. The apparent Km value of DNA polymerase α for dTTP was 5.5 μM; the Ki for PAA was approximately four times higher than the Km. A similar pattern of inhibition was observed with DNA polymerase β; however, higher concentrations of PAA were required for inhibition (Figure 6). The apparent Km value of DNA polymerase β for dTTP was 14 μM; the Ki for PAA was approximately 18 times more than the Km. When the experiments were repeated using, alternatively, radioactive dATP, dCTP, or dGTP as the rate limiting substrates, similar results were obtained.

Effect of the Concentration of Activated DNA on PAA Inhibition

As shown in Figure 7, the double reciprocal plots of DNA synthesis vs. template concentration at two concentrations of PAA yielded parallel lines indicating that the inhibition was uncompetitive with the template DNA. Experiments with DNA polymerase β yielded similar results.

PAA Inhibition with Synthetic Primer Templates in the Assay

The extent of inhibition by PAA when different synthetic primer templates were used in the assay was tested. These studies showed that change of templates did not have a profound effect on the nature of PAA inhibition. However, the difference in sensitivity to PAA between DNA polymerase α and DNA polymerase β was greater when the synthetic primer templates were used in place of activated DNA (Data not presented).

Effect of PAA on Growth of L1210 Cells and Type C Virus Production

The effect of PAA on the growth of L1210 cells and the production of type C virus was examined. As shown in Figure 8, PAA at 50 μg/ml did not have any noticeable effect on cell growth; however, higher concentrations of PAA reduced growth considerably. PAA had a more profound effect on the type C virus production than on cell growth; for example, at 50 μg/ml on day 3, the virus production was inhibited more than 50% while cell growth was affected only by 16%.

DISCUSSION

The discovery of the potent antiviral activity of this chemically simple compound has led to studies on the mode of action at

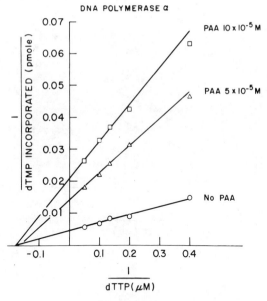

Figure 5

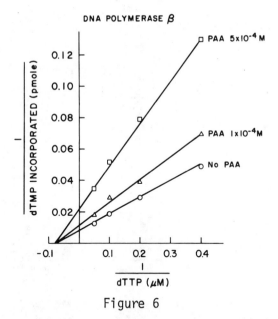

Figure 6

<u>Figures 5 and 6</u>: Effect of PAA on the reaction rate in the presence of different concentrations of dTTP as the rate limiting substrate with DNA polymerase α (Figure 5) and DNA polymerase β (Figure 6) of L1210 cells.

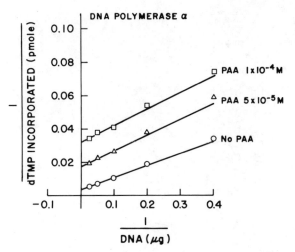

Figure 7: Effect of PAA on the reaction rate in the presence of different concentrations of activated DNA.

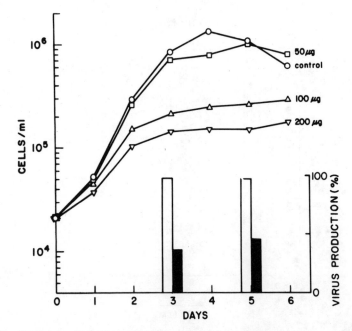

Figure 8: Effect of PAA on the growth of L1210 cells. The cell growth was monitored daily using a Coulter counter. The concentrations (μg/ml) of PAA added are shown. The type C virus production was monitored by estimating the reverse transcriptase activity of the 100,000 g pellet of the culture supernatant as described previously (Allaudeen and Bertino, 1977). Solid bars represent the decrease in the virus production in the presence of 50 μg/ml of PAA.

the molecular level. Mao et al (1975) and Mao and Robishaw (1975) originally reported that PAA suppresses DNA replication of the herpes simplex viruses type 1 and type 2 by inhibiting the virus induced DNA polymerase. It has since been shown that the compound can also inhibit the DNA polymerases induced by a number of other herpes viruses such as human cytomegalovirus (Huang, 1975), Epstein-Barr virus (Miller et al., 1977), equine herpes virus (Allen et al., 1977), and chicken Marek's disease virus (Leinbach et al., 1976). However, the compound is not specific to herpes virus induced DNA polymerase as originally reported by Mao and Robishaw (1975). We found that the DNA polymerase α purified from human AML leukocytes and mouse L1210 cells is just as sensitive as the herpes virus induced DNA polymerase. The cellular DNA polymerase α purified from HeLa cells (Bolden et al., 1975), duck embryo fibroblasts (Leinbach et al., 1976), and horse tumor cells (Allen et al., 1977) was also inhibited. However, the DNA polymerases β and γ of L1210 cells required approximately seven to ten times more PAA than that required for the DNA polymerase α for a 50% inhibition. Similar results were reported by Bolden et al (1975). These studies indicate that it is essential to separate the individual species of the cellular DNA polymerases for a comparison of their sensitivity to PAA. At higher concentrations, the compound can also inhibit the activities of reverse transcriptases from SSV and L1210 virus as well as TdT from CML leukocytes.

Kinetic analysis with the DNA polymerases α and β of L1210 cells showed that the compound is a noncompetitive inhibitor with dNTP substrate and uncompetitive inhibitor with activated DNA. These results are consistent with the mode of PAA inhibition observed with herpes virus induced DNA polymerases (Mao and Robishaw, 1975; Leinbach et al., 1976). The inhibition pattern was similar when different primer templates were used in the enzyme assays indicating that the template is not the likely site of action.

The effect of PAA on type C virus production was more pronounced than on L1210 cell growth. However, the reverse transcriptase isolated from the type C virus particles was less sensitive than the cellular DNA polymerase α to PAA inhibition. Presumably, the compound can also interfere with other step(s) in the replication of the type C virus.

Acknowledgment. This research was supported by grant CH-47 of the American Cancer Society and CA 08010 and 08341 of the United States Public Health Service.

REFERENCES

1.   Allaudeen, H. S., and Bertino, J. R., 1977, Presence of type C particles containing reverse transcriptase in L1210 leukemia, J. Natl. Cancer Inst. 59:227.

2.   Allaudeen, H. S., and Bertino, J. R.,   Inhibition of activities of DNA polymerase α, β, γ, and reverse transcriptase of L1210 cells by phosphonoacetic acid, Submitted to Biochim. Biophys. Acta for publication.

3.   Allen, G. P., O'Callaghan, J., and Randall, C. C., 1977, Purification and characterization of equine herpesvirus-induced DNA polymerase , Virol. 76:395.

4.   Bolden, A., Aucker, J., and Weissbach, A., 1975, Synthesis of herpes simplex virus, vaccinia virus, and adenovirus DNA in isolated HeLa cell nuclei, J. Virol. 16:1584.

5.   Bollum, F. J., 1975, Mammalian DNA polymerases. In "Progress in Nucleic Acid Research and Molecular Biology". (David, J. N., and Cohn, W. E., eds) Academic Press, New York, 15:109.

6.   Huang, E. S., 1975, Human cytomegalovirus. IV Specific inhibition of virus-induced DNA polymerase activity and viral DNA replication by phosphonoacetic acid, J. Virol. 16:1560.

7.   Jofre, J. T., Schaffer, P. A., and Parris, D. S., 1977, Genetic resistance to phosphonoacetic acid in strain KOS of herpes simplex virus type 1, J. Virol. 23:833.

8.   Leinbach, S. S., Reno, J. M., Lee, L. F., Isbell, A. F., and Boezi, J. A., 1976, Mechanism of phosphonoacetate inhibition of herpesvirus-induced DNA polymerase, Biochemistry 15:426.

9.   Mao, J. C. -H., and Robishaw, E. E., 1975, Mode of inhibition of herpes simplex virus DNA polymerase by phosphonoacetate, Biochemistry 14:5475.

10. Mao, J. C. -H., Robishaw, E. E., and Overby, L. R., 1975, Inhibition of DNA polymerase from herpes simplex virus-infected Wi-38 cells by phosphonoacetic acid, J. Virol. 15:1281.

11. Overby, L. R., Robishaw, E. E., Schleicher, J. B., Rueter, A., Shipkowitz, N. L., and Mao, J. C. -H., 1974, Inhibition of herpes simplex virus replication by phosphonoacetic acid, Antimicrob. Agents Chemother. 6:360.

12.   Shipkowitz, N. L., Bower, R. R., Appell, R. N., Nordeen, C. W., Overby, L. R., Roderick, W. R., Schleicher, J. B., and von Esch, A. M., 1973, Appl. Microbiol. 26:264.

13.   Weissbach, A., 1977, Eukaryotic DNA polymerases. In "Ann. Rev. Biochem." (Snell, E. E., Boyer, P. D., Meister, A., and Richardson, C. eds) Ann. Rev. Inc., California 46:25.

14.   Weissbach, A., Hong, S. L., Aucker, J. and Muller, R. 1973, Characterization of herpes simplex virus-induced DNA polymerase, J. Biol. Chem. 248:6270.

15.   Yajima, Y., Tanaka, A., and Nonoyama, M., 1976, Inhibition of productive replication of Epstein-Barr virus DNA by phosphonoacetic acid, Virology 71:352.

SOME CHARACTERISTICS OF REVERTANT CELLS PERTINENT TO IN VIVO GROWTH OF A SARCOMA VIRUS TRANSFORMED NON-PRODUCER 3T3 CELL

P. Ebbesen and L. Olsson

Department of Tumor Virus Research
Institute of Medical Microbiology
30 Juliane Maries Vej
DK-2100 Copenhagen, Denmark

The effect of malignant transformation and reversion on various cell characteristics was studied in cloned Moloney and Kirsten sarcoma virus infected, non-virus producing mouse FL (Swiss) and BALB 3T3 cells. Fully transformed cells as defined by morphology, in vitro and in vivo growth differed from normal uninfected cells with regard to one or more of the following characteristics: surface charge, interferon production, in vitro growth rate, and in vitro migration; however, revertant cells always shared one or more particular characteristics with transformed cells. Testing for cell line specific, reversibly acting DNA inhibitor activity in a 20-60 000 molecular weighy cell extract, the transformed BALB cells were found characterized by, 1) low production of and 2) low susceptibility to the inhibitor, 3) some change in specificity with change in expression of the sarcoma genome, and 4) production also of a DNA stimulator. Furthermore we found a protective effect of admixing a BALB revertant (4111) to transformed BALB cells before grafting to syngeneic recipients, whereas admixture of normal cells had no influence on the in vivo growth of the transformed cells. Inoculation of the "protective" revertant cells at a site separate from the transformed cells had no influence on growth of the trans- formed cells. In vitro test showed the revertant BALB cells slightly more susceptible to the cytotoxic effect of peritoneal macrophages than normal as well as transformed 3T3 cells.

In cloned cultures of sarcoma virus transformed cells there is a spontaneous emergence of cells with the morphology of non-infected cells and without in vivo malignancy, the so-called revertant cells (Rabinowitz and Sachs, 1972; Stephenson et al. 1973; Fischinger et al. 1974). In most cases the sarcoma genome is retained in such revertants, while there is a change in viral and/or cellular gene functions necessary to maintain transformation (Deng et al. 1974; Smith and Gallo, 1976). However, a total loss of the sarcoma genome may also occur (Frankel et al. 1976).

In our experiments FL (Swiss) and BALB mouse cells, normal, murine sarcoma virus transformed and revertant 3T3, kindly supplied by Dr. Nomura (Nomura et al. 1974), were used. Some characteristics of the BALB cells are given in Table 1.

Table 1   Some characteristics of normal, transformed and revertant BALB/c 3T3 cells

Nomura et al. 1974	Normal BALB/c 3T3	Transf. K-BALB	Rev. 12121	Rev. 4111
Morphology	Flat	Rounded	Flat	Flat
in vivo malignant	0	+	0	0
Contact inhibition	+	0	+	+
Saturation density $10^4/cm^2$	13	56	6	6
Sarcoma virus production after leukemia virus inf.	0	+	0	0
Group specific virus antigen	0	0	0	0
Chromosome number	4N	4N	4N	4N
Con A agglutination	+	+	+	+
Cloning, agar (%)	0.04	28	0.4	14
Cloning, liquid (%)	32	45	15	31
Ebbesen et al. 1977				
Interferon prod.	+	0	+	+++
Chalone in cells	+	0	+	+
Chalone in medium	+	+	+	+
Net outer charge	"Neutral"	Negative	Negative	Negative
in vitro doubling(h)	15	15	21	23
in vitro migration 0% serum	+	+	++	++
2% serum	+	+	+++	+++

Table 2 Significant inhibitory and stimulatory effect on DNA-synthesis activity of the various target cell extract combinations

Extract from → Target ↓	Swiss mouse							BALB/c mouse			
	3T3-554(N)	3BII(T)	SR448(R)	2143(R)	3382(T)	F13I(R)	F27I(R)	B-3T3(N)	K-B-23(T)	KSR I2I2I(R)	KSR 4III(R)
Swiss mouse											
3T3-554(N)	●										
3BII(T)		●	x	x	x						
SR448(R)	○	x	●	x	○			x		x	x
2143(R)		x	x	●	x						
3382(T)		x	○	x	●	○		○			
F13I(R)	x	○			x	●	●		x		
F27I(R)	x	x	○	○	x	○	●	x		○	○
BALB/c mouse											
B-3T3(N)	○		○	○	○		○	●		○	○
K-B-23(T)											
KSR I2I2I(R)	○							○		●	○
KSR 4III(R)	○							○		○	●

○ = inhibition

● = strongest inhibition obtained with a given extract

x = stimulation

N = normal

R = revertant

T = transformed

One of the results given in Table 1 is our finding of a cell-line specific, reversibly acting (MW 20-60 000) inhibitor of DNA synthesis extractable from our cells in subconfluence. This chalone-like activity is measured as the inhibition of in vitro incorporation of tritiated thymidine in DNA of cells of various types. Subsequently we made a cross-board study. The extracts from each cell line were tested on all cell lines (Table 2).

Table 2 shows that the transformed BALB cells were character-ized by low production and low susceptibility to the inhibitor extract. A given extract always exerted maximum effect on its cell of origin, suggesting a link between a certain degree of specificity and expression of the sarcoma genome. Furthermore some evidence for the presence of a stimulator primarily produced by the transformed BALB cell was obtained. SDS-polyacrylamide electrophoresis work in progress by Dr. R.A. Newman, Department of Immunobiology, University of Cologne, shows that the extracts contain one major glycoprotein band containing 90 per cent of the protein in the extracts.

Testing for an in vivo interaction between normal, revertant, and transformed cells we used the BALB cell lines and grafted, syngeneic, newborn mice, as shown in Table 3.

Table 3   Influence of admixing revertant cells to transformed cells prior to grafting to syngeneic, newborn BALB recipients

Cell types grafted and number of cells	Mice with tumor takes/ total number of mice
K-BALB-23 transformed 10^2	27/31
4111 revertant 10^6	0/23
12121 revertant 10^6	0/27
3T3 normal 10^6	0/22
K-BAKB-23 10^2 mixed with 4111 10^6	5/29
K-BALB-23 10^2 separate from 4111 10^6	19/26
K-BALB-23 10^2 mixed with 12121 $1o^6$	22/31
K-BALB-23 10^2 separate from 12121 10^6	15/20
K-BALB-23 10^2 mixed with 3T3 10^6	21/27
K-BALB-23 10^2 separate from 3T3 10^6	29/35

Table 4 ^{51}Cr-release from labeled cells cultivated on adherent peritoneal cells for 20 h.

The values are expressed as $\dfrac{\text{cpm 20 h} - \text{cpm 0 h}}{\text{cpm 3T3 total} - \text{cpm 0 h}} \pm$ SEM

Target cells	Origin of attacking mononuclear phagocytes							
	Normal Balb/c-3T3	P[a,b]	Activated Balb/c	P[a]	Normal AkR	P[a]	Activated AkR	P
Normal Balb/c-3T3	1.26 ±0.08	-	1.49 ±0.12	-	1.06 ±0.08	-	1.19 ± 0.07	-
Transf. K-Balb-23	1.16 ±0.06	NS	1.42 ±0.08	NS	1.05 ±0.06	NS	1.07 ± 0.08	NS
Revertant K^{SR}-4111	1.42 ±0.09	NS	1.85 ±0.13	NS	1.38 ±0.11		2.25 ± 0.16	P < 0.001
Revertant K^{SR}-12121	1.58 ±0.09	0.05 <P< 0.02	1.79 ±0.11	NS	1.13 ±0.09		1.02 ± 0.09	NS

a Value of Normal Balb/c-3T3 versus target cell line in question in the same group of attacker cells

b Student-t-test

NS = Not significant

These findings indicate that the presence of the revertant 4111 in intimate contact with the transformed cells may have an antineoplastic effect. As grafting of the "protective" revertants at some distance from the transformed cells is without influence we speculate that either the revertants themselves influence the transformed cells, or the revertants make other locally residing cells react against them. The malignant cells might as innocent bystanders be killed by the non-specific cytotoxicity of activated macrophages (Hibs, 1974; Prehn, 1974; Tuttle and North, 1975). Shared surface antigens on revertants and transformed cells could also make a local specific immune response against revertants effective against the transformed cells.

Working along this line we have so far tested the outcome of in vitro cocultivation of normal, revertant, and transformed BALB 3T3 cells with syngeneic and allogeneic peritoneal macrophages from untreated and BCG-pretreated donor mice (Hibs, 1974) (Table 4).

The BALB revertants appear more susceptible to the cytotoxic effect of macrophages than normal and transformed BALB 3T3 cells, although the difference was statistically significant only for revertant 4111 incubated with activated, allogeneic attacking cells. The possible relevance of this and other immunologic characteristics for the antineoplastic effect of the revertant cell line 4111 awaits further studies.

References

Rabinowitz Z and Sachs L
The formation of variants with a reversion of properties of trans-
formed cells   VI   Stability of the reverted state
Int J Cancer 9:334-343, 1972

Stephenson J R, Reynolds R K and Aaronson S A
Characterization of morphologic revertants of murine and avian
sarcoma virus transformed cells
J Virol 11:218-222, 1973

Fischinger P J, Nomura S, Tuttle-Fuller N and Dunn K J
Revertants of mouse cells transformed by murine sarcoma virus
III   Metastable expression of virus functions in revertants
retransformed by murine sarcoma virus
Virology 59:217-229, 1974

Deng C-T, Boethinger D, MacPherson I and Varmus H E
The persistence and expression of virus-specific DNA in revertants
of Rous sarcoma virus-transformed BHK-21 cells
Virology 62:512-521, 1974

Smith R G and Gallo R C
Prospects for biologic and pharmacologic inhibition of ribonucleic
acid tumor viruses
Biochem Pharmacol 25:491-495, 1976

Frankel A E, Haapala D H, Neubauer R L and Fischinger P J
Elimination of the sarcoma genome from murine sarcoma virus
transformed cat cells
Science 191:1264-1266, 1976

Nomura S, Dunn K J, Mattern C F T, Hartley J W and Fischinger P J
Revertants of mouse cells transformed by murine sarcoma virus:
Flat variants without a rescuable sarcoma virus from a clone of
BALB/3T3 transformed by Kirsten MSV
J Gen Virol 25:207-218, 1974

Ebbesen P, Olsson L, Rudkøbing O, Haahr S and Kristensen G
Correlation of some cell functions to transformation/reversion
studied with cloned Moloney and Kirsten sarcoma virus transformed
mouse 3T3 cells I In vivo malignancy, net outer charge, in vitro
migration, interferon activity, in vitro growth rates and chalone-
like activity
Cancer Res 37:4285-4291, 1977

Hibbs J B Jr
Discrimination between neoplastic and non-neoplastic cells in vitro
by activated macrophages
J Natl Cancer Inst 53:1487-1492, 1974

Prehn R T
Destruction of tumor as an "innocent bystander" in an immune response
specifically directed against non-tumor antigens
Israel J Med Sci 9:375-379, 1973

Tuttle R L and North R J
Mechanisms of antitumor action of Corynebacterium parvum: Nonspecific
tumor cell destruction at site of an immunologically mediated sensitivity reaction to C parvum
J Natl Cancer Inst 55:1403-1411, 1975

THE DEVELOPMENT OF NEW ANTIVIRAL AGENTS BASED ON VIRUS-MEDIATED CELL MODIFICATION

Luis Carrasco

Translation Laboratory, Imperial Cancer Research Fund

London WC2A 3PX

The infection by an animal virus of its host cell, often involves interference with cellular functions (1-5). The mechanisms by which the virus is able to take over the cellular metabolism still remain unknown. Several theories have been proposed during the years to explain the so called shut-off phenomenon (5-8), but to date none of them has been firmly established as correct. We proposed recently that one factor in the strategy for viral take-over is the modification of the plasma membrane caused by the insertion of viral proteins (5). This modification of the membrane will distort the gradient of ions in such a way that sodium will leak in whereas potassium ions leak out the cytoplasm. The net result should be an increase in the concentration of monovalent ions inside the cell, this gradual change of ions in the cytoplasm will affect differentially viral and cellular protein synthesis (see Figure 1).

In support of this interpretation we have observed that monovalent ions affect differentially viral and cellular protein synthesis both in vivo and in vitro. An increase of sodium chloride in the culture medium preferentially inhibited cellular as compared to viral protein synthesis, whereas a hypotonic medium inhibited the translation of the viral mRNA (Figure 2). This result was perfectly reproduced in vitro, when we translated viral or cellular mRNAs in the presence of increasing amounts of sodium chloride (Figure 3) (9).

According to these results, we must then distinguish two different aspects in the regulation of protein synthesis observed after viral infection:

The inhibition of total protein synthesis. This could be explained by several facts all produced by a modification of the membrane: a) The disbalance in the concentration of ions in the

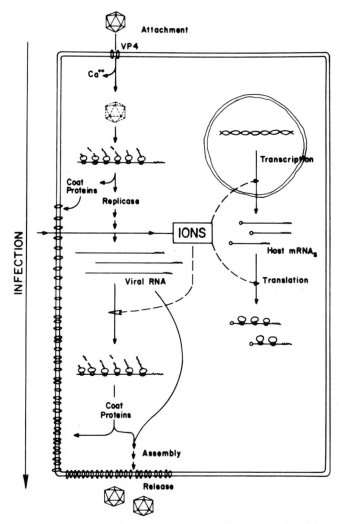

Fig. 1. Schematic representation of the membrane-leakage model. The insertion of a viral coat protein into the membrane causes the modification of the permeability properties of the plasma membrane. At the end of viral infection the assembly process will take place under ionic conditions different from those existing in a normal cell.

cell; b) the inhibition in the transport of amino acids and c) the decrease in the pool of aminoacids and nucleotides in the cytoplasm due to membrane leakiness.

On the other hand we can explain the specific regulation of translation that is, the inhibition of cellular mRNA but not viral

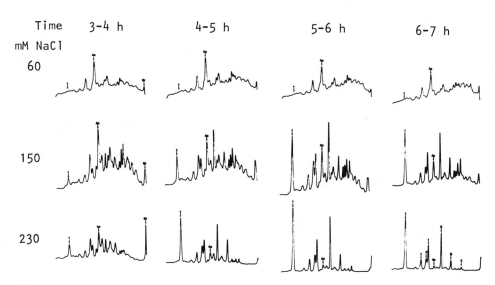

Fig. 2. Protein synthesis in EMC-infected 3T6 cells under different concentrations of sodium in the culture medium. Cells were labelled with (^{35}S)methionine as described (11).

mRNA translation by a) the specific discrimination that the increase in monovalent ions in the cytoplasm has in favor of viral (Figures 2 and 3) and b) the intrinsic higher affinity of viral mRNAs to bind to native ribosomal subunits as compared with cellular mRNAs (8). Of course, these two factors are closely related, because ions influence differentially the affinity of cellular and viral mRNAs for the smaller ribosomal subunit.

MEMBRANE LEAKINESS AND ANTIVIRAL AGENTS

The finding that virus-infected cells differ from normal cells in their different permeability properties, allowed us to design specific inhibitors for infected cells. The approach we proposed was the use of inhibitors which interphere with any viral function following the induction of membrane leakiness, irrespective of whether it involves cellular enzymes or not. The most important characteristic that the antiviral compound must satisfy is to be impermeable for normal uninfected cells. In addition it has to have a low molecular weight and a high activity in its in vitro inhibitory properties.

The first compound we tested that met those characteristics was GppCH$_2$p, a GTP analog that blocks protein synthesis in vitro

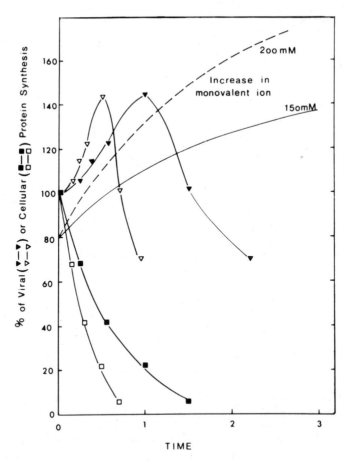

Fig. 3. Representation of the changes in the total concentration of monovalent ions in the cytoplasm under normal salt conditions (150 mM) and in a hypertonic medium (200 mM). Time 0 is taken as the beginning of membrane leakiness. The data on the behaviour of viral and cellular protein synthesis were taken from our in vitro results (9).

(10). The addition of this nucleotide analog to the medium of mock-infected cells had no effect on cellular protein synthesis, whereas it clearly blocked this process in EMC-infected 3T6 cells at a time after infection when viral protein synthesis was maximal (11).

This result is interpreted to mean that the specific inhibition of GppCH2p on infected cells is because this compound is able to pass through the membrane and reach the protein synthesising apparatus only in infected cells. A schematic representation of this interpretation is shown in Figure 4.

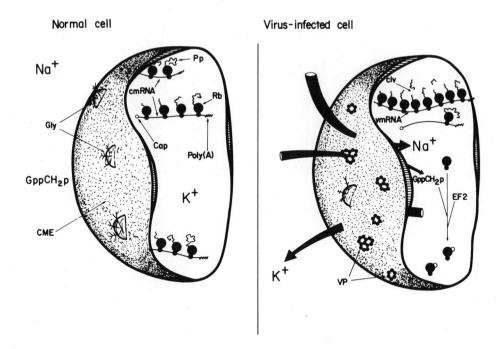

Fig. 4. Schematic representation of the approach we followed to test membrane leakiness. CME: cellular membrane, cmRNA: cellular mRNA, Gly: glycoproteins, Rb: ribosome, Pp: polypeptide, clv: cleavage, vmRNA: viral mRNA, VP: viral proteins.

Using the GppCH$_2$p assay we then observed that the bulk of viral proteins are synthesized in cells which have a leaky membrane. In addition, gene expression at the translational level was necessary for the induction of membrane leakiness and it is probable that a viral function is involved in making the membrane permeable to GppCH$_2$p (11).

ACTIVITY OF OTHER INHIBITORS IMPERMEABLE TO NORMAL CELLS

After we demonstrated that protein synthesis can be specifically inhibited in picornavirus-infected cells by means of an inhibitor impermeable to normal cells, we decided to do a detailed screening with a number of inhibitors of protein synthesis. It was soon found, that three out of nineteen inhibitors tested were powerful and specific inhibitors of protein synthesis in virus-infected cells. These inhibitors were: gougerotin, edeine and blasticidin S

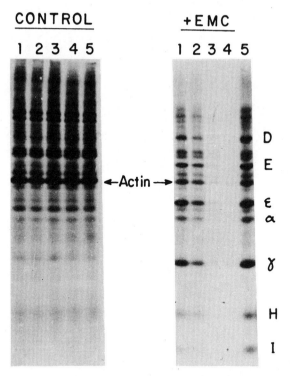

CONTROL **+EMC**

Fig. 5. Effect of hygromycin B on protein synthesis in normal and EMC-infected 3T6 cells. The assay was carried out as previously described (11). 1: 10^{-5} M hygromycin B, 2: 5 x 10^{-5} M, 4: 2 x 10^{-4} M and 5: control, 3: 10^{-4} M hygromycin B.

(12). In subsequent studies it was observed that although these inhibitors do not cross the plasma membrane when they are incubated for a few hours with the cells, they do penetrate suddenly after a lag of a few hours (Contreras and Carrasco, unpublished results). Although we have not yet done a detailed study of the delayed entry of these compounds in normal cells, it resembles me to the uptake of estreptomycin by sensitive cells (13). The retarded permeability that these three inhibitors show make then unsuitable to be used as antiviral agents, however, these studies fulfilled two purposes: a) to support the membrane-leakage model (5) and b) to draw our attention to the general structural properties that an inhibitor impermeable for cells has to meet.

According to those properties, we found a new inhibitor of protein synthesis, that in addition to be a very powerful in vitro inhibitor of translation it was very impermeable for uninfected 3T6 cells, even during long incubation periods. This inhibitor is known as hygromycin B (14,15), its effects on protein synthesis both in

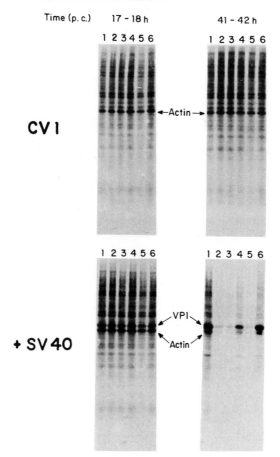

Fig. 6. Effect of different protein synthesis inhibitors in normal and SV40 infected CV1 cells at different times after infection. 1: control, 2: 5 x 10-4 hygromycin B, 3: 10-3 M hygromycin B, 4: 1 mg/ml edeine complex, 5: 3 mg/ml edeine complex and 6: 10-4 gougerotin.

normal and EMC-infected 3T6 cells are shown in Figure 5. It can be observed that hygromycin B had no effect on normal cells even when high concentrations of inhibitor were used. In contrast, those concentrations of hygromycin B completelly blocked translation in EMC-infected 3T6 cells.

Could hygromycin B be used as an antiviral agent in whole organisms?. Experiments are now in progress to test this question, but the fact that this compound is not toxic for mammals points to hygromycin B as a first candidate to be checked as an antiviral agent.

The future design of antiviral agents following this direction looks to me rather promising, because we can now either, to screen

much more known inhibitors that should be impermeable for normal
cells according to their structural formula, or to modify the most
powerful inhibitors of protein synthesis that we know, in order to
make them impermeable, whithout altering their inhibitory properties.

GENERALITY OF MEMBRANE LEAKINESS IN VIRAL INFECTION

Very few antiviral agents have been developed up to date and
none of them is a wide spectrum antiviral agent (for reviews see
16-19). We have proposed that membrane leakiness is a general
mechanism shared by all cytolitic viruses (5). This first
suggestion was supported by experiments in which we tested membrane
leakiness, measured by the $GppCH_2p$ assay, in mengovirus-infected 3T6
cells and in BHK cells infected with Semliki Forest virus (11).

Our earlier experiments done with CV1 cells infected with SV40
were unsuccessful when we used the nucleotide analog $GppCH_2p$. However,
with the availability of the new set of more powerful inhibitors,
impermeable to normal cells, we got clear-cut results. Figure 6
shows the analysis on polyacrilamide gels of the proteins
synthesised by normal and SV40-infected CV1 cells at different
times after infection in the presence of different inhibitors of
protein synthesis. It is observed that hygromycin B has no effect
on normal cells or in SV40-cells, soon after the beginning of the
late phase, but it readilly prevented translation when the synthesis
of the late protein VP1 was maximal. Thus indicating, that the bulk
of the synthesis of late proteins in SV40 occurs in a cell with a
leaky membrane.

These results are in agreement with recent findings indicating
that CV1 cells infected with SV40 become stainable by the
impermeable dye trypan blue (20). Moreover, we have found that the
translation of the 16S mRNA coding for VP1 is more efficient in
vitro in the presence of a high concentration of monovalent ions,
similarly occurs with other late viral mRNAs, indicating that the
translation of those mRNAs occurs in a cell which has a leaky
membrane (Carrasco, Smith, Harvey and Blanchard, unpublished
results).

The modification of the cell surface after viral infection has
been illustrated in many virus-cell system (21,22). In many
instances, this modification can lead to changes in the permeability
properties of the plasma membrane and these changes can be brought
about by viral proteins. It is also well known that the synthesis
of many viral proteins occurs in close association with membranes,
in such a way that after synthesis, they stay integrated in the
membrane. Some of then can thus serve two purposes: a) to modify
the membrane and b) to signal the specific sites in the plasma
membrane in which the morphogenesis of new viral particles will
take place.

ACKNOWLEDGEMENTS

I want to express my acknowledgement to Dr. A.E.Smith for his suggestions and to the Fundación Juan March for financial support. L.C. present address: Instituto de Bioquímica de Macromoléculas, C.B.M. y Dpto. de Microbiología, U.A.M. Canto Blanco, Madrid 34, Spain.

REFERENCES

1. Baltimore, D. (1969) in: The Biochemistry of Viruses (Levy, H. B., ed.), pp. 103-176. Marcel Dekker, New York.
2. Roizman, B. and Spear, P.B. (1969) Curr.Top.Develop.Biol. 4, 79-108.
3. Bablanian, R. (1975) Prog.Med.Virol. 19, 40-83.
4. Smith, A.E. and Carrasco, L. (1978) in: MTP Inter.Rev.Sci. Biochem. Series II (in press).
5. Carrasco, L. (1977) FEBS Letters 76, 11-15.
6. Kaufmann, Y., Goldstein, E. and Penman, S. (1976) Proc.Natl. Acad.Sci. USA 73, 1834-1838.
7. Nuss, D.L. and Koch, G. (1976) J.Virol. 19, 572-578.
8. Golini, F., Thach, S.S., Birge, C.H., Safer, B., Merrick, W.C. and Thach, R.E. (1976) Proc.Natl.Acad.Sci. USA 73, 3040-3044.
9. Carrasco, L. and Smith, A.E. (1976) Nature 264, 807-809.
10. Vázquez, D. (1978) in: MTP Inter.Rev.Sci.Biochem. Series II (in press).
11. Carrasco, L. (1978) Nature (in press).
12. Contreras, A., Vázquez, D. and Carrasco, L. (manuscript submitted for publication).
13. Plotz, P.H., Dubin, D.T. and Davis, B.D. (1961) Nature 191, 1324-1325.
14. Davies, J. and Davis, B.D. (1968) J.Biol.Chem. 243, 3312-3316.
15. Cabañas, M.J., Vázquez, D. and Modolell, J. (1978) Eur.J. Biochem. (in press).
16. Prusoff, W.H. and Goz, B. (1973) Fed.Proc. 32, 1679-1687.
17. Shugar, D. (1974) FEBS Letters 40, S48-S62.
18. Hoffmann, C.E. (1976) Ann.Rep.Med.Chem. 11, 128-137.
19. Diana, G.D. and Pancic, F. (1976) Angew.Chem.Int.Ed.Engl. 15, 410-416.
20. Norkin, L.C. (1977) J.Virol. 21, 872-879.
21. Rifkin, D.B. and Quigley, J.P. (1974) Ann.Rev.Microbiol. 28, 325-351.
22. Burns, W.H. and Allison, A.C. (1977) in: Virus Infection and the Cell Surface (Poste, G. and Nicolson, G.L., eds.), pp. 213-248. North-Holland Pub.Co.

SECTION VI

Human interferons: Effects on tumor viruses and on human

cancer

Convenor

Dr. William A. CARTER

Dep. of Medical Viral Oncology

Roswell Park Memorial Institute

666 Elm Street

Buffalo, New York 14203

U.S.A.

THE EFFECT OF INTERFERON ON TUMOUR VIRUSES, AND ITS POSSIBLE

ROLE IN THE TREATMENT OF HUMAN CANCER

DEREK C. BURKE

Biological Sciences, University of Warwick, Coventry,

CV4 7AL, England

It is now well established that interferon inhibits the
replication of a number of DNA and RNA viruses by inhibition of
viral translation. Whether cells are infected with an RNA virus,
such as Semliki Forest virus, or a DNA virus, such as vaccinia
virus the effect on virus multiplication is the same and appears
to be due to inhibition of virus protein synthesis, with little
effect on virus RNA synthesis. It is true that some effects
have been reported on the primary transcription of virion RNA by
infection with viruses carrying an RNA polymerase, but the
effects are usually not sufficient to explain the much larger
effect on virus multiplication and may well be due to either
artefacts of the system, or to the induction of a new nuclease
in the interferon-treated cells (see review by Friedman, 1977).
The main conclusion of these experiment with virus infected
cells has been amply born out by results with cell-free
translation systems obtained from interferon-treated cells, for
there is no question that translation of viral mRNAs is
substantially inhibited in such systems. Further analysis has
shown that there are a number of ways in which such systems
prepared from interferon-treated cells differ from control preparations. There is an inhibition of initiation, which is due to
the inactivation of one of the initiation factors by a low molecular weight substance - formed from ATP when double-stranded RNA
is added to cell extracts. The double-stranded RNA probably arises
as a by-product of virus infection, and since it would only be
present in infected cells, this inhibition of translation would
be limited to such infected cells. In addition, the production of
a new endonuclease which degrades viral mRNA has been reported
in interferon-treated cells, as well as an effect on virus mRNA
methylation. Finally, cell-free extracts which have been

dialysed or passed through Sephadex to remove low molecular
weight materials, lost their capacity to support translation by
inactivation of one of the rare leucyl-t RNAs. It is not clear
how these effects are related; presumably all of them stem from
a common source peculiar to interferon-treated cells, but no
unifying mechanism has been suggested.

The effects of interferon I have so far described are those
exerted on autonomously replicating viruses in a lytic infection.
However when one considers the effect of interferon on viruses
which are able to integrate into the host cell's genome - the
so-called transforming viruses - the results are rather different
(see Oxman, 1973). Interferon treatment inhibits SV 40 virus
multiplication, and also the formation of the SV 40 coded T
antigen, in lytic infection of permissive cells. Investigation
showed that interferon depressed early viral RNA synthesis in
lytic infection, and suggested that interferon was inhibiting
viral transcription. However further experiments suggest that the
inhibition of SV 40 replication might be due to an effect of
interferon on virus uncoating, rather than on virus transcription,
and it is also clear that when interferon is added to cells
producing SV 40, it does have an inhibitory effect on further
virus production which is almost certainly due to an effect on
virus translation. Thus SV 40 multiplication shows the normal
sensitivity to interferon's effect on translation, but in
addition, has a second early interferon-sensitive stage,
possibly uncoating.

However, SV 40 T antigen production is unaffected by interferon
in transformed cells, and if cells are infected with an SV 40-
adenovirus hybrid, SV 40 T antigen synthesis is considerably less
sensitive to interferon than when the cells were infected with SV
40. Indeed, synthesis of both SV 40 and adenovirus T antigen is
as resistant to interferon as adenovirus T antigen synthesis in
cells infected with adenovirus alone.

These observations show that the sensitivity of SV 40 T antigen synthesis to interferon is reduced when the SV 40 DNA is
covalently attached to another DNA - either cellular or viral.
This means that interferon may be considerably less effective in
inhibiting expression of an integrated viral genome than inhibiting
productive infection, and has implications for the use of
interferon for treatment of virus-transformed cells in vivo.

Surprising results were also obtained when interferon was
tested against RNA tumour virus infection. Interferon inhibits
the multiplication of C-type RNA tumour viruses in exogenously,
endogenously or chronically infected cells. However in detailed
studies with murine leukaemia virus (MLV) it was found that
interferon had little effect on the production of virus RNA or
proteins. Electron microscope pictures clearly showed that the
number of completed virus particles associated with the cell
membrane increased on interferon-treatment, suggesting that

interferon blocks either a late stage in virus assembly or the
final release of virions from the cell surface (see review by
Friedman, 1977). However in addition the released virus has
lowered infectivity, implying a fault in maturation which may
prevent release of cell-associated virus and/or lead to the
release of non-infective virus. A second site at which interferon
may act is on the induction of latent RNA tumour viruses by the
halogenated pyrimidines, since there have been two reports that
interferon inhibited the induction of a xenotropic MLV. It is
not clear whether interferon inhibits either induction or viral
protein synthesis as well as a terminal event, but some second
site of action in addition to the terminal event is possible.
Indeed, there is some recent evidence that the effect of interferon
on the terminal event in MLV replication is unusual, for ouabain,
an inhibitor of Na^+-K^+-dependent ATPase, did not block the
inhibitory effect of interferon on MLV replication (Tomita &
Kuwata, 1978) although it did block the inhibitory effect of
interferon on VSV replication (Kuwata et al., 1977). Ouabain
treatment is known to cause decreased $\overline{K^+}$ ion concentration and
increased Na^+ ion concentration inside the cells, and hence to
disturb protein synthesis. Since it is possible that the selective
effect of interferon on virus protein synthesis might be due to a
disturbance of Na^+ and K^+ balance, it is not difficult to see how
ouabain could reverse its effect. The fact that ouabain does not
prevent interferon exerting its effect on a terminal process of
MLV replication is consistant with the observation that this late
event is not a block in protein synthesis, and that it is
distinct from interferon's normal action. There is now direct
evidence for an effect of interferon on an early stage in
replication, possibly early protein synthesis, analogous to the
effect of interferon on other virus systems. Aboud, Shaw &
Salzberg (1978) found that interferon did inhibit MLV RNA
synthesis in exogenous infection and that a similar effect was
also shown by cycloheximide, suggesting that interferon might be
acting by inhibiting virus protein synthesis. Morris & Clegg
(1978) clearly showed an effect of interferon on the transformation
of 3T3 cells by MSV, by using a stock of MLV/MSV which had an
excess of MSV so that cells could be infected with MSV alone.
This meant that the effect of interferon on the early events
leading to transformation could be studied without any complications
due to effects at other, later sites, since MSV will not replicate,
but only integrate, and then transform in the absence of MLV.
Cycloheximide will also inhibit the integration of MSV showing
that protein synthesis, and presumably virus protein synthesis
is needed for this step, and suggesting that interferon too may
be acting by inhibition of virus protein synthesis. In subsequent
work, A. Morris has shown that when cells are infected with high
multiplicities of MLV/MSV, immediately cloned in the presence of
interferon and then passaged in the absence of interferon the

resultant clones are stably untransformed, do not produce MLV nor
do they contain MSV. Thus the block must be prior to integration
of the virus genome into the cellular genome.

Interferon can also affect the expression of an integrated
MLV genome, for addition of interferon to cells chronically
infected with MLV inhibited virus production. However, the effect
was reversible, since when the interferon was removed, virus
production resumed. This suggests that for the successful
treatment of an established C-type virus infection, interferon
would have to be present throughout.

Thus in summary, interferon inhibits MLV/MSV replication at
two points - prior to integration, possibly by an inhibiting a
process that requires virus protein synthesis, and late in
infection when some process that is essential for production of
infectious virus is inhibited. The first process is less
sensitive to interferon than the second, which explains why the
latter is normally the only one detected. Evidence for more than
one site of action also stems from the observation that when a
glucocorticoid-stimulated murine mammary tumour cell line was
treated with interferon, an inhibition of reverse transcriptase
activity as well as of virus release was detected (Strauchen
et al., 1977).

However, there are other processes affected by interferon
which will also determine the outcome of treatment of a tumour
virus infection with interferon. First, MLV stocks often contain
MSV, and MSV depends for its multiplication upon coinfection with
MLV, so that any effect on MLV multiplication will also affect the
yield of MSV. This effect can be minimised either by using cloned
MLV (free of MSV) or by using MSV in excess of MLV for studying
the effect of interferon on transformation to study the effect on
MLV multiplication, as described above. Second, interferon could
work, not by preventing integration but by slowing the growth of
transformed cells, since interferon has a well-documented effect
on cell growth. Morris & Clegg (1978) showed that a 24 h interferon treatment, sufficient to block transformation, did not
block focus or colony formation by cells already stably
transformed by MSV, but that if interferon were continuously
present, focus formation and growth in agar were inhibited. This
effect of prolonged treatment with interferon may play a role
in vivo, and this point is developed further below. Third,
interferon can either stimulate or depress the host immune system
and this is certainly going to affect the outcome of in vivo
experiments. Finally, some of the effects observed may have been
due to impurities present in the crude interferon. Purified
mouse interferon is now available and should be used for future
studies.

Turning to in vivo experiments, interferon has been clearly
shown to block tumour formation, both by DNA and RNA viruses
(see reviews by Gresser, 1977 and by Krim & Sanders, 1977).

The effects involve inhibition of virus multiplication, and on cell growth in addition to effects mediated via the immune system, and are reviewed by Gresser elsewhere in this volume.

The successful use of interferon to prevent multiplication of tumour viruses in vitro, and to inhibit tumour formation in vivo, has prompted serious consideration of the use of interferon in controlled trials against tumours of possible viral origin in man. However, it must be stressed that we do not know whether the interferon is acting as an antiviral agent, as an anti- cellular agent, or as an antitumour agent. The work carried out by Hans Strander and his group in the Karolinska Hospital in Stockholm is now well-known, and is described elsewhere in this volume. The protection, although striking, is not yet statistically significant, and since the interferon-treated patients are all in Stockholm and the controls in hospitals elsewhere in Sweden, the trial may indeed show a difference between patients and controls, but be unable to say whether this difference was due to interferon or some other difference between the centres, e.g., diagnosis or other treatment.

The Stockholm trial has prompted workers elsewhere to consider setting up trials against human cancers. Two things are necessary for such a trial: an adequate supply of interferon and a disease condition which is satisfactory for such a trial. The Stockholm trial has used interferon prepared in human leukocytes by Cantell and his collaborators in Helsinki. Indeed this material, at various stages of purity, has been used for all clinical trials so far. In Britain, the Scottish Blood Transfusion Service are considering setting up such a production unit in their Protein Fractionation Centre, along the lines so successfully used in Helsinki. The Wellcome Foundation has also pioneered a process using human lymphoblastoid cells in culture. These cells grow in suspension and produce high yields of interferon after induction with Sendai virus. The interferon is, like the material made in Helsinki, leukocyte rather than fibroblast interferon, and yields can be increased by pre-treatment of the cells with BUdr. The cells used, Namalwa cells, contain copies of the EB virus genome and have an abnormal karyotype. There are therefore safety problems to be taken into careful consideration, but the process is comparatively cheap and is easy to scale up. A suitable disease condition is not easy to find: there must be sufficient patients not already in a trial, there must be sound ethical reasons for treatment and there must be good parameters for following the course of treatment. These questions have been considered by the MRC working party in cancer therapy in collaboration with workers at ICRF, and protocols are now being drawn up for trials against ALL (acute lymphocytic leukaemia) and AML (acute myeloblastic leukaemia) in remission. ALL in remission has been chosen, since although relapses are so rare that the answers would be slow to emerge, there is some evidence for specific inhibition by interferon of lymphocyte proliferation. Such a trial might also discover whether viral infections during remission are reduced by interferon. AML in remission was chosen because it might be of viral origin, is reasonably common and relapses are sufficiently common for answers to emerge within a year or two. Myelomatosis in patients presenting without renal failure was chosen as a third target because it is common and since it can be readily monitored for an effect of the interferon. By late 1978 we should have enough interferon to start a multi-centre controlled trial. We plan to follow the course of treatment with suitable parameters - the level of circulating interferon in the serum, the in vitro sensitivity to interferon of the patients leukaemic cells, both before and after relapse, the interferon producing capacity of the patients' leukaemic cells (since the presence of exogenous interferon may act as a primer for interferon production) and possibly the interferon susceptibility of the patient's normal fibroblasts. Other conditions have been considered but interferon supply will be rate-limiting for some time to come. We await these experiments with considerable interest.

REFERENCES

Friedman, R.M. (1977) Antiviral activity of interferons. Bact. Rev. 41, 543-567.

Oxman, M.N. (1973) Interferon, tumours and tumour viruses. In Interferons and Interferon Inducers pp. 391-480. Ed. N.B. Finter, North Holland Publishing Co., Amsterdam & London.

Tomita, Y. & Kuwata, T. (1978) Suppression of murine leukaemia virus production by ouabain and interferon in mouse cells. J. Gen. Virol. 38, 223-230.

Kuwata, T., Fuse, A. & Morinaga, N. (1977) Effects of ouabain on the anticellular and antiviral activities of human and mouse interferon. J. Gen. Virol. 34, 537-540.

Aboud, M., Shoor, R. & Salzberg, S. (1978) Effect of interferon on exogenous murine leukaemia virus infection. Virology, 84, 138-141.

Morris, A.G. & Clegg, C. (1978) The effect of mouse interferon on the transformation of NIH/3T3 mouse cells by murine sarcoma virus. Virology, in press.

Strauchen, J.A., Young, N.A. & Friedman, R.M. (1977) Interferon-mediated inhibition of mouse mammary tumor virus expression in cultured cells. Virology, 82, 232-236.

Krim, M. & Sanders, F.K. (1977) Prophylaxis and therapy with interferons pp. 153-201. In Interferons and their Actions. Ed. W.E. Stewart II, CRC Press Inc., Cleveland, Ohio.

Gresser, I. (1977). Antitumor effects of interferon, pp. 521-551. In Cancer, a comprehensive treatise. Ed. F. Becker, Vol. 5, Chemotherapy, Plenum Press, New York.

INTERFERON INDUCTION BY SYNTHETIC POLYNUCLEOTIDES :

RECENT DEVELOPMENTS

Eric de Clercq

Department of Human Biology, Division of Microbiology
Rega Institute, University of Leuven
B-3000 Leuven, Belgium

STRUCTURAL REQUIREMENTS

Double-stranded (ds) RNAs surpass all other interferon inducers in activity when assayed on a weight basis. These dsRNAs may be of either synthetic or natural (viral) origin. The fact that synthetic homopolymer pairs such as (I)n.(C)n show as good an interferon response as do their natural counterparts has offered the opportunity to critically assess the structural parameters that govern the induction of interferon by dsRNAs. (I)n.(C)n is the prototype of the synthetic polynucleotide inducers of interferon. The salient characteristics of its structure are the ribose-phosphate backbone on the outside and the cytosine-hypoxanthine base pairs in the interior of the double helix (Fig. 1). The interferon inducing activity of (I)n.(C)n depends on a variety of structural requirements. These structural requirements have been reviewed previously (1-4) and are summarized in Table 1. To act as an interferon inducer, the polynucleotide molecule should contain a double-helical configuration of sufficient length and stability, and be endowed with free hydroxyl groups at C-2' of the sugar moieties and with intact pyrimidine-purine base pairs in the interior of the double helix. For (I)n.(C)n, the prerequisite of strand continuity appears to be more stringent in the (I)n than in the (C)n strand, as clearly established by Carter and his colleagues (5).

A large variety of synthetic polynucleotides have now been compared for their interferon inducing activity in a highly sensitive interferon production system, that is human skin fibroblasts (HSF) "primed" with interferon and "superinduced" with

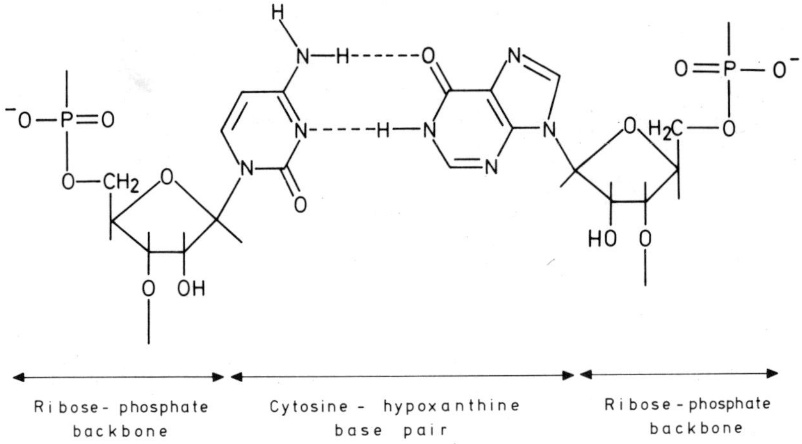

Fig. 1. $(I)_n \cdot (C)_n$ nucleotide pair.

TABLE 1. Interferon Induction by Synthetic Polynucleotides :
Structural Requirements

1. Sufficiently high molecular size (> 4 S for full activity)

2. Double-strandedness, as opposed to either single- or triple-strandedness

3. Sufficiently high thermal stability $\left(T_m > 60° \text{ (in 0.15M Na}^+)\right.$ for full activity$\left.\right)$

4. Adequate, but not necessarily complete, resistance to degradation by nucleases

5. Presence of free 2'-hydroxyl groups in both strands of the double-stranded RNA complex

6. Intact purine-pyrimidine base pairs in the interior of the double helix

metabolic inhibitors (cycloheximide and actinomycin D). To obtain
an interferon response in this "optimized" interferon induction
system, the requirements appear to be less stringent than those
originally established for other systems.

The interferon inducing activity of (I)n.(C)n depends on the
molecular size of its constituent homopolymers. A significant
decrease in interferon induction may be expected if the molecular
size of either (I)n or (C)n falls beneath 4-5 S (1). However, in
HSF cells "primed" with interferon and "superinduced" with metabolic inhibitors, (I)n.(C)n preparations composed of a low molecular weight (I)n (2.5 S) and of a low molecular weight (C)n
(3.1 S) proved almost as effective in inducing interferon as an
(I)n.(C)n preparation composed of a high molecular weight (I)n
(12.5 S) and a high molecular weight (C)n (13.2 S) (Table 2) (6).

To induce interferon, the polynucleotide should be double-
stranded, and not single- or triple-stranded. Since both natural
and synthetic dsRNAs, whether homopolymer pairs such as (I)n.(C)n
or alternating copolymers such as (A-U)n.(A-U)n, are known to
induce interferon formation, it would appear that the exact
nature and sequence of the base pairs has little or no influence
on the interferon inducing capacity of the dsRNA complex (1-4).
Even "pure" (I)n preparations have been obtained which, by virtue
of a "locked-in" double-stranded like configuration, are nearly
as efficient as (I)n.(C)n in inducing interferon in human diploid
cells (Table 2) (7-9). No cytosine residues were detected in the
active (I)n preparations. Hence, the presence of a double-
stranded (I)n.(C)n contaminant in these preparations could be
excluded. Yet, the active (I)n samples partially behaved as a
double RNA helix in that some 1 % of the total sample reacted
with antibody specific for dsRNA (8). The possibility that the
interferon inducing ability of the active (I)n preparations
resided with a subpopulation of dsRNA molecules representing 1 %
of the total population could be eliminated, since the whole (I)n
preparation was found to react poorly with anti-(I)n antiserum.
We have postulated that the interferon inducing (I)n molecules
contain local regions of double-helical configuration which are
recognized by both anti-dsRNA antibody and the cellular receptor
site for interferon induction (8). It would appear, therefore,
that dsRNA molecules need not necessarily to be double-stranded
over their whole length in order to trigger the formation of
interferon.

One may even wonder whether as short a segment as one helical
turn (about 10 base pairs long) would not suffice to elicit an
interferon response. Recently, we have found that the incorporation of a non-complementary (mismatched) base such as U in the
(I)n strand of (I)n.(C)n did not affect the interferon inducing

TABLE 2. Interferon Induction by Synthetic Double-
Stranded Polynucleotides in Human Fibroblast Cells
"Primed" with Interferon and "Superinduced" with
Cycloheximide and Actinomycin D

	Interferon titer[*] ($\log_{10}$ interferon units/ml)
(I)n.(C)n (standard preparation)	4.0
$(I)_{12.5} \cdot (C)_{13.2}$	4.6
$(I)_{12.5} \cdot (C)_{3.1}$	4.5
$(I)_{2.5} \cdot (C)_{13.2}$	4.0
$(I)_{2.5} \cdot (C)_{3.1}$	4.0
(I)n.(br^{5}C)n	4.2
(I)n.(s^{2}C)n	3.7
(dIz)n.(C)n	4.1
(dIcl)n.(C)n	4.0
(A)n.(U)n	4.0
(A)n.(rT)n	4.2
(G)n.(C)n	<1.0
(I_{50},U)n.(C)n	3.9
(I_{10},U)n.(C)n	3.8
(I_2,U)n.(C)n	<1.0
(I)n samples with double-stranded like configuration	up to 4.0
Other (I)n samples	<1.0

* Obtained with a polynucleotide dose of 10 µg/ml.

ability of the latter, provided the ratio of U to I did not exceed
1:10 (Table 2) (10). In interferon induction systems which are
less sensitive than ours (5), the interferon inducing activity of
(Ix,U)n.(C)n may be lost at U/I ratios as low as 1:21 or 1:39. In
contrast with the U residues of (I)n.(Cx,U)n complexes, which
could be accommodated intrahelically, the U residues in (Ix,U)n.
(C)n would be located extrahelically and lead to a helix-with-

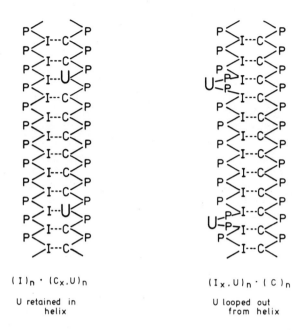

$(I)_n \cdot (C_x.U)_n$ $(I_x.U)_n \cdot (C)_n$

U retained in   U looped out
helix   from helix

Fig. 2. Mismatched $(I)_n \cdot (C)_n$ analogues.

loops structure (Fig. 2) (11-13). Since $(I_x,U).(C)_n$ complexes
with x > 10 retain full interferon inducing activity (in "primed"
and "superinduced" HSF cells : Table 2), one may conclude that
one extrahelical mismatch per ten I residues does not distort the
proper alignment of the double helix and/or that an intact helical
segment of 10 bases (on an average) may contain the necessary
information for recognition by the interferon induction receptor.

If double-strandedness is a prerequisite for interferon
induction, then it follows that the double helix must be intact
under the assay conditions employed. Hence, the thermal stability
(Tm) of the dsRNA complex should be sufficiently high. Experimentally, it has been observed that the most active interferon
inducers have Tm's greater than or equal to 60° (1-4). With a
series of partially thiolated $(I)_n.(C)_n$ analogs, thermal stability
progressively decreased as the degree of thiolation of the
cytosine residues increased, and this decrease in Tm was accompanied by a decrease in antiviral activity (14). For the duplexes
$(A)_n.(br^5U)_n$, $(A)_n.(U)_n$ and $(A)_n.(rT)_n$, the interferon inducing
activity also increased commensurately to their Tm (2→3) values
(45°, 49° and 53°, respectively) (15). Note that the strandwise
(2→3) rearrangement is a factor to be considered only for

duplexes that can form triple helixes. (I)n.(C)n and many of its analogues cannot do so.

In human diploid cells ("primed" with interferon and "super-induced" with metabolic inhibitors), (A)n.(U)n and (A)n.(rT)n equalled (I)n.(C)n in interferon inducing activity (Table 2) (6). (G)n.(C)n, the most stable of all dsRNA complexes $\left(\text{Tm } (2{\to}1) : 136°\right)$, failed to induce any interferon in this system (Table 2). Yet, (G)n.(C)n has been reported to stimulate interferon production in some conditions, viz. in chick embryo cells, in the presence of DEAE-dextran (16,17). As the (G)n.(C)n preparation used in our experiments had been properly purified and characterized (6), the question as to whether (G)n.(C)n is an efficient interferon inducer remains unresolved.

To some extent, the criterion regarding a sufficiently high Tm is reflected by another requirement, that is adequate resistance of the dsRNA to degradation by nucleases. The double-helical RNA should indeed survive premature degradation by extra- and/or intracellular nucleases in order to reach the receptors for interferon induction. Due to extensive "breathing" of the double helix, duplexes with a low Tm are readily attacked by nucleases wherever they present single-stranded sequences. Typical examples of such duplexes which are less stable to heat, and consequently degraded at a faster rate than (I)n.(C)n by the single-strand endonucleases T_1 ribonuclease or pancreatic ribonuclease, are the

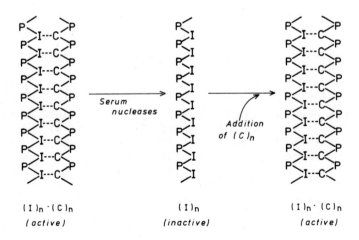

Fig. 3.   Influence of serum nucleases on interferon-inducing activity of $(I)_n \cdot (C)_n$.

copolymers (I)n.(C$_{20}$,G)n and (I)n.(C$_{13}$,G)n (5) and the 2'-modified
RNA complex (dIz)n.(C)n (18). The increased susceptibility of
these dsRNA analogs to degradation by nucleases may not necessarily affect their interferon inducing activity in cell culture but
it may do so in the intact animal (18). On the other hand, increase of nuclease resistance above a certain threshold level may
not improve the compound's in vitro potentials (compare the
interferon inducing activity of (I)n.(br^{5}C)n and (I)n.(s^{2}C)n in
human diploid cells to that of (I)n.(C)n (Table 2)) but may ensure
higher in vivo activity (e.g. in monkeys and humans). Human
serum contains a ribonuclease that specifically degrades the (C)n
strand of (I)n.(C)n (half-life of 1 μg/ml of (I)n.(C)n when
incubated with 50 % human serum at 37° : approximately 3 min)
(19). The resulting product ((I)n) is obviously inactive in
inducing interferon but its activity can be restored completely
upon addition of (C)n (Fig. 3) (19). The resistance of (I)n.(C)n
to hydrolysis by primate serum is markedly increased when (I)n.
(C)n is mixed with poly(L-lysine) and carboxymethylcellulose. The
resulting mixture ("PICLC") proved efficacious in inducing interferon in monkeys under conditions where (I)n.(C)n failed to do so
(20). PICLC has also been shown to protect rhesus monkeys against
simian hemorrhagic fever (21) and to suppress the viral markers
associated with chronic hepatitis B virus infection in chimpanzees (22).

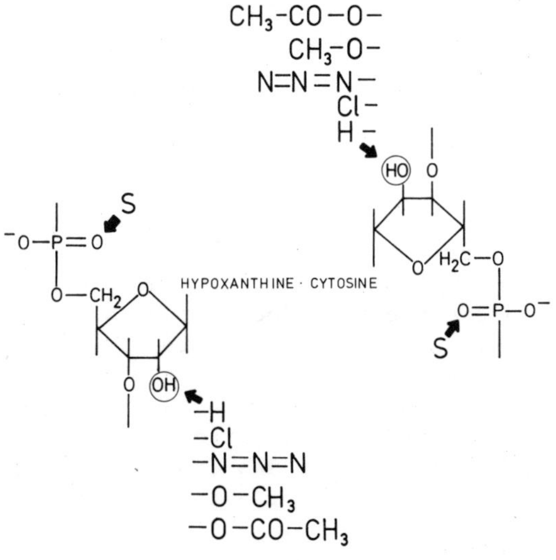

Fig. 4. Chemical modifications of ribose-phosphate moieties
of (I)$_n$·(C)$_n$.

The presence of intact 2'-hydroxyl groups in both strands of
the dsRNA complex has been considered to be an absolute requirement for the interferon inducing ability of synthetic polynucleotides, since various attempts to replace the 2'-OH groups in one
or both strands of (I)n.(C)n or (A)n.(U)n by one or another substituent have invariably produced duplexes with little, if any,
interferon inducing activity (1-4). These modifications included
2'-hydrogen, 2'-chloro-, 2'-azido-, 2'-O-methyl and 2'-O-acetyl
in either the (I)n or the (C)n strand of (I)n.(C)n (Fig. 4).
Whereas most 2'-modified (I)n.(C)n complexes were entirely inactive in inducing interferon (1-4, see also 18,23-25), two particular complexes [(dIz)n.(C)n and (dIcl)n.(C)n in which the 2'-OH
groups of (I)n were replaced by 2'-azido or 2'-chloro, respec-
tively] equalled the parent compound (I)n.(C)n in interferon inducing activity, at least in human diploid cells (Table 2) (18,
23). These results suggest that (i) the presence of free 2'-OH
groups in both strands is not an absolute requirement for the
interferon inducing capacity of dsRNA complexes and that (ii) the
receptor site for interferon induction does not specifically
recognize the 2'-OH groups of the dsRNA molecules but rather the
steric configuration conferred by the presence of these 2'-hydro-
xyls. Apparently, the steric configuration resulting from substitution of 2'-azido or 2'-chloro for 2'-OH in the (I)n strand of
(I)n.(C)n is recognized by the interferon induction receptor.
Since (dIz)n.(C)n and (dIcl)n.(C)n are efficient interferon inducers under conditions were (I)n.(dCz)n and (I)n.(dCcl)n are not
(18,23), it appears as though the (I)n strand is more tolerant to
2'-substitutions than is the (C)n strand. A similar conclusion
has been reached for partially 2'-O-methylated analogues of
(I)n.(C)n (25).

The interferon inducing capacity of dsRNAs also depends on
the nature of the heterocyclic bases in the interior of the double
helix. Substitution of CH for N-1, N-3, N-7 or N-9 and substitution of N for CH-2 in the purine ring of (I)n.(C)n (Fig. 5) led
to a significant, if not complete, reduction of interferon inducing activity (26-30). For some of these analogues [e.g. (aza^{2}I)n.
(C)n], the lack of activity may seem related to the low Tm of the
complex (30), but this contention does not hold for most other
complexes; e.g. (L)n.(br^{5}C)n failed to stimulate interferon production, despite its high Tm (72°) (27). Of all modifications
carried out at the purine ring, substitution of CH for N-7 proved
to be the least deleterious. The resulting (c^{7}I)n.(C)n was still
effective as an interferon inducer and its activity could be
further increased by introduction of a bromine at C-5 of the
pyrimidine strand (26,28).

In contrast with the purine modifications referred to above,
two pyrimidine modifications, that is, substitution of bromine at

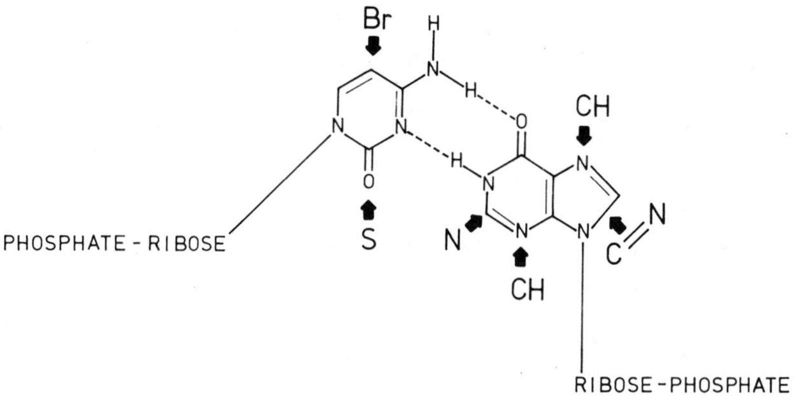

Fig. 5. Chemical modifications of base moieties of $(I)_n \cdot (C)_n$.

C-5 (26,28) and substitution of sulfur at C-2 (31) (Fig. 5), did
not markedly disturb the interferon inducing capacity of
(I)n.(C)n. The resulting (I)n.(br^{5}C)n and (I)n.(s^{2}C)n proved as
effective as (I)n.(C)n in inducing interferon in human fibroblast
cell cultures (Table 2). Both complexes also fulfilled the
necessary requirements for interferon induction in the sense that
they were even more thermostable and more resistant to hydrolysis
by nucleases than their parent compound (I)n.(C)n (26,31).

    For the development of a polynucleotide inducer having
greater therapeutic efficacy than (I)n.(C)n, two different strategies could be followed (Table 3). First, one may take full advantage of the structural requirements that underlie the interferon inducing activity of polynucleotides, and construct a duplex
with perfectly matched base pairs, maximal molecular size,
supreme resistance to enzymatic breakdown, etc. Typical examples
of such approach are (I)n.(s^{2}C)n, (I)n.(br^{5}C)n and "PICLC"
[(I)n.(C)n + poly(L-lysine) + carboxymethylcellulose]. Whether
these nuclease-resistant congeners of (I)n.(C)n offer any advantage (e.g. an increased therapeutic index) over (I)n.(C)n, remains
to be seen. By virtue of their increased resistance to enzymatic
degradation, complexes such as (I)n.(s^{2}C)n, (I)n.(br^{5}C)n and
"PICLC" may be expected to persist longer in biological fluids
than (I)n.(C)n, thus having greater probability of eliciting toxic

TABLE 3. Strategies in the Development of New (I)n.(C)n
Analogues of Greater Interferon Inducing Efficacy

Approach 1 : <u>(I)n.(C)n analogues with increased resistance to
degradation by nucleases</u>

  Examples :   - (I)n.(br^{5}C)n
                    - (I)n.(s^{2}C)n
                    - (I)n.(C)n + poly(L-lysine) + carboxy-
                          methylcellulose

Approach 2 : <u>(I)n.(C)n analogues with decreased resistance to
degradation by nucleases</u>

  Examples :   - mismatched (I)n.(C)n analogues : e.g.
                        (I)n.(Cx,U)n or (Ix,U)n.(C)n
                    - 2'-modified (I)n.(C)n analogues : e.g.
                        (dIz)n.(C)n
                    - (I)n derivatives with a double-stranded
                        like configuration

---

side effects. A second approach for designing polynucleotide
inducers of interferon which are superior to (I)n.(C)n rests upon
the premise that the kinetics for the induction of interferon and
the kinetics for the induction of the other, undesirable, biologic
effects may not be identical (32,33). On this basis, polynucleotides could be developed which would persist long enough in
biological fluids so as to permit the induction of interferon but
would not persist so long as to elicit any toxic side effects.
Mismatched analogues of (I)n.(C)n such as (I)n.(C$_{13}$,U)n and
(I)n.(C$_{20}$,G)n (5,32,33) and some other (I)n.(C)n analogues such
as (dIz)n.(C)n (18), and some (I)n derivatives with a "locked-
in" double-stranded like configuration appear to at least partially fulfil the conditions of the second approach. The mismatched (I)n.(C)n analogues, while comparable in their interferon
inducing properties to (I)n.(C)n, showed indeed less pronounced
secondary effects (32,33). To the extent, however, that prophylaxis or therapy with interferon inducers requires the maintenance
of a high plasma interferon level, these "self-destructive"
(I)n.(C)n analogues may not be ideal since they would have to be
administered repeatedly, hereby defeating the purpose of their
short plasma half-life.

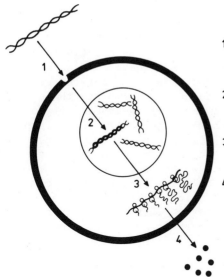

1. Interaction of $(I)_n \cdot (C)_n$ with cellular receptor site, presumably located at outer cell membrane.

2. Transfer of message from the outer cell membrane to the genome. Derepression of the interferon gene.

3. Transcription and translation of the interferon mRNA.

4. Post-translational modification and release of the interferon molecules.

Fig. 6. Interferon induction by $(I)_n \cdot (C)_n$.

MECHANISM OF INTERFERON INDUCTION

Very schematically, the process of interferon induction by synthetic polynucleotides could be divided into four parts (Fig. 6) (2,4), the first step being the interaction of the inducer with a specific cellular receptor site, presumably located at the cell's outer membrane. This interaction would generate a message which would be transmitted into the interior of the cell, leading to a derepression of the interferon gene, transcription, translation of the interferon mRNA into the interferon protein, and, eventually, glycosylation and secretion of the interferon molecule. There is circumstantial evidence for all these steps, except the second one (transfer of the message from the receptor site to the cellular genome).

Although the mechanism of interferon induction as depicted in Figure 6 accommodates most, if not all, established facts on the interferon induction process, some alternative hypotheses have been proposed. Ng and Vilcek (34) suggested that the interferon inducer $[(I)n.(C)n]$ may bind directly to a repressor of interferon mRNA, thus freeing the interferon mRNA for translation. According to De Maeyer-Guignard et al. (35), interferon might

even serve as its own receptor and/or repressor. Guided by the
specific binding of (mouse) interferon to some polynucleotides
((I)n and (U)n), De Maeyer-Guignard et al. speculated that all
cells would be able to synthesize interferon constitutively and
that the appearance in the cell of some RNA sequences (such as
(U)n and (I)n) that bind to interferon, would prevent the latter
from exerting its normal function, and hence stimulate the cell
to synthesize more interferon. This interesting hypothesis does
of course not explain why only double-stranded RNAs (e.g. (A)n.
(U)n) and not single-stranded RNAs (e.g. (U)n) or triple-stranded
complexes (e.g. (A)n.2(U)n) act as interferon inducers. If the
induction of interferon only depends on the appearance of (U)n
sequences in the cell, one may expect all (U)n-containing complexes, whether single-, double- or triple-stranded, to be
equally effective in inducing interferon. This is clearly not the
case (15,36). To account for the selectivity of (A)n.(U)n as an
interferon inducer (as opposed to (U)n and (A)n.2(U)n) one may
assume that there exist an additional receptor, which specifically recognizes the double-stranded RNA configuration and which
determines which (U)n (or (I)n)-containing complexes are further
processed for interferon induction and which are not. The latter
possibility would obviously fit in well with the scheme of
interferon induction presented in Figure 6.

Since antibodies to dsRNA recognize many of the structural
features that are responsible for the interferon inducing capacity
of dsRNAs, it has been postulated that the cellular receptor site
for polynucleotide inducers of interferon may be protein in
nature (37). Is this (putative) receptor site located at the outside of the cell or inside the cell ? Previous studies with
(I)n.(C)n covalently coupled to insoluble supports (sepharose
(38-40), cellulose, sephadex (41) or cellophane (42)) suggested
that the receptor site for interferon induction by (I)n.(C)n may
be located at the cell surface. However, with all insolubilized
(I)n.(C)n preparations employed so far one observes considerable
leakage of polynucleotide material from the matrix into the
surrounding medium during incubation of the matrix-bound (I)n.(C)n
with the cells. This leakage precludes an unequivocal answer to
the question as to whether penetration of the polynucleotide into
the cell is not required for the induction of interferon.

Some recent observations indicate that (I)n.(C)n may in fact
be able to trigger an interferon response without penetrating into
the cell (43). With a particular sepharose-coupled (I)n.(C)n preparation, no uptake of (I)n.(C)n material by the cells could be
witnessed, even after a 4-hour incubation period of the cells with
the immobilized (I)n.(C)n (Fig. 7). Under the same conditions,
free (I)n.(C)n became gradually associated with the PRK (primary
rabbit kidney) cells (Fig. 7). In these cells, equivalent inter-

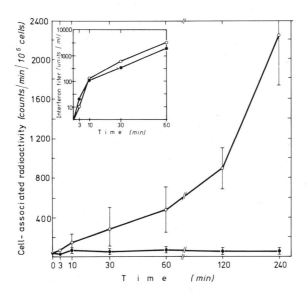

Fig. 7.   Interferon induction by and cellular uptake of free
          $(I)_n \cdot [^{14}C](C)_n$ (o) and sepharose-bound $(I)_n \cdot [^{14}C](C)_n$
          (•) upon different times of exposure of PRK cells to
          the polynucleotide (at 1 µg/ml).

feron titers were obtained with the uncoupled and sepharose-
coupled (I)n.(C)n, as shown in Figure 7 (inset).

     After the receptor has been triggered by the interferon
inducer, a signal is transmitted to the cellular genome and, as
a result, the interferon gene is switched on (Fig. 6). Direct
evidence for this stage of the interferon induction process is
lacking. The fact is that within 2 hours after exposure of the
cells to (I)n.(C)n most of the interferon mRNA has been transcribed (44). Indirect evidence for the existence of interferon
mRNA stemmed from studies with metabolic inhibitors (actinomycin
D, cycloheximide) (45). Direct proof for the existence of interferon mRNA was first provided by De Maeyer and his colleagues
(46,47) who demonstrated that mRNA extracted from mouse cells
which had been induced by NDV (Newcastle disease virus) or
(I)n.(C)n, could be translated into mouse interferon in heterologous (chick embryo) cells. Later on, the translation of mouse
interferon mRNA has also been described in various other recipient
cells (e.g. VERO and HeLa cells (48)) as well as Xenopus laevis
oocytes (49) and cell-free protein synthesis systems (wheat germ
extract (50) and rabbit reticulocyte lysates (49)). Similarly,
translation of human interferon mRNA (extracted from human fibro-

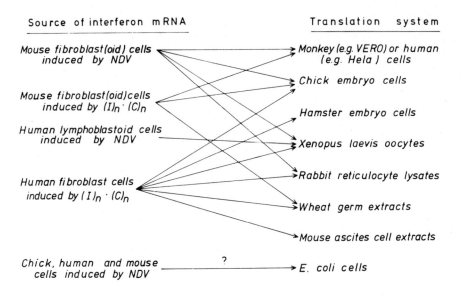

Source of interferon mRNA

Mouse fibroblast(oid) cells induced by NDV

Mouse fibroblast(oid) cells induced by $(I)_n \cdot (C)_n$

Human lymphoblastoid cells induced by NDV

Human fibroblast cells induced by $(I)_n \cdot (C)_n$

Chick, human and mouse cells induced by NDV

Translation system

Monkey (e.g. VERO) or human (e.g. Hela) cells

Chick embryo cells

Hamster embryo cells

Xenopus laevis oocytes

Rabbit reticulocyte lysates

Wheat germ extracts

Mouse ascites cell extracts

E. coli cells

Fig. 8.   Translation of interferon mRNA in heterologous cell
          systems.

blast cells induced with $(I)n.(C)n$] has been obtained in chick
embryo cells (51), hamster embryo cells (52), Xenopus laevis
oocytes (53-57), rabbit reticulocyte lysates (53), wheat germ
extracts (54) and mouse ascites cell extracts (53,58). Quite
surprisingly, intact bacterial cells would also be able to trans-
late mouse, human and chick interferon mRNA (59).

A synopsis of the protein synthesis systems which have been
employed for the translation of heterologous interferon mRNA is
presented in Figure 8. In no instance, interferon mRNA was detected in non-induced cells. In some conditions, even two forms of
interferon mRNA were detected, for example for the RNA extracted
from mouse fibroblastoid (C-243) cells induced with NDV (47) and
for the RNA extracted from human lymphoblastoid (Namalva) cells
induced with NDV (56). Based on the translation products obtained
in Xenopus laevis oocytes, Cavalieri et al. (56) concluded that
human cells may contain (at least) two structural genes for
interferon : fibroblasts would only synthesize one species of
interferon; lymphoblastoid cells would synthesize both species of
interferon.

For the interferon mRNA extracted from NDV-induced L-929
cells, a rather sharp sedimentation profile was obtained when the
total cytoplasmic RNA was analyzed in a formamide-sucrose gradient

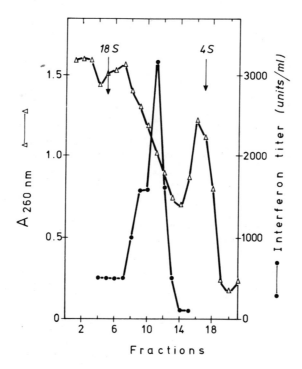

Fig. 9.   Sucrose gradient analysis of mouse interferon mRNA
          extracted from NDV-induced L cells.

(Fig. 9) (49). The mouse interferon mRNA sedimented at approximately 11 S, as may have been expected from a messenger that codes
for a 20,000 dalton protein. A similar sedimentation pattern has
recently been observed for human interferon mRNA extracted from
human fibroblasts induced with (I)n.(C)n (R.Derynck, W.Fiers,
J.Content & E.De Clercq, unpublished data).

    The Xenopus laevis oocyte system permits a direct quantita-
tion of functional interferon mRNA (49,55,56). Hence, the Xenopus
system may be employed to monitor the levels of interferon mRNA
at different stages of the interferon induction process. When
compared to the amounts of interferon that are actually produced
by the intact cells, interferon mRNA measurements may provide a
better insight in the mechanism by which the cell regulates
interferon synthesis. In human fibroblasts exposed to (I)n.(C)n,
interferon production becomes detectable by 1 hour, rises to a
peak by 3 hours and is shut off by 6-8 hours (44) (Fig. 10). This
rapid cessation of interferon production can be prevented by the

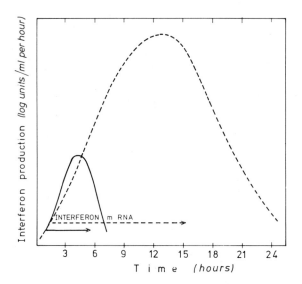

Fig. 10.   Interferon production and interferon mRNA activity
            in human fibroblast cells induced by $(I)_n \cdot (C)_n$,
            in the presence (---) or absence (——) of metabolic
            inhibitors (idealized).

judicious treatment of the cells with inhibitors of RNA and/or
protein synthesis (e.g. actinomycin D, 5,6-dichloro-1-β-D-ribo-
furanosylbenzimidazole and cycloheximide) (44,45,60-62). As a
result, interferon production is increased and prolonged ("superinduction") (Fig. 10). The shut-off of interferon production may
be due to a repressor protein induced coordinately with interferon. According to Sehgal and Tamm (62), this repressor would
inactivate interferon mRNA in an irreversible manner. In the
presence of the appropriate metabolic inhibitor (at the proper
dosage and time) no repressor would be synthesized and the interferon mRNA would remain functional for a much longer time (15
hours, as compared to 3 hours in the absence of metabolic inhibitors) (61) (Fig. 10). The recent findings of Cavalieri et al. (57)
seem to support the latter contention. They found that on induction with (I)n.(C)n human fibroblasts accumulated interferon mRNA
for 1-1.5 hours after which time the mRNA was rapidly degraded.
Treatment of the cells with cycloheximide prolonged the period of
accumulation to 3 hours and decreased the rate of mRNA inactivation, and treatment with actinomycin D decreased the rate of
inactivation still further (57). Thus, the increased interferon
titers obtained in "superinduced" cells may be entirely explained
in terms of the amounts of functional interferon mRNA available
(55).

Most interferons, viz. these interferons that are derived
from fibroblast(oid) cell cultures, can be considered as glycoproteins (63,64). Thus, the interferon protein should be glycosylated before it is released by the cell. In fact, the synthesis
of biologically active human fibroblast interferon is suppressed
by two inhibitors of glycosylation, 2-deoxy-D-glucose and D-
glucosamine (65), and the interferon synthesized in the presence
of partially inhibitory concentrations of 2-deoxy-D-glucose or
D-glucosamine has a molecular weight of 16,000 (as compared to
20,000 for the regular human fibroblast interferon) (66). From
these data, Havell et al. (66) concluded that the carbohydrate
moiety would account for at least 20 % of the total molecular
weight of human fibroblast interferon. The role of the carbohydrate moiety of interferons remains obscure. For mouse fibroblastoid interferon, an intact carbohydrate portion may not be
required for biological activity, as fully active mouse interferon
is synthesized in cell-free systems (e.g. rabbit reticulocyte
lysates) which do not permit glycosylation (49). By electrophoresis on sodium dodecyl sulphate-polyacrylamide gel two polypeptide
bands were obtained for mouse interferon, migrating at molecular
weights 35,000 and 22,000, respectively. Both had antiviral
activity, but only the 35,000 molecular weight band stained with
periodic acid-Schiff (PAS) (64). Hence, the 22,000 molecular
weight component may be considered as a "pure" polypeptide; possibly it would correspond to the deglycosylated part of the
35,000 molecular weight component. Whether the carbohydrate portion of human fibroblast interferon is also of minor importance,
is not as yet clear. Human fibroblast interferon mRNA is translated with high efficiency in Xenopus laevis oocytes (53-57).
However, the oocytes may accomplish the necessary post-translational modifications, including glycosylation. In cell-free
systems which do not perform glycosylation (or other post-translational modifications), human fibroblast interferon is synthesized at a much lower efficiency, or not at all (53-55,58, and
R.Derynck, W.Fiers, J.Content & E.De Clercq, unpublished data).
Thus, for human fibroblast interferon proper glycosylation (or
other post-translational modifications) may indeed be required to
endow the interferon molecule with maximal biologic activity.

The demonstration of interferon mRNA activity in cells induced with either virus or dsRNA undoubtedly represents a major
breakthrough in the current research concerning the mechanism of
interferon induction. Since interferon mRNA directs the synthesis
of biologically active interferon in a number of heterologous
cell systems (e.g. Xenopus laevis oocytes) as well as cell-free
extracts (e.g. rabbit reticulocyte lysates), measurements of
interferon mRNA activity could be considered as a useful tool to
identify some of the regulatory events involved in the expression
of the interferon gene. By monitoring interferon synthesis in

heterologous translation systems it may also be possible to
determine the post-translational modifications that are needed to
generate a fully active product. Furthermore, if the interferon
mRNA can be obtained in a sufficiently pure form, one may appeal
to cell-free translation systems to prepare a highly specific
radiolabelled interferon, or even envisage the transcription of
interferon mRNA to cDNA. Whereas the radiolabelled interferon
preparations may prove useful to investigate the interaction of
interferon with the cell, the interferon cDNA may be employed in
DNA recombinant studies, aimed at cloning the interferon gene in
bacterial systems.

Acknowledgments. The original investigations reported herein
were supported by grants from the F.G.W.O. (Fonds voor Geneeskun-
dig Wetenschappelijk Onderzoek), Krediet nr. 3.0048.75 and the
Geconcerteerde Onderzoeksacties, Conventie nr. 76/81-IV. The
editorial assistance of Janine Putzeys is gratefully acknowledged.

Abbreviations. (A)n, polyadenylic acid; (U)n, polyuridylic
acid; (C)n, polycytidylic acid; (G)n, polyguanylic acid; (I)n,
polyinosinic acid; (rT)n, poly(ribo)thymidylic acid; (br^{5}U)n,
poly(5-bromouridylic acid); (br^{5}C)n, poly(5-bromocytidylic acid);
(s^{2}C)n, poly(2-thiocytidylic acid); (I)$_{12.5}$, (I)n with a sedimentation value (s$_{20,w}$) of 12.5 S; (I)$_{2.5}$, (I)n with s$_{20,w}$ = 2.5 S;
(C)$_{13.2}$, (C)n with s$_{20,w}$ = 13.2 S; (C)$_{3.1}$, (C)n with s$_{20,w}$ = 3.1 S;
(Ix,U)n, copolymer of inosinic acid and uridylic acid, with I/U =
x; (Cx,U)n, copolymer of cytidylic acid and uridylic acid, with
C/U = x; (C$_{13}$,U)n, copolymer of cytidylic acid and uridylic acid,
with C/U = 13; (C$_{20}$,G)n, copolymer of cytidylic acid and guanylic
acid, with C/G = 20; (c^{7}I)n, poly(7-deazainosinic acid); (L)n,
polylaurusin (= polyformycin B); (aza^{2}I)n, poly(2-azainosinic
acid); (dCz)n, poly(2'-azido-2'-deoxycytidylic acid); (dCcl)n,
poly(2'-chloro-2'-deoxycytidylic acid); (dIz)n, poly(2'-azido-2'-
deoxyinosinic acid); (dIcl)n, poly(2'-chloro-2'-deoxyinosinic
acid); (A-U)n.(A-U)n, alternating copolymer of adenylic acid and
uridylic acid; ds, double-stranded; PRK, primary rabbit kidney;
HSF, human skin fibroblst; Tm, melting temperature (at the mid-
point of the absorbancy change). Noncovalent associations are
indicated by a central dot, for example (I)n.(C)n.

REFERENCES

1. De Clercq, E. (1974) Topics in Current Chemistry, _52_, 173-
    208.
2. De Clercq, E. (1977) _In_ Structure and Properties of Biopoly-
    mers, Proceedings of the First Cleveland Symposium on Macro-
    molecules (A.G.Walton, ed.) Elsevier Scientific Publishing
    Company, Amsterdam, pp. 217-243.

3. De Clercq, E. (1977) Texas Rep. Biol. Med., 35, in press.
4. Torrence, P.F. and De Clercq, E. (1977) Pharmacol. Therapeutics, part A, 2, 1-88.
5. Carter, W.A., Pitha, P.M., Marshall, L.W., Tazawa, I., Tazawa, S. and Ts'o, P.O.P. (1972) J. Mol. Biol., 70, 567-587.
6. De Clercq, E. and Torrence, P.F. (1977) J. Gen. Virol., 37, 619-623.
7. Thang, M.N., Bachner, L., De Clercq, E. and Stollar, B.D. (1977) FEBS Letters, 76, 159-165.
8. Stollar, B.D., De Clercq, E., Drocourt, J.L. and Thang, M.N. (1978) Eur. J. Biochem., in press.
9. De Clercq, E., Stollar, B.D. and Thang, M.N. (1978) J. Gen. Virol., in press.
10. Torrence, P.F. and De Clercq, E. (1978) To be published.
11. Wang, A.C. and Kallenbach, N.R. (1971) J. Mol. Biol., 62, 591-611.
12. Lomant, A.J. and Fresco, J.R. (1975). Progr. Nucleic Acid Res. Mol. Biol., 15, 185-218.
13. Topal, M.D. and Fresco, J.R. (1976) Nature, 263, 285-289.
14. O'Malley, J.A., Ho, Y.K., Chakrabarti, P., DiBerardino, L., Chandra, P., Orinda, D.A.O., Byrd, D.M., Bardos, T.J. and Carter, W.A. (1975) Molec. Pharmacol., 11, 61-69.
15. De Clercq, E., Torrence, P.F. and Witkop, B. (1974) Proc. Nat. Acad. Sci. USA, 71, 182-186.
16. Colby, C. and Chamberlin, M.J. (1969) Proc. Nat. Acad. Sci. USA, 63, 160-167.
17. Novokhatsky, A.S., Ershov, F.I., Timkovsky, A.L., Bresler, S.E., Kogan, E.M. and Tikhomirova-Sidorova, N.S. (1975) Acta Virol., 19, 121-129.
18. De Clercq, E., Torrence, P.F., Stollar, B.D., Hobbs, J., Fukui, T., Kakiuchi, N. and Ikehara, M. (1978) Submitted for publication.
19. De Clercq, E. (1978) To be published.
20. Levy, H.B., Baer, G., Baron, S., Buckler, C.E., Gibbs, C.J., Iadarola, M.J., London, W.T. and Rice, J. (1975) J. Infect. Dis., 132, 434-439.
21. Levy, H.B., London, W., Fuccillo, D.A., Baron, S. and Rice, J. (1976) J. Infect. Dis., 133 (suppl.), A256-A259.
22. Purcell, R.H., Gerin, J.L., London, W.T., Wagner, J.A., McAuliffe, V.J., Popper, H., Palmer, A.E., Lvovsky, E., Kaplan, P.M., Wong, D.C. and Levy, H.B. (1976) Lancet, ii, 757-761.
23. De Clercq, E., Hobbs, J., Torrence, P.F. and Ikehara, M. (1978) To be published.
24. Hutchinson, D.W., Johnston, M.D. and Eaton, M.A.W. (1974) J. Gen. Virol., 23, 331-333.
25. Merigan, T.C. and Rottman, F. (1974) Virology, 60, 297-301.

26. Torrence, P.F., De Clercq, E., Waters, J.A. and Witkop, B.
     (1974) Biochemistry, 13, 4400-4408.
27. Torrence, P.F., De Clercq, E., Waters, J.A. and Witkop, B.
     (1975) Biochem. Biophys. Res. Commun., 62, 658-664.
28. De Clercq, E., Edy, V.G., Torrence, P.F., Waters, J.A. and
     Witkop, B. (1976) Molec. Pharmacol., 12, 1045-1051.
29. De Clercq, E., Torrence, P.F., Fukui, T. and Ikehara, M.
     (1976) Nucleic Acids Res., 3, 1591-1601.
30. De Clercq, E., Huang, G.-F., Torrence, P.F., Fukui, T.,
     Kakiuchi, N. and Ikehara, M. (1977) Nucleic Acids Res., 4,
     3643-3653.
31. Reuss, K., Scheit, K.-H. and Saiko, O. (1976) Nucleic Acids
     Res., 3, 2861-2875.
32. Ts'o, P.O.P., Alderfer, J.L., Levy, J., Marshall, L.W.,
     O'Malley, J., Horoszewicz, J.S. and Carter, W.A. (1976)
     Molec. Pharmacol., 12, 299-312.
33. Carter, W.A., O'Malley, J., Beeson, M., Cunnington, P.,
     Kelvin, A., Vere-Hodge, A., Alderfer, J.L. and Ts'o, P.O.P.
     (1976) Molec. Pharmacol., 12, 440-453.
34. Ng, M.H. and Vilcek, J. (1972) Adv. Protein Chem., 26, 173-
     241.
35. De Maeyer-Guignard, J., Thang, M.N. and De Maeyer, E. (1977)
     Proc. Nat. Acad. Sci. USA, 74, 3787-3790.
36. Torrence, P.F., De Clercq, E. and Witkop, B. (1976)
     Biochemistry, 15, 724-734.
37. Johnston, M.I., Stollar, B.D., Torrence, P.F. and Witkop, B.
     (1975) Proc. Nat. Acad. Sci. USA, 72, 4564-4568.
38. Wagner, A.R., Bugianesi, R.L. and Shen, T.Y. (1971) Biochem.
     Biophys. Res. Commun., 45, 184-189.
39. Taylor-Papadimitriou, J. and Kallos, J. (1973) Nature, New
     Biol., 245, 143-144.
40. Bachner, L., De Clercq, E. and Thang, M.N. (1975) Biochem.
     Biophys. Res. Commun., 63, 476-483.
41. Pitha, P.M. and Pitha, J. (1973) J. Gen. Virol., 21, 31-37.
42. Hutchinson, D.W. and Merigan, T.C. (1975) J. Gen. Virol.,
     27, 403-407.
43. De Clercq, E. and Thang, M.N. (1978) To be published.
44. Vilcek, J. and Havell, E.A. (1973) Proc. Nat. Acad. Sci.
     USA, 70, 3909-3913.
45. Vilcek, J. (1970) Ann. N.Y. Acad. Sci., 173, 390-403.
46. De Maeyer-Guignard, J., De Maeyer, E. and Montagnier, L.
     (1972) Proc. Nat. Acad. Sci. USA, 69, 1203-1207.
47. Montagnier, L., Collandre, H., De Maeyer-Guignard, J. and
     De Maeyer, E. (1974) Biochem. Biophys. Res. Commun., 59,
     1031-1038.
48. Kronenberg, L.H. and Friedmann, T. (1975) J. Gen. Virol.,
     27, 225-238.
49. Lebleu, B., Hubert, E., Content, J., De Wit, L., Braude, I.A.
     and De Clercq, E. (1978) Submitted for publication.

50. Thang, M.N., Thang, D.C., De Maeyer, E. and Montagnier, L. (1975) Proc. Nat. Acad. Sci. USA, 72, 3975-3977.

51. Reynolds Jr., F.H. and Pitha, P.M. (1974) Biochem. Biophys. Res. Commun., 59, 1023-1030.

52. Greene, J.J., Dieffenbach, C.W. and Ts'o, P.O.P. (1978) Nature, 271, 81-83.

53. Reynolds Jr., F.H., Premkumar, E. and Pitha, P.M. (1975) Proc. Nat. Acad. Sci. USA, 72, 4881-4885.

54. Raj, N.B.K. and Pitha, P.M. (1977) Proc. Nat. Acad. Sci. USA, 74, 1483-1487.

55. Sehgal, P.B., Dobberstein, B. and Tamm, I. (1977). Proc. Nat. Acad. Sci. USA, 74, 3409-3413.

56. Cavalieri, R.L., Havell, E.A., Vilcek, J. and Pestka, S. (1977) Proc. Nat. Acad. Sci. USA, 74, 3287-3291.

57. Cavalieri, R.L., Havell, E.A., Vilcek, J. and Pestka, S. (1977) Proc. Nat. Acad. Sci. USA, 74, 4415-4419.

58. Pestka, S., McInnes, J., Havell, E.A. and Vilcek, J. (1975) Proc. Nat. Acad. Sci. USA, 72, 3898-3901.

59. Orlova, T.G., Kognovitskaya, A.I., Georgadze, I.I. and Soloviev, V.D. (1977) Acta Virol., 21, 353-358.

60. Sehgal, P.B., Tamm, I. and Vilcek, J. (1975) Science, 190, 282-284.

61. Sehgal, P.B., Tamm, I. and Vilcek, J. (1976) Virology, 70, 532-541.

62. Sehgal, P.B. and Tamm, I. (1976) Proc. Nat. Acad. Sci. USA, 73, 1621-1625.

63. Davey, M.W., Sulkowski, E. and Carter, W.A. (1976) Biochemistry, 15, 704-713.

64. De Maeyer-Guignard, J., Tovey, M.G., Gresser, I. and De Maeyer, E. (1978) Nature, 271, 622-625.

65. Havell, E.A., Vilcek, J., Falcoff, E. and Berman, B. (1975) Virology, 63, 475-483.

66. Havell, E.A., Yamazaki, S. and Vilcek, J. (1977) J. Biol. Chem., 252, 4425-4427.

HUMAN FIBROBLAST INTERFERON IN THE CONTROL OF NEOPLASIA

W.A. Carter, S.S. Leong and J.S. Horoszewicz

Medical Viral Oncology, Roswell Park Memorial Institute

666 Elm Street, Buffalo, New York   14263

Mammalian interferons are naturally occurring proteins whose most widely recognized function is antiviral activity (1). This mechanism of action is through selective blockage in the translation of viral messengers (2) and possibly also through inhibition of viral transcription (3). The antiproliferative (4) and immuno-modulatory (5,6) activities of interferons have also been demonstrated. As a cell regulatory macromolecule, interferon can modulate macrophage function, as shown by the enhancement of phagocytic activity of macrophages in murine in vitro and in vivo systems (7). However, the crude biologic preparations available usually contain many other mediators, thus making it difficult to arrive at firm conclusions regarding pharmacologic action.

Therefore, in our studies of the possible clinical efficacy of human interferon, it was necessary to first establish a large-scale purification facility. Human fibroblast interferon (HFIF) is a glycoprotein and, like the interferons from lower mammals, we have observed that this protein has antiproliferative (8) and immunomodulatory (9), as well as antiviral, activities. We describe herein the recent development of a large-scale production-purification facility for the purpose of obtaining sufficient quantities of purified and safety tested human fibroblast interferon for clinical investigation. Each of these 3 biological functions (inhibition of viral and cell growth, immunomodulation) is being evaluated in our patients with various neoplastic diseases. Certain human tumors apparently have a preferential sensitivity to the antiproliferative effect of HFIF.

The patient with neoplastic disease may possess, in addition to his tumor, a variety of immunologic lesions as well as a predeliction for viral infections. Thus, each of the 3 biological functions of HFIF might favorably alter either the primary neoplastic disease or some of its serious secondary effects.

(1) LARGE-SCALE PRODUCTION OF HUMAN FIBROBLAST INTERFERON HFIF

Mass production of HFIF from human foreskin fibroblasts for clinical investigation was initiated in our laboratories in the spring of 1976. The interferon is "superinduced" by treating the cells with $rI_n \cdot rC_n$, actinomycin D and cycloheximide. Since May 1977, we have been producing up to 10^9 reference units of crude HFIF per month (see Fig. 1). The detailed description of our methods to produce HFIF, characterization of the isolated cell strains, as well as our overall quality control scheme, are provided in a recent publication (10).

Several cell strains for HFIF production have been established in our laboratory and ample stocks of cells at 6th passage levels are kept frozen in liquid nitrogen (90-100 ampules with 2×10^6 cells per cell strain). A total of 12 cell strains which meet the U.S. Food and Drug Administration (F.D.A.) requirements are available in our cell bank and are ready to be used for large-scale production of HFIF. Our calculations indicate that the size of our cell stock should provide an adequate supply for full-scale operation at the present level for many years to come.

Twelve strains of human fibroblasts (derived from the foreskins of normal 3 day old males) are elaborating, on the average, 26-30,000 reference units of interferon per ml of harvested medium. Properties of these cell strains are typical of normal diploid human fibroblasts. Namely, they have fibroblast morphology, are fully contact inhibited, and produce smooth and uniform monolayers; the saturation density on minimal Eagle's medium (MEM) + 10% fetal calf serum is $6-7 \times 10^4$ cells/cm^2. The in vitro life span of these cells is between 55 and 67 population doublings. Karyotypic analysis indicates that the distribution of the chromosome number is normal diploid for human male karyotype, i.e., 46, XY. These cell strains are free of detectable adventitious agents such as viruses, mycoplasma, bacteria and fungi.

Use of the best strain of foreskin fibroblasts available assures us of maxium yields of HFIF with the highest efficiency. Further improvements for increasing HFIF yield in the superinduced cell cultures, to reduce cost, such as double harvesting, modification of production medium, superinduction procedures, etc., are being regularly introduced.

For large-scale interferon production, every ten weeks one fresh ampule of cell seed stock is removed from liquid nitrogen storage tanks and propagated by 2:1 (twice a week) subcultures up to the 18th passage level, when sufficient numbers of cells become available to form monolayer cultures in 128 large roller bottles (1585 cm^2 growth

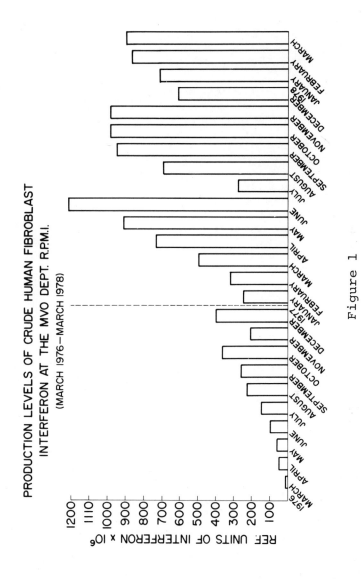

Figure 1

area). From this time on, for the next twelve weeks, interferon production takes place (4X a week the contents of sixteen bottles are
induced). Also, 4X a week, cells from sixteen bottles are subcul-
tured (2:1) in order to maintain a constant number of vessels with
approximately 1×10^8 cells which are 7 days old and suitable for interferon "superinduction". The cells are phased out of production
between the 30th and 33rd passage (population doubling level). At
this time, a cell stock newly built up, at the 18th passage level,
enters the clinical production cycle.

Confluent monolayer cultures in roller bottles are "superinduced" (11,12) as follows: the culture medium in each bottle is aspirated and 100 ml of MEM containing 75 µg/ml of $rIn \cdot rCn$ and 60 µg/ml
of cycloheximide is added per bottle. The cultures are rolled for
220 mins at 34°C prior to the addition of actinomycin D to a final
concentration of 0.75 µg/ml. After 110 mins, the induction medium is
removed and cells are washed three times with 200 ml of pre-warmed
Eagle's balanced salt solution (EBSS). Next, the production medium
(MEM plus 5% heat inactivated human or fetal bovine serum) is added
(100 ml), and cultures are incubated for an additional 22 hrs at
34°C. At this time, the cell culture medium containing interferon is
harvested, pooled, centrifuged and frozen at -90°C. The average yield
of the crude HFIF is approximately 30,000 international reference
units/ml of harvested medium. Interferon titers are expressed in
reference units/ml (ref. U according to standard G-023-901-527,
Research Resources Branch, NIH).

(2) LARGE-SCALE PURIFICATION OF HFIF

Purification of large amounts of HFIF involves utilization of
concanavalin A-Sepharose (13,14) and Phenyl-Sepharose CL-4B column
chromatography (15). A crude preparation of 5 to 7 liters (weekly
production output) of HFIF is charged simultaneously on a battery
of Con-A columns (1.6 x 10 cm) previously equilibrated in 0.02 M
phosphate buffer, pH 7.4, containing 0.15 M NaCl. The HFIF is
bound to the matrix of the column together with some contaminating
glycoproteins by means of carbohydrate recogniation and hydrophobic
interaction. Over 90% of the total proteins pass through in the
breakthrough fraction. After the material is applied, the column is
washed with PBS (0.02 M phosphate buffer, 0.15 M NaCl, pH 7.4), followed by elution with 0.1 M α-methyl-d-mannoside (α-MM) which removes
most of the glycoproteins. Displacement of the HFIF from the
column is achieved with 50% ethylene glycol in 0.1 M α-MM (v/v).
This procedure gives an average 2,000-fold purification resulting in
specific activity between 1-3 x 10^7 units/mg of protein. In the
second step of our large-scale purification procedure, the HFIF (in
40% ethylene glycol) is now applied to a Phenyl-Sepharose CL-4B
column (0.9 x 7 cm). The HFIF binds to Phenyl-Sepharose CL-4B by
hydrophobic interaction, and, following an extensive wash with 50%
ethylene glycol, is displaced by 75% ethylene glycol in PBS. Such a

procedure results in a highly purified and concentrated preparation with a specific activity up to 5×10^7 ref. U/mg protein.

Following the addition of human serum albumin (3 mg/ml) for enhancement of IF stability and extensive dialysis against phosphate buffer-saline, pH 7.4, the HFIF preparation is filtered (0.22 μ), freeze-dried and stored for further use. This product undergoes extensive testing in vitro and in experimental animals to meet F.D.A. requirements for biological products intended for human use. Alternatively, the product obtained from Phenyl-Sepharose column is stored in 25-50% ethylene glycol at -90°C in polypropylene containers. We found that under these conditions only minimal losses of activity occurred over a 2-month period.

An important advantage of the purification procedures developed by our own group is the absence of exposure of the interferon glycoprotein to any denaturing (partial or complete) condition which might affect its native conformational state. Thus, any exposure to chaotrophic salts (as thiocyanates) or detergents (as sodium dodecyl sulfate [SDS]) has been carefully avoided throughout the purification of HFIF. Exposure, even transient, to such denaturing agents carries the theoretical concern for irreversible alteration of the protein molecule. Such alteration could result in unexpected biological effects, such as modification of antigenicity, on repeated administration, as well as undesirable biochemical changes, such as molecular aggregation.

(3) QUALITY CONTROL AND SAFETY OF HFIF AFTER PURIFICATION

During the second half of 1977, our laboratories purified over 850×10^6 ref. U of HFIF to a specific activity 2×10^7 ref. U/mg protein using the above described procedures. After lyophilization, this product was evaluated following the F.D.A. requirements on general safety, pyrogenicity, sterility and toxicity for young rats and mice. Our HFIF did pass these tests.

In addition, we determined that intradermal injections of 90,000 ref. U. in 0.2 ml in nine human volunteers produced only mild reactions limited to faint erythema without detectable induration (8). Specifically, no delayed type hypersensitivity reactions similar to those reported by DeSomer were observed (15).

These tests are the final steps in our scheme of quality control of HFIF (10). Thus, we have in practice completed the entire quality control scheme which started with the evaluation of suitable cell strains, through production and purification of interferon and extending to the safety testing of HFIF in animals and human skin.

Current interpretation of F.D.A. guidelines indicates that human interferon obtained from leukocyte or lymphoblastoid cultures may not

be allowed widespread clinical application – particularly in non
life-threatening situations – because of possible contamination with
slow viruses or with fragments of the EB virus genome. Hence it is
generally agreed that the interferon, derived from normal diploid
fibroblasts, may be unique in meeting all safety requirements. Table
1 summarizes the different forms of human interferon which are potentially available for clinical study.

TABLE 1

Induction of Human Interferons

Interferon Type	Inducer	Comments	References
Fibroblast	$rI_n \cdot rC_n$	Production enhanced by inclusion of cycloheximide and Actinomycin D in induction scheme.	(10,11)
Leukocyte	Sendai virus Newcastle disease virus	–	(16)
Immune	PHA	Production enhanced by inducing lympho-cytes in presence of macrophages.	(17,18)
Immune	Specific antigen	Lymphocytes must be previously sensitized to specific antigen.	(19)
Lymphoblastoid (Namalva)	Sendai virus	–	(20)

(4)   ANTIPROLIFERATIVE EFFECTS OF HIGHLY PURIFIED HFIF

     The antiproliferative activity _in vitro_ of highly purified HFIF
against several established human tumor cell lines was tested as
described (4), in collaboration with Drs. R. Buffett and M. Ito.

     These cell lines were obtained from Dr. J. Fogh of the Memorial
Sloan Kettering Institute. The proliferation of 5959 (osteogenic
sarcoma), RT-4 (transitional cell carcinoma) and DAUDI (Burkitt's
Lymphoma) cell lines was inhibited more than 50% by 100 ref. U/ml of
purified HFIF. In contrast, a concentration of over 1000 ref. U/ml
of HFIF was required for 50% growth inhibition of cell lines A204
(rhabdomyosarcoma), HT-29 (adenocarcinoma of the colon) and MeWo

(malignant melanoma). This lower susceptibility to the antiproliferative effect of HFIF was also observed when normal human diploid
fibroblasts were tested. Thus, it is apparent that HFIF has selective antiproliferative activity in vitro against certain (osteogenic
sarcoma, transitional cell carcinoma and Burkitt's Lymphoma) established human tumor cell lines.

In addition we have found that HFIF can modulate [H³]TdR incorporation in cultures of epithelial and fibroblastic cells derived
from benign prostatic hyperplasia. HFIF (100-1600 U/ml) added for
48 hrs to actively proliferating prostatic epithelial explants, or
subconfluent monolayers of prostatic fibroblasts, resulted in a strong
dose dependent reduction in the number of [H³]TdR labeled nuclei (by
autoradiography) as well as decline in the total radioactive counts
incorporated. Prostatic epithelial cells were found to be between 2
and 10 fold more susceptible to inhibition of [H³]TdR incorporation by
HFIF than prostatic fibroblasts. These observations suggest a selective antiproliferative effect, hitherto undetected, of HFIF
against epithelial vs. fibroblastic cells.

Our studies on the antiproliferative effects of HFIF were then
extended to the use of athymic nude mice as hosts for human malignant
cells. Nude mice (6-10 animals per group) were injected subcutaneously with DAUDI, MeWo, A-204 or RT-4 cells (5 x 10⁶ cells per animal).
These mice were treated daily with 20,000 ref. U of HFIF or a corresponding amount of diluent over a period of 6 weeks. A comparison
of the mean tumor volumes in mice treated with HFIF or diluent served
as indices of HFIF effectiveness in vivo. The growth rate of tumors
induced by injection of RT-4 cells was significantly reduced (over 4
fold) in HFIF treated mice. Tumors induced by injection of MeWo,
A-204 and DAUDI cells did not respond to HFIF treatment (TABLE 2).

TABLE 2

Human Tumors in Nude Mice Treated with HFIF

Injected cell line	Tumor	Tumor volume at 30 days as % of controls ("mock" treated mice) ∓ S.E.
RT-4	Bladder cancer	24.9 ∓ 7.5
MeWO	Melanoma	78.6 ∓ 31.2
DAUDI	Burkitt's lymphoma	87.0 ∓ 14.2
A-204	Rhabdomyosarcoma	151.5 ∓ 39.2

Surprisingly, HFIF was not found to be effective against DAUDI tumors in the nude mice despite the demonstrated susceptibility of these cells to the antiproliferative activity of HFIF in vitro. However, the in vivo susceptibility of RT-4, MeWo and A-204 tumors to HFIF correlated well with the in vitro antiproliferative activity of HFIF for these cells.

Finally, in collaboration with Drs. E. Holyoke and C. Karakousis, the highly purified HFIF $(5 \times 10^5$ ref. U daily) was injected directly into the cutaneous or subcutaneous metastatic lesions of 2 patients with malignant melanoma. A vehicle control with the same pH, osmolality and human albumin content was injected into other lesions of similar size. In the first patient, the cutaneous lesion (5 mm in diameter) injected with HFIF for 14 consecutive days, disappeared grossly. Most interestingly, no tumor cells were evident upon microscopic examination of serial histological sections of the entire excised area. Uninjected lesions and lesions injected with vehicle control contained typical masses of melanoma cells. The second patient with multiple subcutaneous melanoma metastatic nodules was treated for 30 days. All untreated nodules, as well as a control nodule injected with the vehicle, continued to grow and doubled their volumes within a month. In contrast, the lesion treated daily with HFIF was reduced to ¼ of the original volume; however upon microscopic examination tumor cells were still present. In both patients the metastases injected with HFIF were heavily infiltrated with lymphocytes. No such infiltrations were observed in control lesions. No fever or any other side effects associated with HFIF injections were observed. Currently, we are obtaining similar results with intralesional injections into subcutaneous metastatic lesions of breast carcinoma.

In summary, our current results obtained with HFIF tested against human malignant cells in vitro, in the nude mice and in patients, strongly suggest that this glycoprotein may find shortly a practical application in therapy of selected malignancies.

(5) FUTURE DIRECTIONS: COMPARATIVE CLINICAL AND BIOLOGICAL PROP-
ERTIES OF FIBROBLAST, LEUKOCYTE AND IMMUNE INTERFERONS

Recent clinical study by Dr. Merigan et al. with human leukocyte interferon strongly suggests its efficacy both in treatment of herpes zoster in patients with cancer (21) as well as in varicella in children with cancer (22).

It will be particularly valuable to compare human fibroblast and human leukocyte interferons for therapeutic efficacy in various human neoplastic and viral diseases, as well as in disorders of the immune system. Production of immune interferon is still too low for any clinical studies; however, in model systems, such as murine osteogenic sarcoma, it shows strong therapeutic activity, possibly due in part to other lymphokines which are also present (23). Since human

interferons from leukocytes and fibroblasts differ in certain physical (24), antigenic and possibly biologic characteristics, certain
diseases may be more responsive to a specific molecular form of human
interferon. Some of the different binding properties of various
human interferons are illustrated in TABLE 3.

TABLE 3

Binding of Human Interferons on Immobilized Ligands[a]

Chromatographic system	Nature of binding	Interferon type (inducer)		
		Fibroblast ($rI_n \cdot rC_n$)	Leukocyte (NDV)	Immune (PHA)
L-tryptophan-agarose	Hydrophobic	+	−	±
Phenyl-Sepharose CL-4B	Hydrophobic	+	+	
Con A-agarose	Hydrophobic: Carbohydrate recognition	+	−	±

[a]+, complete binding; ±, partial binding; −, no binding.

Historically, comparison of characteristics of various interferons consisted mainly of measuring their relative stabilities at pH
2 and sensitivities to heating (56°C). These techniques have now
been largely replaced by various affinity probes which can measure
the properties of specific interferon components rather than those
common to the biologic mixture of different interferons. The interferons can be characterized by their degree of interaction with a
variety of hydrophobic ligands and immobilized lectins as noted above.
Such studies have provided the first insight into the relative hydro-
phobicities of various interferon molecules, as well as into their
glycoprotein nature. In addition to suggesting the existence of certain amino acid residues on the molecular surface of interferon, we
feel that the hydrophobic ligands may give clues indicating the mode
of interaction between interferons and cellular receptors. Table 3
outlines some of the various differences between binding properties
of human interferons. L-tryptophan-agarose and Phenyl-Sepharose Cl-4B
are both hydrophobic ligands, and, on Concanavalin A (Con A)-agarose,
both carbohydrate recognition and hydrophobicity contribute to the
binding interaction. Each of these three major types of human interferon has a different elution profile. For example, fibroblast interferon, when applied in phosphate-buffered physiologic saline binds to

L-tryptophan-agarose and requires the addition of a hydrophobic solute, ethylene glycol, for its elution. Leukocyte interferon, applied under the same conditions, appears in the breakthrough fraction (25). However, immune interferon displays molecular heterogeneity suggesting three major subcomponents: the first component appears in the breakthrough fraction, a second in fractions eluted in the presence of 1 M NaCl, and a third is eluted with ethylene glcol (26). Chromatography on Phenyl-Sepharose CL-4B allows the binding of all three major types of interferon through a strong hydrophobic interaction. However, the elution profile for each is, once again, different and this can be demonstrated in a facile manner by the development of the column with an ethylene glycol gradient. Leukocyte interferon is eluted with 50% ethylene glycol, fibroblast interferon is eluted with approximately 70% ethylene glycol. Immune interferon displays three molecular subcomponents which appear in the fractions eluted with 20, 50 and 70% of the polarity reducing agent, ethylene glycol (27). On Con A-agarose, fibroblast interferon binds through both hydrophobic interaction and carbohydrate recognition. The presence of D-mannose residues in fibroblast interferon is evidenced, for example, by the ease of eluting the interferon molecule with the displacing sugar α MM.

In order to determine a "molecular profile" of the various interferons elaborated in man, we have used in the past as our principal probe, L-tryptophan-agarose. First, we determined that the interferon molecules made in those few untreated patients who produced measurable interferon levels in response to infection had the typical affinity characteristics of leukocyte, fibroblast, and immune interferons (28). Patients treated with $rI_n \cdot rC_n$ also had the same 3 forms of interferon, albeit in much higher amounts. The relative concentrations of these 3 molecular forms of interferon suggest that leukocytes, in particular, lymphocytes, are probably preferential sites of interferon synthesis.

An opportunity of these clinical studies is also to determine the possible immunomodulation properties of purified fibroblast interferon as compared with human leukocyte interferon (29). To this end, a close collaboration has been developed with Drs. Ernest Borden and Joyce Zarling of the Immunology Research Center, University of Wisconsin Cancer Center, Madison. We have recently determined that purified HFIF augments T killer cell activity in vitro (9). Special excitement exists for extending these observations to the clinic. For example, we are evaluating T and B cell function, following interferon therapy, in patients with chronic viral infection (e.g., hepatitis B) as well as in patients with various neoplasias. Such comparative studies may eventually allow us to determine more clearly the therapeutic potential of the particular biological property of the interferon molecule.

An alternative approach to the use of exogenous interferon is the use of interferon inducers. The inducers generate endogenous production of all 3 forms of human interferon simultaneously. Of the

interferon inducers, the best studied thus far, is the well-regis-
tered double-stranded RNA, polyriboinosinic·polyribocytidylic acid
($rI_n \cdot rC_n$). In collaboration with Dr. Paul O.P. Ts'o and his colleagues at Johns Hopkins University, we have systematically analyzed
the antiviral and other biologic effects of both $rI_n \cdot rC_n$ and certain
analogs (termed mismatched polymers or "self-destruct" inducers).
These inducers were synthesized by inserting mismatched bases at
infrequent intervals in the rC_n strand prior to annealing it with rI_n
(30). This subtle change in the polynucleotide duplex resulted in a
profound shift in many biologic properties of the inducer without
altering its intrinsic ability to induce interferon (30,31,32). For
example, in various in vitro and in vivo systems, the mismatched
analogs of $rI_n \cdot rC_n$ provided similar antiviral effects as $rI_n \cdot rC_n$ and
produced much less toxicity on marrow and various organs in the reticuloendothelial system (spleen, thymus, circulating lymphocytes, etc.)
(33).

These preclinical studies have been of such success that we will
now include mismatched interferon inducers in our clinical investiga-
tive program. It will be of immediate interest to monitor the molecular forms of human interferon which are generated and the secondary
biologic effects encountered when the induction process is triggered
by the very brief signal of a mismatched inducer.

ACKNOWLEDGMENTS

We are grateful to L. A. Di Berardino, D. Donovan, L. Fletcher
and R. Heinaman for their excellent technical assistance.

This work was supported in part by Public Health Service grants
CA-14801-05 in Viral Chemotherapy from the National Cancer Institute
and CA-15502 from the National Cancer Institute, National Institutes
of Health, Department of Health, Education, and Welfare.

REFERENCES

1. FINTER, N.B. (1973): Interferons and inducers in vivo: I. Antiviral effects in experimental animals. In Interferons and
   Interferon Inducers, Vol. 2, (N.B. Finter, ed.), pp. 295 & 363.
   American Elsevier Publishing Co., Inc., New York.
2. LEVY, H.B. & W.A. CARTER (1968): J. Mol. Biol. 31, 561.
3. MARCUS, P.I., D.L. ENGLEHARDT, J.M. HUNT & M.J. SEKELLICK (1971):
   Science 174, 593.
4. BUFFETT, R. F., M. ITO, A.M. CAIRO & W.A. CARTER (1978): J. Natl.
   Cancer Inst. 60, 243.
5. DE CLERCQ, E. & W.E. STEWART, II (1973): In Selective Inhibitors
   of Viral Functions, (W.A. Carter, ed.), p. 81, CRC Press,
   Cleveland.
6. JOHNSON, H.M. & S. BARON (1976): I.C.R.S.J. Med. Science 4, 50.
7. HUANG, K. & R.M. DONAHOE (1975): In Effects of Interferon on
   Cells, Viruses and the Immune System, (A. Geraldes, ed.), p.
   381, Academic Press, London, New York, San Francisco.

8. HOROSZEWICZ, J.S., S.S. LEONG, M. ITO, R. BUFFETT, C. KARAKOUSIS, E. HOLYOKE, L. JOB, J. DOLEN & W.A. CARTER (1978): Cancer Treatment Reports, in press.
9. ZARLING, J.M., J. SOSMAN, E.C. BORDEN, J.S. HOROSZEWICZ & W.A. CARTER (1978):J. Immunology, in press.
10. HOROSZEWICZ, J.S., S.S. LEONG, M. ITO, L.A. DI BERADINO & W.A. CARTER (1978): Infection and Immunity 19, 720.
11. HAVELL, E. & J. VILCEK (1972): Antimicrob. Agents Chemother. 2, 476.
12. BILLIAU, A., M. JONIAU & P. DESOMER (1973): J. Gen. Virol. 19, 1.
13. DAVEY, M.W., E. SULKOWSKI & W.A. CARTER (1976): Biochemistry 15, 704.
14. DAVEY, M.W., J.W. HUANG, E. SULKOWSKI & W.A. CARTER (1974): J. Biol. Chem. 249, 6354.
15. DESOMER, P., V.G. EDY & A. BILLIAU (1977): Lancet July, p. 47.
16. MOGENSEN, K.E. & K. CANTELL (1977): Pharmac. Ther. C 1, 369.
17. EPSTEIN, L.B., M.J. CLINE & T.C. MERIGAN (1971): J. Clin. Invest. 50, 744.
18. WHEELOCK, E.F. (1965): Science 149, 310.
19. GREENE, J.A., S.R. COOPERBAND & S. KIBRICK (1969): Science 164, 1415.
20. OXMAN, M.N. (1973): In Interferons and Interferon Inducers, Vol. 2, (N.B. Finter, ed.), p. 391, American Elseveir Publishing Co., Inc., New York.
21. MERIGAN, T.C., K.H. RAND, R.B. POLLARD, P.S. ABDALLAH, G.W. JORDAN & R.P. FRIED (1978): New Eng. J. Med. 298, 981.
22. ARVIN, A., S. FELDMAN & T.C. MERIGAN (1978): Antimicr. Agents and Chemother. 13, 605.
23. GLASGOW, L.A., J. L. CRANE, E.R. KERN & J.S. YOUNGER (1978): "personal communication", Interferon Scientific Memoranda April.
24. JANKOWSKI, W.J., M.W. DAVEY, J.A. O'MALLEY, E. SULKOWSKI & W.A. CARTER (1975): J. Virol. 16, 1124.
25. SULKOWSKI, E., M.W. DAVEY & W.A. CARTER (1976): J. Biol. Chem. 251, 5381.
26. O'MALLEY, J.A. & W.A. CARTER (1978): J. of Reticuloendothelial Society 23, 299.
27. O'MALLEY, J.A., G.E. PANAGOS, B.J. GROSSMAYER, E. SULKOWSKI & W.A. CARTER (1977): 17th Interscience Conference on Antimicrobial Agents and Chemotherapy, ASM, New York, #33.
28. CARTER, W.A., G.E. PANAGOS, J.A. O'MALLEY & A.I. FREEMAN (1977): Am. Soc. Clin. Res. 25, 488A.
29. HERON, I., K. BERG & K. CANTELL (1976): J. Immunology 117, 1370.
30. CARTER, W.A., P.M. PITHA, I.W. MARSHALL, I. TAZAWA, S. TAZAWA & P.O.P. TS'O (1972): J. Mol. Biol. 70, 567.
31. O'MALLEY, J.A., S. LEONG, J. HOROSZEWICZ, W.A. CARTER, J.L. ALDERFER & P.O.P. TS'O (1978): Molec. Pharmacol., in press.
32. TS'O, P.O.P., J.L. ALDERFER, J. LEVY, L.W. MARSHALL, J. O'MALLEY, J. HOROSZEWICZ & W.A. CARTER (1976): Mol. Pharmacol. 12, 299.
33. CARTER, W.A., J. O'MALLEY, M. BEESON, P. CUNNINGTON, A. KELVIN, A. VERE-HODGE, J.L. ALDERFER & P.O.P. TS'O (1976): Mol. Pharmacol. 12, 440.

THE CLINICAL USE OF FIBROBLAST INTERFERON

A. Billiau, V. G. Edy and P. de Somer

Department of Human Biology, Division of Microbiology
Rege Institute, University of Leuven
B-3000 Leuven, Belgium

INTRODUCTION

Whereas leukocyte interferon has since several years been available for clinical experiments (1-7), fibroblast interferon has only recently been prepared in sufficient amounts to test its effects in man (8). As a result little published information is available as yet. In the past two years large quantities of fibroblast interferon have been produced at the Rega Institute. This interferon has been used to do pilot experiments and to perform controlled trials as well. In this paper we will summarize our experiences and we will also mention results obtained by other groups in so far as the information is available in published or unpublished form (8-13).

The human fibroblast interferon, used in our studies, was prepared on diploid embryonic skin muscle cells by a priming and poly(I).poly(C) superinduction method as described previously (14,15). It was purified either by fractional precipitation with ammonium sulphate (AS-method), by adsorption on controlled pore glass (CPG-method) (16) or by affinity chromatography on zinc iminodiacetate-sepharose (Zn-method) (17). The interferon was titrated by inhibition of vesicular stomatitis virus replication in human diploid cells using a dye uptake method and was calibrated against the Medical Research Council 69/19 standard of human leukocyte interferon. The approximate specific activity, before addition of human serum albumin as a stabilizer, were 50,000 units/mg of protein for the AS-type, 1 million units (MU)/ mg for the CPG-type and 30 MU/mg for the Zn-type of interferon.

Purified leukocyte interferon (PIF-grade) was included in some studies for comparison. It was courteously given by Drs. K. Cantell and H. Kauppinen (State Serum Institute and Finnish Red Cross Transfusion Service, Helsinki, Finland).

PROPHYLACTIC STUDIES

Interferon is designed by Nature to protect uninfected cells against exogenous virus. For this reason it is more logical to use interferon as a prophylactic than as a therapeutic agent against virus infection. However, very few clinical situations are such that the exact time of a viral infection can be predicted. One such situation occurs in patients receiving immunosuppressive therapy for organ transplantation. About 80 % of all renal transplant patients show a seroconversion against one or more viruses within 3 months after transplantation. More than half of these seroconversions are against herpes simplex virus (HSV) or cytomegalovirus (CMV). Both of these are thought to result from activation of latent infection, existing since early life-time. The pathogenesis of this activation is not known. Cellular immunity rather than circulating antibody seems to be the most important factor keeping latent infection in check. It is not known in which cells the viruses are residing during latency : in animal models HSV can be reactivated from the sensory ganglia. Furthermore, it is not clear whether exacerbation involves only activation of virus activity in cells which are latently infected or whether adjacent cells are also infected de novo. Finally, it is not known whether interferon can prevent activation of HSV in latently infected cells. In any case it seems safe to assume that the situation of herpetic infections in renal transplant patients differs from that occurring in the animal model systems where the prophylactic effect of interferon on exogenous virus infection has been demonstrated.

A double-blind clinical trial employing fibroblast interferon, prepared at the Rega Institute, in renal transplant patients has recently been completed by Weimar et al. (13) at the Eramus University of Rotterdam (The Netherlands). The trial was started in February 1976 and included 16 non-diabetic, HBsAg negative patients between 18 and 45 years of age, receiving a cadaver kidney at the Dijkzigt Academic Hospital. The immunosuppressive regimen consisted of prednisone (35 mg daily) and azathioprine (1-2 mg/kg daily). The study was set up in a double-blind, placebo-controlled fashion, in consecutive pairs to allow early detection of possible side-effects of the interferon therapy. In each pair the patients received either placebo or fibroblast interferon (3 MU, twice weekly) for 3 months, starting 1-2 hours before transplantation. The patients were observed for

TABLE 1. Viral Infections in Renal Transplant Patients Treated Prophylactically with Fibroblast Interferon*

Numbers of	Treatment	
	Mock-interferon	Interferon
Patients in group	8	8
Proven viral infections :		
- clinical	4	4
- seroconversion	9	10
Patients with proven viral infections : - clinical	4	4
- seroconversion	6	6
Life-threatening viral infections	0	2 (CMV and rubella)
Patients with herpes virus infections : - clinical	3 (severe)	1 (minor)
- seroconversion	4	1

* Double-blind placebo-controlled trial performed by Weimar et al. (13); serology done for HSV, CMV, rubella virus, influenza virus, respiratory syncytial virus and varicella zoster virus. Treatment regimen : 3 MU of AS-concentrated fibroblast interferon, twice weekly, intramuscularly, for 6 weeks, starting on the day of transplantation. Follow-up period : 6 months.

6 months. Haematological and liver function parameters of interferon-treated patients did not differ from those of placebos. The virological observations are summarized in Table 1. No differences were seen between interferon and placebo-treated patients in the total number of clinically apparent viral infections nor in the total number of seroconversions. Two life-threatening infections occurred in the interferon-treated group, none in the group receiving placebo. The only indication for a beneficial effect of interferon was in the occurrence HSV infections. In the placebo-treated group seroconversions occurred in 4 out of 8 patients; 3 of these had severe orofacial eruptions. Of the 8 patients which received interferon, only one showed a seroconversion against HSV; this was accompanied by a minor fever blister.

THERAPEUTIC STUDIES ON PATIENTS WITH CHRONIC
ACTIVE LIVER DISEASE (CALD)

In a small number of infected patients, hepatitis B (HB) virus persists in the liver cells in an as yet undefined form. Its activity is manifested by the presence of large amounts of hepatitis B surface (HBs)-antigen in the blood and sometimes by the presence of virion-associated DNA polymerase. In some patients the virus persistence leads to CALD. This condition ultimately leads to portal cirrhosis of the liver. Children born from mothers who carry infectious HB virus during pregnancy are invariably infected and develop a chronic carrier state. The prognosis of this condition is not fully known as yet, except that a small percentage of such children develop hepatoma.

The idea to treat these patients with interferon stems from three considerations.
  a) Although active virus replication takes place in DNA polymerase-positive patients, no endogenous interferon seems to be produced. Under these conditions exogenous interferon is more likely to be beneficial than in acute infections where sizable amounts of endogenous interferon are generated by the infection itself.
  b) In some chronically infected cells interferon inhibits virus replication, despite the fact that the viral genome is integrated in that of the cell. Specifically cells which are chronically infected with Retroviridae show a reduced release of virus particles after treatment with small amounts of interferon (18,19). However, more recent investigations, as reviewed by Friedman (20), have shown that the synthesis of the major viral proteins and of viral RNA is not inhibited. The inhibition of particle release is thought to result from minor disturbances in terminal processing of viral components. Similarly, in SV40-transformed cells the production of T-antigen is unaffected by interferon.
  c) The presence of HBs-antigen and of DNA polymerase in the serum enables one to quickly detect an inhibitory effect of interferon therapy on viral functions.

The first, and so far most convincing evidence of an effect of interferon on viral activity in chronic HB virus infection has come from workers at Stanford University. Greenberg et al. (4) treated four CALD patients with leukocyte interferon. Three of them had constant and high levels of particle-associated DNA polymerase in the serum. Doses of 0.3 to 3 MU day were associated with a rapid and reproducible fall in DNA polymerase activity, hepatitis B core antigen (HBcAg) and DNA particle-associated DNA in the serum. The effect was transient when the interferon was given for

TABLE 2. Viral and Disease Parameters in 9 Patients with CALD, Treated with Interferon

Patient Code Nr	Consecutive treatments*	Concurrent favorable evolution of			Follow-up
		Polymerase levels	Transaminase levels	HBcAg in hepatocytes	
031	F_a	+[+]	No	Yes	Normalized transaminases; permanent decrease in hepatocyte HBcAg
003	F_b	Yes	Yes	Yes	Polymerase remains undetectable; transaminases normalized; arthritis
019	F_c & L_d	Yes (L)	Yes (F/L)	?	Polymerase lowered during interim period (F_c,L_d), remaining undetectable in follow-up
018	F_e,F_c & L_d	Yes (F/L)	Yes (F)	?	Improvement transient
020	F_c & L_d	Yes (F/L)	Yes (F)	?	Improvement transient
033	F_f	Yes	No	?	Improvement transient
034	F_f	No	Yes	?	Improvement transient
002	F_g,F_h & L_f	No	No	?	Polymerase lowered 10-fold during interim period (F_g,F_h); no change during follow-up
017	F_e	No	No	?	No change

* F = fibroblast interferon; L = leukocyte interferon; a = 7 x 10 MU in 2 weeks; b = daily injections for 4 weeks, 7 x 0.1 MU, 7 x 0.3 MU, 7 x 1 MU & 7 x 3 MU; c = 14 x 2.2 MU in 2 weeks; d = 14 x 3 MU in 2 weeks; e = 3 x 2 MU, 3 x 4 MU & 3 x 8 MU in 3 consecutive weeks; f = 7 x 3 MU in 1 week; g = daily injections for 3 weeks, 7 x 0.3 MU, 7 x 1 MU & 7 x 3 MU; h = daily injections for 2 weeks, 7 x 3 MU & 7 x 10 MU.

+ e-antigen undetectable before treatment.

10 days or less but appeared to be more permanent when the interferon administration was prolonged for one month or more.

Two research groups have so far used fibroblast interferon
to treat patients with CALD. As of this writing, 9 such patients
have received fibroblast interferon prepared at our Institute
(Table 2). Four of these patients (nrs. 017, 018, 019, 020) were
followed by Weimar et al. (10-12) at the Dijkzigt Hospital
(Erasmus University, Rotterdam, The Netherlands and 5 (nrs. 002,
003, 031, 033, 034) by Desmyter et al. (8,9) at the Academic
Hospital of the University of Leuven. Some of the patients received more than one treatment course, including leukocyte interferon for comparison. In 3 out of 9, no changes occurred in the
viral parameters; in 6 out of 9, a favorable evolution of viral
parameters occurred during or shortly after one of the treatment
courses; in 3 of these 6 patients the improvement was permanent
for the time of follow-up. The evolution of patient nr. 031 has
been described in detail elsewhere. During or shortly after the
treatment, a decrease in HBcAg-staining of hepatocytes was observed. Over 2 years following treatment this patient has evolved
into a chronic HBsAg-carrier : at the time of this writing no
HBcAg was detectable in the hepatocytes and serum transaminase
levels were normalized.

Patient nr. 003, a 50 year-old man, had known CALD since 2
years before interferon treatment. Serum transaminases were elevated (GOT $\sim$ 80 units/liter; GPT $\sim$ 70 units/liter) with two
episodes of aggressive disease (5 and 15 months before treatment
with interferon) characterized by peaks in serum transaminase
levels up to 1500 (GPT) and 2000 (GOT) units/liter. For this the
patient was being treated with prednisone (15 to 30 mg per day).
The decision to administer interferon was taken on the basis of a
high particle-associated DNA polymerase level in the serum.
Increasing doses (Fig. 1) were given over a period of 4 weeks and
serum samples were taken daily. All samples were assayed simultaneously. It appeared that DNA polymerase levels had already been
decreasing before the treatment was started. During the three
first weeks of treatment (0.1 to 1 MU/day) no further decrease
was seen. However, in the last week of treatment (3 MU per day)
DNA polymerase became undetectable. Simultaneously, an increase in
HBcAg level was observed. HBsAg levels were decreasing steadily as
were also the levels of serum transaminases. In the follow-up
period (7 months, at the time of this writing) DNA polymerase
remained undetectable, HBcAg decreased and transaminases normalized. It may be important to note that a nondestructive arthritis
developed in the course of this period.

The third patient (code nr. 019) in whom a favorable evolution occurred during interferon treatment was a 35 year-old woman

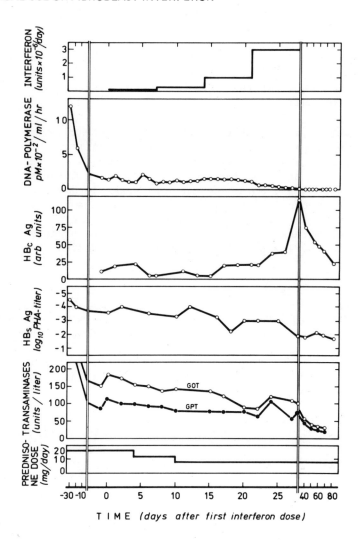

FIGURE 1. Evolution of viral and clinical parameters in a patient
with CALD (code nr. 003) during and after treatment with fibroblast interferon.

with confirmed CALD since 5 years. She received 14 daily injections of 2.2 MU of fibroblast interferon and 14 daily injections
of 3 MU of leukocyte interferon, with an interval of 2 months.
During the treatment with fibroblast interferon the DNA polymerase
level did not change, but the transaminase levels were transiently
decreased. In the interval between the two treatments the DNA
polymerase levels decreased and e-antigen became undetectable.

During the second treatment course (leukocyte interferon) DNA
polymerase levels remained low and transaminases decreased.
Shortly after the treatment DNA polymerase became undetectable
and transaminases continued to normalize. At the time of this
writing (3 months after the last interferon dose) transaminase
levels were normal.

In 4 patients (018, 020, 033 and 034) the changes in viral
and liver function parameters were ambiguous. A transient decrease
in transaminase levels occurred in 3 out of the 4 patients during
treatment with fibroblast but not with leukocyte interferon. Also
in 3 out of the 4 patients the DNA polymerase levels showed a
transient and unconvincing decrease with both interferons. Finally, in 2 patients (002 and 017) fibroblast interferon had no
effect on polymerase or transaminase levels. One of these refrac-
tory patients (002) also received leukocyte interferon without
effect.

Fibroblast interferon has also been used by Kingham et al.
(21) to treat two patients with documented CALD. The patients
received 10 MU daily for two weeks. Both patients were e-antigen
negative before treatment. The HBsAg levels showed a transient
decrease during treatment. The most striking finding was a 64-fold
fall in HBcAg occurring during treatment and being maintained
during the follow-up period. Furthermore, the transaminase levels
normalized in one patient.

PILOT STUDIES IN VARIOUS ACUTE VIRAL INFECTIONS

Drug trials involving relatively large numbers of patients
are usually preceded by pilot tests with single patients. Undoubtedly, a number of patients with various affections have received
interferon, but were never reported on in the literature because
no effect was seen. As fibroblast interferon became available in
large quantities, we have treated a few patients with various
diseases of proven or presumed viral etiology. The purpose of
these studies was to obtain preliminary indications which could
orient us to concentrate more effort on one or other disease. The
results of these investigations are summarized in Table 3. The
diseases treated included acute and fulminant hepatitis by HB
virus infection, cutaneous, laryngeal and venereal papillomas,
osteosarcoma and neuroblastoma. No spectacular changes were seen
in any of these conditions. We were encouraged, however, by the
regression of the small verrucae planae in a renal transplant
carrier (patient nr. 005) with multiple cutaneous warts and by
the partial regression and subsequent necrosis of a laryngeal
papilloma (patient nr. 032) which had been recurring after repeated surgical resections.

TABLE 3. Pilot Trials with Fibroblast Interferon in Patients with Various Diseases of Proven or Presumed Viral Etiology

Patient (Code Nr)	Age (yrs)	Sex	Diagnosis	Interferon treatment			Outcome
				Nr. of injections	Avg. dose (MU)	Duration (days)	
025	43	F	Acute hepatitis	14	2.0	14	Recovery as expected, HBsAg positive for ± 3 months
026	40	F	Acute hepatitis	14	2.0	14	Recovery as expected, HBsAg positive for 3 months
027	48	F	Acute hepatitis	14	2.0	14	Recovery as expected, HBsAg positive for 2 months
024	20	M	Fulminant hepatitis	10	3.5	15	Recovery, HBsAg positive for 3 months
028	40	F	Fulminant hepatitis	6	6.0	6	Died on day 7
029	25	F	Fulminant hepatitis	6	3.5	6	Recovery
030	31	F	Fulminant hepatitis	5	4.4	5	Died on day 5
032	45	F	Papilloma of larynx	13	3.5	18	Partial regression, followed by rejection
005	35	F	Multiple warts in renal transplant carrier	14	5.9	24	Regression of small verrucae planae, not of large warts
037	25	M	Multiple warts	8	3.5	14	No effect
038	18	F	Multiple plantar warts	8	3.5	14	No effect
035	23	F	Condyloma accuminatum	8	3.5	14	No effect
036	80	F	Condyloma accuminatum	8	3.5	14	No effect
001	40	M	Osteosarcoma	15	3.5	15	No effect
006	13	M	Osteosarcoma	42	3.5	90	Transient delay in progression (?)
007	3	F	Neuroblastoma	18	1.7	28	No effect

TABLE 4. Fever Reaction in Patients Given Intramuscular Injections of Fibroblast Interferon

Patient (Code Nr)	Age (yrs)	Sex	Diagnosis*	Interferon treatment			Fever+
				Purification method	Number of injections	Avg. dose (MU)	
031	42	M	CALD	AS	7	10.0	+
009	35	M	Renal transplant	AS	26	3.0	-
010	31	M	Renal transplant	AS	26	3.0	-
011	24	F	Renal transplant	AS	26	3.0	-
012	37	M	Renal transplant	AS	26	3.0	-
013	37	F	Renal transplant	AS	26	3.0	+
014	26	F	Renal transplant	AS	26	3.0	-
015	34	F	Renal transplant	AS	26	3.0	+
016	19	M	Renal transplant	AS	26	3.0	-
017	57	F	CALD	CPG	9	4.6	-
018	21	F	CALD	CPG	16	4.5	-
002	36	M	CALD	CPG	37	3.6	+
003	50	M	CALD	CPG	28	1.2	-
019	35	F	CALD	CPG	14	2.2	-
020	39	M	CALD	CPG	14	2.2	+
025	43	F	Acute hepatitis	CPG	14	2.0	-
026	48	F	Acute hepatitis	CPG	14	2.0	-
027	40	F	Acute hepatitis	CPG	14	2.0	-
024	20	M	Fulminant hepatitis	CPG	10	3.5	-
023	36	M	Renal transplant	CPG	26	3.0	-
001	40	M	Osteosarcoma	CPG	15	3.5	+
006	13	M	Osteosarcoma	CPG	42	3.5	+
005	35	F	Multiple warts	CPG	14	5.9	+
004	30	F	Multiple sclerosis	CPG	7	4.7	-
008	6	M	Avian tuberculosis	CPG	37	1.5	+
022	9	M	SSPE	CPG	12	4.6	+
007	3	F	Neuroblastoma	CPG	18	1.7	+

* : CALD = chronic active liver disease; SSPE = subacute sclerosing panencephalitis.
+ : peaks exceeding 38.0°C.

SIDE-EFFECTS OF SYSTEMIC ADMINISTRATION OF FIBROBLAST INTERFERON

Human fibroblast interferon purified by the CPG-method has been reported to have three types of side-effects in man : pyrogenicity, skin reactivity and transitory lymphopenia.

Pyrogenicity of Interferon

Fever and malaise occurring shortly after each injection were reported in early studies involving systemic administration of leukocyte interferon in man (1-5,7). These reactions were thought to be rather aspecific and were assigned to trivial contaminants of the interferon. As purer preparations became available, less fever and malaise seemed to occur. More recently it has become clear that fever does occur in some patients with relatively pure preparations of leukocyte interferon (6) and with fibroblast interferon as well (22).

We followed body temperature in 27 patients who received several intramuscular injections of > 2 MU of interferon belonging to 17 different batches purified either by the AS- or the CPG-method (Table 4). In 10 patients injections with one or more different batches resulted in fever reactions with peaks exceeding 38°C. Patients who received injections of several batches of interferon did not develop fever with all of these. This suggests that the pyrogenic substance was not interferon itself. Also some batches were pyrogenic in one patient but not in another, indicating that patients differed in sensitivity.

Figure 2 illustrates the fever reaction of a 40 year-old male patient with metastasized osteogenic sarcoma and bronchogenic carcinoma (patient nr. 001). Seven daily injections of 3.5 MU were given without prophylactic use of aspirin. After each injection the temperature rose to peak values averaging 39.5°C at about 90 min. At this time aspirin was given. The temperature then fell to about 37.8°C and subsequently rose slightly to reach a plateau of about 38.0°C between 8 and 10 hr. This biphasic response was more obvious on individual curves; since the second fever peak did not always occur at the same time it appears as a plateau on the average temperature curve. At 8 subsequent days aspirin was given 15 min before injection of the interferon. With this regimen the first fever peak was less high (38.9°C) and delayed (3.5 hr).

Human fibroblast interferon purified by the Zn-method was much less pyrogenic than the CPG-purified batches, when tested in the same patients on consecutive days (Table 5). Also, in the

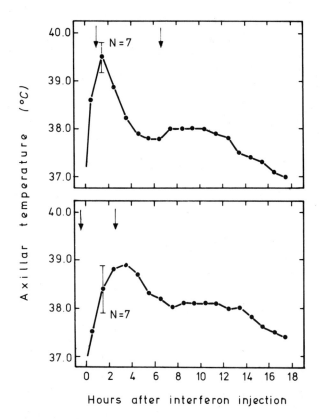

FIGURE 2. Averaged daily temperature curves in a patient injected intramuscularly with human fibroblast interferon. A 40 year-old male patient (nr. 001) with metastatic osteogenic sarcoma and bronchogenic carcinoma received 14 intramuscular injections of 3.5 MU of CPG-purified interferon on 14 consecutive days. Aspirin (500 mg) was given at times indicated by arrows. Vertical bars indicate 95 % confidence limits.

hands of other investigators fibroblast interferon has been reported to be non-pyrogenic in man. This is additional evidence that the pyrogenic substance in our CPG-purified preparation was not interferon itself but an impurity. Although certain leukocyte interferon preparations were reported to be pyrogenic, a present-day preparation of purified leukocyte interferon, injected at the same dosage and in the same patient as fibroblast interferon was not pyrogenic (Table 5). Possibly, leukocyte interferon preparations, used formerly, contained the same pyrogen as CPG-purified fibroblast interferon.

TABLE 5. Fever Reaction in Patients Injected Intramuscularly with Different Interferon Preparations

Patient Nr	Interferon preparation	Dosis (MU)	Nr of injec- tions	Mean body temperature[*] (± 95 % conf. limits)
002	Fibroblast-CPG	3.0	7	37.70 ± 0.18
	Fibroblast-CPG	11.0	7	38.31 ± 0.26
	Leukocyte-PIF	3.0	7	36.70 ± 0.07
	Fibroblast-Zn	3.0	1	36.90
	None	-	12	36.50 ± 0.18
022	Fibroblast-CPG	2.2	7	37.55 ± 0.26
	Fibroblast-CPG	7.0	7	38.20 ± 0.15
	Fibroblast-Zn	3.0	1	36.90
	None	-	12	36.98 ± 0.27

* For each day an average value was calculated from the axillar
temperatures measured at hourly intervals from 1 to 14 hr
after injection of interferon or twice daily on days when no
interferon was given.

The severe fever reaction seen in man cannot so far be
studied in animal model systems. Rabbits injected intramuscularly
with CPG-purified interferons at dosages of 50,000 units/kg (i.e.
an equivalent of 3.5 MU in man), either developed moderate fever
(<0.8°C temperature increase) or showed no temperature elevation
at all.

Haematological Effects

A second side-effect of interferon seen in our studies was
transient lymphopenia. Within several hours after the intramuscular injection of CPG-purified interferon the relative lymphocyte
count decreased to about 2/3 of its value before the injection
(Fig. 3). The total white blood cell count was not significantly
altered. By rosette-assay, both B- and T-cell populations appeared equally affected. Twenty-four hours after the injections the
leukocyte formula had returned to normal. The phenomemon was not
accompanied by complement depletion.

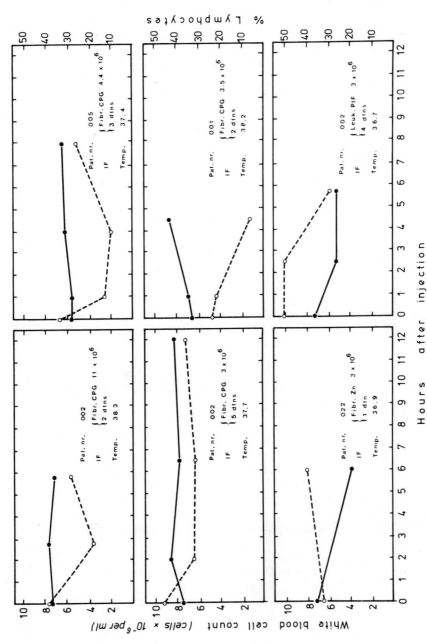

FIGURE 3. Transitory lymphopenia in patients injected intramuscularly with human fibroblast interferon. ● = white blood cell count; o = % lymphocytes. Fever reactions are calculated as indicated in footnote to Table 2.

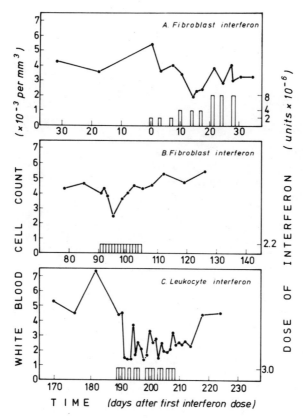

FIGURE 4. Leukopenia in a single CALD patient (code nr. 018) after intramuscular injections of either fibroblast or leukocyte interferon.

Purified leukocyte interferon gave a similar reaction. Zn-purified fibroblast interferon, on the contrary, did not significantly influence the white blood cell count nor the relative number of lymphocytes. It would, therefore, appear that fibroblast interferon preparations contain an additional substance which influences the physiology of lymphocytes. This impurity might resemble leukocyte interferon or a substance present in leukocyte interferon preparations.

A more severe haematological reaction was seen in one CALD patient (nr. 018). After each injection of fibroblast (2.2 MU CPG-purified) or leukocyte (3 MU) interferon the total white blood cell count dramatically decreased, sometimes below 3000 cells/mm^2 (Fig. 4). The remarkable similarity in reaction of this patient to fibroblast and leukocyte interferon virtually excludes the

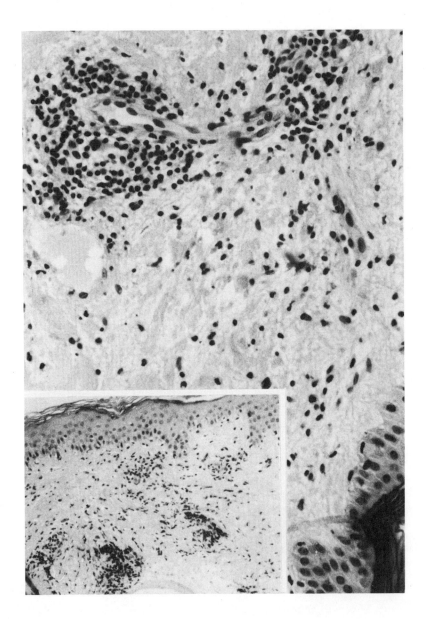

FIGURE 5. Histopathology of skin lesion induced by intracutaneous
injection of CPG-purified fibroblast interferon in man; reaction
48 hr after injection of 100,000 units in 0.1 ml.

possibility that the reaction was due to a trivial impurity and indicates that a molecule closely resembling or associated with interferon is responsible for this side-effect.

Skin Reactivity

The intradermal injection of > 20,000 units of CPG-purified fibroblast interferon resulted in an inflammatory response as previously described (22,23). This consisted of a mild erythema, followed by swelling and induration. The reaction did not itch but was slightly tender. It started about 6 hr post-injection and reached its maximum at about 24 hr. In most cases it was still visible after 48 hr and only faintly visible after 72 hr. The diameter of the reaction was dose-dependent; it reached 1 to 2 cm with a dose of 20,000 units and 3-4 cm with a dose of 80,000 units. The intensity of the reaction varied from one person to another but was constant within single individuals. Histopathologically (Fig. 5), there were no epidermal alterations. The dermal reaction was mainly characterized by perivascular cuffing with a dense mononuclear infiltrate. Most cells in the infiltrate appeared as mature lymphocytes; a few histiocytes and mastocytes were also present. Furthermore, scattered mononuclear cell infiltrates occurred throughout the derma. No alteration of the vascular walls or endothelia was apparent. There were no signs of oedema.

It cannot at present be ascertained whether this skin reaction is due to the interferon molecule. When tested on single volunteers, purified leukocyte interferon as well as Zn-purified fibroblast interferon, consistently gave lesser reactions than CPG-purified fibroblast interferon at the same dosages. This suggests that other substances are involved. If so, it would seem that these are released as a result of the interferon induction process. Indeed, mock-interferon preparations produced and purified in an identical way as CPG-purified interferon, but with omission of poly(I).poly(C), failed to induce reactions when tested in parallel with interferon in single individuals.

The histopathology as well as the time course of the skin reaction are suggestive of a delayed hypersensitivity mechanism. However, the reaction occurred in patients with a defective cellular immune response (DNCB and/or candidine-negative patients) as well as in healthy persons. It also occurred in patients with low mitogen-induced lymphocyte responses due to cancer, extensive tuberculosis or immunosuppressive therapy. This indicates that the reaction does not require the integrity of the cellular immune reactivity.

The skin reaction followed the species specificity pattern of human interferon. Mice and guinea pigs injected with human fibroblast interferon (100,000 units in 0.1 to 1 ml) under the skin of the abdomen showed no reaction. Rabbits and monkeys showed a mild reaction resembling that in man : within 24 hr local swelling and erythema developed. Histopathological examination of the lesions in rabbits revealed a diffuse infiltrate, without oedema or vascular damage. The cellular infiltrate consisted mainly of mononuclear cells but also contained polynuclear cells and eosinophils. In some rabbits, there was a tendency to perivascular cuffing as seen in man. In a BCG-immunized rabbit the interferon-induced lesion resembled the lesion induced by PPD, although the latter contained more polynuclear cells.

DISCUSSION AND CONCLUSIONS

In using the fibroblast interferon produced at our Institute we have tried to answer four basic questions pertaining to its clinical applicability.

The first question was to see whether the systemic administration of interferon would have a prophylactic effect against acute virus infections. To test this we chose renal transplant patients. In a double-blind, placebo-controlled study involving 8 pairs of patients, no effect was seen on the over-all incidence or severity of viral infections occurring during 6 months after transplantation. There was certainly no effect on CMV infections. However, the results suggested that interferon treatment might be able to reduce the incidence and severity of orofacial herpes. This study was started at a time when only relatively small amounts of fibroblast interferon were available, so that the doses had to be limited. On the other hand, the patients were treated for 6 weeks while it appeared from our study that all viral infections occurred in a time interval from 3 to 6 weeks after transplantation. In future trials of this kind it might, therefore, be advisable to heighten the doses and to limit treatment to the critical 3 week period. It seems not excluded that better results might then be obtained.

The second question which we addressed ourselves to, was to see whether systemic interferon might influence the progression of a chronic disease of proven viral origin and in which no endogenous interferon is being produced. Like others, working with leukocyte interferon, we chose patients with CALD. Up to this date, 9 patients have received various regimens of short-term treatments with fibroblast interferon. In 2 out of the 9 patients no effect was seen. Favorable evolutions in viral or disease parameters occurred in the 7 other patients; in 4 out of these the clinical and virological status continued to evolve favorably after the treatments. In four patients leukocyte interferon was given for comparison : no evidence for a better effect with this interferon could be found.

These results do not allow a definitive answer to the question whether fibroblast interferon can influence viral or clinical parameters in CALD. In considering the results of our studies, Weimar et al. (11) have emphasized the unpredictability of trends in DNA polymerase levels in CALD patients and have stressed the necessity to perform controlled trials. However, a sudden and definitive reversal in evolution of established CALD, as seen in 3 out of 9 patients, is a rare event in itself. Therefore, it seems unlikely that the favorable evolutions in these patients after treatment with interferon were mere coincidence.

On this basis, and on the basis of the fact that chronic infections with HB virus is a severe medical and social condition, we deem it justified that further efforts be devoted to test the therapeutic value of interferon in this disease.

A third question was to see whether interferon would have an immediate therapeutic effect in life-threatening or invalidating diseases which are of viral or presumed viral origin and for which no effective cure exists. A number of pilot trials on small groups of patients were done to answer this question. No immediately apparent beneficial effects were seen in either acute or fulminant hepatitis, in osteosarcoma or in neuroblastoma. A slight effect was noted in an immunosuppressed patient with multiple cutaneous warts, in that the small verrucae planae disappeared. Furthermore, a favorable evolution following interferon treatment was also seen in a patient with papillomatosis of the larynx. No effect was seen in patients with venereal warts. In conclusion, these experiments have not allowed us to broaden the clinical spectrum of fibroblast interferon application beyond the two conditions that were discussed earlier.

Finally, we addressed ourselves to the question of the side-effects of interferon therapy. Fibroblast interferon purified by the CPG-method had three types of side-effects in man : pyrogenicity, skin reactivity and transitory lymphopenia. From our data as well as from those reported in the literature (Table 6) it appears that these effects were reduced or eliminated by alternative purification methods. This indicates that the effects are not due to the interferon molecule but rather to one or more impurities.

TABLE 6. Summary of Side-Effects Seen with Different Types of
Human Interferon Preparations

Type of interferon preparation	Pyrogenicity	Skin reactivity	Lymphopenia
Fibroblast–CPG	++	++	++
Fibroblast–Zn	±	+	–
Fibroblast* (?)	–	++	n.d.
Fibroblast–mock	n.d.**	–	n.d.
Leukocyte–PIF	±	+	+

* As reported by Kingham et al. (21), and Scott et al. (23).
** Not determined.

The biological significance of the fever inducing sub-
stance(s) is not clear at present. It is not excluded that they
are also released during interferon induction in the intact
animal and that they are responsible for fever reactions during
acute viral infections. Evidence exists that interferon stimulates the production of prostaglandin E in cultured cells (24).
Since prostaglandin E is known to cause fever, it is tempting to
speculate that fever reactions to interferon preparations are
mediated by prostaglandin.

The significance of the transitory lymphopenia is likewise
unclear. In one patient (nr. 005) it was accompanied by a decrease
in lymphocyte stimulation by phytohemagglutinin. Such immunosuppression is a common finding in measles virus infection. However,
neutropenia rather than lymphopenia occurs during measles. Yet,
it is interesting to speculate that many symptoms of acute virus
infections are caused by interferon or by molecules produced by
cells in association with interferon. A similar suggestion has
come from Ida et al. (25) who found that interferon stimulated
the release of histamine from basophilic leukocytes of allergic
individuals.

The histopathology and time course of the interferon-induced
skin reaction were suggestive of a delayed hypersentivity-type
response. Some of the skin alterations during such reactions have
been ascribed to a lymphokine called SRF (skin reactive factor)
(26). Moreover, these reactions are accompanied by the production
of an interferon termed "immune interferon" (27). Thus, immune
interferon and SRF are considered as effector molecules of the
delayed hypersensitivity reaction. Fibroblast interferon preparation might contain substances similar or identical to immune

interferon and/or SRF. This would explain our observation that even patients with strongly reduced cellular immunity showed positive reactions towards intradermal interferon.

Carrying this hypothesis one step further, we propose that, under certain circumstances, fibroblasts release effector substances resembling those released by stimulated lymphocytes. In analogy to the term lymphokines, these substances might be called "fibrokines". Fibroblast interferon might be just one of these; fever, skin reaction, lymphocyte depletion and other possible effects might be due to other fibrokines. This would account for the observation that the side-effects may be present or absent depending on the purification method.

Acknowledgments. The production of the interferon used in this study was made possible by grants from the Belgian A.S.L.K. (General Savings and Retirement Fund), from the Belgian Ministries of Economic Affairs and of Science Administration (OOA). The authors are indebted to many colleagues from St. Rafaël Academic Hospital (Leuven, Belgium), Academic Hospital (Gent, Belgium) and Dijkzigt Hospital (Rotterdam, The Netherlands), who cooperated in the clinical trials.

REFERENCES

1. Åhström, L., Dohlwitz, A., Strander, H., Carlström, G. and Cantell, K. (1974) Lancet, I, 166-167.
2. Emödi, G., Just, M., Hernandez, R. and Hirt, H.R. (1975) J. Nat. Cancer Inst., 54, 1045-1049.
3. Emödi, G., Rufli, T., Just, M. and Hernadez, R. (1975) Scand. J. Infect. Dis., 7, 1-5.
4. Greenberg, H.B., Pollard, R.B., Lutwick, L.I., Gregory, P.B., Robinson, W.S. and Merigan, T.C. (1976) New Engl. J. Med., 295, 517-522.
5. Jordan, G.W., Fried, R.P. and Merigan, T.C. (1974) J. Infect. Dis., 130, 56-62.
6. Merigan, T.C., Jordan, G.W. and Fried, R.P. (1975) In Perspectives in Virology, M. Pollard (ed.), IX, pp. 249-267. Academic Press, New York.
7. Strander, H., Cantell, K., Carlström, G. and Jakobsson, P.Å. (1973) J. Nat. Cancer Inst., 51, 733-742.
8. Desmyter, J., De Groote, J., Desmet, V.J., Billiau, A., Ray, M.B., Bradburne, A.F., Edy, V.G., De Somer, P. and Mortelmans, J. (1976) Lancet, II, 645-647.
9. Desmyter, J. et al. (1978) In preparation.
10. Weimar, W., Heijtink, R.A., Schalm, S.W. and Schellekens, H. (1978) Gastroenterology (abstract), submitted.

11. Weimar, W., Heijtink, R.A., Schalm, S.W., van Blankenstein, M., Schellekens, H., Masurel, N., Edy, V.G., Billiau, A. and De Somer, P. (1977) Lancet, II, 1282.

12. Weimar, W., Heijtink, R.A., Schalm, S.W., van Blankenstein, M., Schellekens, H., Masurel, N., Edy, V.G., Billiau, A. and De Somer, P. (1978) Eur. J. Clin. Invest. (abstract) in press.

13. Weimar, W., Schellekens, H., Lameijer, L.D.F., Masurel, N., Edy, V.G., Billiau, A. and De Somer, P. (1978) In preparation.

14. Billiau, A., Joniau, M. and De Somer, P. (1973) J. Gen. Virol., 19, 1-8.

15. Havell, E.A. and Vilcek, J. (1972) Antimicrob. Ag. Chemother., 2, 476-484.

16. Edy, V.G., Braude, I.A., De Clercq, E., Billiau, A. and De Somer, P. (1976) J. Gen. Virol., 33, 517-521.

17. Edy, V.G., Billiau, A. and De Somer, P. (1977) J. Biol. Chem., 252, 5934-5935.

18. Billiau, A., Sobis, H. and De Somer, P. (1973) Int. J. Cancer, 12, 646-653.

19. Friedman, R.M. and Ramseur, J.M. (1974) Proc. Nat. Acad. Sci. USA, 71, 3542-3544.

20. Friedman, R.M. (1977) Bacteriol. Rev., 41, 543-567.

21. Kingham, J.G., Ganguly, N.K., Shari, Z.D., Mendelson, R., Cartwright, T., Scott, G.M., Richards, B.M. and Wright, R. (1978) Gut, in press.

22. De Somer, P., Edy, V.G. and Billiau, A. (1977) Lancet, II, 47-48.

23. Scott, G.M., Butler, J.K., Cartwright, T., Richards, B.M., Kingham, J.G., Wright, R. and Tyrrell, D.A.J. (1977) Lancet, II, 402-403.

24. Yaron, M., Yaron, I., Gurari-Rotman, D., Revel, M., Lindner, H.R. and Zor, U. (1977) Nature, 267, 457-459.

25. Ida, S., Hooks, J.J., Siraganian, R.P. and Notkins, A.L. (1977) J. Exp. Med., 145, 892-906.

26. Bloom, B.R. (1971) Adv. Immunol., 13, 101-208.

27. Green, J.A., Cooperband, S.R. and Kibrick, S. (1969) Science, 164, 1415-1417.

THE ANTITUMOR EFFECTS OF INTERFERON IN EXPERIMENTAL ANIMALS

Ion Gresser

Institut de Recherches Scientifiques sur le Cancer

7, rue Guy Mocquet - 94800 Villejuif, France

In reviewing the antitumor effects of interferon in experimental animals I would like to list first the different systems that have been used, try to draw some inferences as to the relative effectiveness of interferon as an antitumor drug, and then suggest possible explanations for these effects. The first point to emphasize however is that virtually all the experiments on the antitumor effects of interferon have been perpetrated on mice. There are a few exceptions-experiments with polyoma virus in hamsters, Rous virus in chickens, and fibroma virus in rabbits. For obvious reasons mice have been the animal of choice but in the future it certainly would be worthwhile to investigate the antitumor effects of interferon in other species.

I have divided the various experimental systems arbitrarily into three categories : First : the effect of interferon on neoplasia induced in animals by DNA or RNA viruses. Second : the effect of interferon on mice inoculated with transplantable tumors. Third : the effect of interferon in mice developing a "spontaneous" neoplastic disease - exemplified by the lymphoid leukemia in AKR mice and the mammary carcinoma in RIII mice.

What can we say about the effectiveness of interferon as an antitumor substance in these various experimental systems ? I will confine my remarks to the therapeutic use of interferon and will not be concerned with prophylaxis. I will be referring only to the use of exogenous interferon and not to inducers of endogenous interferon.

It seems clear that when sufficient interferon, is administered, it is effective in delaying the evolution of the neoplastic
process in all these systems. For example, in mice inoculated
with the Friend or Rauscher viruses, repeated daily interferon
treatment is associated with a marked inhibition in the evolution
of the leukemic process, inhibition of the development of hepatosplenomegaly and an increase in animal survival. Less virus is
detected in the organs of interferon treated mice than in untreated viral infected mice. In most instances the animal is not
cured by treatment with the exogenous interferon preparations
currently available, but the evolution of the leukemia is
definitely inhibited, even when treatment is initiated well after
viral infection at a time when the signs of well established
disease are already apparent. (For example in our studies when
interferon treatment was begun one week after inoculation of
Friend virus at a time when spleens were already enlarged, or
as in the studies of Dr. F. Wheelock, one month after inoculation of Friend virus).

As to the second category-interferon treatment of mice
inoculated with transplantable tumor cells: Interferon has proven
effective in inhibiting the growth of allogeneic and syngeneic
tumors, that were originally derived from mice inoculated with
oncogenic viruses or chemical carcinogens or were of spontaneous
origin. Interferon has proven effective against ascitic as well
as solid tumors. Here also it is clear that interferon treatment
is associated with an inhibition of the growth of the tumor.
The effects are often quite impressive. Again, I am concerned
with therapeutic effects ; that is treatment initiated days or
weeks after inoculation of the tumor cells. The efficacy of
interferon does seem to be related to the tumor load. If the
tumor load is not overwhelming, interferon treatment can effect
cures. For example, the mean survival time of untreated mice
inoculated with 10^4 Ehrlich ascites cells (equivalent to approximately 5,000 LD_{50}) was 18 days, and all mice were dead by the
60th day. In mice treated with interferon (treatment beginning
24 hours after tumor inoculation and continued daily for 1
month) all mice were alive by the 30th day and 90 % survived
beyond the 6th month. The tumor does not appear to develop in
interferon treated mice or grows for a few days and then is
completely inhibited by daily interferon treatment. These mice
can be considered cured.

I must emphasize that this is not just one injection of
interferon - it is a repeated daily inoculation of interferon
for a month or several months. Therefore in contrast to endo-
toxin, B.C.G., and similar substances ; interferon does not
seem to have a significant antitumor effect when administered

prior to inoculation of tumor cells. It is effective only when
it is administered repeatedly during the test period. It is
therefore active therapeutically rather than prophylactically.

Dr. Chirigos has also found that the tumor load is important
and has suggested the use of interferon together with conventional
chemotherapeutic drugs. He found that interferon was most effective in mice whose tumor load had already been reduced by prior
treatment with BCNU. In fact combination treatment was more
effective than treatment with interferon or BCNU alone. Likewise,
treatment of lymphomatous AKR mice with interferon and cyclophosphamide proved more effective than either interferon or
cyclophosphamide alone.

I should now like to turn to the use of interferon in the
treatment of a solid tumor of mice. The Lewis lung carcinoma
transplanted subcutaneously in mice, metastasizes to the lung,
and these metastatic foci can be counted macroscopically. This
tumor was considered by Dr. G. Zubrod of the National Cancer
Institute as a good model for the assay of potentiel anticancer
chemotherapeutic substances. This tumor is however unresponsive
to antimetabolites ; somewhat affected by alkylating agents
and natural products, and rather unresponsive to present
antitumor agents. Table 1 shows the inhibitory effect of daily
interferon treatment on the growth of the primary 3LL tumor and
on the development of pulmonary metastases in C57B1/6 mice. Note
that an inhibitory effect was observed even when treatment was
initiated 6 days after tumor inoculation.

Table 1   Inhibition of the primary 3LL tumor and
               pulmonary metastases by interferon

Treatment	N° of mice	Primary tumor (weight in g)	Mean number of pulmonary metastases
None	19	4.7 g	30.0
Interferon day +1 to 20	20	2.6 g	7.7
Interferon day +6 to 20	20	2.9 g	6.1

Reprinted from Gresser and Bourali – Nature 236,
78, 1972.

I want now to say a few words about the effect of interferon
on the development of 2 spontaneously appearing malignancies
in mice. The mean survival times for male and female AKR mice
in our Institute are 270 and 230 days respectively and 95 %
of these mice die with manifestations of lymphatic leukemia.
In contrast, the mean survival times for male and female AKR
mice treated with interferon preparations daily for 1 year
since birth were 385 and 310 days respectively, and only 63 %
of these mice had macroscopic signs of leukemia at autopsy.
Moreover, 17 % of interferon treated male mice were still alive
at the 500th day. Drs Came and Moore showed that the development
of mammary tumors was delayed in RIII mice treated with interferon at 6 weeks of age, but a less marked effect was observed
when treatment was initiated at 22 weeks of age. Interferon has
thus proved effective not only in delaying the appearance of
tumors and increasing survival in animals inoculated with
oncogenic viruses or transplantable tumors but it has also
proven effective in mice with spontaneously appearing malignant
disease. Our recent results are of perhaps more relevance to the
clinician. We have found that interferon treatment of AKR mice
begun after diagnosis of lymphoma increased the average survival
time by 100 %. In fact interferon appeared as effective in this
experimental system as the most effective standard anti-cancer
drugs.

The oncologist wants to know from the animal data how .
effective is interferon in an animal with an established malignancy ? What kind of therapeutic effects can be observed ?
It is evident that in many instances in which sufficient interferon is given, an inhibitory effect has been observed. For the
most part this represents a delay in the evolution of the neoplastic process. To my knowledge, complete regression of a well
established tumor mass with cure of the interferon treated animal
has not been observed.

Now, I would like to say a few words about the possible
mechanisms of action of the antitumor effect of interferon. In
the experimental viral leukemias, (the Friend and Rauscher
leukemias) there is good evidence that although the virus multi-
plies throughout the course of the disease, the evolution of
the leukemia is probably in great part due to the proliferation
of the transformed cells themselves. I have come to believe
that the inhibitory effect of interferon on the evolution of
these leukemias may not be mediated by the antiviral effect
of interferon. This is speculation but I think that a good case
can be made that the effect of interferon on the evolution of
these viral leukemias is at least in part a non-antiviral effect.
This leads then to the question of how does interferon affect
the growth of a transplantable tumor ? I think there are probably

several explanations or several mechanisms, and it may depend
on the experimental system used. I think that there is an
inhibitory effect on the multiplication of the tumor cells
themselves. I don't believe this to be a lytic effect, but
rather a slowing in the multiplication of the tumor cells.
There is also another possibility. Interferon may induce modifications in the cell so that they are operationally less
malignant. For example, we have found that interferon inhibits
the multiplication of L1210 tumor cells in vitro, and that these
treated cells are far less tumorigenic when inoculated into
the animal. They also display a reduced capacity to form
colonies in agarose. Thus treatment of L1210 cells in vitro with
interferon has markedly changed the behavior of these tumor
cells. Other studies in vitro suggest that the surface of L1210
tumor cells may be altered by interferon treatment. I think it
is entirely possible that the tumor in the animal undergoes
changes because of its contact with interferon.

There is also another possibility. Aside from a direct effect
of interferon on the tumor cell, either by affecting its multiplication or by affecting biologic properties of the tumor cell,
interferon may act on the host. This hypothesis is supported by
the results of experiments in which mice inoculated with L1210
cells derived from a cell line resistant to interferon were
still protected by interferon treatment. We feel therefore that
there is an effect of interferon on the host but the nature of
this host mediated component is for the moment still obscure.

If the antitumor effect of interferon is not primarily mediated by the antiviral action of interferon, it follows that in
thinking about the usefulness of interferon in the treatment of
patients with different malignancies, we should not confine our
choices to those malignancies suspected of being viral associated, but rather envisage its use in a variety of different
types of neoplasia. From a practical point of view, interferon
appears to be most effective when the tumor load is reduced.
I think we should envisage combining interferon therapy with
surgical, radiation, and chemotherapy. Lastly, I wonder whether
by using the experimental systems available, we are not really
stacking the cards against ourselves. These are all highly
artificial systems and highly virulent. For example, in the
various transplantable tumor systems we have used, one tumor
cell can prove lethal.

Before ending, I want to emphasize a point which seems to
me of primary importance. Although in some experiments mice
have been inoculated with 1,000,000 units of interferon - this
interferon preparation may contain only a tenth of a microgram
of interferon protein or less. Interferon is thus an extremely

active protein. Are we already giving optimal amounts of interferon or will we achieve even more significant effects if we
inject 10 or 100 or 1000 fold these amounts ?

Despite all these difficulties and unknowns, interferon
does exert a pronounced antitumor effect and affords a very
significant degree of protection with increased animal survival.
The efficacy of interferon in many of these systems appears
to be as pronounced as in animals treated with several standard
chemotherapeutic substances. Based on the results of experiments
on animals I think there is every reason to be optimistic that
interferon will prove of considerable value in the treatment
of patients with different types of malignancy.

References to work cited in the text may be found in
Gresser, Advances in Cancer Research 16, 97-141, 1972 and Gresser,
Cancer - A comprehensive treatise, vol. 5, 521-571, 1977, Ed. F.
Becker, Plenum Press, New York.

The work from our laboratory has been supported by grants
from the C.N.R.S., D.R.M.E., D.G.R.S.T. and I.N.S.E.R.M.

ILMBIS: A ONE-YEAR-OLD EXPERIMENT

CO-OPERATIVE INTERFERON RESEARCH

Mathilde Krim, Ph.D.

Sloan-Kettering Institute for Cancer Research

1275 York Avenue, New York, N.Y. 10021

The "International Laboratories for the Molecular Biology of Interferon Systems" (ILMBIS) were conceived in 1975, as a basic re- search unit for the "Interferon Evaluation Program" of the Sloan- Kettering Institute for Cancer Research in New York. It was to include eventually, also an interferon production laboratory and collabor- ative clinical trials. The whole "Program" was then housed in a small office, furnished with two desks, and occupied by Kingsley Sanders and myself. It was not until the fall of 1976 that the first group of workers, which included C. Colby, W.E. Stewart II, F.K. Sanders and myself, could move into laboratories which were, however, still bare. In early 1977 two more investigators, F.C. Bancroft and S.L. Gupta, joined us. Together with our supporting staff, we now constitute ILMBIS. I have chosen to draw attention to our mode of organization because it is unusual in academic research laboratories and because it has, in itself, I believe, enabled the group rapidly to reach high scientific productivity. I will also report on some of the data obtained by ILMBIS over this last year insofar as they illustrate not only the abilities of its research staff but also the merit of its particular organization.

The creation of ILMBIS was a sort of "happening".

My own active interest in interferon research started in 1970, when, as a member of a U.S. Senate Committee deliberating the merits of a National Cancer Program, and writing a part of its report, I looked with increasing fascination into the then scarce literature regarding mouse interferon's surprising, if not then impressive, antitumor effect. About that time I also became aware

703

of its remarkable lack of toxicity and of its many effects on cell functions, including the expression of cell surface antigens. I came to realize that this material could be regarded as an <u>induced inducer</u> (1), a regulator of eukaryotic cell function and one, moreover, that could be produced in quantity and easily (in fact, uniquely) be quantified by means of one of its biological activities. Ever since, I have been convinced that the interferon field was heading towards a bright future.

During those same years, between 1970 and 1975, a group of young interferon investigators working thousands of miles apart, and as different as could be from each other in temperament and even in specific research interests, were meeting as they did, once a year, at one of those "interferon meetings" "benignly neglected" by the rest of the biomedical community. Colby, Stewart and Tan were walking along a beach in Portugal one day, talking of experiments, dreaming of super-producer cells, rapid microtests and pure interferons, while bemoaning not to be able to share such talk every day.

An opportunity to do so, it appeared to them, presented itself at the Sloan-Kettering Institute in New York in 1975. That year, as participants in the International Workshop on Interferon in the Treatment of Cancer (2), they had heard oncologists and immunologists speak with enthusiasm of the clinical promise of their field; molecular biologists and biochemists spoke then of interferons with the respect implied by referring to them as molecular entities. Finally, they also met the organizer of the Workshop, myself, who obviously had worked hard to make it all happen.

A few weeks after the Workshop, in a letter approved by them all, Stewart first proposed to me that a group of young researchers be given an opportunity to work intensively at the Sloan-Kettering Institute for a period of five years, as a team in interferon research. He also proposed that I be the Coordinator for the group.

A propitious moment came to submit the idea to our Director, Robert A. Good. His immediate comment was "great idea" and he proceeded to tell me that an adjacent building, a former hospital, was going to be converted into new laboratories for the Memorial Sloan-Kettering Cancer Center. I glanced through his office window, and said that we would take the tenth floor, which happened to be the highest full-sized floor. And so, for better or for worse, interferon research acquired a foot-hold in our Center, and ILMBIS acquired a home.

Over the following months, dreams gave place to reality; competition, intramurally for space and autonomy, extramurally for

resources, put us through some gruelling moments. Something like
the survival of the fittest thinned our ranks. We had to defend
not only our research interests and plans through several critical
peer reviews, but also had to convince individual granting agencies
of our individual and collective merit. This drove us to much
self examination and a critical appraisal of our needs and plans
for the group as a whole. Little by little there emerged not only
a specific research program but a specific organizational scheme
which has been implemented and which by now has been put to the
test. It can be considered an experiment in itself.

I felt it worth describing it to you because I believe that
it has served us well and could be equally useful to others working
with other biologically active, though elusive, cell products.
Indeed, any such field of research shares now, or will soon share,
several basic similarities with the interferon field. The first
is that the materials under study need to be produced in large
scale cell culture systems; the higher the specific activity of the
product, the less of it is needed in nature and therefore also the
less is produced in terms of amount per cell; the larger, therefore, the cell culture systems required to produce sufficient
amounts of it for purification and physicochemical studies, as well
as antigenic characterization.

The major impediment to rapid advances in interferon research
has been, and still is, the total lack of funding ear-marked
specifically for production. Grants obtained for interferon
research do not take into account the time, efforts, and costly
supplies that must go into the production of cells and interferons
before experiments can actually start. In addition, various biological systems are also needed for assays. As a result, the early
interferon literature in replete with papers - particularly among
those reporting in vivo studies - on work conducted with ridic-
ulously low-activity preparations (3). Their authors, nevertheless,
draw emphatic conclusions concerning the activity of interferons,
when much less than one part in a million of their preparations
may have been interferon itself. No wonder many such papers
reported negative or inconclusive results. It will be a long time
before the field as a whole can live down the reputation for
ineffectiveness that they gave to interferons. In addition,
purification efforts have suffered greatly from the quantitative
inadequacy of the initial crude preparations used (4).

Well aware of the problems that had to be faced for both
physicochemical and biological studies with interferons, we
determined, very early in the planning of ILMBIS, either to produce, sub-contract, or else procure against payment, the various
interferon preparations ILMBIS needed, and to do so at levels fully

appropriate to the kind of work planned. Thus, ILMBIS was conceived from the start as a group that would be supported by
adequate production facilities. Space, personnel and supply funds
were set aside from the beginning for this purpose.

In addition to in-house production involving mainly human and
mouse fibroblast interferons, we have implemented plans for the
large-scale production of human leukocyte interferon preparations,
since these are the only interferon preparations which can be rapidly
approved for clinical use. Our facility is based on an international collaborative partnership in production and research
between the Sloan-Kettering Institute, New York,and the University
of Bern, Switzerland, with the cooperation of the Central Laboratory of the Swiss Red Cross. The facility's staff is headed by
Victor Edy, an investigator from the Sloan-Kettering Institute,
occupying space at the Theodor Kocher Institute at the University
of Bern, and working with leukocytes provided by the Swiss Red
Cross. To begin with, human leukocyte interferon will be prepared
according to the method of Mögensen and Cantell (5). The existing
facility has a potential production capacity similar to that of
Dr. Kari Cantell in Helsinki, Finland, presently the sole source
of this material in substantial amounts. Partial purification (to
an extent suitable for clinical use) will be carried out in Berne.
The material produced will be used for both laboratory and clinical
investigations on a collaborative international basis, to begin
late in 1978.

Another important decision which was dictated by the nature
of the system under study (which, when contemplated in its entirety,
ranges from molecular studies of interferon induction and action
to in vivo experimentation in animals and man) was that the members
of the group would be selected for their collective expertise
covering all aspects of the system. By the same token, we decided
that no one aspect would be given a priori more emphasis than any
other; none of the investigators, whatever his academic rank, ought
to be solely responsible for the overall direction of the research.
This would be shared equally and be determined during frequent,
informal group discussions involving all those to be called "core
members" of ILMBIS. These are, today, Carter Bancroft, Bud Colby,
Sohan Gupta, and Bill Stewart, together with Kingsley Sanders and
myself, who are also, respectively, the Associate Coordinator and
Coordinator for the group. This arrangement, which embodies the
concept that a broad and complex research field can be tackled
more effectively, in terms of research strategies, with a critical
mass of complementary scientific expertise and technical skills, is
new to biological research conducted in an academic environment.
It is not new to industrial research, where effeciency is at a
premium, nor to research in the physical sciences, where teams of

investigators sharing a telescope or an accelerator are by now the rule. Needless to say, when a similar arrangement was proposed for our group it was greeted with doubts and prophecies of doom; it has also been difficult to fit into the administrative organization of our Institute, which is accustomed to deal with single "heads of laboratories". For this reason, as well as for administrative convenience, one of us was appointed administrative head of the group. In the event, this has simplified communications with the Institute's central office as well as with the outside world. It has also been an added convenience to the others who now can concentrate almost exclusively on research. Thus, while effectively scientific co-directors of research, they have achieved an enviable status in this age of increasing bureaucratization of research, that of being spared a considerable amount of responsibility and chores related to dealing with a central administration and funding agencies.

ILMBIS's organizational structure can be accurately pictured as an upside-down pyramid. The Coordinator and Associate Coordinator with their staff are at the bottom because their task is to create the conditions in which unhampered research can be carried out. They join the group at the top in discussions on research direction and allocations of resources. The latter are pooled and allocated by common agreement.

Each investigator, in addition to his own supporting staff, has access to personnel and facilities common to the group as a whole. These consist of laboratories for the production of cells and interferons; a virus production and assay laboratory; a biochemistry laboratory in which is located at present all the equipment needed for routine interferon purification; an instrumentation laboratory; glassware washing and media preparation rooms. Each of these common facilities has its own permanently assigned, specialized personnel. Shared basic facilities have many advantages: they reduce the cost of research for each individual investigator; they make it possible for personnel attached to them to concentrate on a limited number of standard methods to which they dedicate their whole time, using the same standard reagents for all the laboratories they serve. This ensures efficiency, high reproducibility, and it results in data that can be used by more than one investigator, or data from different laboratories that lend themselves to valid comparisons.

In the assay laboratory, two titration methods have been selected for the routine measurement of antiviral activity: the assays are always carried out in exactly the same way for interferon samples from the same species. These methods are:

1. For rapidity, simplicity and economy of samples and materials: inhibition of virus-induced cytopathology in semi-micro-titration trays in which titer is measured as a 50% end point (6). With this, two technicians can assay thousands of samples each week with virtually a 100% rate of success.

2. For greater accuracy and sensitivity, an infectious-yield reduction assay is used, measured after a single cycle of viral replication (7). The latter is a more laborious, time consuming and expensive procedure. It is used more often by those who need to measure variations in activity within one log, usually in preparations of lower titer.

Both procedures are carried out completely by technicians; the results are usually verified by the investigators since the micro-test assay, in particular, requires some subjective judgement.

It has become amply clear to us that ILMBIS could not have reached a high level of productivity within a short time without these shared facilities, whether for administration, production, assays or other supporting functions. As an illustration, Drs. Stewart and Lin now start each purification run with a 20-liter volume of crude material. This is the product of 400 roller bottles or 200 buffy coats, and represents from 2.10^8 units of activity for human, to 10^9 units for mouse L-cell, interferons. It is only the availability of such large starting batches that has made possible physico-chemical purification schemes to be used routinely for the first time to yield preparations with specific activities as high as 10^9 units per mg protein (8). This can now be achieved consistently for each of these three interferons.

However appropriate our organizational structure, I do not wish to imply that it would have been useful had not the people involved also had the wisdom not to let it stand in the way of personal creativity. The members of ILMBIS have used well their closeness and the opportunities for exchanges it offered them, whether for ideas, technical information or materials. They are, however, also collaborating extensively with individuals in laboratories outside the Institute, and not only in the U.S.A. A rapid review of their achievements, during the short period they have worked at ILMBIS, may be more convincing of the value of these arrangements than my personal evaluation.

Since joining ILMBIS, Bud Colby has pursued extensively the biological and biochemical characterization of a mutant cell resistant to a number of unrelated viruses. Following exhaustive testing (7) he could conclude that these cells arose from a mutation(s) in genes regulating interferon biosynthesis (9).

Although no measurable interferon was ever detected in the growth medium of these cells, he determined that the antiviral activity could be transferred from them to sensitive mouse lines by co-cultivation; the presence in the medium of antiserum directed against mouse interferon eliminated transfer of resistance to sensitive cells, and reversed the resistant phenotype of the mutant cells themselves to a sensitive one. Thus, the mutants must be semi-constitutive producers of interferon. In collaboration with Peter Lengyel and Andrew Ball, he then proceeded to look for bio-chemical markers in his mutant cells, known to be associated with interferon action. It was found that cytoplasmic extracts, both from interferon-treated parental cells, and from the untreated virus resistant mutant, contain high levels of an enzyme respon-sible for the synthesis of the low molecular weight oligonucleotide inhibitor of cell-free protein synthesis, first found by Ian Kerr; they also contain a protein-kinase, a dsRNA-dependent enzyme responsible for catalyzing the phosphorylation of a 67,000 daltons protein (10).

These mutant cells are proving to be very valuable tools for analyzing not only the biochemical, but also the genetical characteristics of the regulation of interferon biosynthesis. Genetic experiments have been done to determine whether interferon synthesis is under positive or negative control, i.e. whether the mutation is of a dominant or recessive nature. Somatic cell hybri-dization was used between virus resistant cells and a 3T3 mutant cell-strain normal for interferon production and response, but temperature-sensitive for growth, and resistant to ouabain. Hybrids all had the virus resistant phenotype; they could render inter-feron-sensitive cells resistant to viruses upon co-cultivation; and, in addition, antiserum against mouse interferon eliminated this transfer and reversed the virus-resistant phenotype of the hybrid itself (11). It could thus be concluded that since the mutation which results in semi-constitutive synthesis of inter-feron is dominant in somatic cell hybrids, interferon synthesis must be under positive control.

Bud Colby's laboratory has also begun to study whether a double-stranded replicative intermediate derived from viral RNA plays a part in the expression of the antiviral state induced by interferon. He has confirmed recently that a variety of dsRNA-activated enzyme activities appear in, and are apparently restricted to, interferon-treated cells (one endonuclease, two protein kinases, one of them phosphorylating a 67,000 dalton, and the other a 35,000 dalton protein, as well as an activity which converts ATP into the low molecular weight, heat stable inhibitor of cell-free protein synthesis, already mentioned). These obser-vations have raised the intriguing possibility that viruses infecting interferon-treated cells may actively help to inhibit

their own replication. This hypothesis is now being tested experimentally by comparing the infectivities of the single-stranded
virion RNA with that of the double-stranded replicative form of a
picornavirus (polio virus) in cells treated identically with interferon.

Evidence that human chromosome 21 specifies a cell surface
receptor rather than an intracellular "antiviral protein" has come
from M. Revel and F. Ruddle. Recently, the Stewarts, at ILMBIS,
have confirmed that chromosome 21 does code for an interferon
receptor component (12). They compared the relative sensitivities
of human fibroblasts mono-, di- and trisomic for chromosome 21 and
found these not only to increase in sensitivity, in that order,
but also to be capable of binding increasing amounts of interferon.
An interferon from a heterologous species (mouse) was also respectively much more, and somewhat more, active in trisomic and di-
somic, than in monosomic cells. These data suggest that the
heterologous and homologous interferons may share common receptor
component(s) coded by chromosome 21. The highly sensitive trisomic
cell strain GM258 is now routinely used by ILMBIS to assay human
interferons.

Sohan Gupta, a former associate of Peter Lengyel, joined the
ILMBIS group as core member in May 1977. His previous expertise
with molecular approaches to the analysis of interferon action as
well as his more recently acquired skills in immunology and immuno-
genetics, have led him to attempt to identify the cell surface
components specified by chromosome 21 and involved in the human
cellular response to interferons. In collaboration with Frank
Ruddle, he is using antibodies raised in mice against man-mouse
hybrid cells (in which the parental mouse cell is syngeneic with
the animal producing the antibodies). Such antisera block the
response of the hybrid cells, as well as that of human fibroblasts,
to human fibroblast interferon. Using an immunoprecipitation
technique with lysates prepared from cells labelled with ^{125}I
(lactoperoxidase technique) and the analysis of the immunoprecipi-
tates in SDS-PAGE - a technique he has already used successfully
for the identification of other cell surface antigens (13) - Gupta
has analyzed the cell surface components recognized by antibodies
which block the interferon response. He is now trying to establish
which of these components are specified by human chromosome 21, by
correlating their presence with the presence of chromosome 21 in
man-mouse hybrids.

Sohan Gupta has already initiated studies directed towards an
understanding of the shut-off mechanisms which limit interferon
production in induced and superinduced cells. The rate limiting
events are being studied under various inducing and superinducing
conditions, utilizing protein synthesizing cell-free extracts as

well as the frog oocyte system.

Carter Bancroft joined ILMBIS in 1977 to apply to interferons his experience in the study of the biosynthesis of other secretory proteins, i.e. growth hormone and prolactin. Now, he is carrying out a number of projects in both fields.

He has recently made several notable contributions concerning the structure and processing of rat pregrowth hormone, a short-lived precursor of growth hormone previously discovered in his laboratory (14, 15). In collaboration with Günter Blobel, he was able to carry out a radiosequence analysis of rat pregrowth hormone coded for by growth hormone mRNA in a wheat germ cell-free system. This revealed that the "pre" portion, or signal sequence (16), is 25 amino acids long. The analysis yielded a partial amino acid sequence for the signal portion, composed largely of hydrophobic amino acids. Furthermore, cell-free translation of rat growth hormone mRNA in the presence of heterologous microsomal membrane fractions led to cleavage of pregrowth to growth hormone. Sequence analysis of the latter showed that it contained the unique amino terminal sequence of authentic rat growth hormone.

Bancroft has also pursued the study of growth hormone and pro-lactin producing rat pituitary tumor cells, and of one of their variants, which produces growth hormone, but little or no prolactin. Experiments involving injection of variant cell mRNA into frog oocytes showed both that the relative levels of their mRNA's correspond to the amounts of hormone secreted and that oocytes process the preproteins to their mature products.

He also showed that his rat pituitary cells could grow in athymic nude mice. When at least 10^6 rat tumor cells were injected, virtually all mice developed slow-growing non-metastasizing tumors at the injection site. The differentiated function of the cells was retained even through repeated passages in the animals. In immature nude mice, which proved sensitive to the rat growth hormone, the latter's somatotropic effect was clearly evidenct since mice with a final body weight of 60 g were regularly produced (17).

However, the portion of Bancroft's work which has a major bearing on ILMBIS' central effort has been his purification of rat growth hormone mRNA to a degree sufficient to allow him, in collaboration with workers in Dr. James Darnell's laboratory, to synthesize DNA complementary to it, to insert the latter in a bacterial plasmid, and to show that the cloned cDNA can be employed for hybridization of growth hormone mRNA newly synthesized by the hormone-producing pituitary cells. The present availability of virtually unlimited amounts of growth hormone cDNA will now be used to study gene transcription in growth hormone producing cells.

The above results are invaluable not only for providing novel research tools but also because the experience gained with the purification of growth hormone mRNA and cloning of its cDNA can be used in attempts to purify the interferon mRNA and ultimately synthesize and clone a DNA sequence complementary to it (18).

The interferon system presents particular difficulties in this area, the first one being that in induced cells, the ratio of interferon mRNA to total cytoplasmic mRNA is much lower - perhaps by a factor of 100x - than for growth hormone mRNA to total mRNA in growth hormone producing cells. So far, the frog oocyte system has remained the only translation system which appears sensitive enough to use in studies of interferon mRNA purification. Further experiments are in progress, however, to obtain interferon mRNA-enriched cellular fractions, with the hope that these can be purified sufficiently for eventually constructing a cDNA for cloning. This could then be used in the large scale purification of interferon mRNA and in investigations on the transcription of the interferon structural gene(s), an area that has not,so far, been amenable to experiment.

Studies that ILMBIS intends to expand in the future but has so far had to put on the back burner for lack of sufficient resources, have been in vivo work concerning the all-important antitumor effect of interferons, and its mechanisms. In preparation for such studies Kingsley Sanders of ILMBIS has devised an innovative technique for titrating the antitumor activity of interferon preparations. Evidence from animal experiments and human studies indicates, so far, that interferons cannot be expected to cause advanced tumors to regress. Rather, they seem both to slow or arrest early tumor development and to prevent tumor "takes" or metastases (3). In view of this, the kind of tests used routinely in the screening of potential chemotherapeutic agents for cancer do not appear suitable. Sanders has attempted to establish whether an "oncogenic potential" - a concept akin to "virulence" in pathogenic microorganisms or viruses - could be established and measured for tumor cells. The oncogenic potential of a given cell type can be defined as the mean number of cells which must be inoculated into a suitable host in order to give rise to tumors of a certain size within a certain time. By applying a mathematical formula derived for the purpose, to sets of data on numbers of cells inoculated and time needed to achieve a critical tumor size, reproducible figures for the oncogenic potential of different cell types can be obtained. An effective antitumor agent decreases the capacity of tumor cells to form tumors, and the extent to which it does so can be quantitated in terms of the increased number of tumor cells needed to negate its effect. Use of this test with interferons in various mouse syngeneic systems may greatly facilitate investigations of the antitumor mechanisms involved, and hence, perhaps contribute to future rational antitumor therapy.

Evidence in the literature suggests that the macrophage system may be involved in the antitumor activity of interferons (19,20). An effect of interferons on macrophages may provide the basis for an in vitro assay for a property which correlates directly with their antitumor effect. Kingsley Sanders has found that mouse interferon appears to be able to activate mouse peritoneal macrophages to prevent the growth of mouse ascites and virus transformed cells as well as heterologous tumor cells at a macrophage target cell ratio of ≤ 10/1. On such cells, a similar concentration of human interferon is without effect. The response of macrophages to interferons appears to differ from that initiated by lymphokines in that, although the final result is non-specific (macrophages treated with interferon attack neoplastic cells irrespective of their species of origin) the interaction between interferon and macrophages itself is specific (i.e. it is necessary to use mouse and not human interferon to activate mouse macrophages). This macrophage-activating capacity of interferon preparations can be quantitated, and a micro-method for its assay has been developed.

Stewart has carried forward considerably, over the last year, his studies on the purification as well as the physical, chemical and biological characterization of human and mouse interferons. With Leo Lin, he demonstrated that human leukocyte interferon is physically more heterogeneous than had been demonstrable by sodium dodecyl sulfate gel electrophoresis (SDS-PAGE) which separates only two size components. Ion exchange chromatography (DEAE Biogel A chromatography) reveals two charge components. However each of these (when analyzed again by SDS-PAGE) was shown to contain two size components. Human leukocyte interferon preparations thus appeared to contain at least four distinct molecular populations (21). Furthermore, when analyzed by isoelectric focusing, they found the preparations to resolve into at least ten major peaks of activity distributed from pH 5.5 to 7.0 (22). Human leukocyte interferons also express biological heterogeneity, in terms of their cross-species antiviral activity. Molecular populations from within single preparations were separated according to size by SDS-PAGE, and according to charge by isoelectric focusing. Each population was then analyzed for its activity in human and bovine cells. Different forms of human leukocyte interferons varied markedly in biological activity. The fastest migrating component in SDS-PAGE, with an apparent molecular weight of 13,500 daltons, was 100x more active on bovine than on human cells (23).

Stewart attempted to eliminate the heterogeneity of native human leukocyte interferons by treatment with dilute sodium periodate at low temperature and pH. Both size and charge heterogeneities rapidly disappeared, and all biological activity now migrated in SDS-PAGE as a single, narrow band at 15,000 daltons and was found as a narrow band at pH 5.7 in isoelectric focusing. This change could be due to extensive deglycosylation, or alternatively, periodate treatment could inactivate all other forms of interferons except the smallest. However, when uniform molecular populations, previously separated by SDS-PAGE or isoelectric focusing were treated, each of them had the same stability to periodate as the smallest, 15,000 dalton species. This suggested that deglycosylation and conversion from larger to smaller forms had indeed occurred (22).

With mouse interferons, a major native interferon with a molecular weight of 38,000 daltons was progressively and quantitatively converted by periodate treatment into a 22,000 daltons molecular weight form, which is only a very minor component in the original mouse interferon preparation (24). Furthermore, a new band of interferon activity appeared following periodate treatment at about 15,000 daltons, a region where none can be observed in native mouse interferon preparations (25).

Since it appeared from these results that interferons could be deglycosylated without losing biological activity, Bill Stewart then attempted to induce mouse cells to produce interferon in the presence of inhibitors of glycosylation (D-glucosamine or 2-deoxyglucose). Yields of interferon activity were normal, but the interferons produced contained little or no activity at either 38,000 or 22,000 daltons. However, a 15,000 dalton component, smaller than any native mouse interferon, was produced, representing more than 90% of the total antiviral activity. It was christened "interferoid" (26). It appears to be a carbohydrate-free protein having both the biological activity and the hydrophobic properties of native interferons (in preparation).

In similar studies with human lymphoblastoid and fibroblast interferons, the former behaved very much like human leukocyte interferon, i.e. reduction of molecular size with increased activity on bovine cells. Fibroblast interferon behaved differently; it was not altered either in size or in "host-range", but gradually decreased in activity. It was concluded, therefore, that either fibroblast interferon is not a glycoprotein, or else its carbohydrate moiety is necessary for biological activity.

Mild oxidation with sodium periodate has also proved extremely useful in interferon purification procedures. It was noted that 50% of the protein contaminants of human leukocyte interferon could be eliminated from these preparations when periodate treatment was incorporated in purification procedures; these then yielded interferon preparations with very high specific activity, of the order of 10^9 units/mg protein. Analysis of the product by 2-dimensional gel electrophoresis indicated that size and charge heterogeneity had disappeared. The biological activity now appeared in one spot of activity, focusing at pH 5.7 and migrating at 15,000 daltons (8).

In a presentation discussing interferon research, it seems difficult to end on a more positive note than to state that several interferons have at long last been obtained "pure" according to accepted criteria. It is interesting that after so many years, this was achieved in ours and at least one other laboratory (27) at about the same time.

This, together with indications that carbohydrate moieties may have only a limited role in the biological activity of inter-ferons, is sure to open a new era in interferon research. We shall soon witness, I believe, interferons becoming the object of an intense interest on the part of biologists, who will now have the possibility to use highly purified and characterized prepara-tions in animal model systems, and clinicians, who will want to use them for clinical investigations; there will also be molecular biologists who will want to exploit recombinant DNA technology for the industrial scale production at low unit cost of the active polypeptides, and chemists who will attempt the synthesis in vitro of "interferoids" or perhaps, even soon, a smaller "active core". All of us can look forward to exciting times ahead.

REFERENCES

1. Colby, C. The interferon system - An overview, in: Inter-ferons and Their Actions (W.E. Stewart II, ed.), Cleveland, CRC Press, 1977, pp. 1-11.

2. Report of the International Workshop on Interferon in the Treatment of Cancer. Sloan-Kettering Institute, New York, March 31-April 2nd 1975.

3. Krim, M. and Sanders, F.K. Prophylaxis and Therapy with Interferons, in: Interferons and Their Actions (W.E. Stewart II, ed.), CRC Press, Cleveland, 1977, pp. 153.

4. Fantes, K.H. Purification and physical properties, in: Interferons and Interferon Inducers, (N.B. Finter, ed.), North Holland, Amsterdam, 1973, p. 171.

5. Mögensen, K.E. and Cantell, K. Production and preparation of human leukoycte interferon. Pharmacology and Therapeutics 1, 369, 1977.

6. Stewart II, W.E. The Interferon System. Springer-Verlag, 1978.

7. Hallu, J.V. and Youngner, J.S. Quantitative aspects of
    inhibition of virus replication by interferon in chick embryo
    cell cultures. J. Bact. 92, 1047, 1966.

8. Lin, L.S. and Stewart II, W.E. Two-dimensional gel electro-
    phoresis of human leukocyte interferon. Abstract. Amer. Soc.
    Biol. Chem., 1978.

9. Jarvis, A.P. and Colby, C. Regulation of the murine inter-
    feron system: Isolation and characterization of a mutant 3T6
    cell engaged in the semi-constitutive synthesis of interferon.
    Cell, to be puslished, June 1978.

10. Jarvis, A.P., Colby, C., Gupta, S.L., Ball, A., White, C.,
    Sen, G.C. and Ratner, L. Interferon-induced dsRNA-dependent
    enzymes present in extracts of a mutant 3T6 cell engaged in
    the semi-constitutive synthesis of interferon. Submitted to
    Cell.

11. Jarvis, A.P. and Colby, C. A murine cell possessing a
    dominant mutation affecting the regulation of interferon
    production: characterization by intraspecific hybrids.
    Submitted to Somatic Cell Genetics.

12. Wiranowska-Stewart, M. and Stewart II, W.E. The Role of human
    chromosome 21 in sensitivity to interferons. J. Gen. Virol.
    37, 629, 1977.

13. Gupta, S.L., Goldstein, G. and Boyse, E.A. Accessibility of
    plasma membrane antigens. Immunogenetics 5, 379, 1977.

14. Sussman, P.M., Tushinski, R.J. and Bancroft, F.C. Pregrowth
    hormone: Product of the translation in vitro of messenger RNA
    coding for growth hormone. Proc. Nat. Acad. Sci. U.S.A. 73,
    29, 1976.

15. Spielman, L.L. and Bancroft, F.C. Pregrowth hormone:
    Evidence for conversion to growth hormone during synthesis
    on membrane-bound polysomes. Endocrinology 101, 651, 1977.

16. Blobel, G. and Dobberstein, B.J. Transfer of Proteins Across
    Membranes. I. Presence of Proteolytically Processed and
    Unprocessed Nascent Immunoglobulin Light Chains on Membrane-
    Bound Ribosomes of Murine Myeloma. J. Cell Biol. 67, 835,
    1975.

17. Shin, S.-I., Brown, A.L. and Bancroft, F.C. Growth response in athymic nude mice to transplanted growth hormone-secreting rat pituitary tumor cells. Endocrinology, in press (July, 1978).

18. Science, 196 #4286, April 8, 1977.

19. Gresser, I., Maury, C. and Brouty-Boyé , D. Mechanism of the anti-tumor effect of interferon in mice. Nature 239, 167, 1972.

20. Schultz, R.M., Papamatheakis, J.D. and Chirigos, M.A. Interferon: An Inducer of Macrophage Activation by Polyanions. Science 197, 674, 1977.

21. Lin, L.S., Wiranowska-Stewart, M., Chudzio, T. and Stewart II, W.E. Characterization of the human leukocyte interferon heterogeneities. Arch. Virol. in press, 1978.

22. Stewart II, W.E., Lin, L.S., Wiranowska-Stewart, M. and Cantell, K. Elimination of the size and charge heterogeneities of human leukocyte interferons by chemical cleavage. Proc. Nat. Acad. Sci. U.S.A. 74, 4200, 1977.

23. Lin, L.S., Wiranowska-Stewart, M., Chudzio, T. and Stewart II, W.E. Characterization of the heterogeneous molecules of human leukocyte interferons. J. Gen. Virol. in press, 1978.

24. Stewart II, W.E., Legoff, S. and Wiranowska-Stewart, M. Characterization of two distinct molecular populations of type I mouse interferons. J. Gen. Virol. 37, 277, 1977.

25. Lin, L.S. and Stewart II, W.E., personal communication, 1978.

26. Stewart II, W.E., Chudzio, T., Lin, L.S. and Wiranowska-Stewart M. Interferoids: In vitro and In vivo Production of Modified Interferon. Abstract Amer. Soc. Microbiol., 1978.

27. DeMaeyer-Guignard, J.D., Tovey, M.G., Gresser, I. and DeMaeyer, E. Purification of mouse interferon by sequential affinity chromatography on poly(U)- and antibody-agarose columns. Nature 271, 622, 1978.

THE EFFECT OF INTERFERONS ON CELL GROWTH AND THE CELL CYCLE

F.R. Balkwill, D. Watling, and
J. Taylor-Papadimitriou

Imperial Cancer Research Fund
P.O. Box 123, Lincoln's Inn Field
London WC2A 3PX, England

It is now established that the interferons can have a more profound effect on cells than merely establishing a state of resistance to virus infection. Interferons can influence the cell surface, cell growth and division and cellular differentiation (for review of this see ref. 1). All these properties are potentially important in the inhibitory effect shown by interferons on the establishment and growth of tumours. We have studied the growth inhibitory effect of interferon on a range of normal, hyperplastic, and malignant cells derived from the human breast and grown in tissue and report here on the characteristics of this inhibition.

Human lymphoblastoid cell (Namalva) interferon (prepared and partially purified by Dr K. Fantes, Wellcome Research Laboratories, Beckenham, U.K.) inhibited the growth in vitro of all the human breast cells investigated. The effect of interferon on the growth of breast fibroblasts and malignant epithelial cell lines could be tested on monolayer cultures, whereas epithelial cells from milk or benign tumours were tested in a colony forming assay because of the limited number of cells available.

Monolayer Cultures

Interferon at 10^2 and 10^3 1.U/ml caused a significant reduction of growth in monolayer culture of two strains of diploid adult breast fibroblasts ($N_{13}F$ and HumF) and three cell lines derived from pleural effusions of breast cancer patients (MCF-7, MDA-157 & 231) (Fig. 1). No significant effects were seen with 10 1.U/ml. Further experiments showed that in the monolayer cultures of MCF-7 cells, the inhibitory effect of interferon at $10^3$1.U/ml was

719

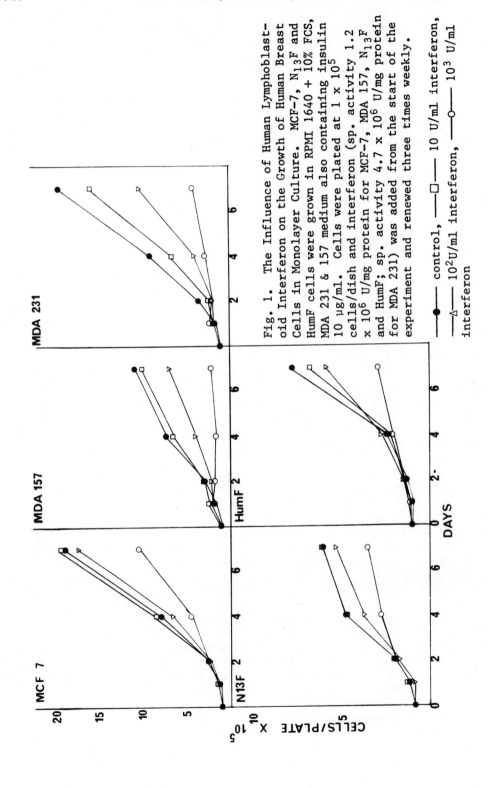

Fig. 1. The Influence of Human Lymphoblastoid Interferon on the Growth of Human Breast Cells in Monolayer Culture. MCF-7, $N_{13}F$ and HumF cells were grown in RPMI 1640 + 10% FCS, MDA 231 & 157 medium also containing insulin 10 μg/ml. Cells were plated at 1×10^5 cells/dish and interferon (sp. activity 1.2 $\times 10^6$ U/mg protein for MCF-7, MDA 157, $N_{13}F$ and HumF; sp. activity 4.7×10^6 U/mg protein for MDA 231) was added from the start of the experiment and renewed three times weekly.

——— control, ——□—— 10 U/ml interferon, ——△—— 10^2 U/ml interferon, ——○—— 10^3 U/ml interferon

Table 1

The Reversibility of the Growth Inhibitory Effects of Interferon on MCF-7 Cells *

Grown in Monolayer Culture

CONTROL		Pre-exposure to Interferon** for 7 days	
No. colonies of >20 cells	<20 cells	No. colonies of >20 cells	<20 cells
120	29	144	31

* After 7 days' culture in monolayer, cells seeded at 10^3 cells/dish in med. RPMI 1640 + 10% FCS and cultured for 14 days.

** Interferon (sp. activity 1.2 x 10^6 U/mg protein) at 10^3 l.U/ml renewed x 3 weekly.

completely reversible.   Cells pretreated with interferon for
7 days, and control untreated cells, were cloned by plating at low
density and cultured for 14 days.   No difference was seen in
colony size or number obtained between control or interferon
treated cells, as shown in Table 1.

Colony Cultures

Human mammary epithelial cells (HumE) derived from milk, or
from fibroadenoma cells can be grown as discrete colonies in
vitro (2).   The development of these colonies over a 14-day
culture period was significantly reduced by the addition of as
little as 10 1.U/ml of interferon, renewed 3 times weekly.   Also,
the inhibitory effects of the interferon were not totally reversible
in the colony forming assay.   A 2-day exposure to 10^3U/ml of
interferon between Day 5 and Day 7 of a HumE cell culture caused a
significant reduction in number and size of colonies obtained even
when the cultures were left for 7 days longer than control
cells (Fig. 2).

MCF-7 cells grown as discrete colonies by plating at a low
density showed the same sensitivity to interferon as the HumE and
fibroadenoma cells and a greater sensitivity than identical cells
grown at higher density in monolayer cultures (data not shown).

Control Experiments

Control experiments were carried out to show that the inhibi-
tions obtained were due to interferon per se and not some contaminant of the preparations.   Interferon batches of purities ranging
from $5 \times 10^5 \rightarrow 3 \times 10^7$ 1.U/mg protein showed the same growth inhibi-
tions on MCF-7 and MDA-157 and MDA-231 cells (data not shown).
Also, the inhibitory effects could be abolished with a specific
antiserum to this interferon (kindly donated by Dr K. Fantes of
Wellcome Research Laboratories).   10µl of this serum completely
neutralised $10^3$1.U/ml interferon as measured by reduction of virus
plaques and also abolished the cell growth inhibitory effects.
2µl of this serum reduced 10^3 1.U of interferon to 10^2 1.U in the
virus plaque assay and reduced the growth inhibitory effects by
equivalent amounts (Table 2).

Cell Cycle Experiments

Analysis was made of DNA synthesis in control and interferon
treated populations of asynchronously growing MCF-7 cells in order
to obtain information on the effects of interferon on different
stages of the cell cycle.   When a 30 min. pulse of tritiated

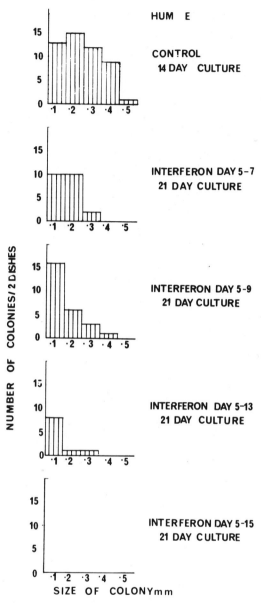

Fig. 2.   The Reversibility of the Inhibitory Effect of Interferon
on Colony Growth of Human Mammary Epithelial Cells.   Interferon
(sp. activity 1.2×10^6 U/ml was added for the stated time
interval, then the cells washed three times and fresh medium
(199 + insulin 10 μg/ml hydrocortisone 10 μg/ml FCS 15% and human
serum 30%), with or without interferon as appropriate, was
renewed three times weekly.   Cells were fixed and stained after
14 days in control cultures and 21 days in the interferon-treated
cultures.   The number of colonies shown in the histograms
represents the sum of two dishes.

Table 2

The Effect of Anti-interferon Serum on the Growth Inhibitory Effects of Interferon on MDA-157 and 231* Cells

Original concentration interferon 1.U/ml	Amount of anti-interferon** or normal rabbit serum added to 10^3 1.U interferon	Remaining interferon 1.U/ml	Cell no. interferon treated	
			Cell no. control cultures x 100%	
			MDA-157	MDA-231
-	-	-	100	100
10^3	-	10^3	30	34
10^2	-	10^2	49	47
10^3	10 µl anti-IF	0	91	112
10^3	2 µl anti-IF	10^2	44	46
10^3	10 µl NRS	10^3	31	34

*   Cells grown for 4 days in med. RPMI 1640 + 10% FCS interferon (specific activity 3×10^7 U/mg protein) with or without sera renewed every 2 days.

** Sera preincubated with interferon for 1 hr 37°C.

thymidine was added to cultures of MCF-7 cells which had been
treated with 10^3 1.U/ml of Namalva interferon for 7 days, the
labelling index was 50% of control values.   However, if the cells
were incubated for 24 hrs with the label, little difference in
the number of cycling cells could be seen between control and
interferon-treated cultures.   We interpreted these data to mean
that interferon did not reduce the number of cells capable of
cycling but that there were fewer cells in S-phase at any one
time in the cell cycle and thus G_1 and/or G_2+M were extended.   To
further clarify the effects of interferon on specific phases of
the cell cycle, the DNA content of control and interferon-treated
cell populations was analysed by cytofluorimetry using a fluores-
cence-activated cell sorter.   DNA histograms were obtained (Fig. 3)
which showed the proportion of cells with $2n(G_0/G_1$ phase) intermediate (S-phase) and $4n(G_2$+M phases) DNA content and thus the
percentage of cells in each phase of the cell cycle could be calculated.   There were no obvious differences between control and
interferon-treated cell histograms, although interferon had caused
a significant reduction in cell number by 7 days (Fig. 3) cell
cycle times computed from the growth curves in Fig. 3, and the
percentage of cells in each phase of the cell cycle, computed from
the histograms in Fig. 3, allowed an estimation of G_1, S, and
G_2+M in control and interferon-treated cultures.   In control cell
cultures the approximate times were G_1 24 hours, S 11 hr, G_2+M 3 hr
and in the interferon-treated cultures G_1 was 102 hours, S 25 hr
and G_2+M 17 hr.

Thus the lengths of G_1 and G_2+M were increased 4-5 fold
while S was extended to only twice its normal length which is consistent with the autoradiographic data.

The data are also in agreement with those of Killander et al
(3) and Matarese and Rossi (4) who observed an extension of G_1
and G_2 in asynchronously growing cultures of L.1210 cells or Friend
leukemic cells treated with interferon.

These experiments have shown that human lymphoblastoid cell
interferon will inhibit the growth of normal, hyperplastic and
neoplastic human breast cells in vitro at concentrations that can
be obtained in vivo.   The greater sensitivity to interferon of
cells growing at low density in an in vitro colony-forming situation
may explain the inhibitory effect that interferons have shown in
vivo on the establishment of metastases in experimental animal
tumours (5) and in osteogenic sarcoma in man (6).

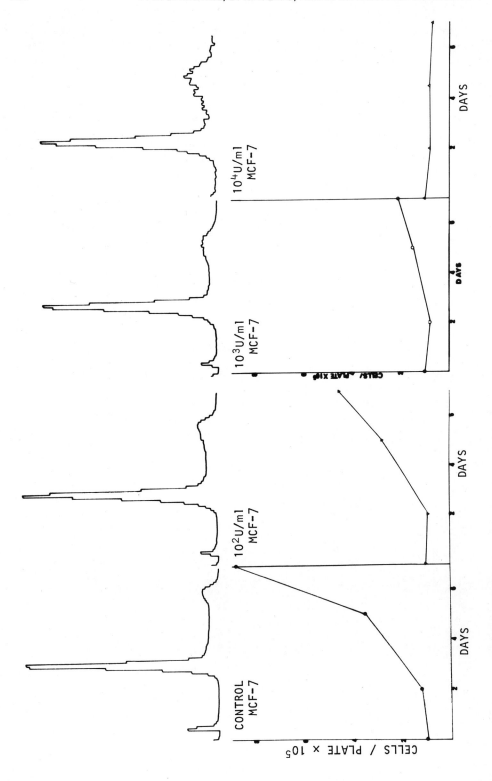

Fig. 3. The Influence of Interferon on the Growth and Cell Cycle Distribution of MCF-7 Cells. MCF-7 cells were plated at 10^5 cells/dish with or without interferon and medium RPMI 1640 + 10% FCS was renewed three times weekly. At 7 days cells were processed for cytofluorimetry and the histograms obtained as shown in the figure. The ordinate represents the number of cells, the abscissa the DNA content.

References

1. Gresser, I.   Cell. Immunol. 34, 406-415 (1977)

2. Taylor-Papadimitriou, J., Shearer, M., Stoker, M.   Int. J.
        Cancer. 20, 903-908 (1977).

3. Killander, D., Lindahl, P., Lundin, P., Leary, P. and
        Gresser, I.   Eur. J. Immunol. 6, 56-59 (1976).

4. Matarese, G.P. and Rossi, G.B.   J. Cell. Biol. 75, 344-354 (1977)

5. Gresser, I., Maury, C., Brouty-Boye, D.   Nature 239, 167-168
                                                           (1972)

6. Strander H. et al.
        Fogarty Int. Centre Proc. (1976).

EFFECTS OF INTERFERON ON THE EXPRESSION OF CELLULAR AND INTEGRATED VIRAL GENES IN FRIEND ERYTHROLEUKEMIC CELLS

A.DOLEI[+], M.R.CAPOBIANCHI[+], L.CIOE[+], G.COLLETTA[++], G.VECCHIO[++], G.B.ROSSI[·], E.AFFABRIS[··] and F.BELARDELLI[··]
[+]Istituto di Virologia, University of Rome, Rome
[++]Cattedra di Virologia Oncologica and Centro di Endocrinologia e Oncologia Sperimentale del CNR, II Facoltà di Medicina, University of Naples, Naples
[··]Cattedra di Microbiologia, University of Rome and Istituto Superiore di Sanità, Rome, Italy

Data collected in the past 2-3 years have provided evidence of widespread pleiotropic effects of Interferon (IF). As reviewed elsewhere (1), inhibitory as well as stimulatory effects of IF on various types of cells have been reported. Cell growth, division cycle and erythroid differentiation of Friend cells (FLC) (2-4) are profoundly inhibited by the administration of high dosages of IF. Low dosages of IF, instead, do not affect cell growth and cycle while stimulating erythroid differentiation of FLC (1,5). High doses of IF also inhibit antibody synthesis in spleen cell cultures (6), the synthesis and activity of tyrosine amino transferase in rat cells (7), the biosynthesis of the steroid-inducible glutamine synthetase in embryonic chick neural retina cells (8) as well as the growth potential of a long list of cell types (1).

IF action on viruses is always of an inhibitory type, and can be evidentiated at low as well as at high dosages, being more pronounced with the latters. As stated by Friedman (9), IF-treatment of cells infected with conventional cytopathic viruses, such as Vesicular Stomatitis Virus or Herpes Simplex Virus type I, rapidly abolishes infectious virus production and intracellular virus antigen expression. In these conditions no indication of survival of the viral genome can be found in the cell.

In cells chronically infected with oncogenic RNA tumor viruses, IF treatment also suppresses extracellular virus production, but does not abolish intracellular virus antigen expression. It has been reported that the pool size of cell-associated viral proteins, such as p30 and reverse transcriptase, are either increased or unaffected by IF treatment of such cell lines (data reviewed in ref.10).

IF EFFECTS ON THE FRIEND SYSTEM

We focused our attention on the effect(s) of IF treatment on Friend erythroleukemic cells and on Friend Leukemia Virus (FLV) life cycle. This system is particularly suitable for this type of analysis since the effects of IF on cell differentiation as well as those on the expression of integrated viral genomes can be studied at the same time.

Effects on Friend Leukemia Cells

The results obtained with high doses of IF on FLC growth, cell cycle and erythroid differentiation have been previously described (1-4) and will only be summarized here. Administration of IF causes a dose-dependent and reversible inhibition of FLC growth, with a cell cycle prolongation, mainly with respect to G_1 and G_2 phases. In conditions where requirements for DMSO-stimulated differentiation were met, DMSO+IF-treated FLC exhibited a 90% reduction of Hb synthesis as opposed to only 30% reduced amounts of globin mRNA. These mRNAs are indistinguishable by base sequence from those detected in DMSO-stimulated FLC. Analysis of size distribution of these molecules by Formamide 99%, polyacrylamide gel electrophoresis seems to indicate that, in the presence of IF, globin mRNA molecules are less degraded than those found in DMSO-treated cells. In addition, these mRNAs, tested in a wheat-germ cell-free protein synthesizing system, proved as able in directing the synthesis of globin-sized products as those obtained from DMSO-treated cells. DMSO-IF-treated FLC do not synthesize appreciable amounts of globin α and β chains in spite of the fact that significant amounts of mRNA were available. This "translational" effect is by far much more pronounced than that observed on transcription. It must be pointed out, however, that a class of protein(s) more cationic than authentic β chains is present in greater amounts in DMSO+IF-treated FLC than in DMSO-treated cells. These proteins are largely immunoprecipitable by a globin monospecific antiserum. Their origin and structure remain to be determined.

In contrast to these results, the administration of low doses (100 U/ml or less) of IF to DMSO-stimulated FLC induces a substantial increase of Hb producing cells (1). In a preliminary test we have also observed that low doses of Interferon have a stimulatory effect on globin mRNA concentration. As a matter of fact, it seems clear that very low doses of IF (25-50 U/ml) stimulate erythroid differentiation, intermediate amounts of IF (100-300 U/ml) have no effects on differentiation, whereas large doses of IF (above 500 U/ml) are inhibitory. Preliminary results, moreover, indicate that also when administered in the absence of DMSO, IF seems to stimulate slightly but significantly erythroid differentiation.

Effects on Friend Leukemia Virus

As for virus replication and production of virus antigens in chronically infected FLC, virus release is impaired by IF, whereas the synthesis of specific FLV proteins is not blocked so that intracytoplasmic accumulation of such proteins occurs (11). These data are consistent with those previously obtained in cells chronically infected by several murine leukemia viruses (reviewed in ref.10).

Under these conditions, quantitative data on the viral proteins being produced in IF-treated cells vary from system to system. Amounts of p30, for example, have been found either unaffected or increased. In addition, a sizable bulk of evidence has accumulated indicating that IF inhibits the terminal events in the replication cycle of murine leukemia virus. It is conceivable that such block occurs at the plasma membrane level.

No data are available concerning the quantitation of virus-specific RNAs in cells chronically infected with murine leukemia viruses and treated with IF. We have approached this problem in the Friend cell system by analyzing viral RNAs extracted from IF-treated FLC, with/without simultaneous treatment with DMSO, by molecular hybridization with cDNA probes.

In addition we have studied the following two parameters in FLC treated with Interferon and/or DMSO: i) intracellular virus-specific antigens, and ii) extracellular virus production.

Total and/or cytoplasmic RNAs were extracted with the chlorophorm-isoamyl alcohol-phenol procedure, treated with RNase-free DNase (25 ug/ml), then reextracted as before and ethanol precipitated. Hybridization procedures were as described in (12). The complementary ^{3}H-DNA to the AKR MuLV RNA was prepared as described in (12) and was kindly provided by Dr. N.Tsuchida, the Wistar Institute , Philadelphia, Pennsylvania. The complementary ^{3}H-DNA to the LLV component of the FLV complex was a gift of Dr. D. Troxler, N.I.H., Bethesda, Md. The AKR probe is protected from S_1 nuclease digestion up to 80% by the homologous purified 70S RNA. The hybridization values with such probe have been normalized by considering the 80% values equal to 100% protection. The LLV-probe, being deprived of SFFV-specific sequences, hybridizes up to 60% to 70S RNA from the FLV complex (personal communication from Dr. Troxler). Two types of IF preparations were used in these experiments: one designated IF_S, was obtained from mouse L929 cells by the routine procedure of induction with Newcastle Disease virus; the second, designated IF_G, a generous gift of I. Gresser, Villejuif, France, was obtained from C_{243-3} cells by the "super-induction" procedure described by Vilcek's group (13), and modified by Tovey et al. (14). Specific activities were 10^4 and 10^7 U/mg protein, respectively. Differences in the specific activity of the IF preparations used did not interfere with the IF effects observed on Friend virus and on growth, cell cycle and erythroid differentiation of FLC.

FLC were grown for 3 days with/without IF, at the indicated doses, and/or DMSO; total RNAs were extracted and increasing amounts of RNA's were hybridized to constant amounts of AKR cDNA probe. The results, shown in Fig.1, indicate that the virus-specific RNA content of IF-treated cells is slightly decreased as compared to untreated FLC. Furthermore, the combined DMSO+IF treatment reduces even more significantly the virus-specific intracellular RNA content. From the analysis of the figure it also appears that the RNA from untreated FLC hybridizes up to 50% with the AKR cDNA probe. This result is in agreement with data previously published and concerning the degrees of homology among different murine leukemia viruses (15).

A detailed analysis of viral RNA sequences present in the cytoplasm of FLC treated with different IF preparations, was carried out with a more specific probe, i.e. the LLV-cDNA.

In Table I are reported the percent values of virus-specific RNA sequences present in cytoplasmic RNAs of FLC in different experimental conditions. While in DMSO-treated FLC there is a significant increase of viral RNAs, in keeping with our previous observations (16), in FLC treated with 25 U/ml of either IF_S or IF_G there is a slight reduction of viral transcripts after 3 days of treatment. These data are in keeping with the results shown in Fig.1, obtained with total RNA and the AKR probe.

As far as the intracellular virus-specific proteins are concerned, it has been previously shown by our group (11) that IF

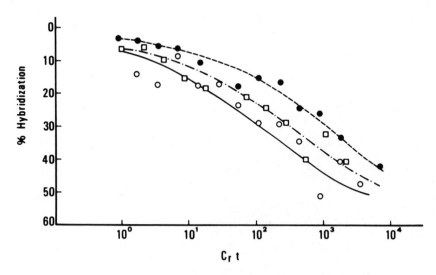

Fig.1. Hybridization of total RNA from control (o), IF-treated (□), and DMSO+IF-treated FLC (●) with cDNA AKR probe. The N-tropic AKR virus was grown in SC-1 cells.

Table I

Viral RNA sequences present in cytoplasmic
RNAs of FLC: $C_r t_{\frac{1}{2}}$ values of hybrids with
LLV probe, and percentages of viral RNAs.

treatment	$C_r t_{\frac{1}{2}}$	%
none	50	0.048
+DMSO 1.5%	18	0.130
+IF$_G$ 25 U/ml	160	0.015
+IF$_S$ 25 U/ml	100	0.024

treatment of FLC results in an accumulation of virus-specific antigens into the cytoplasm, as estimated by immunofluorescence staining. In Table II we report data obtained from FLC treated also
with low doses of IF. Some quantitation was obtained by comparing
the immunofluorescence of fixed FLC stained with increasing dilutions of the antiserum. The FLV-antiserum used was prepared in
C57Bl mice against total FLV, and was absorbed in vivo in DBA/2
mice, in order to eliminate isoantibodies. DMSO-treated FLC are
positive with undiluted and with a 1:2 diluted antiserum whereas
IF-treated FLC, with/without DMSO, are still positive with the
antiserum diluted 1:4. There is no evidence, in these conditions,
of any difference between the two IF preparations.

Finally, we have investigated the extracellular virus release
by assaying the reverse transcriptase activity present in the
supernatant fluids of FLC cultures, 3 days after cell seeding. The
assay was performed in the conditions described by Lieberman et
al. (17), except that aliquots of crude supernatants were added
to the reaction mixture, without pelleting the virus. The incorporation of the labeled precursor was measured in conditions of
linearity of the reaction. As shown in Table III, FLV release was
strongly reduced in FLC treated with either IF$_G$ or IF$_S$. This drastic inhibition of virus release was observed in unstimulated as
well as in DMSO-stimulated FLC.

DISCUSSION

In this paper we have analyzed the effect(s) of IF administration on Friend cells, with respect to both erythroid differentiation and expression of the viral genome.

As far as the effects on differentiation are concerned, it is
clear that IF has a "pendulum" type of action when used at low or
high doses. In the former instance, differentiation is enhanced,

Table II

FLV antigens accumulated in FLC (endocellular immunofluorescence with different FLV antiserum dilutions).

treatment	undiluted	diluted 1:2	diluted 1:4
none	+ $(°)$	+	$\pm$
+IF$_G$ 25 U/ml	+++	++	++$\pm$
+IF$_S$ 25 U/ml	+++	++	++
+DMSO 1.5%	++	$\pm$	−
+DMSO +IF$_G$ 25 U/ml	++++	+++	++
+DMSO +IF$_S$ 25 U/ml	++++	+++	++$\pm$

$(°)$ The symbols, ranging from (−) to (++++), represent the arbitrary quantitation made by the same
individual in a single-blind fashion.

Table III

Reverse transcriptase activity in
supernatant fluids of 10^6 FLC.

treatment	^{3}H-TTP pmoles	% inhibition
none	25.8	−
+IF$_G$ 25 U/ml	1.3	95
+IF$_S$ 25 U/ml	3.8	85
+DMSO 1.5%	32.1	−
+DMSO +IF$_G$ 25 U/ml	3.9	88
+DMSO +IF$_S$ 25 U/ml	6.1	81

whereas, at high doses,IF treatment results in a drastic reduction
of erythroid differentiation. Both the transcription and the translation of globin gene are reduced. However, the magnitude of the
effect on translation (10-fold reduction) exceeds that of the inhibition of transcription (roughly 2-fold). This implies that
globin mRNA molecules are accumulated in the cytoplasm, while they
are not translated. The evidence available so far does not indicate
that degradation of mRNAs is actually taking place in DMSO+IF-
treated FLC; if anything, the analysis of size classes of such
mRNAs shows lesser degradation than in globin mRNA populations obtained from DMSO-treated cells. This suggests that mRNAs somehow
prevented from being translated are not necessarily degraded. It
will be interesting to determine whether there is any appreciable
difference between the two mRNA populations under study with respect to their ability to bind to the polysomes.

The almost complete lack of production of α and β globin chains
in the presence of IF is a clear-cut finding (4). It will be interesting, however, to determine the origin and the nature of the more
cationic protein components which are actively synthesized in IF-
treated FLC. In view of the fact that these materials are heavily
immunoprecipitated by a globin antiserum, it follows that they are
somehow globin-related.

The fact that the IF action on FLC differentiation resembles
that of a "pendulum", in keeping with other observations carried
out on the immune system (18), represents another IF feature which
is also found in polypeptide hormones. One is tempted to speculate
that the clue to IF type of effects may lie in the ratio of IF
molecules to the plasma membrane receptors for IF.

This "pendulum" situation does not seem to apply in the case
of IF-directed effects on virus gene expression. In fact low as
well as high doses of IF consistently block virus release in the
supernatants. Most of the experiments reported in this paper were,
therefore, carried out with low doses of IF. The most interesting
conclusion that can be derived from our as well as from several
other observations (reviewed in ref.10), is that the IF effect on
viruses cannot be explained according to the Marcus & Salb's (18)
model of a Translation Inhibitory Protein (T.I.P.) "induced" by IF
treatment. It is obvious to infer that this discrepancy may be due
to the fact that retrovirus genomes are integrated into the host
cell genomes. There are two possible explanations: either the T.I.P.
is not synthesized in cells chronically infected by retroviruses or
it does not affect the translation of messenger RNAs transcribed
from integrated viral genes. The accumulation of viral antigens
within the cell contrasts with the reduced amounts of virus-specific
cytoplasmic RNAs observed in the experiments presented here. The
magnitude of this reduction is not striking, yet is has been observed with both AKR and the LLV cDNA probes. The combined treatment of FLC with DMSO+IF results in an even greater reduction of
virus-specific RNAs, as compared to FLC treated only with IF. In

the same experimental conditions extracellular virus release was
almost abolished. This set of results can be interpreted as follows:
either IF operates at both an early (transcription) and a late (assembly) step of the virus cycle or, alternatively, the intracellular
levels of virus RNAs are controlled by the accumulated viral pro-
tein(s) in a "feedback"-type inhibition.

In conclusion, we are faced with a mixture of data that, although of some interest, may seem somewhat unrelated to one another,
namely the   "pendulum" type of effect of IF on FLC differentiation
and the peculiar inhibitory action on the life cycle of FLV. There
is, however, a possibility of putting together these apparently
disorderly pieces of evidence. The following unifying interpretation rests on some most recent evidence gathered at this Meeting
that has tempted us to formulate some assumptions.

- Recent evidence, both from the literature (20) and from M.Moore's
  contribution at this Meeting, suggests that the socalled "Lymphatic
  Leukemia helper Virus" of the FLV complex is able on its own to
  induce erythroid leukemias in susceptible newborn mice. This virus
  is also able to apparently induce erythroleukemic transformation
  in vitro when administered to bone marrow cultures set up according to Dexter and Testa (21).

- Should the above results be fully confirmed, one would have to
  reckon the question as to what role the SFFV component of the FLV
  complex is playing in the biology of the Friend system, and, in
  particular, in the as yet unknown mechanism(s) triggering off
  erythroid differentiation in vitro. One possible answer, stemming
  from a suggestion made by H.Eisen at this Meeting, is as follows.

- The one thing that the SFFV component certainly does is to induce
  high levels of polycythemia in susceptible mice. Whether or not
  the SFFV interaction(s) with its target cells results also in bona
  fide leukemic transformations has been debated at length, with no
  firm conclusions reached as yet, and may become irrelevant. It is
  reasonable, however, to assume that its ability to induce polycythemia in vivo may play a critical role in providing the "transforming" leukemia virus component with a much larger subpopulation
  of "erythroid-committed" precursor cells available for the "transforming" event. An erythroleukemia would then ensue as a consequence of a combined and sequential action of the two viruses.
  This would also explain why the SFFV-deprived preparations of
  FLV induce "late" lymphatic leukemias, whereas it does not account
  for the fact that the anemic strain of FLV, which is free of SFFV,
  is also able to cause erythroleukemias, and only these, in vivo.
  Minor, and as yet undetected, differences between the two strains
  of FLV may be responsible for this apparent discrepancy. For instance, CFU-E's from mice injected with the polycythemic strain
  are a mixture of erythropoietin-dependent and erythropoietin-in-
  dependent cells, whereas CFU-E's from mice inoculated with the
  anemic strain are all erythropoietin-dependent (Peschle and Rossi,
  unpublished data).

- In the <u>in vitro</u> system, treatment either with DMSO or with other inducers results in pronounced erythroid differentiation accompanied by increased production of the FLV complex components. It is very important, in this respect, to compare the kinetics of the increased production of SFFV with that of the LLV component in the framework of the "induced" erythroid differentiation. According to Ostertag et al. (22), and also to our observations (23), the stimulation of virus-specific LLV materials by DMSO is quantitatively small (2-5 fold) and occurs late (3 or 4 days) after induction. It seems apparently a follow-up of the erythroid differentiation, whose early parameters (spectrin, 24,25, glycophorin, 26, non-histone chromatin changes, 27,28, etc.) have been detected much earlier. The SFFV increased production, instead, is a very early and much more pronounced phenomenon (22) and seemingly occurs prior to the appearance of the above-mentioned markers of erythroid differentiation. It is again reasonable to suggest that the real "trigger" of differentiation in the Friend system is the burst of SFFV production following the treatment with any of the inducers.
- Needless to say, much work must be done to substantiate the suggested hypothesis that derives its strength partly from available experimental evidence but mainly from its built-in coherence. Such an hypothesis would also help in understanding the effects of IF administration on this system. While it is conceivable that the IF "pendulum" type of action on erythroid differentiation is due to some inherent properties of the IF molecules, one may also proffer an alternative explanation based on interactions between IF and the two components of the FLV complex. Briefly, differences in the susceptibility of viruses to IF have been reported in a number of cases (29). The least and most sensitive viruses may differ in their sensitivity to IF by a factor of 16-128, depending on the cell concerned (30). It follows that the relative sensitivity of the SFFV and the LLV component to IF may be different. In particular we postulate that the LLV component is sensitive even at low doses of IF whereas the SFFV component is sensitive only to the high (above 500 U/ml) doses of IF. If this is so, it would be possible to explain the "pendulum" effect in terms of selective inhibition of some steps of the life cycle of the two viruses. At low doses, in fact, only the LLV component would be inhibited, with a relative enrichment of the SFFV component and consequently with some enhancement of erythroid differentiation. At high doses, instead, also the SFFV component would be blocked with a consequent inhibition of differentiation.

ACKNOWLEDGEMENTS

    This work was supported in part by grants from C.N.R., Progetto Finalizzato Virus (NN. 77.00300.84, 77.00304.84 and 77.00315.84), Rome, Italy and from N.A.T.O. (N.1152).

REFERENCES

1. Cioè, L., Dolei, A., Rossi, G.B., Belardelli, F., Affabris, E., Gambari , R. and Fantoni, A., in "In vitro aspects of erythropoiesis", ed. M.Murphy; Springer-Verlag - New York, (1978), in press.
2. Rossi, G.B., Matarese, G.P., Grappelli, C., Benedetto, A. and Belardelli, F., Nature, 267, 50-52, (1977).
3. Matarese, G.P. and Rossi, G.B., J. Cell. Biol., 75, 344-355, (1978).
4. Rossi, G.B., Dolei, A., Cioè, L., Benedetto, A., Matarese, G.P. and Belardelli, F., Proc. Natl. Acad. Sci., USA, 74, 2036-2040, (1977).
5. Luftig, R.B., Conscience, J.F., Skoultchi, A., Mc Millan, P., Revel, M. and Ruddle, F.H., J. Virol., 23, 799-810, (1977).
6. Gisler, R.H., Lindahl, P. and Gresser, I., J. Immunol., 113, 438-444, (1974).
7. Beck, G., Poindron, P., Illinger, D., Beck, J.P., Ebel, J.P. and Falcoff, R., FEBS Lett., 48, 297-300, (1974).
8. Matsuno, T. and Shirasawa, N., Bioch. Biophys. Acta, 538, 188-194, (1978).
9. Friedman, R.M., Costa, J.C., Ramseur, J.M. and Meyers, M.W., J. Virol., 16, 569-574, (1975).
10. Friedman, R.M., Bact. Rev., 41, 543-567, (1977).
11. Ramoni, C., Rossi, G.B., Matarese, G.P. and Dolei, A., J. Gen. Virol., 37, 285-296, (1977).
12. Shanmugam, G., Bhaduri, S. and Green, M., Biochem. Biophys. Res. Communs., 56, 697-702, (1974).
13. Sehgal, P.B., Tamm, I. and Vilcek, J., Virology, 70, 256-259, (1976).
14. Tovey, M.G., Begon-Lours, J. and Gresser, I., Proc. Soc. Exp. Biol. Med., 146, 809-815, (1974).
15. East, J.L., Knesek, J.E., Chan, J.C. and Domochowski, L., J. Virol., 15, 1396-1408, (1975).
16. Colletta, G., Fragomele, F. and Vecchio, G., manuscript in preparation.
17. Lieberman, D., Voloch, Z., Aviv, H., Nudel, V. and Revel M., Mol. Biol. Rep., 1, 477-481, (1975).
18. Gresser, I., in "Cancer. A Comprehensive Treatise", 5, 521-571, ed. Fred. F. Becker, Plenum Press, New York and London, (1977).
19. Marcus, P.I. and Salb, J.M., Virology, 30, 502-516, (1966).
20. Friend, C., Scher, W., Tsuei, D., Haddad, J., Holland, J.G., Szrajer, N. and Haubenstock, H., in "Oncogenic Viruses and Host Genes", ed. Y. Ikawa, Academic Press, New York, (1977), in press.
21. Dexter, T.M. and Testa N.G., Methods Cell Biol., 14, 387-405, (1976).
22. Ostertag, W., Pragnell, J.B., Swetly, P., Arndt-Jovin, D., Krieg, C. and Clauss, U., Symposium on Interferons and the Control of Cell-Virus Interactions, May 2-6, Rehovot, Israel, (1977), (abstract).

23. Vecchio, G., Colletta, G., Fragomele, F., Sandomenico, M.L. and Laurenza, M., submitted for publication.
24. Eisen, H., Bach, R. and Emery, R., Proc. Natl. Acad. Sci., USA, $\underline{74}$, 3898-3902, (1977).
25. Rossi, G.B., Aducci, P., Gambari, R., Minetti, M. and Vernole P., submitted for publication.
26. Eisen, H., Sassa, S., Granick, D. and Keppel, F., Cold Spring Harbour Symp. Quantit. Biol., (1977), in press.
27. Lunadei, M., Matteucci, P., Ullu, E., Gangari, R., Rossi, G.B. and Fantoni, A., Exp. Cell Res., (1978), in press.
28. Keppel, S., Allet, B. and Eisen, H., Proc. Natl. Acad. Sci., USA, $\underline{74}$, 653-656, (1977).
29. Lockart, R.Z., Jr., in "Interferons and Interferon Inducers", ed. N.B. Finter, North-Holland Publ., Ansterdam, 11-27, (1973).
30. Stewart, W.E. II, Scott, W.D. and Sulkin, S.E., J. Virol., $\underline{4}$, 147-153, (1969).

PARTICIPANTS

Dr. Ahuja, M.R.
Genetisches Institut der
Justus-Liebig-Universität
Heinrich-Buff-Ring 58-62
6300 Giessen
Germany

Dr. Allaudeen, H.S.
Department of Pharmacology
School of Medicine
Yale University
Sterling Hall of Medicine
333 Cedar Street
New Haven, Connecticut 06510
U.S.A.

Dr. Baldwin, R.
Cancer Research Campaign
Laboratories
University of Nottingham
University Park
Nottingham NG 7 2RD
England

Dr. Balkwill, F.
Imperial Cancer Research
Fund Labs
P.O. Box No. 123
Lincoln's Inn Fields
London WC2A 3PX
Engalnd

Dr. Barnes, R.D.
Medical Research Council
Clinical Research Center
Watford Road
Harrow
Middlesex HA1 3UI
England

Dr. Bentvelzen, P.
Radiobiological Institute TNO
Lange Kleiweg
Rijswijk Z.H.
The Netherlands

Bernhardt, U.
Gustav-Embden-Zentrum der
Biologischen Chemie
Abteilung für Molekularbiologie
Klinikum der Johann-Wolfgang-
Goethe Universität
Theodor-Stern-Kai 7
6000 Frankfurt/Main Germany

Dr. Billiau, A.
Rega Institute
Minderbroedersstraat 10
13-3000 Leuven
Belgium

Dr. Blaudin de The, G.
76 Quai Clemenceau
69300 Calurie
France

Dr. Bollum, F.J.
Chairman, Dep. of Biochemistry
Uniformed Services
University of Health Services
4301 Jones Bridge Road
Bethesda, Maryland 20014
U.S.A.

Dr. Bolognesi, D.P.
Duke University Medical Center
Department of Surgery
Box 2926
Durham, North Carolina 27710
U.S.A.

Dr. Burke, D.C.
University of Warwick
Department of Biological
Sciences
Coventry CV4 7AL
England

Dr. Burny, A.
University of Brussels
Department of Molecular Biology
Laboratory of Biological
Chemistry
67, Rue des Chevaux
1640 Rhode St. Genese
Belgium

Dr. Carrasco, L.
Centro de Biologica Molecular
Instituto de Bioquimica
de Macromolecuals
Universidad Autonoma de Madrid
Canto Blanco
Madrid 34 Spain

Dr. Carter, W.A.[x]
Department of Medical Viral
Oncology
Roswell Park Memorial Institute
666 Elm Street
Buffalo, New York 14203
U.S.A.

Dr. Chandra, P. [x]
Gustav-Embden-Zentrum der
Biologischen Chemie
Abteilung für Molekularbiologie
Klinikum der Johann-Wolfgang-
Goethe-Universität
Theodor-Stern-Kai 7
6000 Frankfurt/Main
Germany

Dr. de Clercq, E.
Katholieke Universiteit Leuven
Rega Institute
Minderbroedersstraat 10
3000 Leuven
Belgium

Dr. Ebener, U.
Gustav-Embden-Zentrum der
Biologischen Chemie
Abteilung für Molekularbiologie
Klinikum der Johann-Wofgang-
Goethe-Universität
Theodor-Stern-Kai 7
6000 Frankfurt/Main
Germany

Dr. Ebbesen, P.
Institut for Medicinsk
Mikrobiologi
University of Copenhagen
Juliane Maries Vej 22
2100 Copenhagen
Denmark

Dr. Eisen, H.
Institut Pasteur
25 Rue du Dr. Roux
Paris 75015
France

Dr. Essex, M.
Harvard School of Public Health
Dep. of Microbiology
665 Huntington Avenue
Boston, Mass. 02115
U.S.A.

[x] Section Convenor

Dr. Fischinger, P.
National Cancer Institute
Bldg. 41, Room 400
Bethesda, Maryland 20014
U.S.A.

Dr. Fleischer, B.
Institut für Virologie
der Justus-Liebig-Universität
Fachbereich Medizin
Frankfurter Straße 107
6300 Giessen
Germany

Freudenberg, R.
Gustav-Embden-Zentrum der
Biologischen Chemie
Abteilung für Molekularbiologie
Klinikum der Johann-Wolfgang-
Goethe-Universität
Theodor-Stern-Kai 7
6000 Frankfurt/Main
Germany

Dr. Frisby, D.
Imperial Cancer Research
Fund Labs
P.O. Box No. 123
Lincoln's Inn Fields
London, WC 2A 3 PX
England

Dr. Gallo, R.C. [x]
National Cancer Institute
Laboratory of Tumor Cell
Biology
Building 37, Room 6B04
Bethesda, Maryland 20014
U.S.A.

Dr. Ghione. M.
Montesdison
Divisione Farmaceutici
Viale E. Bezzi, 24
20146 Milano
Italy

Dr. Gresser, I.
Institut de Recherches Scienti-
fiques sur le Cancer
Boite Postale No. 8
94, Villejuif
France

Dr. zur Hausen, H.
Institut für Virologie im
Zentrum der Hygiene
Hermann-Herder-Straße 11
7800 Freiburg
Germany

Dr. Hofschneider, P.H.
Max-Planck-Institut für
Biochemie
8033 Martinsried/München
Germany

Dr. Horoszewicz, J.S.
Dep. of Medical Viral Oncology
Roswell Park Memorial
Institute
666 Elm Street
Buffalo, N.Y. 14263
U.S.A.

Dr. Illiakis, G.
Gesellschaft für Strahlen-
und Umweltforschung m. b. H.
Paul-Ehrlich-Straße 20
6000 Frankfurt/Main
Germany

Dr. Jarrett, O.
Dr. Jarrett, W.F.H.
University of Glasgow
Dep. of Veterinary Pathology
Veterinary School
Bearsden Road
Bearsden, Glasgow G61 1QH
Scotland

Dr. Kiessling, R.
Dep. of Tumor Biology
Karolinska Institute
104 01 Stockholm 60
Sweden

Dr. Kirsten, W.
Dep. of Pathology
University of Chicago
950 East 59th Street
Chicago, Illinois 60637
U.S.A.

Dr. Klein, E.
Dep. of Tumor Biology
Karolinska Institutet
104 01 Stockholm 60
Sweden

Dr. Klein, G. ˣ
Dep. of Tumor Biology
Karolinska Institutet
104 01 Stockholm 60
Sweden

Dr. Kontaratos, A.
School of Engineering
Uni of Patras
Rio-Patras
Greece

Dr. Kornhuber, B.
Zentrum der Kinderheilkunde
Abt. für pädiatrische
Onkologie und Hämatologie
Klinikum der Johann-Wolfgang-
Goethe-Universität
Theodor-Stern-Kai 7
6000 Frankfurt/Main
Germany

Dr. Kottaridis, S.D.
Hellenic Anticancer Institute
Papanikolaou Research Center of
Oncology and Experimental
Surgery, 171 Alexanras Avenue
603 Athens
Greece

Dr. Krim, M.
Sloan-Kettering-Institute
Interferon Program
1275 York Ave
New York, N.Y. 10021
U.S.A.

Dr. Kropp, H.
Zentrum der Kinderheilkunde
Abt. für Onkologie und Hämato-
logie
Klinikum der Johann-Wolfgang-
Goethe-Universität
Theodor-Stern-Kai 7
6000 Frankfurt/Main
Germany

Dr. Kulikowski, T.
Polish Academy of Sciences
Institute of Biochemistry and
Biophysics
Ul. Rakowiecka 36
02-532 Warszawa
Poland

Dr. Kurth, R.
Friedrich-Miescher-Labor
Max-Planck-Gesellschaft
Spemann Straße 37-39
7400 Tübingen
Germany

Dr. Laube, H.
Gustav-Embden-Zentrum der
Biologischen Chemie
Abt. für Molekularbiologie
Klinikum der Johann-Wolfgang-
Goethe-Universität
Theodor-Stern-Kai 7
6000 Frankfurt/Main
Germany

Dr. Minson, A.
Div. of Virology
Dep. of Pathology
Univ. of Cambridge
Laboratories Block
Addenbrookes Hospital
Hills Road
Cambridge   CB 200
England

Dr. McDougall, J.
Cold Spring Harbor Laboratory
Cold Spring Harbor
New York 11724
U.S.A.

Dr. Moore, M.
Sloan-Kettering-Cancer Center
1275 New York Ave
New York, N.Y. 10021
U.S.A.

Dr. Moroni, Ch.
Friedrich-Miescher-Institut
Postfach 273
4002 Basel
Switzerland

Dr. Müller, W.E.G.
Institut für Physiologische
Chemie
Abt. "Angewandte Molekular-
biologie"
Duisbergweg
6500 Mainz
Germany

Dr. Munk, K.
Institut für Virusforschung
Deutsches Krebsforschungs-
zentrum
Kirchner Straße 6
6900 Heidelberg
Germany

Dr. Neth, R.
Molekularbiologisch-Hämatolo-
gische Arbeitsgruppe
Universitäts-Kinderklinik
Martinistraße 52
2000 Hamburg 50
Germany

Dr. Nashed, N.
Klinikum der Johann-Wolfgang-
Goethe-Universität
Zentrum der Biologischen
Chemie
Abt. für Molekularbiologie
Theodor-Stern-Kai 7
6000 Frankfurt/Main
Germany

Dr. van der Noordaa, J.
Laboratorium voor de
Gezondheidsleer
Mauntskade 57
Amsterdam
The Netherlands

Dr. O'Brien, R.E.
Research Director
New England Nuclear Corp.
Boston, Mass.
U.S.A.

Dr. Pontin, J.
Wallenberg Laboratory
75237 Uppsala
Sweden

Dr. Pressler, K.
Asta-Werke AG
Postfach 14 01 29
4800 Bielefeld 14
Germany

Dr. Rapp, F. [x]
The Milton S. Hershey Medical
Center
College of Medicine
Dep. of Microbiology
Hershey, Pennsylvania 17033
U.S.A.

Reiter, H-L.
Gustav-Embden-Zentrum der
Biologischen Chemie
Abt. für Molekularbiologie
Klinikum der Johann-Wolfgang-
Goethe-Universität
Theodor-Stern-Kai 7
6000 Frankfurt/Main
Germany

Dr. Roizman, B.
The University of Chicago
Viral Oncological Labs
910 East 58th Street
Chicago, Illinois 60637
U.S.A.

Dr. Rossi, G.B.
Instituto Superiore di Sanita
Viale Regina Elena 299
Rome
Italy

Dr. Sachs, L.
Dep. of Genetics
Weizmann Institute of Sciences
Rehovoth
Israel

Dr. Sambrook, J.
Cold Spring Harbor Laboratory
Cold Spring Harbor
New York 11724
U.S.A.

Dr. Shugar, D.
Polish Academy of Sciences
Institute of Biochemistry and
Biophysics
Ul. Rakowiecka 36
02-532 Warszawa
Poland

Dr. Sieber, S.
Laboratory of Chemical Pharma-
cology
National Cancer Institute
Building 37, Room 5A 15
Bethesda, Maryland 20014
U.S.A.

Dr. Singh, A.
Klinisch-Chemisches Labor
Nervenklinik der Universität
Ortenbergstraße 8
3550 Marburg/Lahn
Germany

Dr. Spandidos, D.
Dep. of Medical Genetics
University of Toronto
Toronto, Ontario M5S 1A8
Canada

Dr. Steel, L.K.
Gustav-Embden-Zentrum der
Biologischen Chemie
Abt. für Molekularbiologie
Klinikum der Johann-Wolfgang-
Goethe-Universität
Theodor-Stern-Kai 7
6000 Frankfurt/Main
Germany

Dr. Teich, N.
Imperial Cancer Research
Fund Laboratories
P.O. Box. No. 123
Lincoln's Inn Fields
London, WC 2A 3PX
England

Dr. Voss, R.
Dep. of Genetics
Hebrew University
Jerusalem
Israel

Dr. Waksal, S.
Tufts University
School of Medicine
Tufts Cancer Research Center
136 Harrison Ave
Boston, Mass. 02111
U.S.A.

Dr. Weimann, B.
Basel Institute for Immunology
487 Grenzacherstraße
4058 Basel
Switzerland

Dr. Weiss, R.A. [x]
Imperial Cancer Research Fund
Laboratories
P.O. Box No. 123
Lincoln's Inn Fields
London, WC2A 3PX
England

Dr. Witz, I.
Department of Microbiology
Tel Aviv University
Tel Aviv
Israel

Dr. Wolf, H.
Max von Pettenkofer-Institut
Abt. für Molekularvirologie
Pettenkoferstraße 9a
8000 München 2
Germany